DIAGNOSTIC AND SURGICAL ARTHROSCOPY
THE KNEE AND OTHER JOINTS

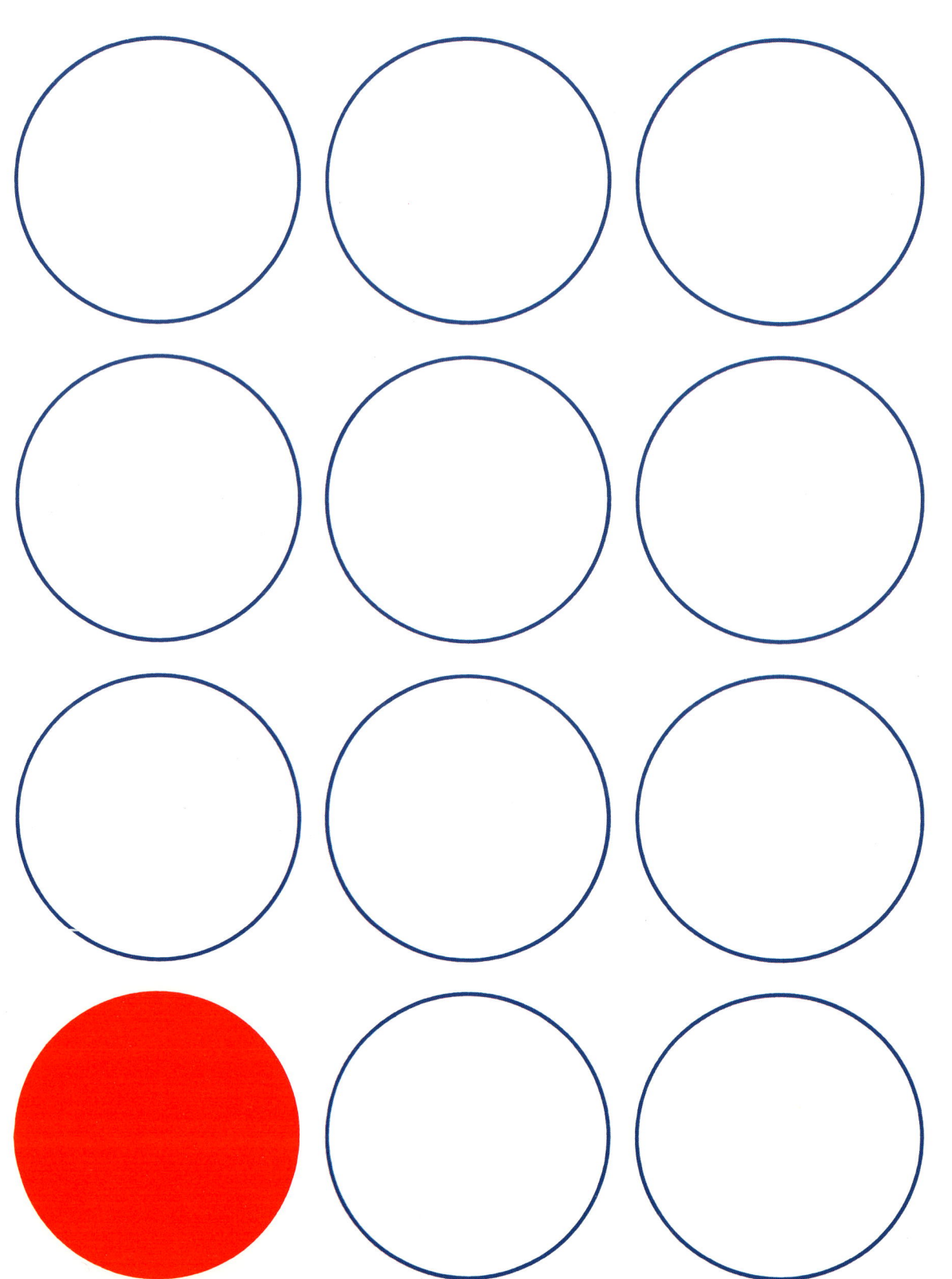

DIAGNOSTIC AND SURGICAL ARTHROSCOPY

THE KNEE AND OTHER JOINTS

Lanny L. Johnson, M.D.
Clinical Professor of Surgery, College of Human Medicine,
Michigan State University, East Lansing, Michigan;
Active staff, Ingham Medical Center,
Lansing, Michigan

SECOND EDITION

with **690** illustrations, including **479** in full color

THE C. V. MOSBY COMPANY

ST. LOUIS • TORONTO • LONDON   **1981**

SECOND EDITION

Copyright © 1981 by The C. V. Mosby Company

All rights reserved. No part of this book may be reproduced in any manner without written permission of the publisher.

Previous edition copyrighted 1977

Printed in the United States of America

The C. V. Mosby Company
11830 Westline Industrial Drive, St. Louis, Missouri 63141

Library of Congress Cataloging in Publication Data

Johnson, Lanny L
   Diagnostic and surgical arthroscopy, the knee and other joints.

   Edition of 1977 published under title: Comprehensive arthroscopic examination of the knee.
   Includes bibliographical references and index.
   1. Knee—Examination. 2. Joints—Examination. 3. Arthroscopy. I. Title. [DNLM: 1. Endoscopy—Instrumentation. 2. Joint diseases—Diagnosis. 3. Knee joint—Physiopathology. WE870 J67c]
RD561.J63   1980   617'.5820754   80-23381
ISBN 0-8016-2535-1

Preface
to second edition

When *Comprehensive Arthroscopic Examination of the Knee* was published in 1977, clinical trials were underway with the Intra-articular Shaver. Since then my practice has rapidly become that of an arthroscopic surgeon. I enjoy general orthopedics and still consider myself an orthropedic surgeon, yet the excitement and advancements in the field of arthroscopy cannot be ignored. I believe it will become a major discipline within orthopedic surgery.

I am concerned about the role of arthroscopic surgery in the care of patients. Arthroscopic surgery should not replace sound clinical judgment. It will not solve all knee problems. Proficiency in these techniques should not allow one to ignore or avoid treating ligamentous instability. Arthroscopy is not the only means to successful clinical results. Every effort has been made in this text to illustrate the role of arthroscopy in clinical management and care of a patient.

In preparation for this edition it was necessary to reread the first edition. It was apparent to me that my dogmatism would have to be tempered with the phrase "at the present time." The developments in arthroscopic surgery have been happening so fast that personal communication is required to keep pace. Even so, every effort has been made, including some last-minute revisions, to have this text reflect the state of the art at publication time. As my experience and knowledge increased, prejudices were broken. Methods and concepts are changing.

Knowledge of the knee joint is essential for a successful diagnostic arthroscopy. Basic arthroscopic skills must be mastered before progressing to even the simplest arthroscopic surgical manipulation. The comprehensive arthroscopic setup and surgical techniques should follow the development of these other skills.

Arthroscopic surgery was, and still is, technically difficult; but it is not impossible. It is not the summation of many tricks that leads to success, but rather sound surgical principles. These principles are just being applied in a different discipline from what we have been accustomed to, that is, endoscopic techniques and microsurgical instrumentation, as well as television monitoring. The careful integration of established surgical principles such as exposure, asepsis, hemostasis, and gentleness to this new medium will yield clinical success. This text is dedicated to the demonstration of a rationale for this method of treatment, an exploration of technical details, and encouragement. Arthroscopic surgery is a means of treatment that produces less morbidity and results equal to, if not better than, previously established methods.

Preface to second edition

Arthroscopic surgical techniques are best learned by observation of a surgeon experienced in these methods. Repeat visits are recommended after personal experience has been gained. The surgeon should not enter into this adventure halfway. Purchase of all the necessary equipment is essential for success. Perhaps most important is an abundance of patience. The yields in knowledge and understanding make one forget the toil of plowing, planting, and harvesting.

This text is not intended to be a "consumer's report." The instruments shown are those which were available and most fitting at the time the techniques were being developed. There are many good arthroscopes and instruments that are not mentioned in this book. It was not economical to purchase duplicates of each tool from various companies. Therefore no attempt has been made to evaluate or make comparisons of companies producing various products. The equipment demonstrated has produced satisfactory results in my experience.

This text is truly a composition. The term "we" clearly reflects the team effort so essential in arthroscopic surgery. The acknowledgments identify the many contributors. Many of the concepts and maneuvers outlined might seem simple and obvious to you; they did to us also after we had thought of them.

I have come to understand that what I called training and experience was often just prejudicial thinking. The arthroscopic surgical experience has convinced me of that, and I hope this text will challenge you and some of your previous concepts.

Again, P.T.L.

Lanny L. Johnson

Preface
to first edition

Arthroscopy is a dynamic, colorful, and exciting experience for the physician. It is best appreciated by performing the procedure. A one-on-one method of teaching is ideal, but because of time and logistics, it is just not possible. The second-best method of experiencing arthroscopy or learning the technique is by movie photography or television.

In this book, an attempt has been made to duplicate the experience of arthroscopy by logos, photographic selection, diagrams, and design. The color illustrations were carefully chosen to be representative rather than comprehensive.

This book is written for the physician who desires the practical details necessary to successfully accomplish a complete inspection of the knee joint. A description of technical details is necessarily labored. The role of the assistant is included to help the inexperienced arthroscopist.

The physician who perseveres will be rewarded with increased knowledge from arthroscopy. The patient will benefit in better diagnostic judgments and therapeutic designs.

I acknowledge and am exceedingly grateful to my assistant, Mrs. Ruth L. Becker, LPN, who has contributed many of the details of this technique. Her contribution has been recognized by the many visiting physicians as being the most essential ingredient in my ability to perform arthroscopy so easily. I agree.

I appreciate the encouragement I received from Dr. David Shneider, who has been able to completely duplicate this technique with great facility and finesse. Using these methods, he has made observations that have added to my understanding.

Gloria Aveiro typed manuscript and revisions at times undoubtedly inconvenient for her; for this I am grateful. For most of the black-and-white photographs, I thank Tom A. Cannel.

Most of all I appreciate Mary Ann, my wife, and our daughters, Charlotte Ann and Autumn Lynn, who have been faithful in many adventures, including this book.

P.T.L.

Lanny L. Johnson, M.D.

Acknowledgments

As mentioned in the preface, this book is truly a product of the input from many people. As the author of this book I have merely compiled the information that I have received. I have benefited from the encouragement of supporters and certainly from reexamination of our experience by those who are unsympathetic to arthroscopy and arthroscopic surgery.

All physicians have many demands on their time. I wish to thank my wife, Mary Ann, and daughters, Charlotte and Autumn, who have been willing to accept rain checks even on sunny days, so that this manuscript might be completed. I can now validate those certificates.

Dave Shneider's encouragement, counsel, and ideas permeate this text. I want not only to acknowledge him, but also to express my sincere appreciation.

Michael Austin's support and personal technical accomplishments have been gratifying.

More than anything else, Ruth Becker's day-by-day contributions have made the publication of this book possible.

I am especially appreciative of the engineering input and assistance in the development of the Intra-articular Shaver. Without the thoughts, efforts, and energy of Leonard Bonnell, Douglas Sjostrom, and Edward McHugh, this system for arthroscopic surgery might not have become a reality.

Many of the ideas concerning the technical dimensions of arthroscopic surgery were solved by operating room personnel at the time a specific problem arose. Their awareness of materials from other disciplines was generously offered. Although their motive may have been just to "get finished," I am most appreciative of the contributions of every one of them. Foremost was Judy Stout, who both willingly and unwillingly participated as the circulating nurse in the early developmental days of the Intra-articular Shaver System and arthroscopic surgical adventure.

A thank-you is not enough for the patience given and accommodations made by anesthesiologists Bert Bez, Suk Chang, Y. Chi, and Darryl Smith during the early days.

I appreciate Ingham Medical Center's administrative support and foresight in developing a surgical suite specifically for arthroscopic surgery. This has provided an environment that has not only made arthroscopic surgery possible, but has also greatly facilitated its execution and further development. A provision has also been made for ongoing educational experiences within the institution.

Anyone who has attempted solo arthroscopic surgery knows it is facilitated by a team effort. Lacking either a dedication to this discipline or a vision of its

Acknowledgments

potential value in the care of patients, a surgical assistant in arthroscopic surgery will be bored, disgusted, or even angry. This is not the case with those with whom I have had the pleasure of being associated professionally. At the present time the original staff of our Arthroscopic Surgical Center includes Larry Andrews, R.N., Cindy Kosowan, R.N., Mary Jo Ferris, R.N., Robin Marshall, L.P.N., Julie Hatfield, C.S.T., Jean Fox, C.S.T., Sharon Lenon, orderly, Sharon Sider, unit secretary, and Helene Whitford, R.N. (recovery room). I thank each one of them for forgiving my shortcomings and for making each one of my days more pleasant (even possible on some occasions).

My thanks also go to Cheri Swanson for her enthusiasm in assisting with the compiling of this text and running down and juggling all the photographs.

Contents

PART ONE
DIAGNOSTIC ARTHROSCOPY OF THE KNEE

1 Development, 3
  Instrumentation, 4
  Technique, 6
    First arthroscopy with local anesthetic, 6
    Clinical value of arthroscopy, 8
    Posteromedial puncture routine, 8
    Posterolateral puncture routine, 8
    Suprapatellar puncture routine, 9
  Documentation, 9
    Slide photography, 9
    Cinephotography, 10
    Television, 10
  New developments in instrumentation, 10
  Summary, 10

2 Instrumentation, 13
  Selection of an arthroscope, 13
  Types of arthroscopes, 14
    Thin-lens system, 14
    Rod-lens system, 14
    Coherent bundle system, 16
    Graded refractory index system, 16
  Light sources, 17
  Light guides, 17
    Halo light, 19
    Light wand, 19
  Accessories, 20
    Cannulas, 20
    Forceps, 21
  Sterilization and disinfection, 22

3 Basic arthroscopic techniques, 25
  Technical concepts, 26
    Light, 26
    Distension, 27
    Placement, 28
    Replacement, 28
    Entry, 29
    Redirection, 31
    Hand control, 31
    Palpation, 32
    Probing, 32
    Manipulation, 33
    Cleansing and vacuuming, 33
    Contrast staining, 35
    Scanning the horizon, 35
    Pistoning, 35
    Rotation, 35
    Scope sweeping, 36
    Free hand activity, 37
  Team approach, 38
    Responsibilities of circulating nurse, 40
    Responsibilities of assistant, 40
    Care of instruments between patients, 41
    Diagnostic arthroscopy procedure, 43
  Arthroscopic compartments, 43
    Anteromedial approach, 43
    Patella and suprapatellar pouch, 46
    Anterolateral compartment, 48
    Intercondylar notch, 48
    Anteromedial compartment, 49
    Posteromedial compartment, 50
    Posterolateral compartment, 53
    Suprapatellar approach, 56
    Transpatellar tendon approach, 57
    Modified Gillquist approach, 58
  Follow-up, 58
  Complications, 58

4 Anesthesia, 61
  Local anesthesia, 61
    Technique, 62
    Patient instruction, 63
    Patient selection for local anesthesia, 65
    Patient monitoring, 65
    Discussion, 66
  General anesthesia, 67
    Technique, 67
    Patient selection, 67
  Complications, 67

5 Diagnostic arthroscopy in clinical practice, 69
  Enhancement of clinical skills, 70
  Effect on patient management, 70

Contents

Differential diagnosis, 71
Arthroscopy versus arthrography, 72
Effect on surgical design, 72
Rehabilitation, 73
Arthroscopy in joints other than the knee, 74
Research, 74
Review of diagnostic arthroscopy
   experience, 75
   Choice of anesthetic, 75
   Classification of patients, 76
   Analysis, 76
   Series I (1972 to 1975), 77
   Series II (1975 to 1976), 81
   Series III: general anesthesia (1975 to 1976), 86
   Series IV (1976 to 1978), 87
   Summary, 92
Patient management routine, 92
Value of diagnostic arthroscopy, 95
Learning arthroscopy, 95

6 Documentation, 97

Dictated narrative, 97
Chart documentation, 99
Still photography, 99
   Camera and adapter, 102
   Film, 104
Movie photography, 106
Television, 108

7 Arthroscopic anatomy, 113

Normal arthroscopic anatomy, 113
Anatomic compartments: technique and pathology, 117
   Anterolateral compartment, 118
   Intercondylar notch, 120
   Anteromedial compartment, 122
   Posteromedial compartment, 124
   Posterolateral compartment, 126
Modified Gillquist technique, 128
   Suprapatellar pouch, 130
   Medial compartment, 132
   Posteromedial compartment, 134
   Intercondylar notch, 136
   Lateral compartment, 138
   Posterolateral compartment, 140

8 Pathology, 142

Pathologic arthroscopic findings of the meniscus, 142
Meniscus in service of the articular cartilage, 145
Condylar disease, 145
Osteochondritis dissecans, 147
Articular disease, 147
Ligamentous injury, 148
Capsular tissue, 148
Synovial disease, 151
Healing of intra-articular tissues, 151
Articular cartilage healing, 154

9 Meniscal disease, 158

Normal meniscus, 158
Torn meniscus, 159
Degeneration of the meniscus, 161
Peripheral detachment, 162
Discoid meniscus, 164
Retained meniscus, 165
Bucket-handle tear, 167
Hypermobile meniscus, 168
Postoperative evaluations, 168

10 Patellar disease, 170

Chondromalacia, 171
Dislocation, 173
Subluxation, 175
Osteochondritis dissecans, 175
Acute fracture, 175
Old fractures, 176
Ruptured tendon, 176
Contusion of the knee, 177
Postoperative evaluation, 177
   Patella baja, 177
   Metallic prosthesis, 177
   Subtotal patellectomy, 177
   Patellectomy, 179
Bipartite patella, 179
Peripatellar synovitis, 179

11 Condylar disease, 180

Fractures, 180
Degenerative changes, 182
Loose bodies, 182
Degenerative synovitis, 182
Osteochondritis dissecans, 184
Osteochondral defects, 184
Preoperative evaluations, 184
Postoperative evaluations, 185

12 Extrasynovial lesions, 186

Torn ligaments, 186
   Anterior cruciate, 186
   Tibial collateral, 190

Posterior cruciate, 192
Lateral complex injury, 192
Chronic instability, 192
Cysts, 194
Ankylosis, 195
Osgood-Schlatter disease, 195
Preoperative evaluations, 196

13 Synovial disease, 197

Synovial plica, 198
Rheumatoid arthritis, 201
Degenerative arthritis, 203
Pigmented villonodular synovitis, 204
Osteochondromatosis, 206
Gout, 206
Pseudogout, 207
Reiter syndrome, 208
Hemangioma, 208
Psoriatic arthritis, 209
Hemorrhagic synovium, 209
Alkaptonuria, 209
Foreign bodies, 212
Pedunculated nodular synovitis, 212
Infection, 212
Postoperative evaluations, 212

PART TWO
ARTHROSCOPIC SURGERY OF THE KNEE

14 Surgical instrumentation, 215

Development of powered instrumentation, 215
History, 215
Intra-articular Shaver System, 217
Further improvements, 219
Summary, 221
Surgical equipment and instruments, 221
Visual equipment, 221
Positioning equipment, 223
Surgical Assistant, 223
Saline inflow, 225
Outflow, 225
Draping, 227
Other equipment, 227
Needle, 227
Surgical hand tools, 227
Hand cutting instruments, 233
Operating arthroscopes, 235
Intra-articular Shaver System, 235
Golden Retriever, 239

15 Basic principles of arthroscopic surgery, 241

How to learn, 241
Triangulation, 242
Concepts of joint irrigation, inflows, and outflows, 243
Expectations, 244
Patient selection and preparation, 244
Surgical techniques, 246
Technical concepts, 246
Team approach, 248
Basic setup for patellar shaving, 249
Patient positioning and preparation, 249
Circulating nurse, 250
Control of the extremity, 251
Outflow system during operation, 255
Lateral release technique, 258
Comprehensive arthroscopic surgical technique, 263
Patient positioning and preparation, 264
Placement of the inflow cannula, 269
Positions for arthroscopic surgery, 271
Placement of the arthroscope, 272
Preoperative arthroscopic diagnostic examination, 275
Probing, 278
Puncture sites for surgical instrumentation, 279
Patella and patellofemoral shaving, 283
Summary, 284

16 Meniscal surgery, 285

Meniscectomy, 285
Surgical principles of arthroscopic meniscectomy, 288
Types of tears, 293
Medial meniscus tears, 295
Lateral meniscus tears, 302
Postoperative management, 311
Complications, 311
Case reports, 312

17 Patellar surgery, 317

Standard procedures, 317
Intra-articular shaving, 320
Complications of the procedure, 325
Results, 326
Adequacy of resection, 329
Patellofemoral degeneration, 333
Postoperative management, 333
Lateral release, 334
Postoperative management, 334
Complications, 335
Case report, 336

Contents

18 Chondral conditions, 338
    Indications for treatment, 338
    Loose bodies, 340
    Osteochondritis dissecans, 343
    Condylar defects, 347
    Chondronecrosis, 348
    Degenerative arthritis with compartmental loss and deformity, 349
    All-compartment shave, 349

19 Extrasynovial disease, 352
    Acute tear of the anterior cruciate ligament, 352
    Chronic instabilities, 355
    Cysts, 357
    Ankylosis, 357
    Extra ossicles, 358
    Osteophytes, 359

20 Synovial surgery, 360
    Synovial folds, 360
    Medial shelf, 362
    Lateral plicae, 362
    Plica resection technique, 362
    Synovial adhesions, 365
    Localized synovial lesions, 365
    Synovitis, 366
    Arthroscopic synovectomy technique, 366
    Pigmented villonodular synovitis, 368
    Osteochondromatosis, 369
    Synovitis plus chondral abnormalities, 369
        Peripatellar synovitis, 369
        Juxta-articular synovitis, 369
    Foreign body, 370
    Infection, 370

PART THREE
DIAGNOSTIC AND SURGICAL ARTHROSCOPY: OTHER JOINTS

21 Temporomandibular joint, 373
    Technique, 373
    Distension, 374
    Arthroscopic landmarks, 374
    Indications, 374
    Normal findings, 374
    Pathologic findings, 375
    Postoperative developments, 375
    Complications, 375

22 Shoulder joint, 376
    Indications, 376
    Technique, 376
    Identifiable lesions, 382
        Congenital problems, 382
        Rotator cuff injury, 382
        Subluxation or dislocation of the shoulder, 382
        Loose bodies, 383
        Degenerative arthritis, 383
        Ruptured biceps tendon, 383
        Frozen shoulder, 384
        Avulsed and displaced anterior labrum, 384
    Postoperative evaluations, 384
    Rheumatoid arthritis, 384
    Operative arthroscopy, 385

23 Elbow joint, 390
    Technique, 390
    Normal anatomy, 393
        Radial or lateral view, 393
        Ulnar or medial approach, 393
    Findings or conditions, 394
        Degenerative arthritis, 394
        Rheumatoid arthritis, 394
        Fracture, 394
        Osteochondritis dissecans or Panner disease, 395
    Loose body removal, 396
    Operative arthroscopy, 399

24 Wrist joint, 400
    Technique, 400
    Diagnostic problems, 403
    Meniscoid lesion, 403
    Synovitis, 403
    Compression articular fracture, 403

25 Finger joint, 404

26 Hip joint, 405
    Technique, 405
    Findings, 409
        Early degenerative arthritis, 409
        Synovitis, 409
        Trauma, 409
        Osteochondritis dissecans, 409
        Aseptic necrosis, 411
    Evaluation for reconstructive surgery, 411

27 Ankle joint, 412

    Technique, 412
    Findings, 414
        Osteochondritis dissecans, 416
        Loose bodies, 416
        Degenerative arthritis, 416
        Rheumatoid arthritis, 416
        Fibrosis and fibrous adhesions, 416
        Subluxation, 418
        Degenerative change, 418
    Operative arthroscopy, 418

Appendix, 421

PART ONE

DIAGNOSTIC ARTHROSCOPY OF THE KNEE

Chapter 1

Development

Instrumentation
Technique
    First arthroscopy with local anesthetic
    Clinical value of arthroscopy
    Posteromedial puncture routine
    Posterolateral puncture routine
    Suprapatellar puncture routine
Documentation
    Slide photography
    Cinephotography
    Television
New developments in instrumentation
Summary

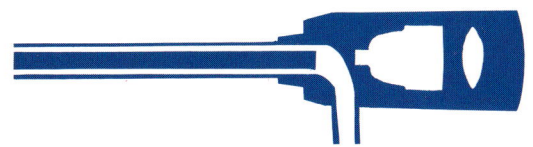

Technologic advances have occurred so rapidly over the past few years that the bulk of arthroscopic history can be found in contemporary innovations. This is no different, of course, from any other area of scientific endeavor. Eikelaar,[9] Joyce,[19] and Jackson[15,16] have presented excellent comprehensive historical reviews of arthroscopy. No attempts have been made to duplicate their efforts; this book concerns the more recent developments in diagnostic arthroscopy and arthroscopic surgery.

The present arthroscopic techniques evolved from the contributions of predecessors. Those of Burman,[5,6] Casscells,[7] Jackson,[15,16] and Watanabe[27-29] are well known. Most orthopedists are well versed in the traditional technique, that is, the large-diameter endoscopes such as the Watanabe 21 placed through a single anterolateral approach, viewing only the anterior chambers of the knee joint. An elaborate irrigation system and the use of general anesthesia were customary.

McGinty[21] and O'Connor[24,25] have adapted modern endoscopes to the classic Watanabe method. Bechtol[2] and Guten[12] have contributed devices and photographic and dye techniques that enhanced arthroscopic inspection.

Learning arthroscopy is an enormous task for orthopedic surgeons. We have not been previously trained or skilled in endoscopic work. Eilert,[10] in the development and production of knee models and instruction techniques, has assisted in introducing orthopedic surgeons to this new field. McGinty[21] advocated the use of video equipment as a teaching aid and has applied photographic techniques to arthroscopy.

Watanabe[27-29] credits himself with the first arthroscopic meniscectomy. O'Connor[24,25] further developed the technique and introduced operative arthroscopy to the United States. Metcalf,[23] through superb technical skills, audiovisual demonstrations, and case experience, supported O'Connor's work. In addition, Metcalf introduced the concept of a lateral release for patellar dislocation and subluxation under arthroscopic control. Guhl[11] has reviewed and reported extensive series of patients with osteochondritis dissecans treated transcutaneously by arthroscopic methods. O'Connor,[25] Jackson and Dandy,[15] and Watanabe, Takeda, and Ikeuchi[28] have all published texts on arthroscopy in the past few years.

The American Academy of Orthopaedic Surgeons regularly sponsors symposiums on arthroscopy and arthrography. These meetings provide the membership with an introduction to arthroscopic techniques. A text published by the Academy contains the material presented in these seminars and includes an extensive bibliography.[1] The first German symposium was edited by Blaugh and Donner.[4]

Arthroscopy is still in its infancy in the United States. The results of a questionnaire for the membership of the American Academy of Orthopaedic Surgeons in 1978 showed that 50% of the Academy members used arthroscopy, usually prior to arthrotomy, 10% performed arthroscopy under local anesthesia, and only 6% of those responding had ever performed arthroscopy on a joint other than the knee. Even a smaller percentage had tried arthroscopic surgery.

The Scandinavians have taken a lead, with Jon Gillquist demonstrating the transpatellar tendon approach to the knee and Nils Oretorp introducing a variety of hand surgical instruments. Einer Erikkson has considerable arthroscopic experience and has chaired the annual Scandinavian seminars. Harold R. Eikelarin of the Netherlands, Hertel, Miekel, and Wilhelm Klein[20] are active in Germany. Henry and Dandy are proponents in England. Jeff Rombouts has considerable case experience in Belgium. Bircher[3] first used air with oxygen and carbon monoxide for arthroscopy. A carbon dioxide method has been popularized by Hinche, a European. Saline is still the medium of choice of most arthroscopists.

Very few arthroscopic reports are published concerning joints other than the knee. These areas are just developing.

No attempts have been made to ignore, duplicate, or reiterate the work of others. Rather, attention is given to my experience with a small-diameter arthroscope in diagnosis and a method of operative arthroscopy. In addition, the development of powered arthroscopic instrumentation and its place in arthroscopic surgery is presented.

INSTRUMENTATION

In 1970 the first self-focusing arthroscope was developed through the joint efforts of the Nippon Sheet Glass Company and the Department of Orthopaedic Surgery of Tokyo Teishin Hospital. This scope, 1.7 mm in diameter, was used through a cannula having an outside diameter of 2 mm and provided a direct field of view of 37° in saline. It was introduced in North America in January, 1972, by Mr. Leonard J. Bonnell. To my knowledge, it was first used for arthroscopy by Drs. Clement Sledge and J. Drennen Lowell at the Robert Brigham Hospital in Boston.

After viewing a single procedure, Mr. Harold L. Neuman assessed the uses of and requirements for such a small-diameter endoscope. The original Watanabe No. 24 arthroscope was redesigned in four ways. The diameter of the endoscope was increased from 1.7 to 2.2 mm, which improved the illumination by a factor of four and resulted in a more rugged assembly. The design was changed to allow for a detachable light guide to improve handling and ease of sterilization. The eyepiece, which required manual focusing, was changed to a fixed-focus lens to reduce confusion and contamination during the procedure. A long lightweight handle was designed for manipulation of the lens so that the physician's head and eye were away from the sterile field and his glove was protected from becoming contaminated.

This three-piece instrument, the Needlescope, was available for marketing in the fall of 1972 (Fig. 1-1). It had a fore-oblique view of 47° in saline but was rejected by many arthroscopists because of its fragility, low illumination, and reduced optical clarity as compared with existing large-diameter endoscopes of different construction. Additionally, the cover lens in the interior was vulnerable to the collection of small dirt particles, which when magnified obscured the view. Therefore the second model of the Needlescope was developed with a nitrogen-sealed optical system, which gave consistently satisfactory viewing.

By June, 1976, the third model of the Needlescope was being tested. It was enhanced by optical design of the terminal lens to increase its field of view in

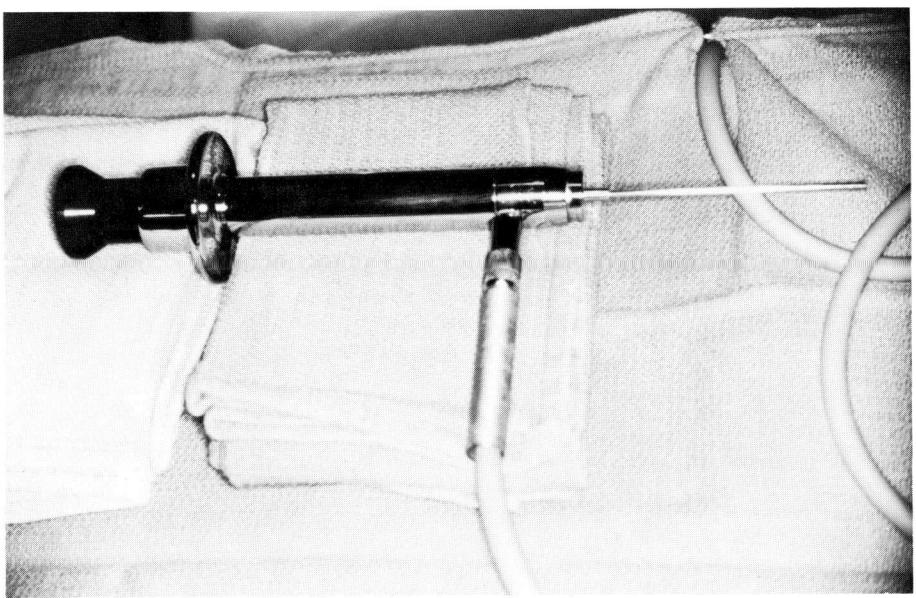

FIG. 1-1. Original model of Needlescope, with three-piece arthroscope. Headpiece screwed onto stainless steel handle. There was a barrier between handle and eyepiece to prevent contamination of the hand by the arthroscopist's head. Eyepiece was inserted manually by a separate maneuver. Disadvantage of this system was that it allowed collection of small dust particles, which when magnified obscured viewing.

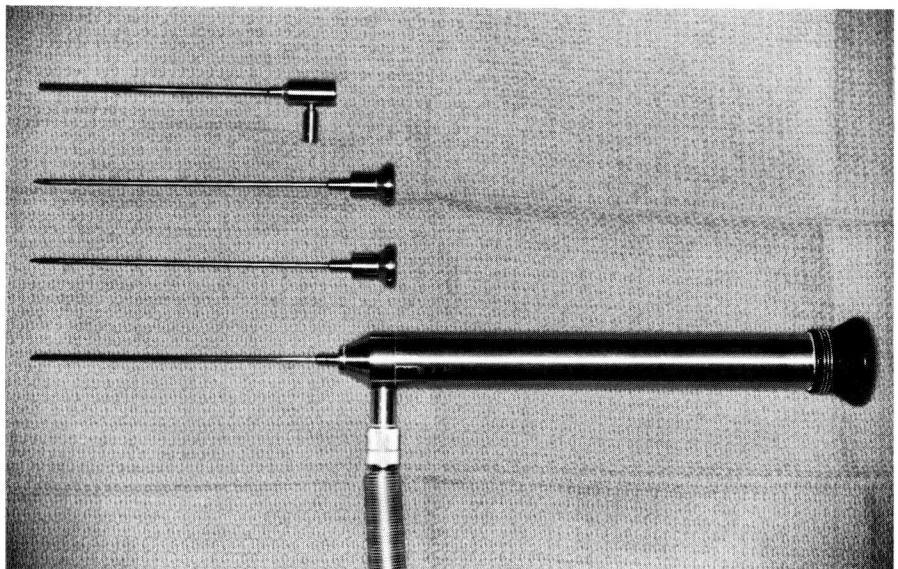

FIG. 1-2. Third model of Needlescope is a closed system with a viewing angle of approximately 70° in saline. Endoscope shown here is 2.2 mm in outside diameter. Cannula, which is superior, has an outside sheath of 2.6 mm in diameter. Sharp and blunt trocars accompany system.

saline to 70°. Another modification improved the light illumination capacity by at least two f-stops. There now was a small-diameter endoscope with an angle of visualization comparable to that of the largest scope and with a facility to document with optical clarity that was competitive with the larger diameter arthroscopes (Fig. 1-2).

TECHNIQUE
First arthroscopy with local anesthetic

The capacity to view the anterior chambers of the knee joint arthroscopically held a great attraction. However, the length of the procedure, the size of the incision including suture closure, and the use of general anesthetic detracted from its practical application. In the late 1960s it was difficult to make a strong argument for an arthroscopic examination when the consensus was that the knee, including its anterior chambers, could be better visualized by arthrotomy in less time and with a less elaborate surgical setup than with a large-diameter endoscope.

I had not been attracted to the Watanabe technique because of the objections just mentioned. However, on October 30, 1972, without having witnessed any arthroscopies, I examined an athlete who had undergone knee surgery but had exacerbation of knee problems with an effusion. The arthroscopic procedure was carried out with the patient under local anesthesia and with tourniquet control. The intra-articular structures were visualized, and cleansing of the joint was possible. A diagnosis of degenerative arthritis with loose bodies was established.

I was excited about the ease with which this examination was accomplished and the observations that could be made. My enthusiasm was not shared by others, however; in fact, the endoscope manufacturer doubted the success of the procedure on the basis of letters received from established arthroscopists. Although limitations in technique and understanding of the arthroscopic image were recognized, I was encouraged to offer this procedure to other patients with knee problems. Ten such arthroscopies were performed in the following month. Experience established confidence and the ability to visualize the interior compartments of the knee joint by arthroscopy with local anesthetic.

Subsequently I learned of the Bircher[3] report of arthroscopic examinations under local anesthesia. Also, Clayton[8] performed arthroscopy in rheumatoid patients with a Watanabe 21 arthroscope under local anesthesia in the late 1960s. In 1976 I reported 400 knee joint arthroscopic examinations under local anesthesia at the annual meeting of the American Academy of Orthopaedic Surgeons. These included multiple punctures without the necessity of preoperative medication. A detailed analysis of the cases was included in the first edition of this book.

McGinty[22] reported his method of outpatient local anesthesia in 1978. He used lidocaine for the skin, subcutaneous tissue, and capsule and 0.5% bupivacaine (Marcaine) intra-articularly for a long-lasting effect. He indicated that this allowed him to perform arthroscopies of up to 1 hour duration. He used a single anterolateral puncture in most instances, occasionally making a posteromedial approach.

Pevey[26] reported arthroscopies under local anesthesia on an outpatient basis with the Needlescope. By 1979 arthroscopy on an outpatient basis was accepted, but still the majority of orthopedic surgeons were performing their diagnostic arthroscopy under general anesthesia (90%).

I purchased a Needlescope on the basis of satisfaction with my first arthroscopic experience. By the time the instrument arrived, the quality of the lens had been improved. Originally, the lens was processed with a thalium salt ionizing procedure. In the interval this was changed to use cesium. Resolution was improved by a factor of 10, further enhancing the diagnostic capacity.

Because the early model of the Needlescope lacked optical quality and had a limited angle of view (47° inclined), it was necessary to compensate technically. The concepts of "pistoning," or moving in and out with the endoscope, and scanning back and forth were introduced. These techniques are applicable to and commonly used with any endoscope but are essential with the Needlescope. In arthroscopy, as in surgery, one learns to work from known to unknown. When unsure of an anatomic relationship, the surgeon goes back to areas of known structure. In the knee the landmark of most common orientation is the tangential view of the femoral condyle, or its "horizon." The horizon is followed by moving from one compartment to the other for orientation during inspection of the knee joint.

By 1973, arguments against the traditional arthroscopic technique were being resolved. The technique was modified to eliminate the use of general anesthetic, prolonged time needed to perform the technique, incision with suture, and the elaborate saline-drainage system. With the patient under local anesthesia it was possible to visualize the interior of the knee joint better through a 2-mm skin puncture than by the largest arthrotomy short of disarticulation.

In September, 1973, *Diagnostic arthroscopy of the knee*[17] was presented at the International Congress. This paper reviewed the first 100 arthroscopies, many of them performed with the patient under local anesthesia, and showed some of the early photographic documentation on slides.

Clinical value of arthroscopy

The clinical value of arthroscopy was now established. Because it could be performed under local anesthesia, patients could be placed in two clinical categories. The first group included those patients for whom diagnosis could not be well established by history, physical or x-ray examination, or arthrography and in whom findings were insufficient to warrant surgical exploration under general anesthesia. Arthroscopy with local anesthesia was recommended.

The second group comprised those patients who showed clear-cut evidence of intra-articular abnormality or ligamentous injury. Arthroscopy was performed immediately preceding an anticipated arthrotomy or arthroscopic surgery. The procedure substantiated that many lesions missed by unicompartmental arthrotomy were visualized by arthroscopy. Arthroscopic examination prior to arthrotomy provides an opportunity for an arthroscopist to correlate these observations with operative findings and to reflect back on his clinical impression. In many cases the preoperative diagnosis was either erroneous or incomplete. Additionally, the surgical design was frequently modified after arthroscopy.

Posteromedial puncture routine

During my first year of arthroscopic experience it was recognized that inspection of the anterior compartments and the suprapatellar pouch was inadequate. Although it was possible to document abnormalities under the meniscus, even in the areas of the coronary ligament, diagnoses of posterior tears of the medial meniscus were going unrecognized. Inspection of the posteromedial compartment was initiated on every patient in whom anterior examination showed that compartment to be normal. It was not surprising to find that a number of these patients had meniscal tears in the posterior compartment or loose bodies not visible from the front. It was also recognized that the posterior cruciate ligament was easily visualized in many patients from the posteromedial approach. Thus this approach became part of the routine examination in 1973; the technique is detailed in Chapter 3.

Posterolateral puncture routine

Many attempts were made to view the knee posterolaterally. Even from an anterolateral approach it was impossible to completely visualize the posterolateral compartment except in patients with ligamentous laxity or under general anesthesia. From that view the popliteus tendon can be seen at its origin on the lateral femoral condyle, but the mass of the meniscus and the tendon will block the view into the sulcus. Various attempts had been made from different angles to achieve access to that space. In September, 1975, it was possible with regularity to enter and completely inspect the posterolateral compartment; the technique is detailed in Chapter 3. Prior to that, it was thought that an adequate view of that compartment could be achieved from an anterior approach, but when direct viewing of the area was possible this proved to be erroneous. Many meniscal lesions in the posterolateral compartment cannot be visualized from the front, even with the small-diameter endoscope. More important, the posterolateral compartment harbors most loose bodies found in the knee joint. Many can be removed through a cannula placed in the compartment. It became apparent that for complete evaluation, posterolateral inspection was required even for patients with normal anterior arthroscopic findings of the lateral compartment.

Suprapatellar puncture routine

With increased experience the suprapatellar puncture has become routine for adequate visualization of the patella and the confines of that compartment. It should no longer be considered an auxiliary or optional portal. The single anterolateral or anteromedial anterior portal often provides a superficial and tangential view of the patella; the plica can also be overlooked if this lower approach is used. Whipple[30] reported the importance of multiple approaches in 1977.

At this time I am satisfied that it is possible to inspect virtually every recess of the joint by direct observation, using the multiple puncture technique.

DOCUMENTATION
Slide photography

The first photographs made to document Needlescope arthroscopic observations were taken with a single-lens reflex camera, using available light from a 300-W source and Kodak high-speed Ektachrome ASA-160 film. The photographs were primitive at best, due to the narrow angle of view of the endoscope, the inability with still photography to create a composition including adjacent areas, and the limited light source. With the improved Model III Needlescope the problems, except for that of composition, have been resolved.

The rod-lens telescope provides a larger cross-sectional area of fiber light and has a larger diameter lens to transmit light; it thus provides an optimal photographic document. In addition, a Storz flash generator produces an excellent photographic image on Kodachrome ASA-64 film. The color balance with this technique is very good.

Available-light photographic slides taken on Ektachrome ASA-400 film at $1/30$ second using a rod-lens type of endoscope are also uniformly excellent documents.

Cinephotography

Because slides are unsatisfactory for developing composition and because of the low light levels, movie photography provides a better means of documentation. In February, 1973, Mr. Harold Neuman matched color film to a light source and provided an optical adapter from the camera to the endoscope. He had built the original 300-W short-arc lamp illuminator, first known as the Blue Max and now marketed as the Dyonics Model 500 Illuminator. The first movies were taken at a rather slow shutter speed with Ektachrome 7241 film. Cinephotography became the medium of choice for documenting technique.

Television

In the spring of 1976, with the technology provided by television, it was possible to document more clearly the observations made with the Needlescope. Video equipment could produce an image at a lower light level than was possible with cinephotography. By this time videocassette recordings were being used as a means of transmitting our findings to the referring orthopedists. This provided not only a narrative but the same visualization of abnormalities as observed during arthroscopy. Subsequently this program has been abandoned because of cost and failure of the referring physician to return the materials.

Currently every case performed under general anesthesia is reviewed and recorded on television. This has proved an easier means of performing the surgery and provides interest for the operating room staff. In addition, a record is available for teaching and research.

NEW DEVELOPMENTS IN INSTRUMENTATION

In conjunction with Dyonics, Inc., studies were initiated in 1977 toward developing a motorized system for the resection of diseased intra-articular tissues. A battery-powered, rotating, cutting, suction device had its first clinical trial in September of that year. It was introduced commercially in December of 1978. The first scientific report was made at the American Academy of Orthopaedic Surgeons at the forty-sixth annual meeting in San Francisco in February, 1979. This report included 72 patients with a 2½-year follow-up. By that time there were almost 400 of these instruments being used in the United States.

In January of 1979 the intra-articular cutter, a modified cutting head, was introduced for the resection of tougher intra-articular tissue, including the meniscus. (See Chapter 14.) At this time the Intra-articular Shaver System is an integral part of most arthroscopic surgeons' armamentarium.

SUMMARY

The comprehensive arthroscopic examination of the knee includes visualization of every recess in the knee joint; posteromedial and posterolateral compartments may be seen, as well as the region beneath the menisci in the area of the coronary ligaments. Furthermore, when there are only diagnostic problems, this examination is easily performed with patients under local anesthesia. The same technique is adaptable for the complete inspection of the knee joint prior to surgical procedures in those patients with an established clinical diagnosis. The technique provides access for synovial membrane biopsy and collection of synovial fluid for microscopic studies. The comprehensive technique includes intra-articular documentation by still and cinephotography or videotape recordings. It has proved to be a simple, efficient, and reliable technique.

Arthroscopic surgery has challenged conventional methods in the field of orthopedics. With time arthroscopic procedures will replace previous accepted techniques.

REFERENCES
1. American Academy of Orthopaedic Surgeons: Symposium on arthroscopy and arthrography of the knee, St. Louis, 1978, The C. V. Mosby Co.
2. Bechtol, R. C.: Diagnostic aids in arthroscopy. In American Academy of Orthopaedic Surgeons: Symposium on arthroscopy and arthrography of the knee, St. Louis, 1978, The C. V. Mosby Co.
3. Bircher, E.: Beitrag zur Pathologie und Diagnose der Meniscusverletzungen (Arthroendoskopie), Brums Beitrage zur Klinischen Chirurgie **127**:239, 1922.
4. Blaugh, H., and Donner, K.: Arthroskopie des Kniegdenkes, Symposium Kiel, Stuttgart, 1979, Georg Thieme Verlag.
5. Burman, M. S.: Arthroscopy on direct visualization of joints: an experimental cadaver study, J. Bone Joint Surg. **13**(4):669, 1931.
6. Burman, M. S., Finkelstein, H., and Mayer, L.: Arthroscopy of the knee joint, J. Bone Joint Surg. **16**:255, 1934.
7. Casscells, S. W.: Arthroscopy of the knee joint: a review of 150 cases, J. Bone Joint Surg. (Am.) **53**:287-298, 1971.
8. Clayton, M.: Personal communication, 1979.
9. Eikelaar, H. R.: Arthroscopy of the knee, Groningen, Holland, 1975, Royal United Printers, Hoitsema B.V.
10. Eilert, R.: Laboratory aid in the teaching of arthroscopy. In American Academy of Orthopaedic Surgeons: Symposium on arthroscopy and arthrography of the knee, St. Louis, 1978, The C. V. Mosby Co.
11. Guhl, J. F.: Operative arthroscopy, Am. J. Sports Med. **7**(6):328, 1979.
12. Guten, G. S.: Methylene blue staining of articular cartilage during arthroscopy, Orthop. Rev. **6**(3):59, 1977.
13. Hencke, H.-R.: Arthroscopy of the knee joint, Berlin, 1980, Springer-Verlag.
14. Jackson, R. W., and Abe, I.: The role of arthroscopy in the management of disorders of the knee: an analysis of 200 consecutive examinations, J. Bone Joint Surg. (Br.) **54**:310, 1972.
15. Jackson, R. W., and Dandy, D. J.: Arthroscopy of the knee, New York, 1976, Grune and Stratton, Inc.
16. Jackson, R. W., and DeHaven, K. E.: Arthroscopy of the knee, Clin. Orthop. **107**:87, 1975.
17. Johnson, L. L.: Diagnostic arthroscopy of the knee: the knee joint, Amsterdam, Excerpta Medica; New York, 1974, American Elsevier Publishing Co.
18. Johnson, L. L.: Arthroscopy of the knee using local anesthesia: a review of 400 patients, J. Bone Joint Surg. (Am.) **58**(5):736, 1976.
19. Joyce, J. J.: Symposium on arthroscopy (foreword), Orthop. Clin. North Am. **10**(3), 1979.
20. Klein, W., and Huth, F.: Arthroskopie und Histopathologie in der Diagnostik von Gelenkerkrankungen, Internislische. Welt. **10**:349, 1979.
21. McGinty, J. B., and Freedman, D. A.: Arthroscopy of the knee, Clin. Orthop. **121**:171, 1976.
22. McGinty, J. B., and Mapza, R. A.: Evaluation of an outpatient procedure under local anesthesia, J. Bone Joint Surg. (Am.) **60**:787, 1978.
23. Metcalf, R.: Personal communication, 1980.
24. O'Conner, R.: Arthroscopy in the diagnosis and treatment of acute ligament injuries of the knee, J. Bone Joint Surg. (Am.) **56**:333, 1974.

25. O'Connor, R. L.: Arthroscopy, Philadelphia, 1977, J. B. Lippincott Co.
26. Pevey, J. K.: Outpatient arthroscopy of the knee under local anesthesia, Am. J. Sports Med. **6**(3):122, 1978.
27. Watanabe, M., and Takeda, S.: The number 21 arthroscope, J. Jpn. Orthop. Assoc. **34**:1041, 1960.
28. Watanabe, M., Takeda, S., and Ikeuchi, H.: Atlas of arthroscopy, ed. 3, Berlin, 1979, Springer-Verlag.
29. Watanabe, M.: Arthroscope: present and future, Surg. Ther. **26**(7):73, 1972.
30. Whipple, T. L., and Bassett, F. H.: Arthroscopic examination of the knee: polypuncture technique with percutaneous intra-articular manipulation, J. Bone Joint Surg. (Am.) **60**(4):444, 1978.

Chapter 2

Instrumentation

Selection of an arthroscope
Types of arthroscopes
    Thin-lens system
    Rod-lens system
    Coherent bundle system
    Graded refractory index system
Light sources
Light guides
    Halo light
    Light wand
Accessories
    Cannulas
    Forceps
Sterilization and disinfection

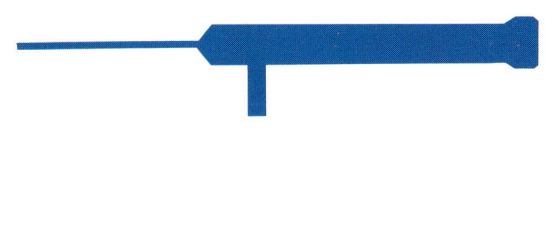

SELECTION OF AN ARTHROSCOPE

The selection of an arthroscope is based on the personality, vision, eye-hand coordination, and technical ability of the arthroscopist. No endoscope is ideal for every arthroscopist or for every situation. A single initial purchase is usually difficult because the limitations of any given scope cannot be anticipated. With the second endoscope a system can be selected that has advantages not possible with the first. All endoscopes or other optical systems have limitations, and trade-offs may be necessary in the purchase of new equipment.

It is possible in selected patients to carry out a complete arthroscopy of the knee with virtually any endoscope, except perhaps the Watanabe No. 21, which is too large with the tungsten light bulb attached. I prefer the 1.7-mm diameter Needlescope, which when housed in its cannula has an outside diameter of 2 mm. This small-diameter endoscope allows an ease of access under the menisci and into the posteromedial and posterolateral compartments that the larger diameter endoscopes do not afford. If multiple punctures are made with a large-diameter endoscope (e.g., 3.5 mm), the joint will deflate because of leakage from previous entry sites; when distension is lost, ease of access into the posteromedial and posterolateral compartments is diminished. In some patients, even a 2.2-mm Needlescope with a 2.7-mm cannula limits access for viewing the posterior horn from an anterior approach. With use of large-diameter endoscopes the view of the knee joint that has normal stability is even more limited, except when the patient is under general anesthesia and the thigh is secured in a Surgical Assistant. Larger arthroscopes are preferred for surgical procedures.

TYPES OF ARTHROSCOPES
Thin-lens system

In the classic thin-lens system (Fig. 2-1) the lenses are thin in comparison with their diameters. Air spaces separate each of the conventional lenses. The objective lens is to the left and transmits the light from the image through the relay lens system to the ocular lens. The ocular lens transmits the image to the observer's eye. This is the classic design for telescopes.

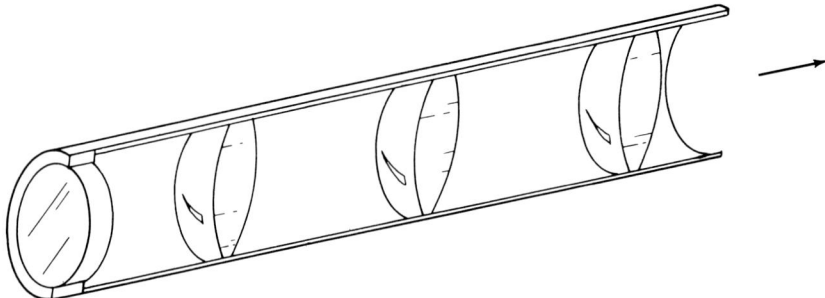

FIG. 2-1. Classic thin-lens system is series of small lenses divided by cylinders of air. Image comes through objective lens from left and is transmitted by relay lens system to ocular lens. Light is transmitted in direction of arrow to arthroscopist's eye. The relay lens system varies in different types of endoscopes.

Rod-lens system

The rod-lens system (Fig. 2-2, A) was designed by Professor H. H. Hopkins of Reading, England. In this system the lenses are thick compared with the diameter. The surfaces are convex, and the air space between the lenses is relatively small. The cylindrical space is glass rather than air, as in the thin-lens relay system. The image is transmitted from the ocular lens to the eyepiece. The Storz-Hopkins rod-lens system (Fig. 2-2, B and C) and Dyonics rod-lens system (Fig. 2-2, D and E) are representative.

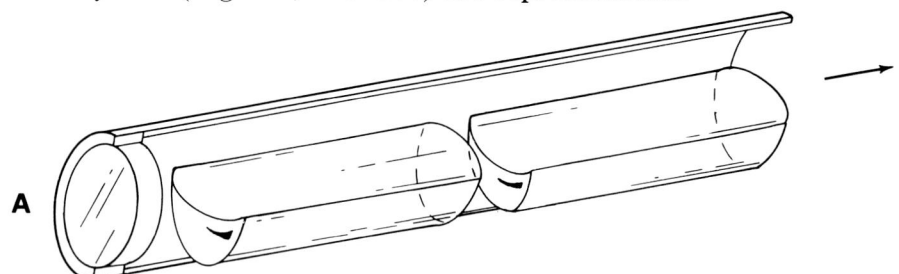

FIG. 2-2. A, Rod-lens system is series of glass cylinders separated by small areas of air, or reverse of thin-lens system. **B,** Storz rod-lens system is available in two sizes, with a 2.7-mm or 4-mm telescope. Both provide excellent optical clarity. **C,** Storz 70° inclined view rod-lens telescope is 4 mm in diameter. Its separate cannula is shorter than standard to accommodate greater degree angle of optics and not cover the view with the metallic sheath. It is used in posterior compartment via the Gillquist method. **D,** Dyonics rod lens affords excellent optical clarity and has trocar and cannula of simpler design and operation than does Storz endoscope. **E,** Left to right, 4-mm diameter Dyonics rod-lens endoscope; 2.2-mm Needlescope seen in end view; 1.7-mm Needlescope; No. 18 needle, shown for relative size comparison.

Instrumentation

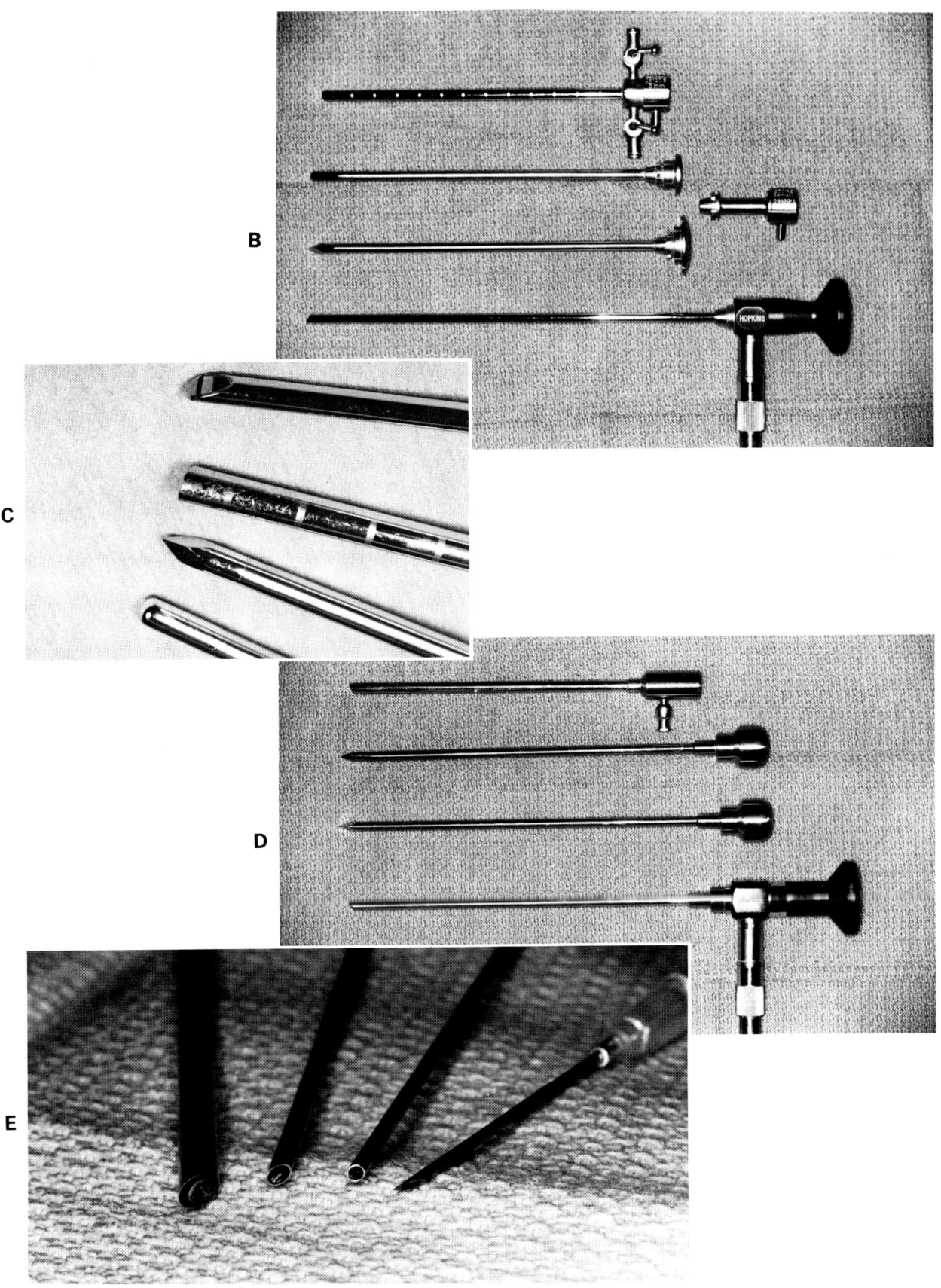

Diagnostic arthroscopy of the knee

Coherent bundle system

The coherent bundle system (Fig. 2-3) has an objective lens that relays the light from the image. It is then transmitted through a bundle of coherent light fibers. The image is transmitted through the ocular lens to the observer's eye. With this system the viewer sees many fine dots, each of which transmits an element of the image that is being viewed. It was marketed as a No. 24–type arthroscope but is no longer available.*

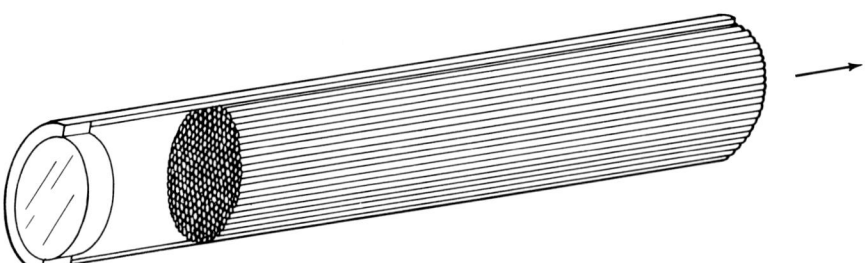

FIG. 2-3. Fused coherent bundle system transmits light by individual fibers. Composition consists of many fine dots, each transmitting an element of image.

Graded refractory index system

A graded refractory index (GRIN) lens system is one in which the entire instrument consists of a slender rod of glass. The refractory index decreases from the center to the periphery according to a specific mathematic relationship. The lens is processed by an ion-exchange treatment utilizing cesium. This endoscope is self-focusing (Selfoc). The rays of light that enter the lens from a particular point in an optic space follow helical patterns and come into focus, periodically along the rod, producing an image.[3,4] The Watanabe No. 24 arthroscope (1.7 mm diameter) was the precursor of the Needlescope (Fig. 2-4).

*Pro-Med Co., Montreal, Canada.

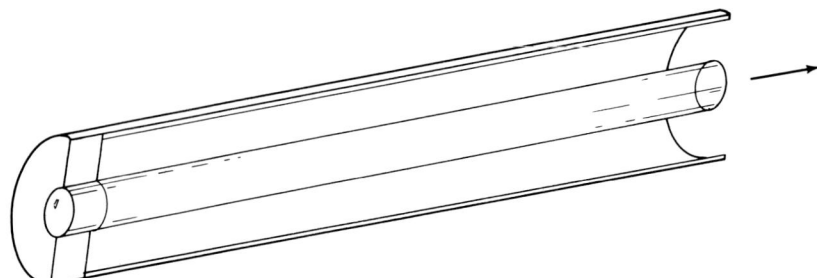

FIG. 2-4. Needlescope system consists of two graded refractory index (GRIN) lenses and an ocular lens. Objective lens, about 3 mm in length and 1 mm in diameter, gives a wide field of view. Relay lens, about 134 mm in length and 1 mm in diameter, transfers image from objective lens back to ocular lens, which magnifies image for viewing.

Instrumentation

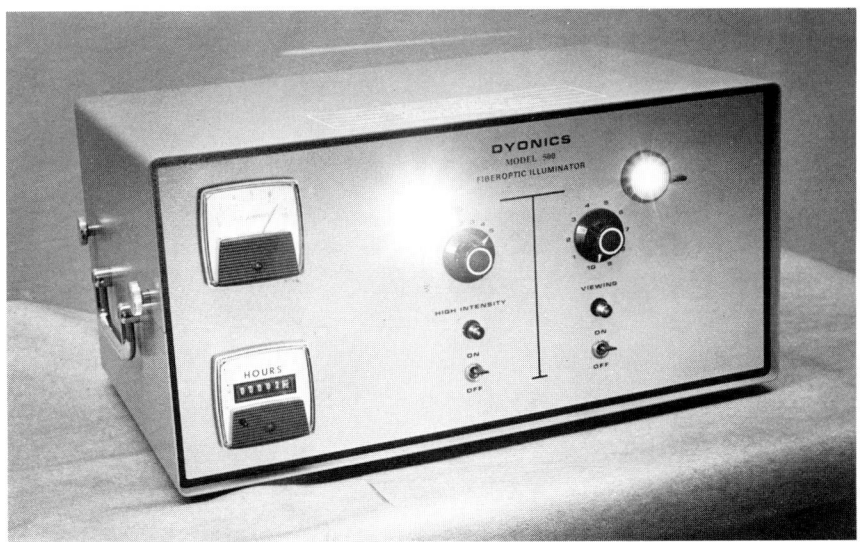

FIG. 2-5. Dyonics Model 500 light source.

LIGHT SOURCES

I have used a variety of light sources, perhaps virtually every one on the market in North America, in demonstrating the technique of the comprehensive arthroscopic examination of the knee. It is my opinion that the Dyonics Model 500 light source (Fig. 2-5) and the Storz xenon arc illuminator are the light sources of choice for the serious arthroscopist. The intensity of the light in these two sources is comparable. The color arc appears different when documented photographically and perhaps would not be apparent to the uninitiated eye. Movie filmstrips of the same patient taken on the same day, changing only the light source, show the Model 500 Illuminator to have a blue-white light, which provides more optical clarity than does the xenon light source, which has a slight yellowish tint. Other light sources that have less intensity can be used, but the depth of field of illumination is limited, as is the clarity, and the photographic capacity is diminished.

The Sylvania 300/16 light bulb is favored as the illumination source. This light is too bright for comfortable direct viewing when set on high intensity, so the shading device is used. The high-intensity setting is essentially for documentation. The light bulb will last many hours, but its maximum intensity starts to decline after 6 hours. The effective light is virtually dissipated by 24 hours of use. The level of loss is not recognized under direct viewing but will result in poor photographic documents. This often surprises the arthroscopist who saw a good image and then finds the photograph very dull. The diminution of light intensity is most easily recognized when recording and viewing are monitored on television.

LIGHT GUIDES

A variety of light guides, or cables, is available. Any manufacturer will make attachments for a competitor's endoscopes, and vice versa. The Silastic covering on the Dyonics cables is more thermal resistant than is that marketed by others and therefore has a potentially longer life. It has been my experience that cables manufactured by Dyonics last for approximately 1 year and in excess of 300 steam autoclavings. Care of the cables is important; they should not be kinked or twisted. As with any other technical equipment, performance of the light cable should be checked periodically so that gradual deterioration does not compromise the arthroscopic examination. The passage of light or usage over many months does not wear out the cables. However, over a period of time (approximately 1 year) multiple fiber breaks develop, and light cannot be transmitted along the entire length of the cable. To check for breaks, first turn off bright overhead lights; then hold one end of the cable up to an available lamp (light bulb). By looking down the other end of the cable, one can visualize darkened or black areas (breaks). Also, that same fiber will emit light at the point of the break along the cable. Each end of the cable must have a polished,

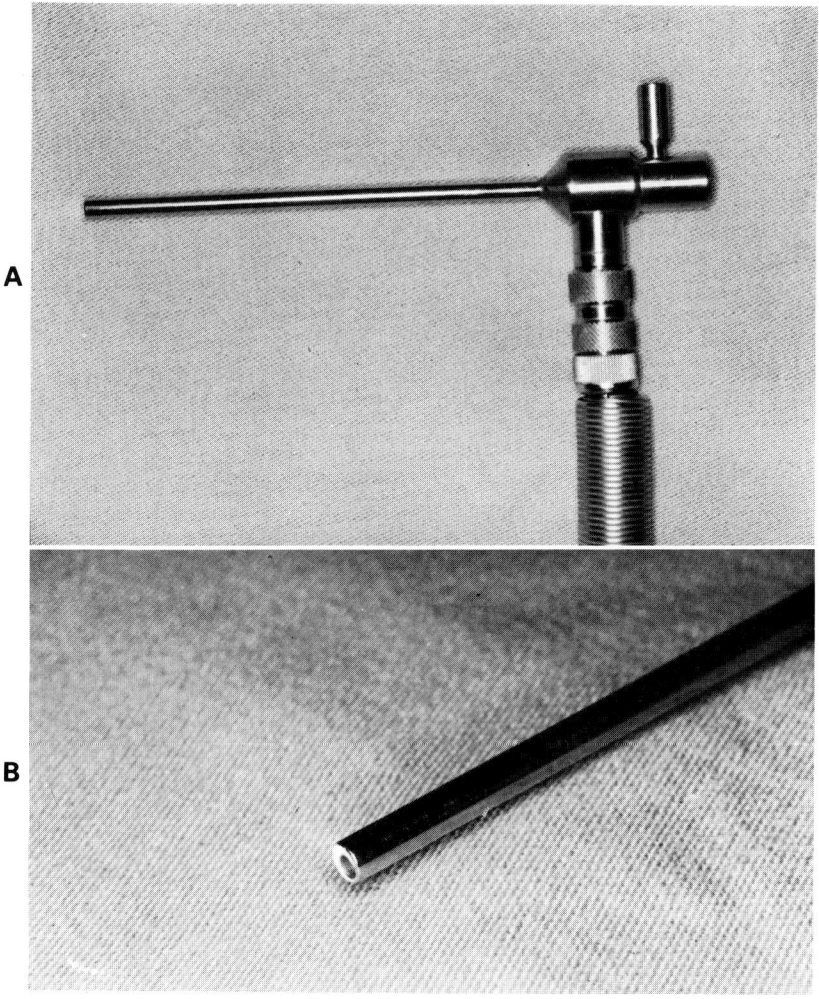

FIG. 2-6. A, Halo light is advantageous for photographic work and for protection of small-diameter endoscope when utilized for training purposes. **B,** End of halo light. Notice central opening that will house 1.7-mm Needlescope. Illumination is up to sixteen times that of endoscope.

Instrumentation

clean surface. Repeated checks and replacements are necessary to ensure optimal transmission of light.

Halo light

Fragility of the small-diameter endoscope (1.7 mm outside diameter) has been a concern, especially in training programs. Therefore the halo light, or teaching cannula, was introduced (Fig. 2-6). This 3.5-mm outside diameter cannula provides sixteen times the illumination of the small-diameter Needlescope. It allows arthroscopists to become proficient with the small-diameter scope and yet have the safety, protection, and photographic capacity of a larger diameter endoscope.

Light wand

A light wand (Fig. 2-7) is helpful in transillumination and photographic work. It is either placed parallel to the view or may transilluminate tissue for examination. Transillumination first showed the engulfing of saline by synovium. Observation of the vascular pattern and morphologic characteristics is enhanced by transillumination effects on photographic film.

A light cable with a small (2 to 3 mm diameter) attached light wand has been useful in arthroscopic surgery. The main cable is attached as usual to the viewing arthroscope. The second portion of the cable with its attached light wand can be placed in the posterior compartment via a separate puncture. This provides back lighting that improves one's visualization and depth of field.

The bifurcated light cable (Fig. 2-8) has one attachment for the endoscope and the second attachment with a metallic light source for separate entry for back illumination and improvement of visualization and depth of field conceptualization.

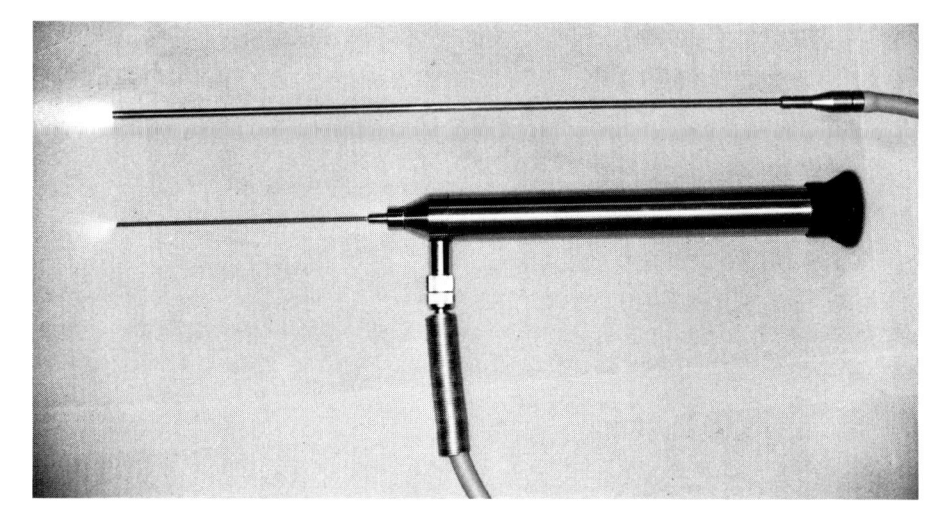

FIG. 2-7. Light wand, shown above Needlescope, can be useful for photographic purposes, especially transillumination. It is brought into knee through a separate puncture wound. Photographs are taken through small-diameter endoscope with a camera attached to ocular lens.

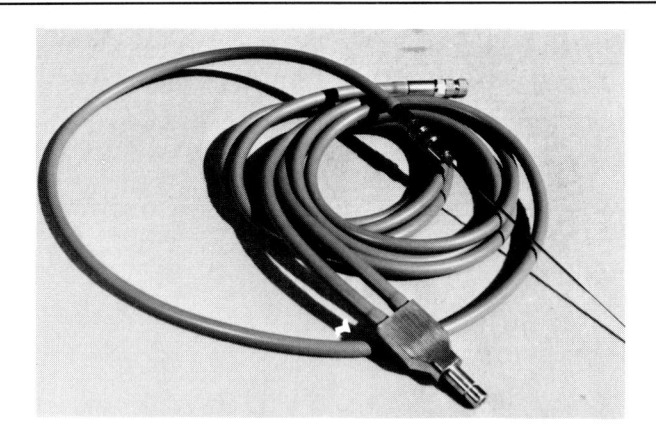

FIG. 2-8. Bifurcated cable.

ACCESSORIES
Cannulas

Cannulas serve various purposes (Fig. 2-9). For the irrigation of joints, a separate cannula is used to provide a source of saline. Suction through a second cannula removes multiple loose bodies. For example, if the posterolateral compartment is being viewed and a large number of loose bodies of small diameter are seen in that compartment, a separate cannula, 2 mm in outside diameter, can be placed anteriorly in the joint to deliver fluid to flush them out. Cannulas up to 6.5 mm outside diameter have been used for the removal of large loose bodies or for the insertion of a modified pituitary forceps for removal of large loose bodies.

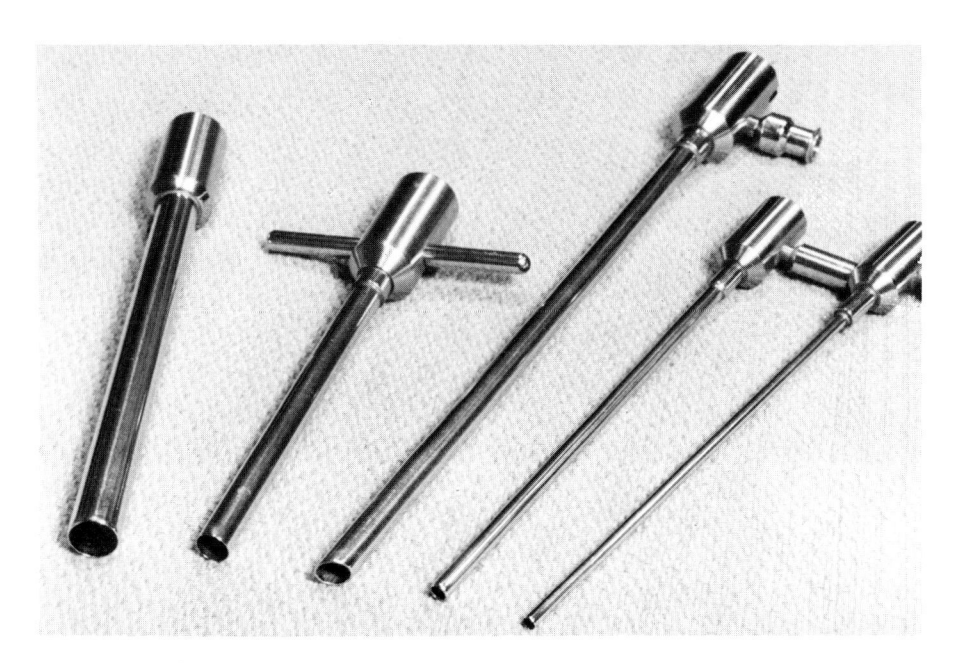

FIG. 2-9. Cannulas varying in size from 8-mm (left) to 2-mm outside diameter (right). Latter holds a 1.7-mm Needlescope.

Instrumentation

Forceps

A regular pituitary forceps was originally used for removal of loose bodies; however, the loose body often pinched out of the forceps like a watermelon seed. A reversed-tooth pituitary forceps was designed, called Jaws (Fig. 2-10). Loose bodies can be gripped percutaneously with this instrument. When the forceps holding the loose body is firmly up against the capsule, a local anesthetic can be placed alongside the instrument shaft. An incision is then made, down to the loose body. Stretching the tissues permits removal of a loose body through an incision smaller than the diameter of the loose body. Rongeuring of partially attached articular cartilage is also possible during arthroscopic examination. The Jaws forceps may be used during open-knee surgery for grasping small tags of menisci that remain after excision of the major fragment.

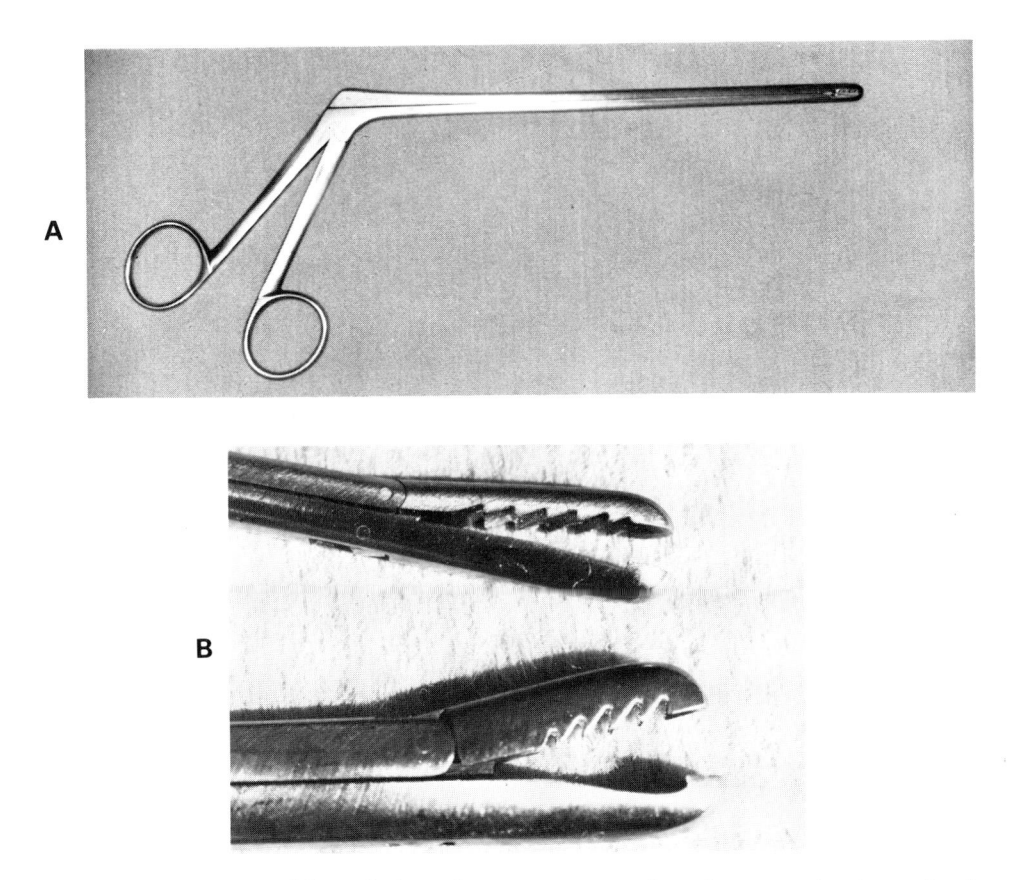

FIG. 2-10. A, Jaws modified pituitary forceps are excellent for removing loose bodies of rather large size, even with patient under local anesthesia. They are useful for grasping fragments of menisci that must be excised when patient requires general anesthesia. **B,** Reverse-tooth Jaws modified pituitary forceps. Notice reversed superior teeth, which guard against slippage of loose body. Scooped-out inferior portion of forceps holds oval-shaped foreign body. Jaws Jr., a smaller instrument, passes through an Intra-articular Shaver System cannula.

Diagnostic arthroscopy of the knee

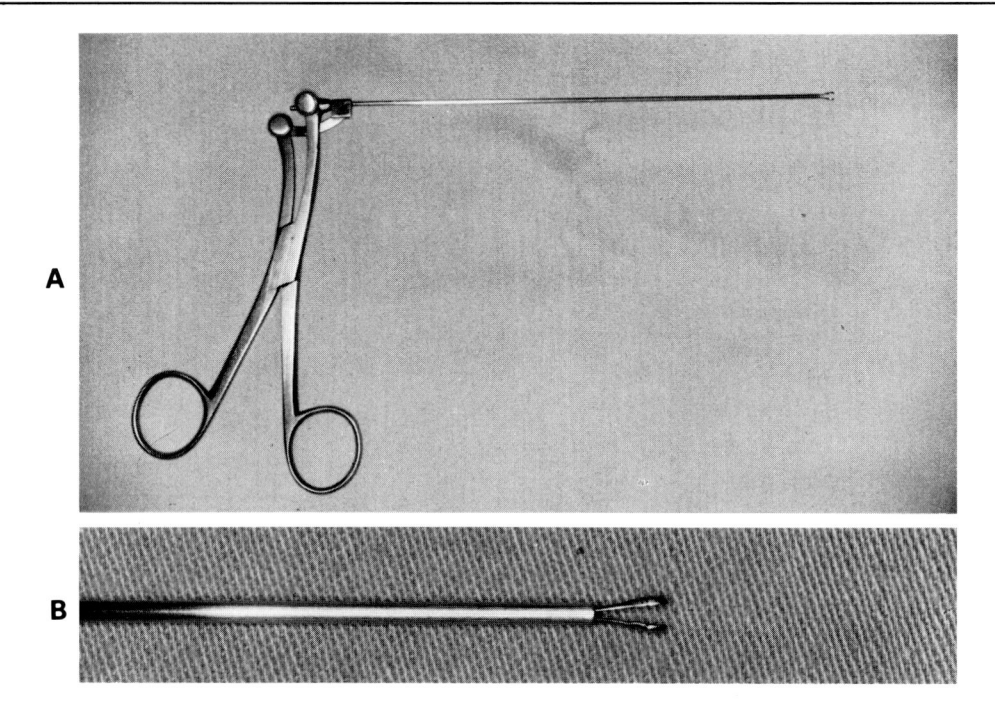

FIG. 2-11. A, Small biopsy forceps can be placed through 2-mm diameter cannula of Needlescope. Biopsy can be done by a separate puncture under direct vision or blindly through existing puncture. **B,** Biting end of miniature biopsy forceps.

A second grasping forceps, Jaws Jr., fits through the cannulas of the intra-articular shaver system. It is best for small loose bodies in the intercondylar areas or in the posterior compartments.

A miniature biopsy forceps (Fig. 2-11) can be placed through a 2-mm outside diameter cannula for synovial membrane or cartilage biopsy. It is possible in cases of diffuse synovitis to excise multiple pieces by this technique without directly visualizing them. A separate puncture will permit biopsy with direct vision. The specimens are of adequate size for histologic evaluation. Schlessinger forceps are preferred for grasping the meniscus.

STERILIZATION AND DISINFECTION

Sterilization of endoscopic equipment has caused considerable concern among orthopedic surgeons and nursing personnel. Sterile technique and the prevention of infection are essential.

No arthroscope will withstand high-pressure steam autoclaving indefinitely. It is estimated that deterioration will be significant after 100 steam autoclavings. The present construction of arthroscopes is such that with this type of sterilization the adhesive seals between the lenses or the chambers eventually break down. Therefore it is recommended that the endoscope be sterilized with ethylene oxide gas. One of the disadvantages of this method of sterilization is that many hospitals do not possess the necessary equipment. In addition, it takes at least 4 hours, sometimes overnight, for complete drying after the sterilization process. This is impractical because the arthroscopist is restricted to one examination per arthroscope per day. One is not likely to purchase a number of expensive instruments so that more than one arthroscopic procedure can be carried out each day. Therefore an alternative method of disinfection, which is both practical and safe, was instituted.

Thackary has developed a small autoclave for arthroscopic sterilization. It uses lower temperatures to protect the adhesives between the lens systems and has a cycle of 1 hour. I have no personal experience with that system. Therefore I clean the endoscope first with alcohol and then place it in an activated dialdehyde solution (Cidex) for 20 minutes. Prior to use it is rinsed with sterile saline; when dry, it is placed on a sterile Mayo stand. Most equipment used for arthroscopy (i.e., cannulas, light cords, catheters, and suction tubes) are either steam autoclavable or are disposable sterile materials.

At the close of each week all the equipment is cleaned, assembled for ethylene oxide sterilization over the weekend, and stored.

In my experience over the past 7 years with nearly 3,000 patients, no infection or hepatitis has resulted from arthroscopy.[2] For one 18-month period in which over 400 patients were arthroscopically examined, either under local or general anesthesia, ethylene oxide sterilization was not used, but the endoscopes were cleansed with Cidex disinfectant only. No patients developed infection. Some patients experienced "unexplained" synovitis either after surgery or arthroscopy. Cultures were taken, but none showed positive findings. Most cases of synovitis were nonspecific, with negative culture findings. Some occurred secondary to articular loose bodies within the joint; cleansing the joint of the loose bodies or synovial debris remedied the synovitis. No case of a spore-producing bacterial infection was recognized. There was no hepatitis.

We reported 3,388 case experiences by five orthopedic surgeons over 4½ years at the Ingham Medical Center in Lansing, Michigan. There was one explained infection following arthroscopy on a loose, infected total-knee joint. There was also an exacerbation of a previous, unrecognized infection.

Our last review at the Ingham Medical Center showed 7,240 case experiences by six orthopedic surgeons between October 30, 1972, and June 30, 1979. There were four patients who had infections following an arthroscopic procedure. One patient had an arthroscopy 2 weeks before his meniscectomy, and 2 weeks after the meniscectomy he developed a superficial wound infection. Separate aspiration of the joint produced a negative culture. The wound was drained, and the patient was immediately given antibiotics.

Two other patients underwent arthroscopy immediately prior to reconstructive surgery. One patient developed a *Staphylococcus aureus* infection at the most extreme posterior portion of the transverse medial arthrotomy. He had no inflammatory signs at his lateral incision where the reconstruction was done. He did have a history of carbunculosis. The wound was drained and healed readily after antibiotic therapy with no joint involvement. The other patient had an arthroscopy immediately preceding the reconstructive procedure and developed a mixed organism infection. The wound opened entirely and required considerable care, but it did heal.

The fourth patient had a loose, infected Waldius prosthesis. He underwent an arthroscopy to inspect the joint and developed an exacerbation of the infection requiring arthrotomy the following day. The bleeding from the arthroscopy provided a culture medium for the low-grade infection in this total-knee patient. Subsequent removal of the total knee was required, but he was able to undergo a revision at a later date. He has maintained the revision for 2 years.

Most arthroscopists use a disinfection method similar to that just described to facilitate doing a series of arthroscopies in one day. There has been no attempt, to my knowledge, to incur the rigors of an Environmental Protection Agency investigation to validate the use of activated dialdehyde solution (Cidex) for cold sterilization in arthroscopy. When this chemical was introduced in 1964, the label indicated that a 3-hour sterilization time was appropriate. This was based on the spore-testing method accepted by the United States Department of Agriculture, which regulated agents such as pesticides and disinfectants and which at the time used stainless steel penicylinders. In 1969 the responsibility for evaluation of pesticides and disinfectants was transferred to the Environmental Protection Agency. That agency employs a loop-suture method for spore testing, which requires that a sterilization solution penetrate the fibers of the loop material as well as the spore itself. Because loop fibers are more difficult to penetrate than is stainless steel, the required sterilization time for Cidex became 10 hours, indicated on the chemical's label. There has been no provision made by the Environmental Protection Agency for a method that would be comparable to soaking arthroscopes or laparoscopes in Cidex for between 10 and 30 minutes. However, no instance of infection as a result of this technique has been reported to the manufacturer. The bulk of clinical evidence supports Cidex disinfecting as safe and practical, and it is the standard of practice of established arthroscopists throughout the United States.

At Ingham Medical Center we continue to use this method of disinfection and recommend it to others in spite of the theoretical arguments and the resistance by operating room head nurses in many hospitals. Experience has shown that this method is best introduced to our hospital by the pathologist and the infection committee. Generally, persuasiveness toward the operating room staff is not fruitful.

REFERENCES

1. Arbrook Inc., Arlington, Texas: Personal correspondence, 1976.
2. Johnson, L. L., Shneider, D., Goodman, F. G., Bullock, J. M., and DeBrun, J. D., Jr.: Cold sterilization method for arthroscopies using activated dialdehyde, Orthop. Rev. **6**(9):75, 1977.
3. Prescott, R.: Optical principles of endoscopy, J. Med. Primatol. **5**(2):133, 1976.
4. Prescott, R.: Optical design and care of the endoscope. In The American Academy of Orthopaedic Surgeons: Symposium on arthroscopy and arthrography of the knee, St. Louis, 1978, The C. V. Mosby Co.

Chapter 3

Basic arthroscopic techniques

Technical concepts
    Light
    Distension
    Placement
    Replacement
    Entry
    Redirection
    Hand control
    Palpation
    Probing
    Manipulation
    Cleansing and vacuuming
    Contrast staining
    Scanning the horizon
    Pistoning
    Rotation
    Scope sweeping
    Free hand activity
Team approach
    Responsibilities of circulating nurse
    Responsibilities of assistant
    Care of instruments between patients
    Diagnostic arthroscopy procedure
Arthroscopic compartments
    Anteromedial approach
    Patella and suprapatellar pouch
    Anterolateral compartment
    Intercondylar notch
    Anteromedial compartment
    Posteromedial compartment
    Posterolateral compartment
    Suprapatellar approach
    Transpatellar tendon approach: Gillquist technique
    Modified Gillquist approach
Follow-up
Complications

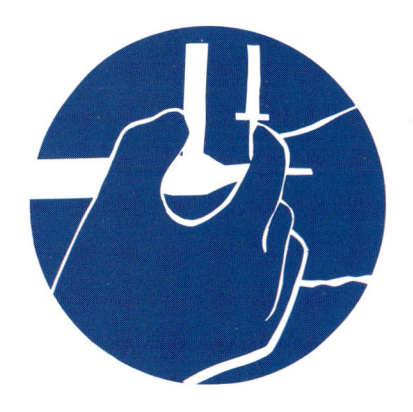

    The comprehensive arthroscopic examination of the knee requires that established principles and disciplines be used to successfully accomplish the technique.
    Although arthroscopy is potentially a simple procedure, a great number of details need attention before the technique is accomplished with ease. As orthopedists, we are accustomed to working with tools. In recent years new operative procedures (e.g., Harrington rod instrumentation or total-hip surgery) have required increased focus of attention on a number of details heretofore not required in the usual orthopedic surgical procedures. Although

arthroscopy does not require that an incision be made or that anatomic pathways be known, there is no decrease in the technical details to be attended to nor any less demand on the technical prowess of the surgeon. The procedure demands mastering the use of fine instruments, the arthroscope and miniature tools.

Preoperative organization and planning will contribute more to the technical skill with which the procedure is accomplished than will any compensatory effort during arthroscopy. It is important that procedures be done in a similar manner each time. Each member of the arthroscopic team performs his or her duties in coordination with the others in a similar manner for every operation. Responsibliities do not overlap, and there is very little improvisation. Each participant has a great deal of individual responsibility, carried out with the support of the other members of the team. Such compulsiveness may bother some personalities, but it eliminates aimlessness during the surgical procedure.

TECHNICAL CONCEPTS

A number of concepts are unique to arthroscopy and must be mastered by any physician desiring to become an accomplished arthroscopist. I have learned many of the technical details by trial and error. The following material is offered so that others may learn more easily.

The absence of adequate light and maximal distension are the two most common faults that hinder an arthroscopic examination. In the absence of excellent light and distension, all the other "tricks" are useless. They are the most essential of all the technical concepts necessary for arthroscopy.

Light

A common requirement for any photography is light. Arthroscopy is photography, with the physician's eye being the camera and the retina the film. Whatever system the physician chooses to act as a telescope between his camera (eye) and the inside of the patient's joint requires adequate illumination. If the arthroscopist chooses an endoscope of small diameter, the amount of fiber light bundles that can be contained in a small endoscope is limited. A powerful light source is required for adequate illumination. For instance, if one performs macroscopic examination during an arthrotomy, then the ambient light in the operating theater is adequate to view the inside of the knee joint. If one were then to take a photograph with a single-lens reflex camera (with a 50-mm lens) of that arthrotomy site, additional light would be required to record an adequate image. When lens size is decreased to 1 mm, as in the Needlescope, the amount of light that can travel through that 1 mm has to be enhanced by another powerful light being projected onto the image. When the cross-sectional diameter of the entire telescope is only 2 mm, then the cross-sectional area of the light-carrying fibers would be approximately 0.7 mm. This necessitates a powerful and forceful source to push the light down a small cross-sectional area of fiberglass for adequate illumination. When the endoscope has a lens diameter of 2 or 3 mm and an outside diameter of 6 mm, then the cross-sectional area is increased by as great a factor as 16. A less powerful light source may suffice as an illuminator.

It is my opinion that the serious arthroscopist should acquire a high quality, powerful light source, not only for regular viewing but also for photographic and video documentation. This is especially so when carrying light through an articulated viewing device, with television monitoring.

Distension

Distension is essential for viewing "inside the balloon," in this case the knee joint. Undistended synovial folds easily block one's view and result in a whiteout. The most common complaint of an inexperienced arthroscopist is "How do you get around the fat pad?" This usually is a result of lack of distension; occasionally it is because of placement. If one uses an inflow cannula of a small diameter, such as a Verres needle, the needle can either be plugged, blocked off, or up against the synovium so that the flow is diminished. In addition, during a lengthy procedure the volume of saline in the system can decrease, and therefore the head of pressure is decreased and distension minimized. When using an inflow adjacent to the arthroscope and a large-diameter endoscope, the side spigots appear to have a diameter of about 4 mm, but the open valve has only a 1-mm diameter. This often becomes clogged or rusted, diminishing even further the potential flow. Therefore a large reservoir (6 liters) suspended above the patient (at least 1 m) is necessary to maintain distension.

If one chooses the vacuuming system outlined later in the chapter, then distension of the joint by compartments is necessary. The use of 60 ml of saline will adequately distend the joint for approximately 3 to 5 minutes. If viewing goes beyond that time, collapse occurs and the arthroscopist must struggle. Further distension is necessary. Therefore many beginning arthroscopists opt for the continuous flow methods rather than repeated distension because their procedures take longer than a few minutes. That system is fine, but then the problems just mentioned with a continuous flow must be considered. Whatever method one uses, attention should be paid to the details that ensure maximal distension for viewing.

Distension of the joint is essential and may be accomplished by filling the knee through a separate needle puncture or after direct entry with the endoscope by the more experienced arthroscopist. Entry should be confirmed by direct visualization prior to the instillation of saline. Whichever method is used for joint distension, extravasation of fluid outside the joint should not be allowed, since it will compress the potential space of the joint. The synovium will absorb approximately 25 ml of saline every 5 minutes. Therefore the distended joint will collapse after a short period of viewing. Instillation of another bolus of 50 ml of saline is required for maximal retraction of the synovium and capsule wall. With close arthroscopic inspection the saline can be seen engulfed in the synovial villae, appearing very much like silver or translucent balls (the saline) within larger balloons (the synovial villae). This commences quickly after instillation of the saline and continues throughout the procedure. Prolonged use

Diagnostic arthroscopy of the knee

of separate drainage tubes for instillation of saline under pressure results in considerable absorption of fluid, increased thickness of the synovium, and capsular edema. There is some decreased mobility and increased morbidity following this method of irrigation.

Distension is paramount in making the posteromedial and posterolateral entries for the comprehensive examination of the joint. The use of the small-diameter endoscope reduces the leakage about the previous puncture sites, and there is less loss of distension.

REMEMBER: LIGHT AND DISTENSION

Placement

Excellent placement of the endoscope is essential to successful arthroscopy. A scope placed too superior does not enter the slot of the intercondylar space, and access for viewing the posterior horn is eliminated. It is possible that a scope placed too inferior could go through or under the meniscus, impeding movement and limiting subsequent viewing (Fig. 3-1). Uninitiated arthroscopists are so intense about initial placement that they fail to see that an incorrect positioning should be redone. It is considered good technique to redirect or replace rather than to waste time twisting and wrestling with a badly positioned arthroscope.

Replacement

In patients who are referred for a second arthroscopic examination after failure of the first attempt, the entrance sites on the patient's knee are usually

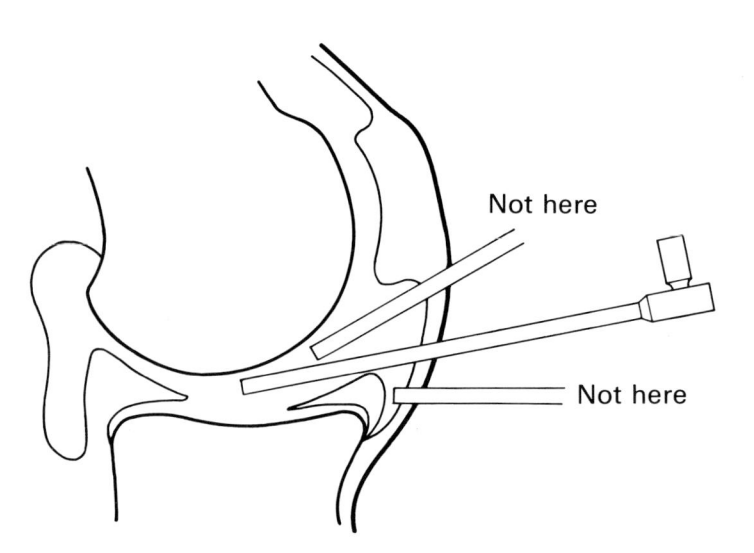

FIG. 3-1. Ideal placement of cannula. If positioned too high, angle of obliquity is such that posterior horn cannot be seen; if too low, it can go through meniscus and limit visualization or mobility. Ideal placement is directly in slot between femur and tibia.

Basic arthroscopic techniques

in such a position that it would be virtually impossible to visualize the inside of the knee. Therefore the arthroscopist should not hesitate even to make another stab wound through the skin to secure adequate intra-articular viewing.

If the surgeon determines that he is close to a position that would allow entry into the joint, then it is not necessary to make another stab wound through the skin. Sliding over on the capsule entrance makes the clear view possible. Then it is not necessary to make another stab wound through the skin. Replacement can be accomplished by pulling the cannula and trocar out through the capsule, then choosing a point 1 or 2 mm above or moving 1 or 2 mm to the side, thus gaining access to the intercondylar slot (Fig. 3-2).

Entry

It is advantageous that the endoscope enter the suprapatellar pouch rather briskly and then be retracted very slowly. Brisk entry allows the synovium to hang up on the shank of the metallic cannula, and slow retraction of the instrument prevents the fat pad from slipping down over the end of the scope, which makes intra-articular viewing impossible (Fig. 3-3).

For the uninitiated arthroscopist it is important that the inside of the joint be visualized before any fluid is instilled, to be certain that entry has been accomplished. Fluid placed outside the capsule only compresses the potential space of the knee joint and impedes subsequent viewing.

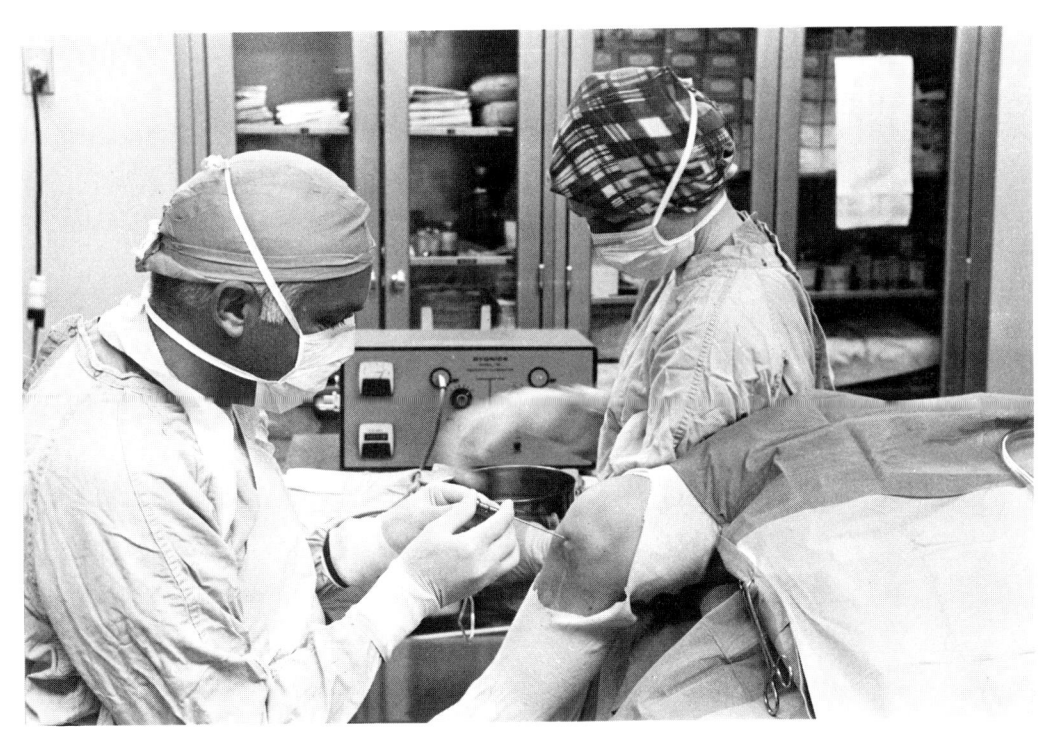

FIG. 3-2. Redirection of endoscope can be of value. It may require withdrawing, reinserting cannula, and moving as little as 1 mm superiorly or laterally to achieve exact position. It is considered good technique to redirect endoscope. This is most often necessary when viewing in medial compartment in a patient who has a scarred or fat knee with a large fulcrum.

Diagnostic arthroscopy of the knee

After entry has been confirmed, the joint is distended (Fig. 3-4), or it may be distended with a separate needle prior to entry. If the joint is not filled with any obscuring synovial fluid or blood, viewing can commence. At this time the operating room lights are turned down; the x-ray viewbox provides sufficient illumination for activity in the room but does not distract the arthroscopist.

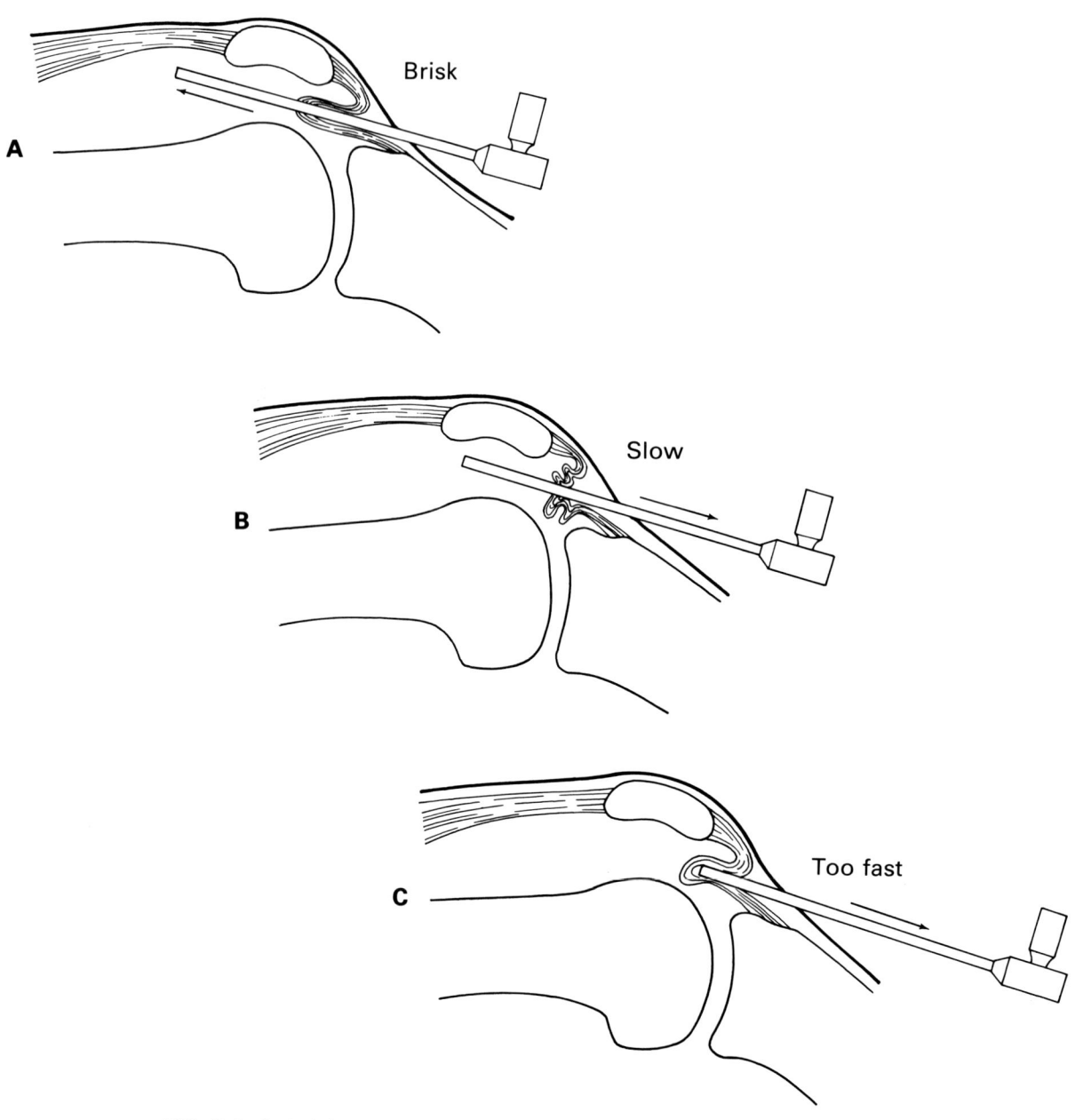

FIG. 3-3. A, Brisk motion will penetrate fat pad and suprapatellar pouch, hanging fat pad synovium on shank of cannula. **B,** Very slow retraction of cannula and endoscope will prevent fat pad from slipping over end of scope. **C,** Fast retraction will pull endoscope into fat pad and obscure viewing.

Basic arthroscopic techniques

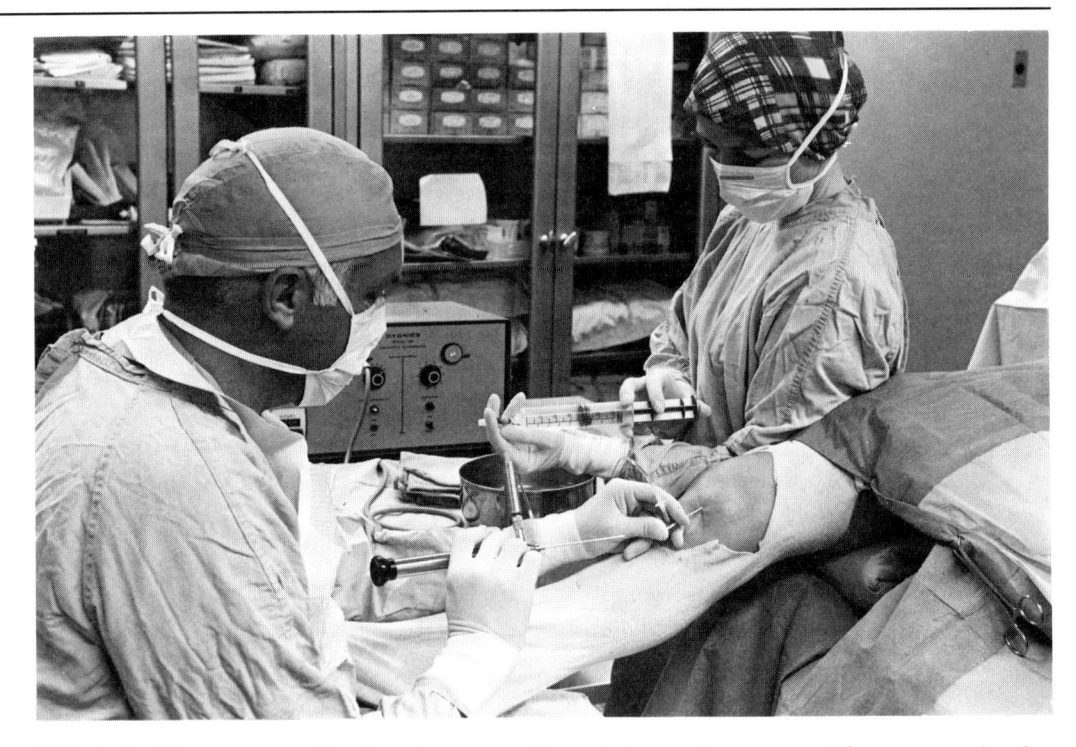

FIG. 3-4. After penetration has been confirmed, trocar is removed from cannula. Arthroscopist places thumb over end of cannula, and assistant forces approximately 60 ml of normal saline through polyethylene catheter into joint. With this maximal distension, viewing can commence.

Redirection

With an anteromedial approach it is important that the initial entry be at a 30° angle toward the lateral side (Fig. 3-2). The opposite is so if the approach is anterolateral. The entry point is just lateral to the tip of the patella, and insertion is directed toward the intercondylar notch, not, initially, up under the patella. In a knee that is fatty (with a large fulcrum) or scarred (with a rigid fulcrum), redirection may be necessary. In unusual circumstances, such as in a tight, fat, or scarred joint, it may be necessary to redirect as many as three times to view a single compartment. In most cases, after viewing in the suprapatellar pouch, lateral compartment, and intercondylar notch through the original placement, the medial compartment can be entered, but bending of the scope may occur. Redirection to the area of the medial meniscus attachment is simple, painless, and nondestructive and facilitates completion of the examination of the anterior and superior chambers.

Hand control

The endoscope is held very firmly with the index finger and thumb (Fig. 3-5), although the wrist and upper arm should be relaxed to facilitate movement of the scope. The firmness of grip allows precise movements and prevents slippage. Dexterity is provided by the combined universal joints of the wrist, elbow, and shoulder. Lack of precision in holding an endoscope, cannula, or

Diagnostic arthroscopy of the knee

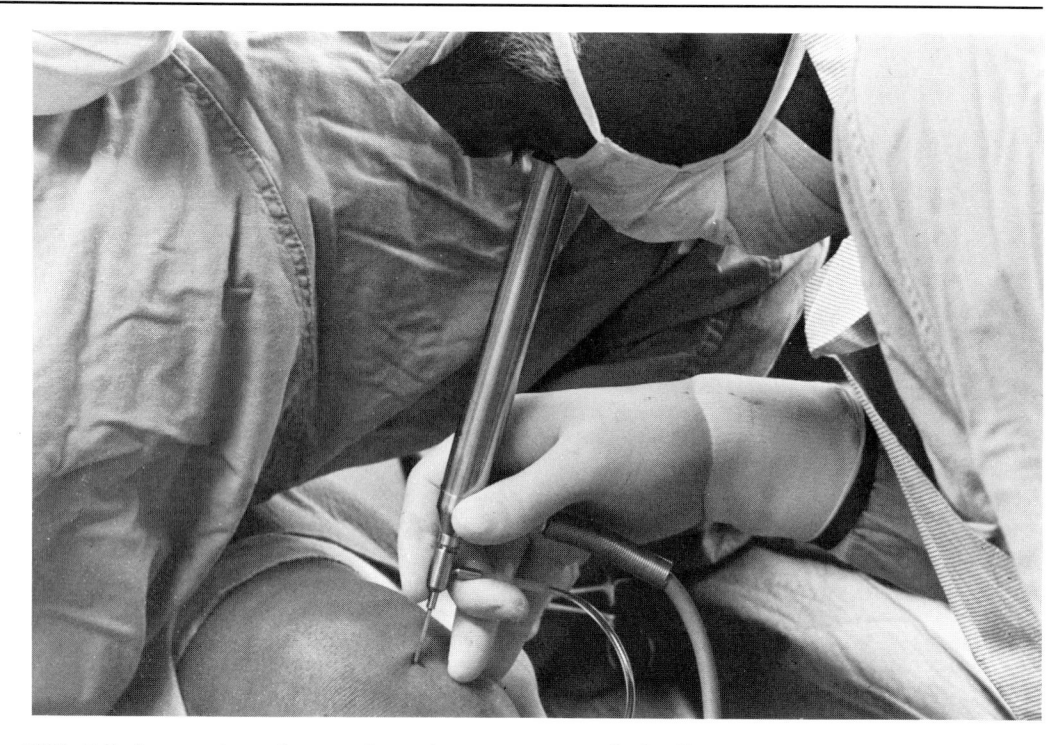

FIG. 3-5. Inspection of anterolateral compartment is facilitated by assistant's hand held to the medial distal femur and valgus force being applied by arthroscopist. Notice safe distance between arthroscopist's hand and viewing eyepiece; this reduces contamination. Endoscope is securely held. Middle finger holds cannula tight against arthroscope, which facilitates manipulation without loosening grip.

trocar will result in quick motions and potential abrasions to the knee joint or injury to the endoscope.

Palpation

Although arthroscopy emphasizes hand-eye coordination, palpation skill is important. As technical skills improve, so does the ability to sense by palpation a location within the knee joint. Visualization follows. For instance, one learns to sense by drag and palpation the different layers of fat, capsule, and synovium that have been penetrated, as well as the position of the endoscope in relation to the patella and the suprapatellar pouch. After some experience, the anterior cruciate ligament can be sensed without direct visualization. The skill of palpation is especially important when one advances to arthroscopic inspection of smaller joints such as the shoulder, elbow, hip, or ankle.

A well-placed scope and an awareness of palpation will result in an excellent arthroscopic examination.

Probing

A simple metallic probe can assist in exploration of the joint. It is especially necessary when a large-diameter (4 mm) endoscope is used because this size does not penetrate easily under or behind the meniscus. The probe can be used to elevate or tug on the meniscus to reveal tears not otherwise recognized.

Basic arthroscopic techniques

> **REMEMBER: PLACEMENT, PALPATION, THEN VISUALIZATION**

Manipulation

Manipulation of the scope in the knee joint is best accomplished with the assistant stabilizing the knee, either with her elbow on the lateral side or her hand on the inner side (Fig. 3-3). Some patients tend to roll, externally rotating the hip; thus stabilization of the thigh is essential to placement and manipulation of the endoscope. With experience, the assistant and the arthroscopist will learn to coordinate their efforts so that a good position is accomplished for endoscope viewing and documentation on film. Stabilization of the thigh by the Surgical Assistant allows the arthroscopist to have complete control by manipulation of the distal part of the extremity; it is only one human variable in this coordinated effort. (See Fig. 14-5.)

Cleansing and vacuuming

It should be emphasized that the best photographic results are obtained in a clean joint. Also, the best arthroscopic view by direct vision is achieved in this manner. Cleansing is accomplished by directly vacuuming out any synovial fluid, debris, or blood that may be in the joint (Fig. 3-6). Jackson[4] initially re-

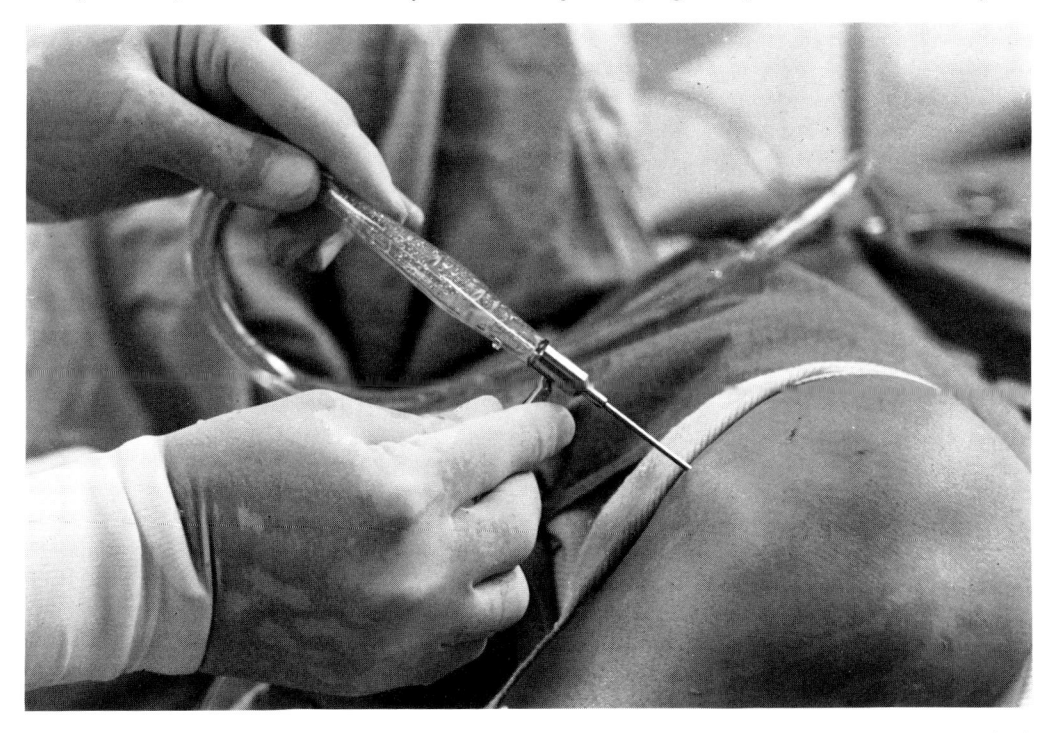

FIG. 3-6. Vacuuming joint to cleanse it of loose bodies and bloody synovial debris is often indicated. Notice that plastic tubing is slightly open and angulated at cannula entrance so as not to create a complete vacuum, bringing synovium up to tip of cannula inside joint. With slight break in suction, it is possible to cleanse joint very well for perfect viewing.

Diagnostic arthroscopy of the knee

ported that hemarthrosis was a contraindication to arthroscopy. Subsequently, Jackson and Dandy[5] reported using arthroscopy in some cases of acutely injured joints. When using an inflow cannula during arthroscopic surgery, it is possible to cleanse a compartment by applying the suction to the valves of the large-diameter endoscope. Usually the space between the cannula and the endoscopes allows fluid and small particles to flow and be vacuumed. The disadvantage is that the larger particles can be suctioned against the end of the arthroscope and block the view.

With drainage tubes and recirculation of fluid, blood in the joint can be gradually diluted, but not enough that visualization is quickly and readily accomplished. The joint with hemarthrosis can be completely cleansed of blood-tinged synovial fluid by vacuuming through the cannula (Fig. 3-7). As the endoscope is moved from one compartment to another, blood may run from one recess of the joint to another and cloud the compartment. Repeat vacuuming with the cannula may be necessary in each compartment to be examined. A bolus of saline will sweep material out of the way for excellent viewing.

It may be necessary to clean proteinaceous material off the end of the scope or to clear an area of syrupy synovial fluid that is interfering with viewing. This can be accomplished by instilling saline through a K-52 catheter placed adjacent to the endoscope.

The alternate method of bringing the distension through the large-diameter arthroscope valves clears the area of debris but also causes a turbulence immediately in front of the arthroscope that can obscure viewing. Therefore I favor the method of vacuuming, cleansing, and maintaining distension without a flow for viewing. Viewing has been crystal clear without either inflow or suction activity.

Hydrodynamics can be used to the arthroscopist's advantage. Vaccuming or forcing loose bodies into view from under the meniscus or within the synovial recess facilitates their removal. This is discussed further in Chapter 15. Good palpation technique is paramount during this visual activity, making it easier to move from one compartment to the other.

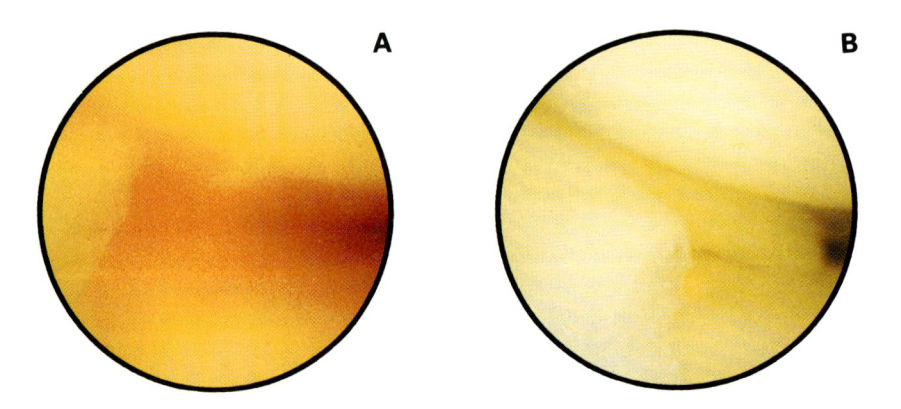

FIG. 3-7. A, Arthroscopic photograph taken prior to cleansing of cloudy synovial fluid in joint. **B,** After vacuuming synovial debris from joint and reinstilling clear bolus of saline, arthroscopic visualization is much clearer.

Vacuuming a joint can be therapeutic if pieces of articular cartilage and synovial debris are removed (Fig. 3-7). The force of the suction removes pieces of softened articular cartilage larger than the diameter of the endoscope because they fold on themselves and are drawn out through the cannula. Larger, firmer pieces that contain bone must be removed by a Jaws modified pituitary forceps. (See Fig. 11-3.)

Contrast staining

The use of contrast dye during arthroscopy was reported by Burman[1] and reviewed recently by Guten.[3] Methylene blue has not produced any complications in over 200 of my patients. It readily clears from the joint and has no permanent sequelae. It can be of benefit in arthroscopy because it demonstrates morphologic characteristics of the articular surfaces or synovium. It has been of special help in diagnosing osteochondritis dissecans (see Fig. 11-3, *A* and *B*) and in the study of synovial diseases (see Fig. 13-1, *C* to *E*). Staining has been most valuable in those patients with diffuse degenerative arthritis, which has a shaggy, woolly arthroscopic appearance. Optically ill-defined borders diminish definition of the contours of the articular cartilage and meniscus. Methylene blue increases contrast in joints with these degenerative changes and enhances diagnostic capabilities.

Scanning the horizon

As in surgery, it is important to work from known to unknown. Where there is no known identifiable structure, the arthroscopist must return to the area that was last identified and then progress to areas yet to be documented. One of the most important landmarks arthroscopically is the tangential horizon of the femoral condyle. It is possible to move from the patellar surface to the lateral femoral condyle and follow it tangentially all the way to the lateral compartment. As the horizon is followed, the edge of the meniscus will come into view. It is then possible by repositioning of the knee and the scope to follow the inner margin of the meniscus all the way to the posterior horn. This may be accomplished by moving the arthroscope or just by rotating the inclined-view arthroscope 180° (Fig. 3-8).

Pistoning

The back-and-forth motion of the endoscope can be described as pistoning. Pistoning can establish location and dimension, and the size of the object being viewed can be conceptualized in relation to other objects.

Rotation

I prefer, as do many arthroscopists, an endoscope with a fore-oblique view, that is, approximately 30° off center (Fig. 3-8). With such a scope it is possible to view directly as well as slightly to the side. This is essential in the knee joint, where after placement of the scope most objects are to the side (i.e., the meniscus) or above or below (i.e., the patella and intercondylar notch). It is not difficult, with a minimum of practice, with a fore-oblique viewing device to

Diagnostic arthroscopy of the knee

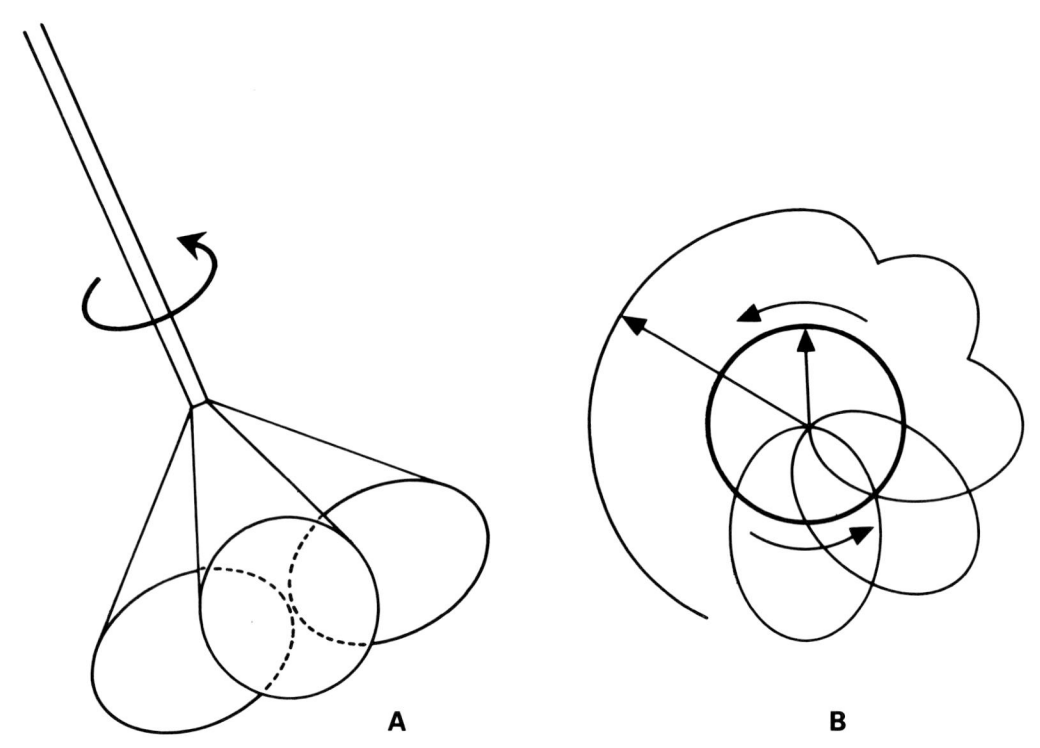

FIG. 3-8. A, Result of rotation of direct-viewing device in center, which is essentially a circle. When circle is rotated, view does not change. When fore-oblique endoscope is rotated, view changes from one side to the opposite side, and effective viewing area is increased. **B,** Comparison of end-on view of diameter of straight-viewing endoscope versus fore-oblique endoscope. Notice considerable increase in area and diameter of view possible with fore-oblique scope when rotated.

become accustomed to this angle of viewing. Its other advantage is that with rotation one may view in a direction opposite from that being observed. Without a change in position the scope can be rotated, moving the image to the right or to the left. Rotation of the fore-oblique scope therefore increases the range of viewing, which is not accomplished as satisfactorily with rotation of a direct-viewing scope with the same optical angle of view.

Scope sweeping

Another basic manipulative principle involves motion of the scope (Fig. 3-9). If a stick 4 inches long has a fulcrum in the middle, there are 2 inches on each side of it. If one end of the stick is displaced 1 inch, the opposite end is also displaced 1 inch. Likewise, when an endoscope is displaced rather rapidly at one end (outside the knee) a rather broad arc is made at the opposite end (inside). The ratio, of course, is not equal because length outside the knee is greater than inside. Gross movements of the scope during repositioning or viewing should be guarded against because the tip of the endoscope may be displaced from ½ to 1 inch within the joint.

When a scope is moved very slowly, a natural sequence of images is observed. Although there is no depth perception because the scope has a single

Basic arthroscopic techniques

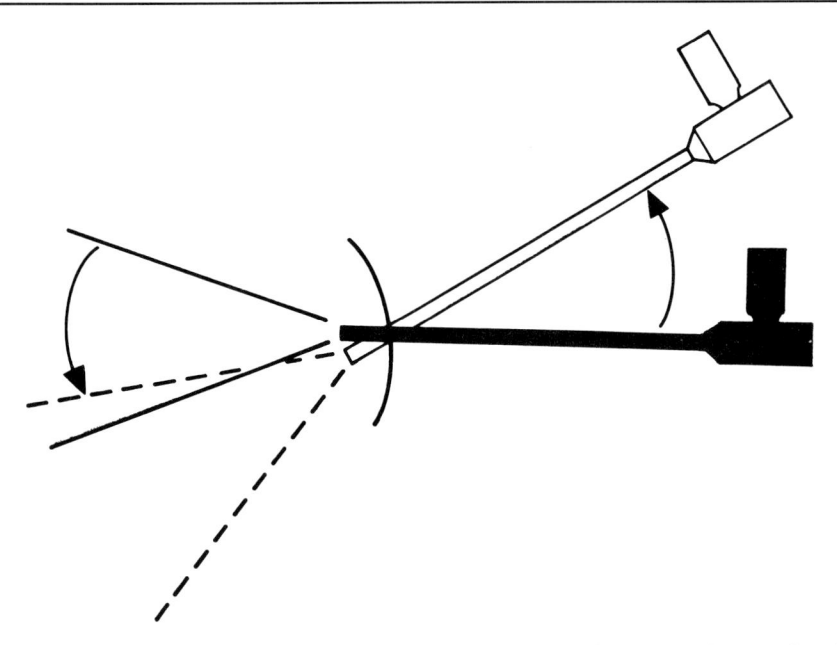

FIG. 3-9. Scope sweeping in wide motion results in considerable change in objective viewed. It is important to realize that rather gross outside motion with endoscope produces marked change in angle of view inside knee; therefore rather gentle scanning motions slowly performed are indicated for best viewing.

ocular lens, slow movements, combined with the manipulative procedures just described, make it possible to fully construct the arthroscopic composite.

Free hand activity

The arthroscopist holds the endoscope in one hand and the patient's ankle in the other (Fig. 3-10). With patients under local anesthesia it is possible to monitor the tightness of the lower extremity by their spontaneous tightening of the Achilles tendon. Varus and valgus strain or rotational stress can be applied to the joint in coordination with the positioning of the endoscope to create a good arthroscopic image.

A technical detail that can be of immense importance is fixing the position of the arthroscope within the compartment. Manipulating the knee moves the anatomic components across the endoscopic view. In fact, too much emphasis has been placed on manipulation of the arthroscope and too little on manipulation of the extremity to crease the arthroscopic composition.

One hand can be freed for scope manipulation, vacuuming, or suctioning by resting the patient's leg against the hip while the assistant supplies support. For lateral viewing or vacuuming, the arthroscopist can use his free hand to bring the patient's foot into his lap and, with support being provided to the inner side by the assistant, push the patient's knee into the varus position.

Another use for the free hand is palpation of, or ballottement on, the posteromedial or posterolateral compartments when viewing from the anterior position. This can push the loose bodies and the fluid up into the anterior compartment for visualization and subsequent removal. In addition, it is possi-

Diagnostic arthroscopy of the knee

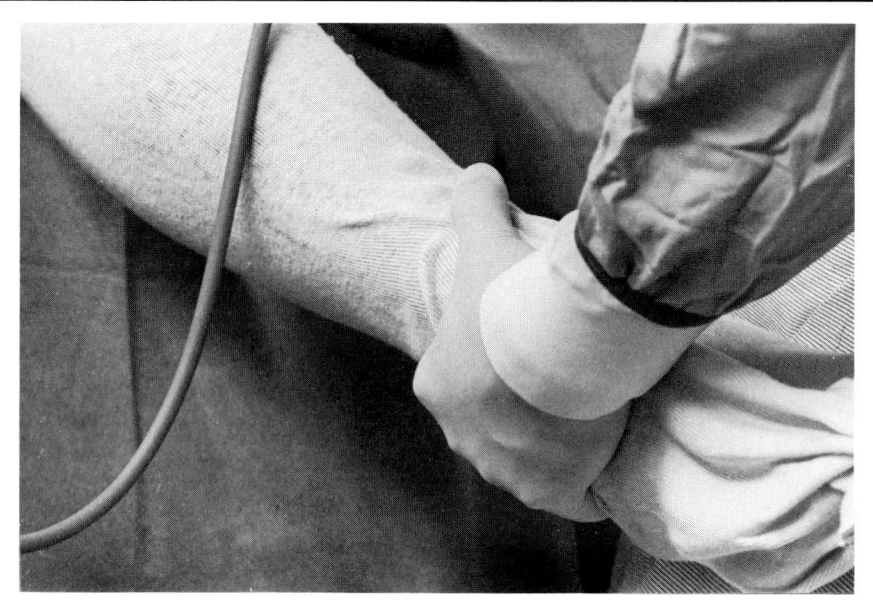

FIG. 3-10. With free hand, arthroscopist can hold patient's ankle and monitor tightening of Achilles tendon. Any tightening of knee or apprehension of patient is quickly discerned through Achilles tendon tenseness, allowing arthroscopist to be sensitive to patient's comfort under local anesthesia. In addition, with internal and external rotation, flexion and extension, abduction and adduction, arthroscopist can compose clear-cut endoscopic picture.

ble to visualize the motion of the meniscus. In a thin person this maneuver brings the posterior horn of the meniscus forward for better inspection.

TEAM APPROACH

Enough cannot be said for the team approach to an arthroscopic evaluation. Recent surveys have shown that most arthroscopists have a *different, untrained* assistant for every case. Every effort should be made, either personally or through the hospital, to secure a well-trained assistant in arthroscopy.

It is important that each member of the arthroscopic team understand his or her delegated responsibilities and participate in a cooperative manner. For example, efforts of the surgeon (e.g., placement of hands for manipulation of the patient's knee) and of the assistant (e.g., positioning of body for support) should be coordinated in a similar manner for each arthroscopy. These patterns, when rigidly observed, result in extreme efficiency. My organizational setup is demonstrated in Fig. 3-11.

All personnel must be familiar with each piece of equipment to be used (see box on facing page), and for all procedures these implements should be placed in the same location on the appropriate table.

If each procedure is carried out in a consistent manner, the results will be more satisfying and success predictable.

Basic arthroscopic techniques

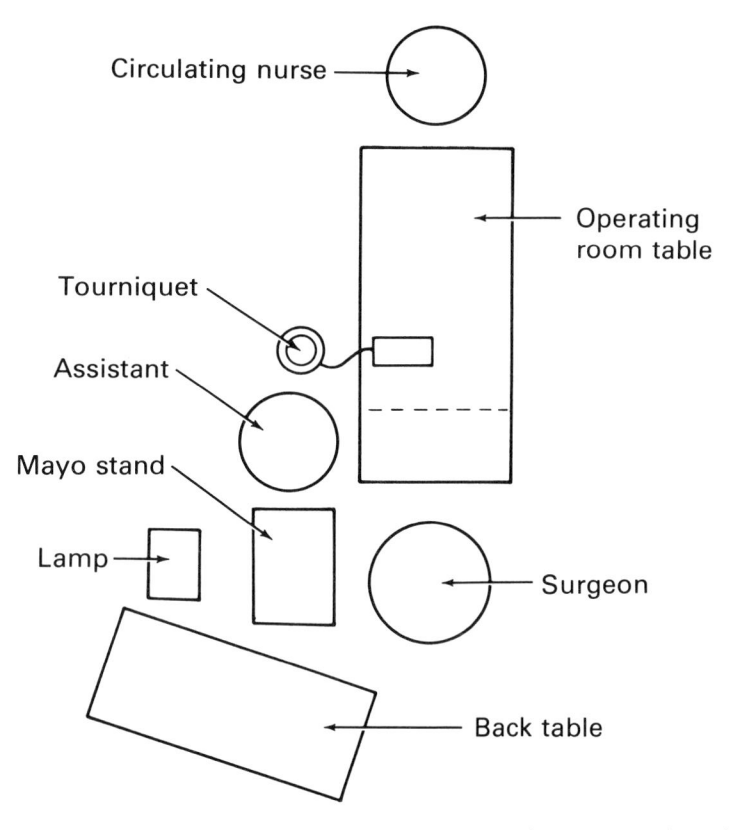

FIG. 3-11. Equipment distribution for diagnostic arthroscopy.

Mayo stand
1 Straight Mayo scissors
1 No. 11 blade
1 No. 3 knife handle
1 Cannula
1 Trocar
1 Obturator
1 K-52 catheter (Novex three-way stopcock with extension tube)
1 Syringe, 60 ml
1 Small metal basin
1 No. 21 needle, 1½ inches
1 Syringe, 12 ml
1 Light cord
1 Arthroscope

Back table
5 Drawsheets
1 Suction tube
  Sponges, 3 × 4 inches
5 Folded towels
1 Mayo cover
1 Polyethylene shield
1 Stockinette, 6 inches
1 Kling, 4 inches
1 Preparation tray
6 Towel clips
1 Sponge stick
  Lidocaine, 1% plain

Head of table
1 Specimen trap
1 Pneumatic tourniquet

Diagnostic arthroscopy of the knee

Responsibilities of circulating nurse

The responsibilities of the circulating nurse follow. Foremost is monitoring of the patient's comfort and vital signs. Conversation with the patient under local anesthesia can contribute to patient assurance and relaxation.

Responsibilities of assistant

Among other advantages, coordinated efforts of the surgeon and the assistant facilitate opening of the compartments of the knee. The assistant can cleanse the joint during the procedure, allowing the physician to concentrate on viewing. She stabilizes the patient's thigh, freeing the surgeon's hands and aiding in the patient's comfort and relaxation. By having the assistant assemble and care for equipment, the arthroscopist is able to interact with the patient or document the procedure between cases, increasing efficiency and productivity. As a result of these efforts I am able to do an arthroscopy, including room change and instrument preparation time, in ½ hour. The duties of the assistant follow.

During setup
1. Set up back table.
2. Set up Mayo stand.
3. Assist in preparing and draping patient.

During arthroscopy
1. Stabilize patient's knee.
2. Handle instruments or pass them to surgeon.

During setup
1. Turn on lights.
2. Set up skin preparation materials.
3. Position suction tubing and collection jars for cell-block preparation.
4. Open main pack.
5. Bring patient into room and position on table so that knees are at edge of table.
6. Check and record patient's pulse, blood pressure, and respiration rate.
7. Check tourniquet and apply to appropriate thigh.
8. Bring in autoclaved instruments; place on opened back table.
9. Hold patient's leg during skin preparation.
10. Inflate tourniquet.
11. Attach light source.

During arthroscopy
1. Record patient's blood pressure.
2. Converse with patient.
3. Collect cell-block specimen and reestablish suction.
4. Control light sources.

After procedure
1. Deflate tourniquet.
2. Record patient's vital signs.
3. Label specimen and records.
4. Take patient to recovery room.
5. Help clean room and set up for next examination.

Basic arthroscopic techniques

    3. Keep syringe filled with saline for delivery on command.
    4. Hand dressings to physician.

After procedure
1. Clean equipment.
2. Ready steam autoclaving tray.
3. Sterilize scope in Cidex.
4. Remove and strip operating room of laundry and waste and prepare for next patient.

At end of day
1. Clean, dry, and place scope in properly secured compartment.

At end of week
1. Prepare arthroscope for gas sterilization.

Care of instruments between patients

After each arthroscopic examination the assistant carefully cleanses the arthroscope with alcohol and places it in activated dialdehyde solution (Cidex). The interior of the cannula is cleaned by forcing saline through it with a K-52 catheter. Other instruments, including all metal tools and the light cable and connectors, are cleaned with saline and alcohol, placed in the sterilization tray, and autoclaved.

Care of endoscopic equipment increases its longevity. With careful handling a Needlescope can last for 3 years and approximately 300 examinations.

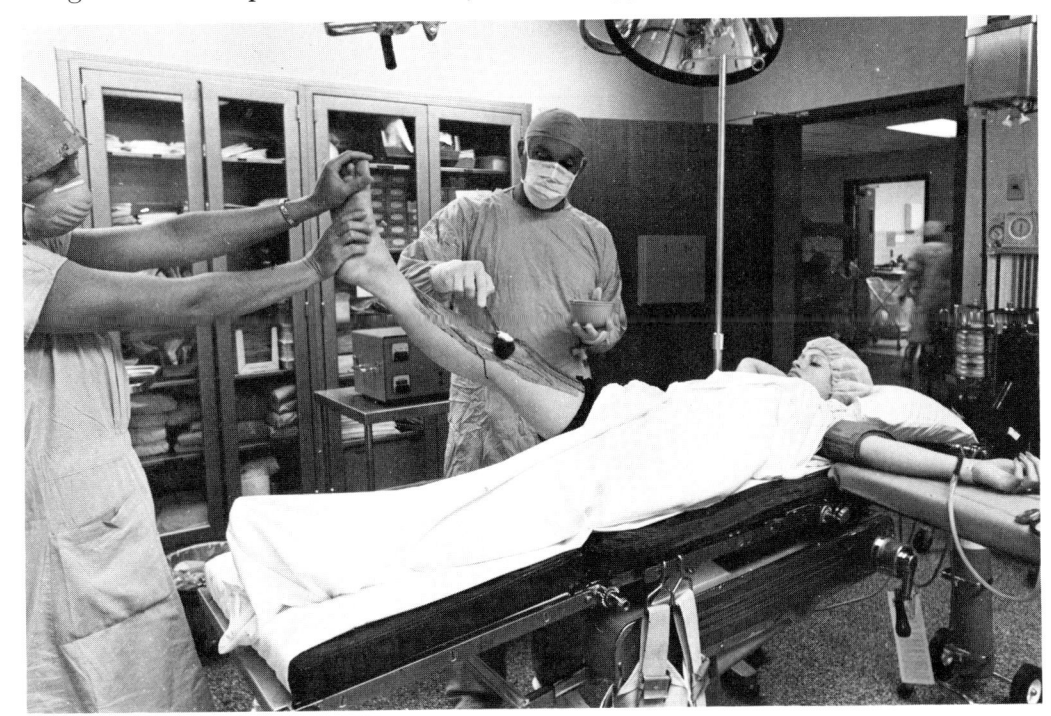

FIG. 3-12. Under local anesthesia, patient is relaxed. Simple skin preparation of povidone-iodine complex (Betadine) is used. Notice that tourniquet is in place but not elevated at this time. With anticipated open surgery, more elaborate skin preparation and draping may be indicated.

Diagnostic arthroscopy of the knee

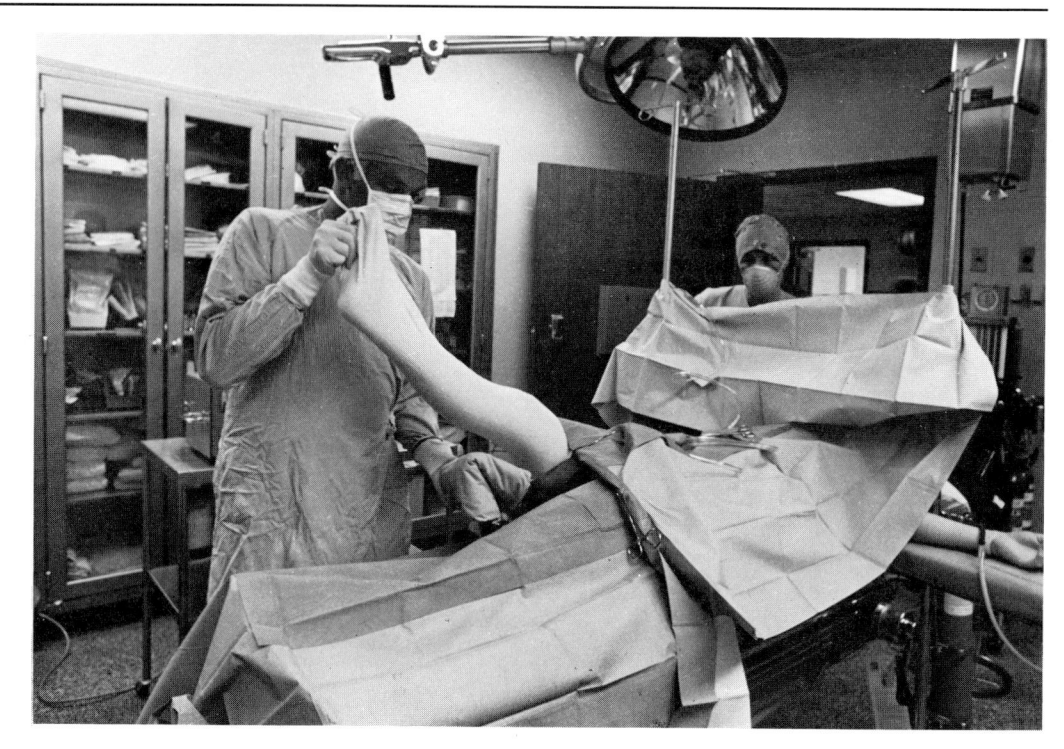

FIG. 3-13. After simple paper drape has been placed on patient's leg, folded towel is placed under knee to provide suspension of knee and greater mobility for arthroscopic inspection.

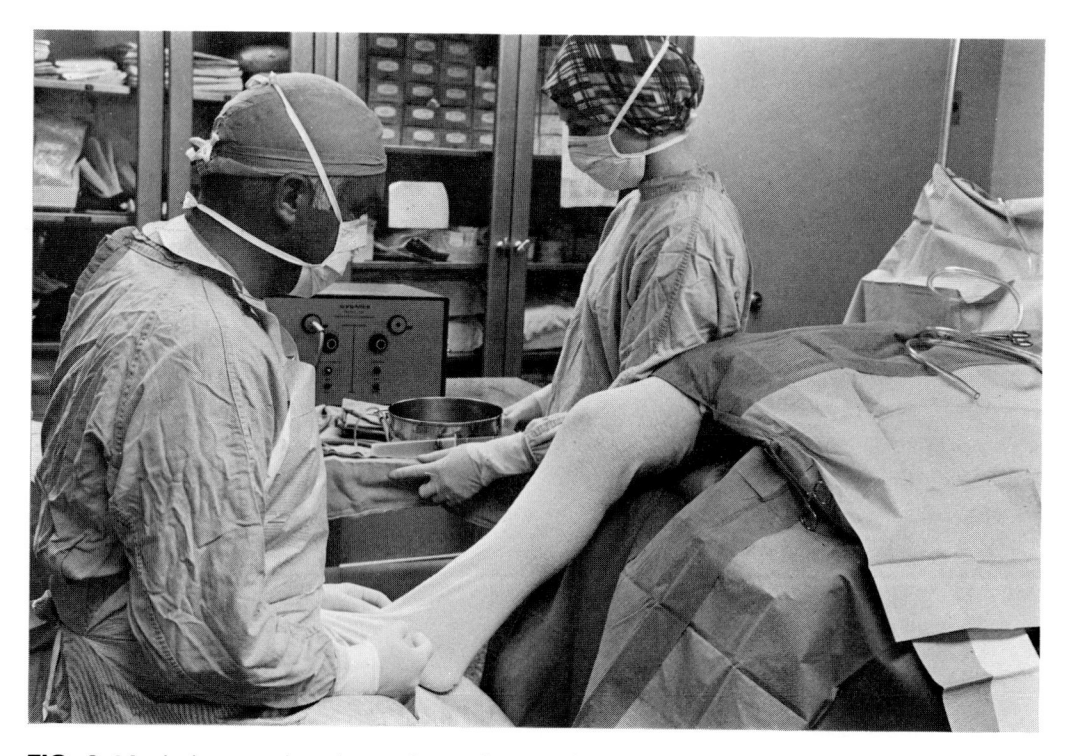

FIG. 3-14. Arthroscopist sits at foot of operating table. Patient is relaxed, with knee hanging freely over end of table. Knee, which would tend to roll into external rotation, is secured by assistant's elbow and weight of body.

Diagnostic arthroscopy procedure

A sequential approach to the arthroscopic examination is important.

The circulating nurse inflates the tourniquet. The patient's skin is prepared and the extremity draped (Fig. 3-12). A folded towel is placed under the distal thigh to suspend the knee above the table and facilitate movement (Fig. 3-13). The foot of the operating room table is lowered so that the patient's legs hang down, with knees flexed. The nurse then moves the illuminator into place and attaches the cord to the light source.

The surgeon stands at the end of the table and rests the patient's foot in his lap, which is covered with a sterile apron. The Mayo stand is positioned next to him (Fig. 3-14).

The assistant takes a position adjacent to the knee to be examined and helps stabilize the patient's thigh. During the procedure she hands instruments to the surgeon and maintains organization and placement of the instruments on the back table and Mayo stand, enabling the arthroscopist to find equipment in the dim light.

ARTHROSCOPIC COMPARTMENTS

I generally make an anteromedial puncture and view the patellar surface and suprapatellar pouch from below, then move in sequence to the anterolateral compartment, the intercondylar notch, and the anteromedial compartment. At the completion of the anterior viewing a suprapatellar puncture may be required to observe this area in patients who have a large fulcrum caused by fat, a tight scarred capsule, or osteophytes around the patella.

Even in patients with normal anteromedial or anterolateral compartments, as viewed in the preceding sequence, the posterior compartments are inspected because of their high yield of lesions and loose bodies not seen anteriorly. (See Chapter 5.)

The posterior approach is not necessary when an abnormality that requires surgical repair is seen in the anterior compartment, if the surgical technique includes an incision that allows routine inspection of the posterior compartment. The presurgical inspection approach is from lateral. Although the sequence may vary, the inspection routine always includes the same elements.

Anteromedial approach

An anteromedial entry allows the arthroscopist to sit squarely in front of the patient's extremity. The site is more central in relation to the knee joint than is a lateral entry, and access to the lateral compartment from the medial side is easier than is viewing posteromedially from an anterior entry. The anteroposterior diameter of the medial condyle is greater than is that of the lateral condyle. Also, with a varus strain on the knee and an anteromedial placement of the endoscope, the knee rotates in such a way that its posterolateral portion comes forward. Viewing is much easier than in the posteromedial compartment, which is tighter and in a normal stable knee has less opening and anterior rotation.

The posterior horn of the medial meniscus has less mobility than the

Diagnostic arthroscopy of the knee

posterior horn of the lateral meniscus; therefore it cannot be moved into view as easily by suction or probing. In addition, the configuration of the tibial spine often causes it to mechanically block the placement of the arthroscope and eliminate adequate viewing when the approach is made from the lateral side. This rarely happens with medial placement, which is near the center line; there is more rotation and mobility of the lateral compartment. A lateral approach allows more mobility if it is slightly higher and opposite the tip of the patella.

In some patients, especially women with genu valgus, it is possible to create enough varus strain in 10° to 15° of flexion to pass a small endoscope into the posterolateral compartment and view the entire superior meniscal surface and posterior attachments of the lateral meniscus. In the most relaxed knee it is possible to pass along the superior aspect of the meniscus to see the popliteus tendon and the sheath as it passes posterior and lateral to the lateral meniscus. When the posterolateral compartment is not seen and the examination is normal from the anterior portal, a separate posterolateral approach is indicated to determine whether there is a lesion in the posterolateral compartment.

Also, the anteromedial approach is more easily blocked with local anesthetic by infiltration of the infrapatellar branch of the saphenous nerve (Fig. 3-15).

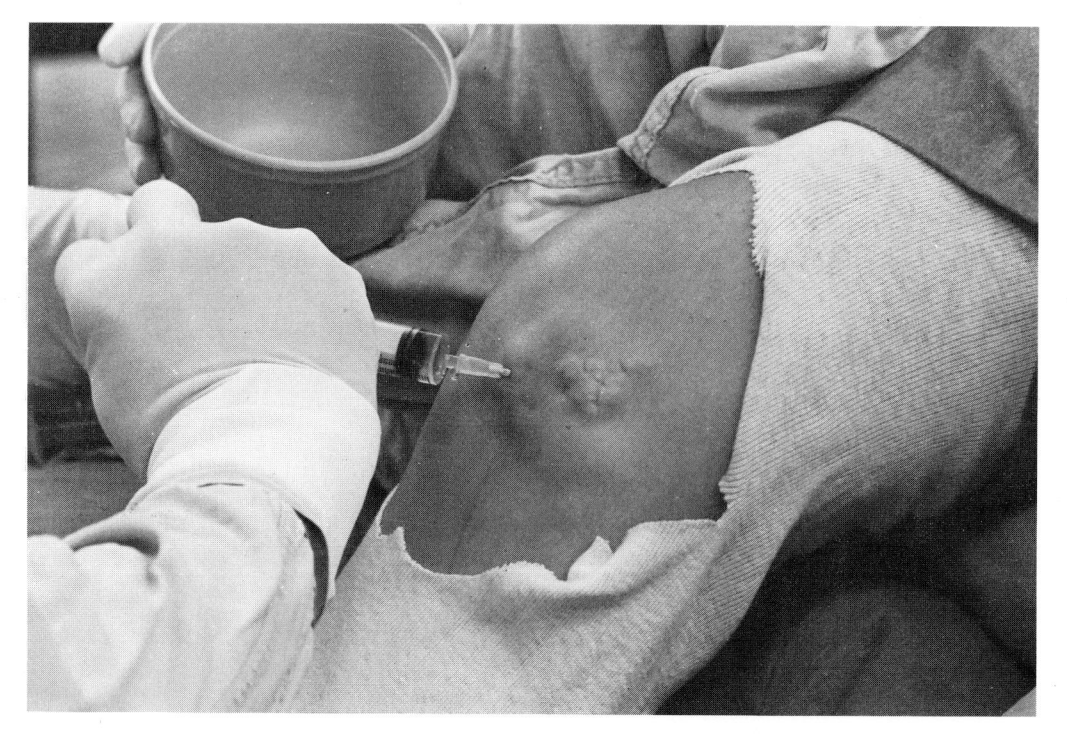

FIG. 3-15. Infrapatellar branch of saphenous nerve is blocked by local infiltration in three to four directions medial from the initial puncture. This decreases proprioception during manipulation of knee and therefore reduces apprehension.

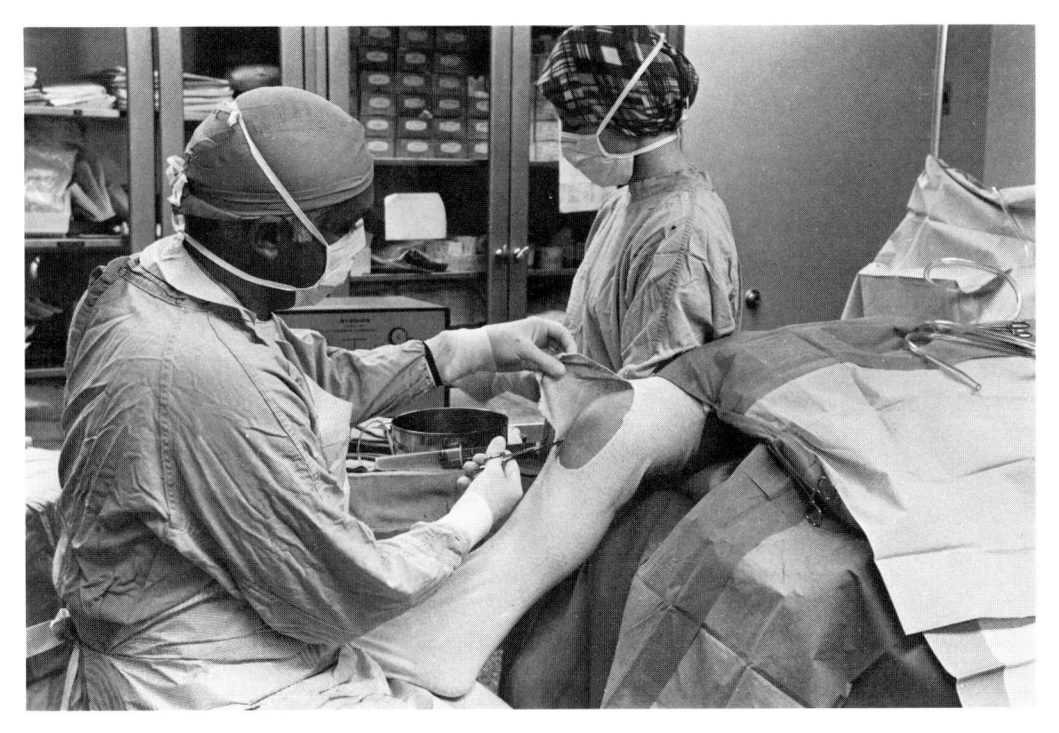

FIG. 3-16. For surgery with local anesthetic, paper barrier drapes and a single stockinette are used. If surgical procedure is anticipated, richer draping system is used.

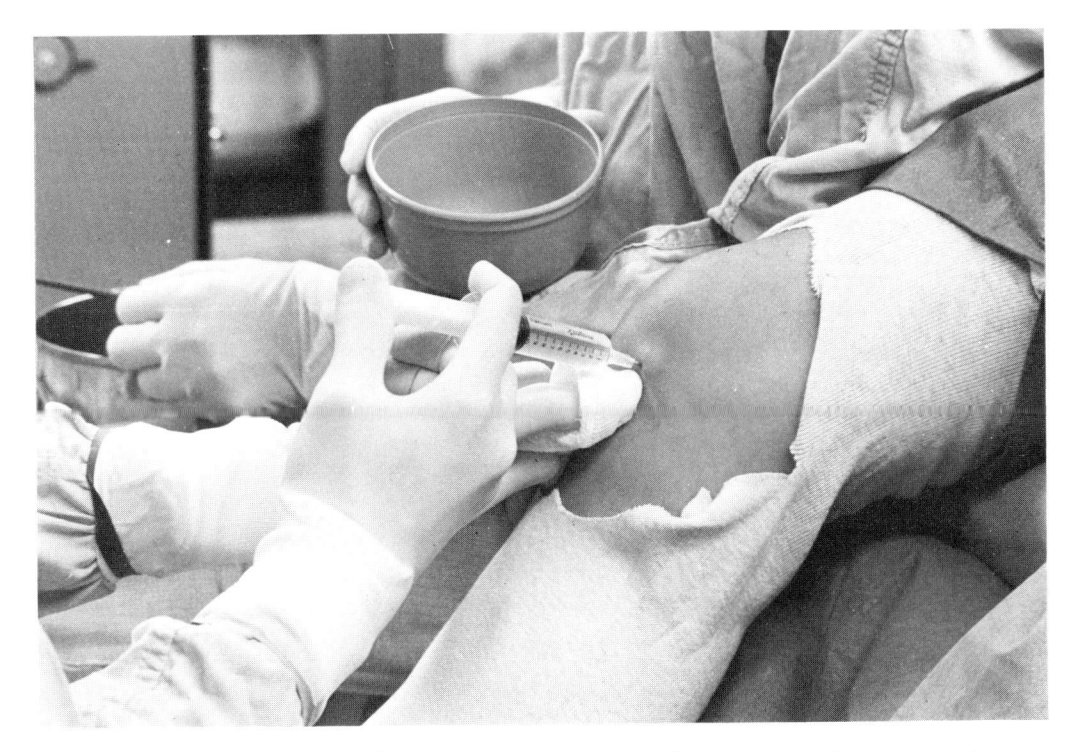

FIG. 3-17. Plain lidocaine, 1%, is placed within knee along course of anticipated penetration of joint. Surgeon places index finger against patellar tendon and onto tibial plateau to palpate for entry one finger breadth above tibial plateau and approximately half a finger breadth medial to inner border of patellar tendon. In some overweight patients, position may be considerably more lateral because knee tends to rotate externally.

Diagnostic arthroscopy of the knee

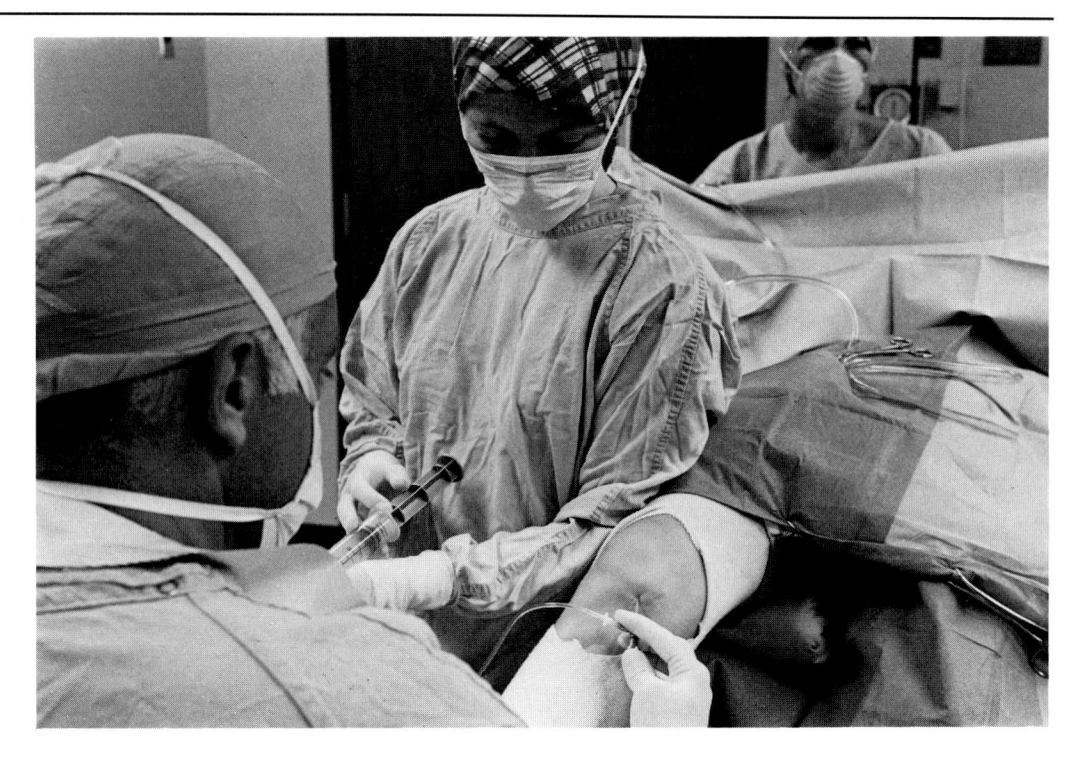

FIG. 3-18. With a blunt trocar in cannula and knee in extension, penetration of suprapatellar pouch is possible. In relaxed patient, patella will float, facilitating entry. Notice that cannula is aligned at an angle of about 30° off center.

With the patient's knee in a position of 90° flexion and resting in the surgeon's lap (Fig. 3-16), a site of entry is selected one finger breadth above the tibial plateau and half a finger breadth medial to the patellar tendon. This is accomplished by the placement of the index finger against the patellar tendon and down onto the tibial condyle (Fig. 3-17). The skin immediately above the palpating index finger is lanced with a No. 11 blade, and the subcutaneous tissue and capsule are penetrated by a cannula with a sharp trocar. The plane is parallel to the tibial condyles and directed 30° toward the lateral side of the joint. The sharp trocar is exchanged for a blunt one, and the patient's knee is brought into extension. The blunt trocar in the cannula can penetrate the suprapatellar pouch by angling laterally and superiorly (Fig. 3-18). It may be difficult to gain access to the suprapatellar space with this maneuver in some patients who have a scar from previous surgery or a fat knee, since the fulcrum may be limited by the firmness of the scar or the depth of the fat or in patients with marked osteochondritic prominences about the patella. A separate suprapatellar puncture is indicated in such patients.

Patella and suprapatellar pouch

The assistant stabilizes the lateral femur with her elbow. The physician extends the patient's leg and moves the cannula and blunt trocar into the suprapatellar pouch under the patella. When the patient is relaxed under local

Basic arthroscopic techniques

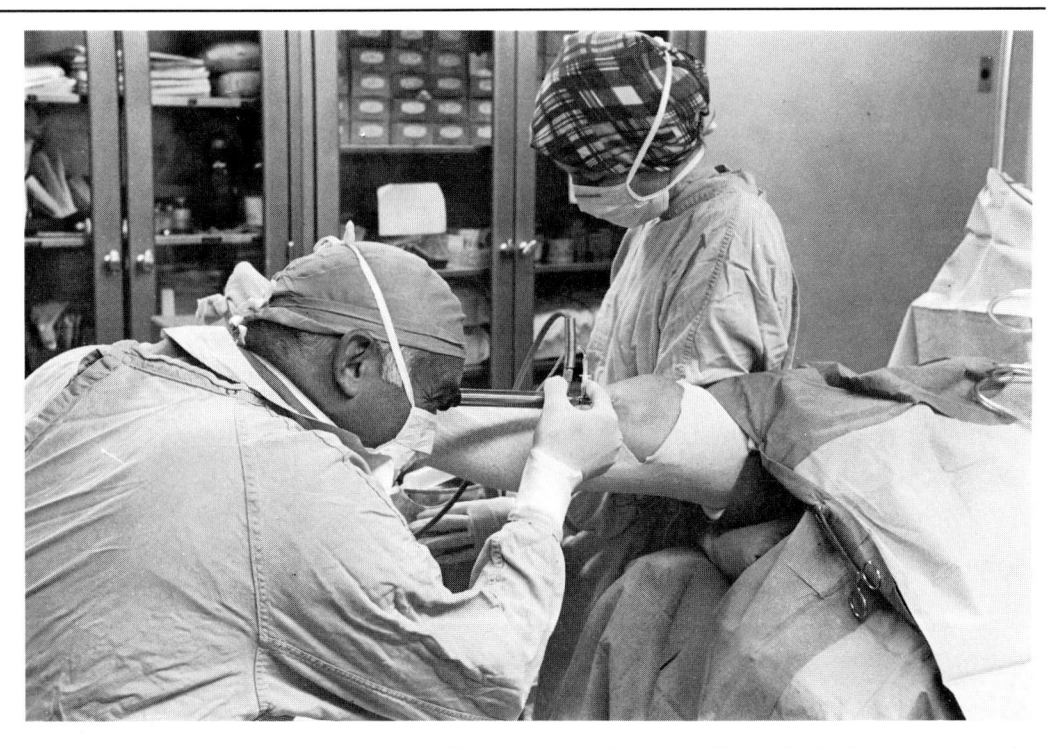

FIG. 3-19. After entry has been confirmed and saline has distended joint, suprapatellar pouch and patellar area may be visualized.

anesthesia, flexion and extension allow the patella to float, facilitating entry to this area.

Viewing is then carried out by slowly retracting the endoscope while the leg is extended (Fig. 3-19). Rotating the scope so the inclined view is superior allows the horizon of the patella to come into view. From that position it is possible to scan the patellar surface. The assistant may manipulate the patella to bring it into various views for inspection. The suprapatellar pouch can be viewed by advancement of the endoscope. Close inspection of the villae is possible. Plicae, loose bodies, or fibrous adhesions can also be observed. In some patients the endoscope can be retracted enough that both the intercondylar notch and patella can be in one view.

The move to the anterolateral compartment can be more easily accomplished by (1) observing the lateral femoral condyle in tangential view down into the compartment; (2) removing the endoscope, replacing the blunt trocar, and carrying the cannula with the trocar down into the lateral compartment by palpation (this may be especially helpful to the inexperienced arthroscopist who is concerned about fragility of the endoscope during manipulation); or (3) bringing the endoscope tip down into the intercondylar notch and then finding the lateral femoral condyle adjacent to the anterior cruciate ligament. In some patients there is a large imperforate fat pad up to the ligamentous mucosa. Either direct penetration through this fibrous membrane or moving above the ligamentum mucosum and down into the lateral compartment is required.

Diagnostic arthroscopy of the knee

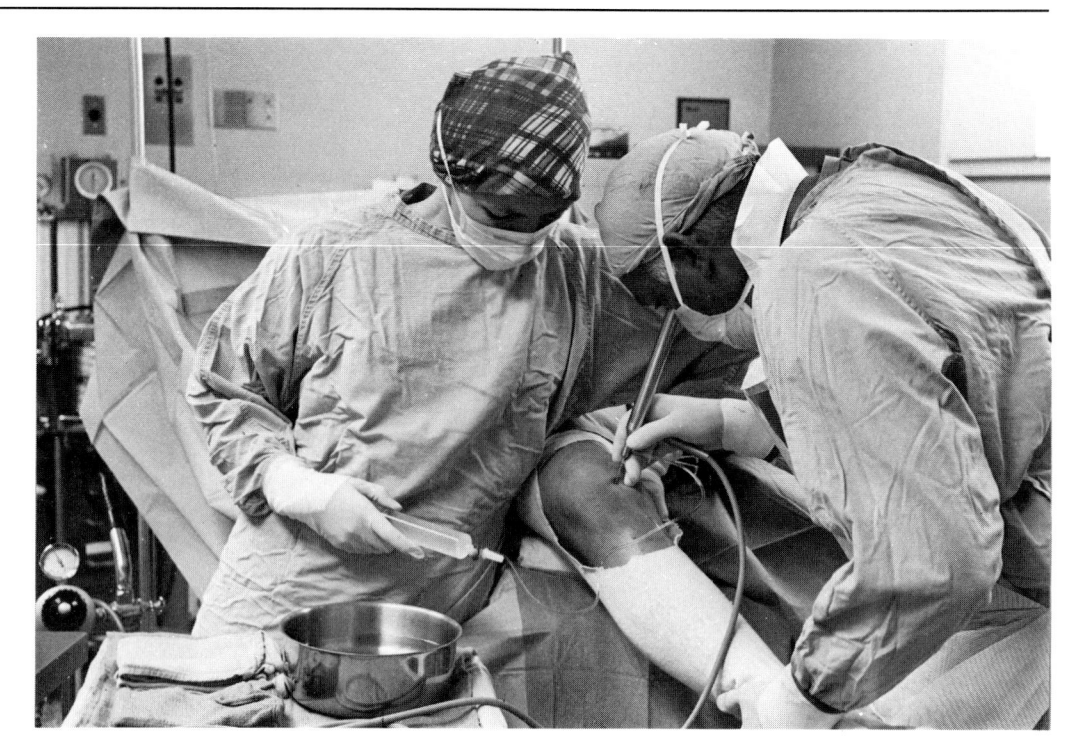

FIG. 3-20. Inspection of anterolateral compartment is facilitated by assistant supporting distal medial femur. Arthroscopist provides varus stress with hand on patient's ankle. Notice that assistant has syringe of saline ready to clear any proteinaceous material from end of scope.

Anterolateral compartment

The anterolateral compartment is best viewed with the patient's knee flexed between 5° and 15° while the assistant provides support to the medial aspect of the distal femur and the surgeon applies varus strain with his hand on the patient's ankle (Fig. 3-20). If this is accompanied by slight internal rotation of the tibia, the lateral compartment will come into view and the entire meniscus can be visualized easily. (See Fig. 7-2, A.) It is possible to pass under the posterolateral corner of the meniscus and view the popliteus tendon as it crosses through the open space in the coronary ligament. This tendon appears cordlike and shows a different color reflection than does the meniscus or the tibial condyle. (See Fig. 7-2, B.) It is important to inspect the lateral reflection of the meniscus at its synovial junction and to follow the tangential view of the condyle at least one meniscus breadth superior to the meniscal-synovial junction. A lesion in this area is pathognomonic of a subluxed or dislocated patella. (See Fig. 7-3, A.)

Intercondylar notch

The intercondylar notch is viewed next, with the patient's knee flexed between 45° and 90° and with the assistant stabilizing the lateral femur with her elbow (Fig. 3-21). In this position the anterior cruciate ligament will be in the midportion of the field. In a well-distended knee the fat pad should not

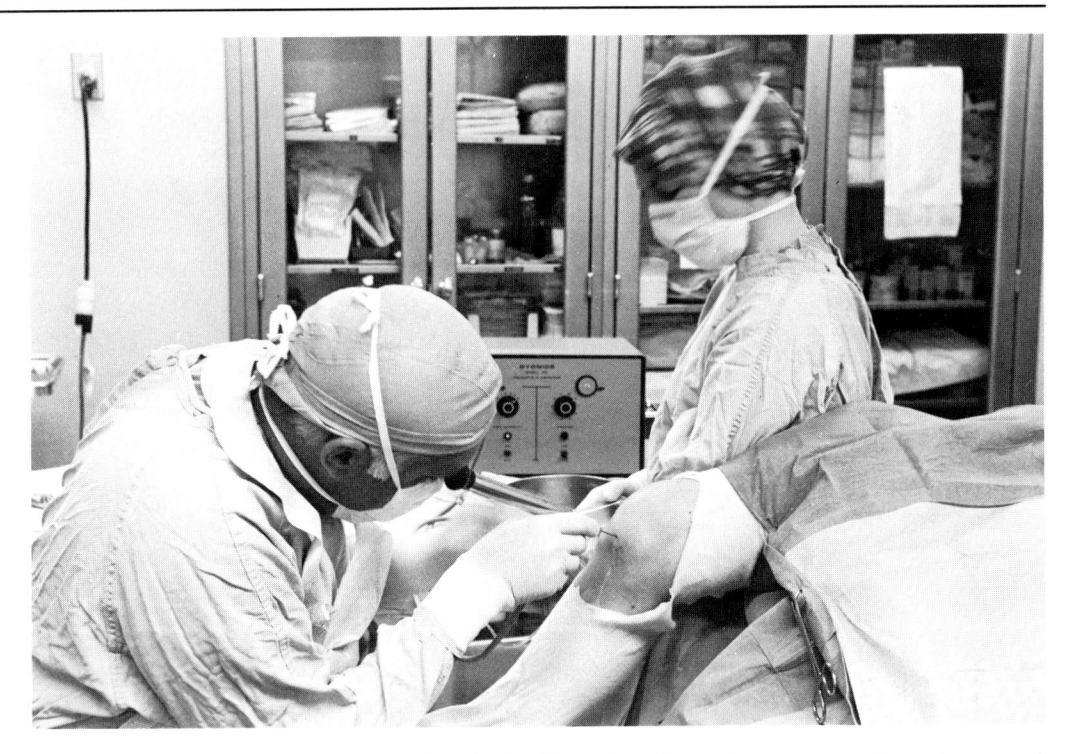

FIG. 3-21. Endocondylar inspection is facilitated with patient's knee flexed approximately 45° to 90°. Arthroscopist sits, and assistant stabilizes patient's knee so that it does not roll externally.

present any problem to entry from the medial side. If the fat pad slips down over the shank of the cannula, a rather smooth but brisk forward motion followed by slow retraction will again hang the fat pad up on the shank of the cannula (Fig. 3-1). Movement across the intercondylar notch is from the femoral condyle on one side around the cruciate ligament to the femoral condyle on the opposite side. (See Fig. 7-4, *A* to *C*.)

It should be noted that at about this point in the procedure there may be some deflation of the distended joint, and instillation of another bolus of saline may be necessary.

Anteromedial compartment

Complete inspection of the anteromedial compartment may be facilitated by redirection of the endoscope. From initial placement 30° laterally the scope is removed and the blunt trocar is reinserted and directed toward the medial meniscus.

The physician stands up and applies valgus strain to the patient's knee while the assistant provides support to the lateral femur (Fig. 3-22). With internal and external rotation of the tibia and with flexion and extension, an excellent composite of the medial compartment can be recorded. In most patients it is possible to pass under the meniscus with a 1.7-mm diameter Needlescope. Horizontal cleft tears back to the area of the coronary ligament

Diagnostic arthroscopy of the knee

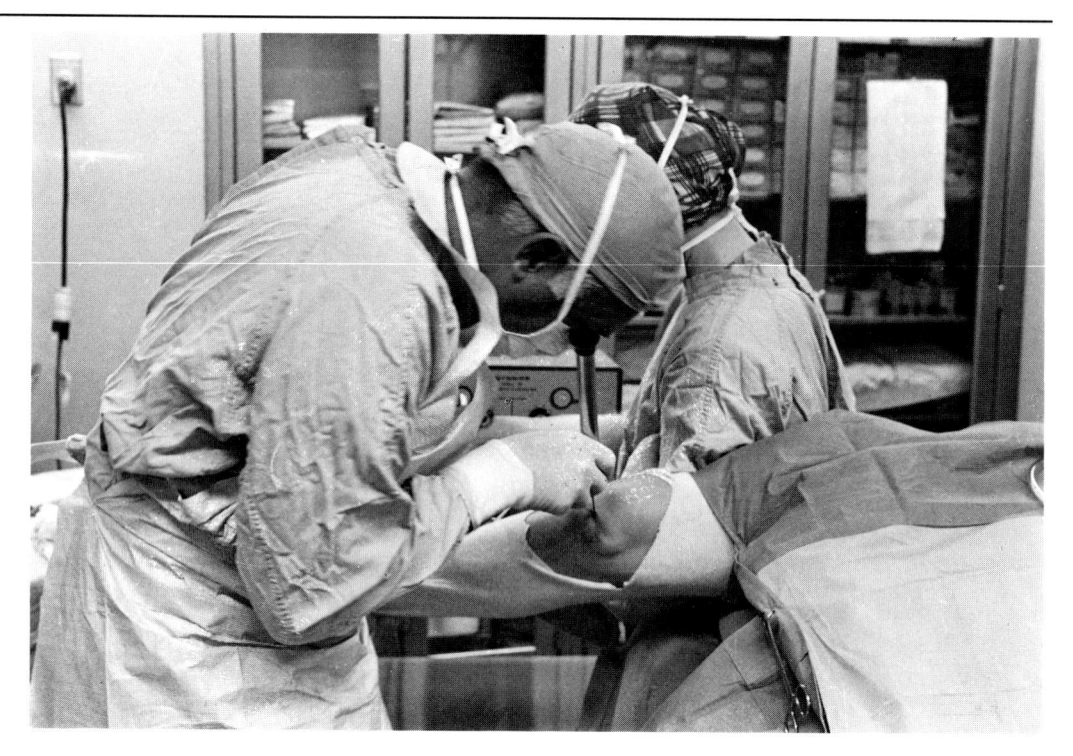

FIG. 3-22. Inspection of anteromedial compartment is facilitated by nurse placing elbow and body against distal lateral femur and arthroscopist applying valgus stress to patient's knee. Notice safe distance between arthroscopist's eye and hand, reducing potential for contamination.

attachment can be inspected. In some patients acute coronary ligament tears have been identified. Examination proceeds from the anterior portion of the posterior horn to the meniscus and its medial substance and then to the anterior horn; a return to the medial substance and up the meniscal surface to the meniscal-synovial junction completes the procedure. In this area the endoscope can be passed forward, adjacent to the attachment to the tibial collateral ligament. (See Fig. 9-1, *H* and *J*.) If an area with no definition is found (whiteout), I recommend moving back to the horizon of the femoral condyle to reestablish location and then proceeding to the unknown areas. Flexion and extension can demonstrate mobility of the meniscus and can improve viewing of any particular area; in fact, it is possible to follow the tangent of the medial femoral condyle all the way into the suprapatellar pouch for complete examination. It is not unusual, with stress on the knee, to see a serpentine border on the inner portion of the meniscus. (See Fig. 7-5, *B*.) Findings of the condylar surface should be recorded.

Posteromedial compartment

After the anterior compartments have been viewed, the endoscope is removed and the *joint is redistended to maximum* with saline to facilitate the posterior compartment inspection.

The patient's hip is rotated externally and the knee is slightly flexed. The

Basic arthroscopic techniques

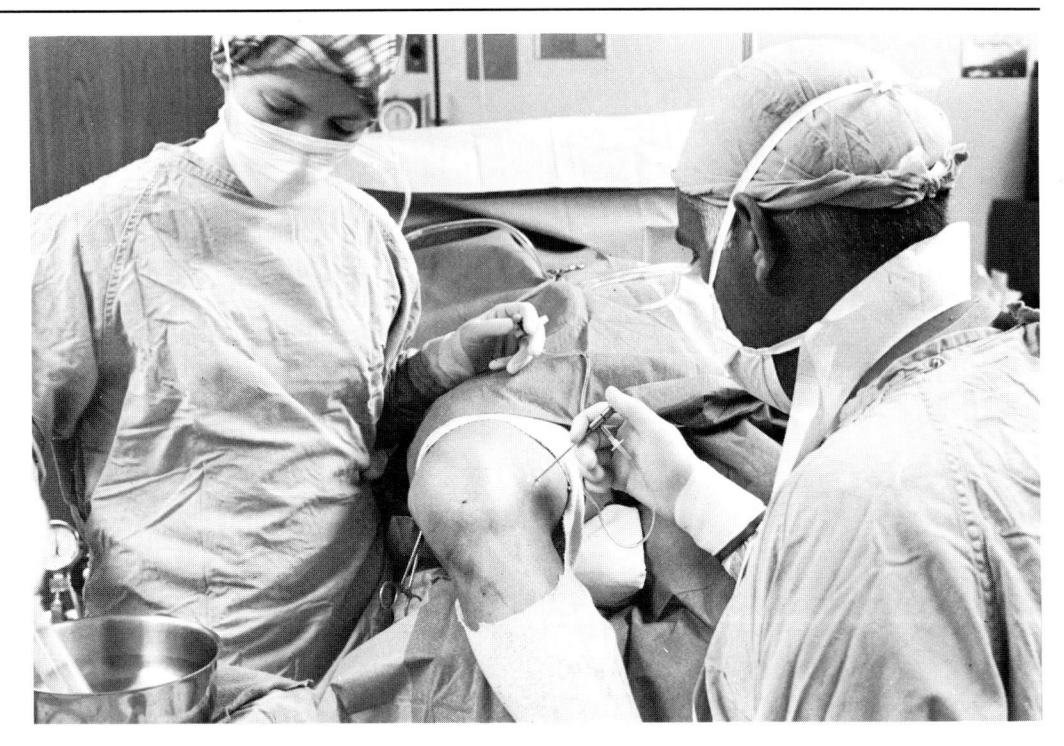

FIG. 3-23. Posteromedial puncture is made with cannula and sharp trocar, parallel to tibial condyles and posterior to meniscus. Arthroscopist can palpate the "soft spot" in maximally distended joint.

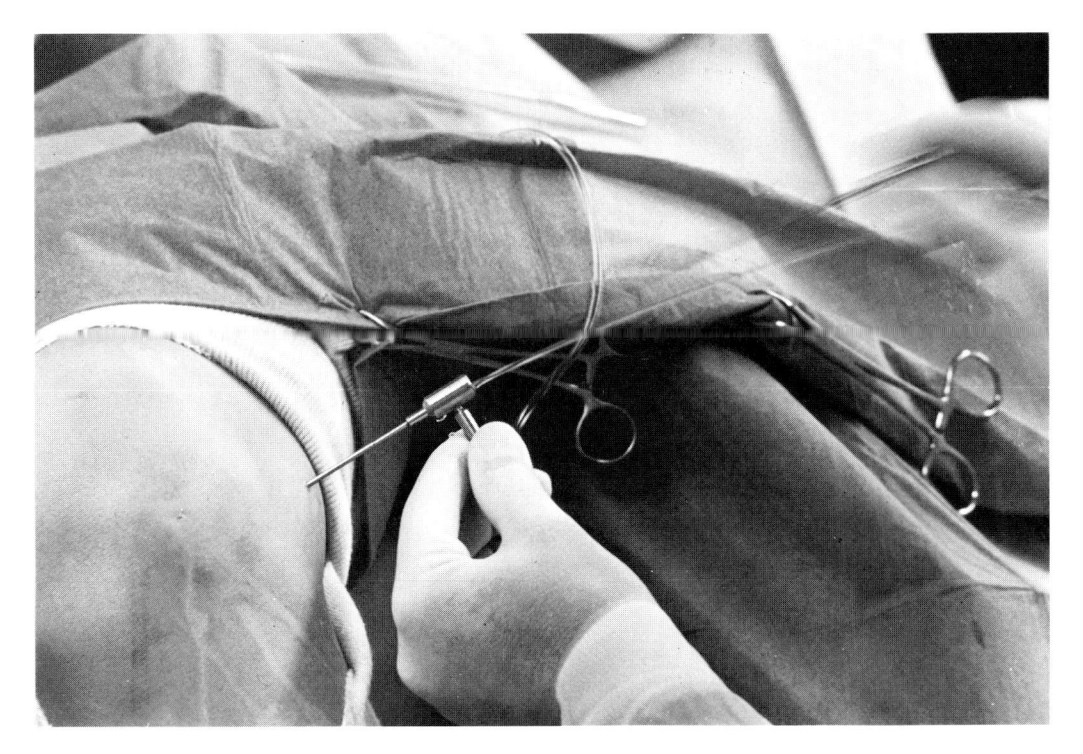

FIG. 3-24. Extrusion of saline from cannula confirms entry of cannula into joint. It is especially important that posteromedial and posterolateral entries be made into maximally distended joint. This facilitates entry and confirms penetration.

Diagnostic arthroscopy of the knee

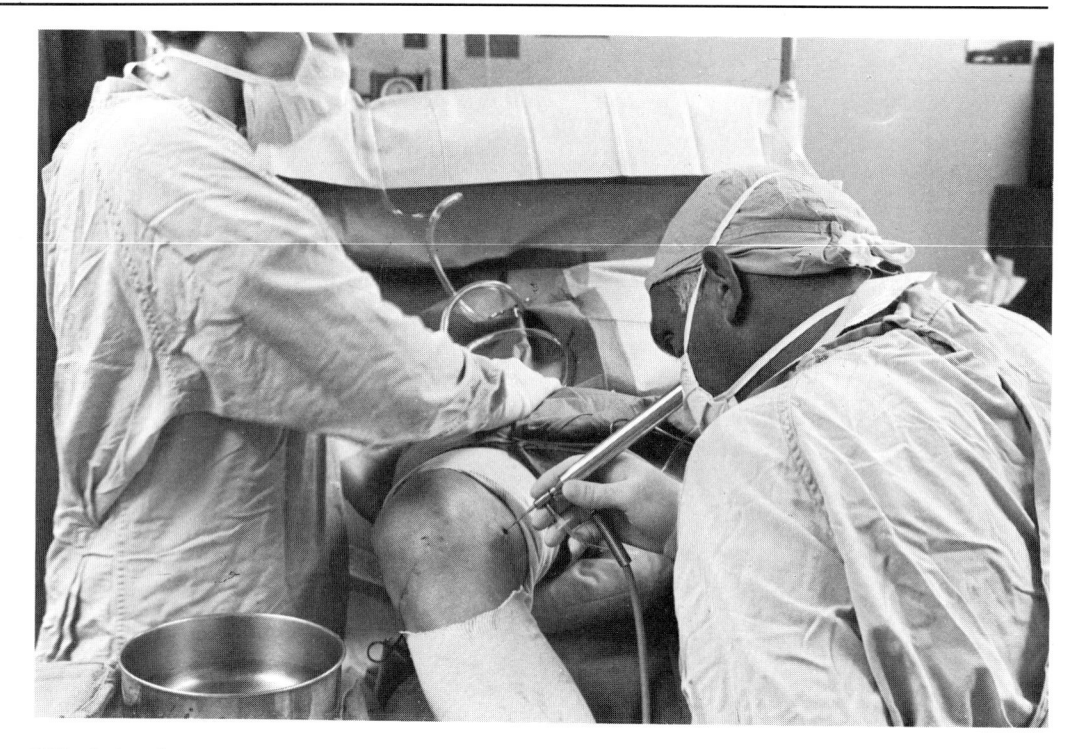

FIG. 3-25. In posteromedial approach, patient's hip is rolled into external rotation and knee is flexed; foot rests in arthroscopist's lap. Thus posteromedial portion of knee joint can be entered with relative ease and freedom.

assistant supports the patient's thigh. The physician sits with the patient's foot in his lap (Fig. 3-23).

The area of entry is posterior to the tibial collateral ligament, superior to the meniscus, and posterior to the medial femoral condyle. In thin patients it is possible to see a bulge in this area when the knee is distended. The cannula and sharp trocar are directed parallel to the tibial condyles and directly into the posterior compartment (Fig. 3-23). With removal of the sharp trocar, extravasation of saline confirms the entry (Fig. 3-24), and visualization is then possible (Fig. 3-25). The landmark for orientation is the junction between the meniscus and the femoral condyle, and with advancement of the endoscope it is possible in many patients to see the posterior cruciate ligament. (See Fig. 7-1, *F*.) Inspection down the posterior aspect of the meniscus will show any vertical rim tears or separation from the attachment. In some patients it is possible to see into a Baker cyst.

Some obese patients, in whom the landmark is difficult to find, also have a large Baker cyst. This can be entered either intentionally or inadvertently. Vacuuming of loose bodies or debris may reduce the morbidity in certain patients and lead to resolution of the symptoms of the posterior area. Simple manual compression over a posteromedial puncture can prevent leakage and thus maintain knee joint distension.

A second position that has proved advantageous is placement of the tibia in marked internal rotation, which drops the meniscus off the femoral condyle.

Basic arthroscopic techniques

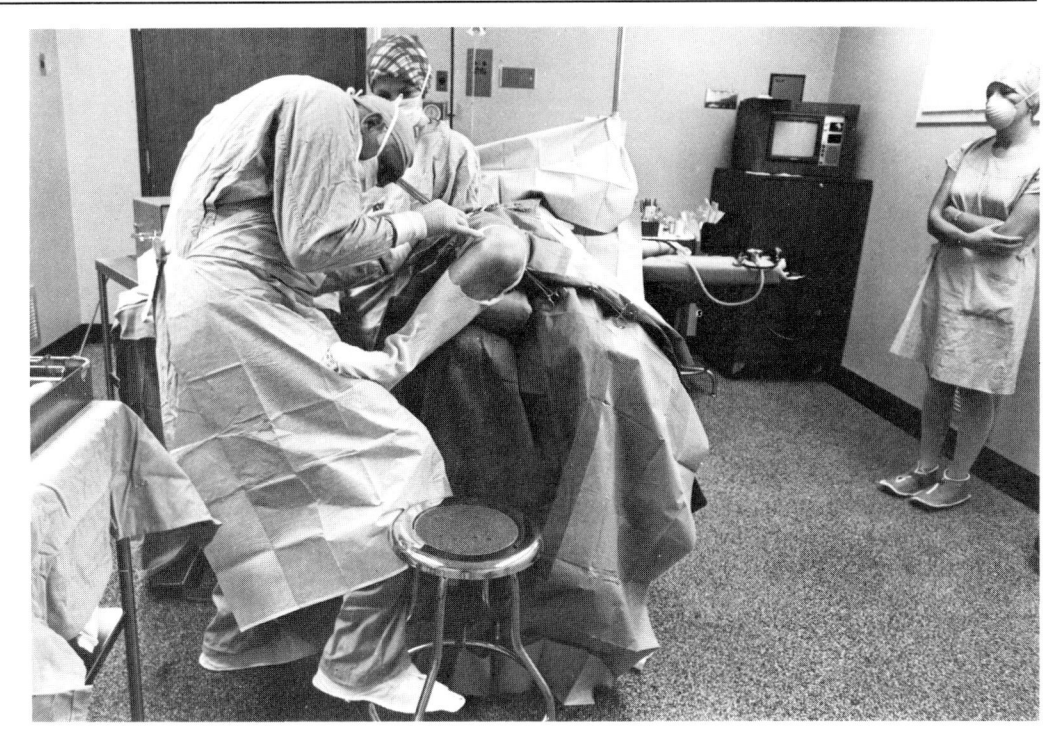

FIG. 3-26. Posterolateral inspection is facilitated by surgeon placing foot on a stool rung so that patient's foot can rest on thigh. This frees arthroscopist's hands for posterolateral inspection of patient's knee. Mayo stand, light source, and assistant are in more proximal positions.

This allows viewing down the superior surface of the medial meniscus, which is not possible anteriorly because the curve of the condyle blocks the view. (See Fig. 7-6, *G* and *H*.)

On completion of this inspection the knee is redistended with saline to facilitate entry to the posterolateral compartment.

Posterolateral compartment

The assistant moves to an area next to the patient's pelvis. The patient's hip is moved into adduction, and the knee is flexed approximately 100°. The arthroscopist stands facing the lateral aspect of the patient's thigh. After placing his foot on a stool rung, the surgeon can rest the patient's leg on his thigh (Fig. 3-26). During this repositioning it is necessary that the circulating nurse move the Mayo stand and the light source to make room for the arthroscopist.

The landmark for the posterolateral puncture is at a point where a line drawn along the lateral intermuscular septum intersects with a second line drawn parallel to the posterior margin of the fibula (Fig. 3-27). At this site the skin is lanced, and a cannula with a sharp trocar is inserted and directed slightly anterior and slightly inferior. With palpation the instrument is placed in the posterolateral compartment. The previous anteromedial puncture and the distended lateral joint line immediately superior to the meniscus can be helpful in orientation.

Diagnostic arthroscopy of the knee

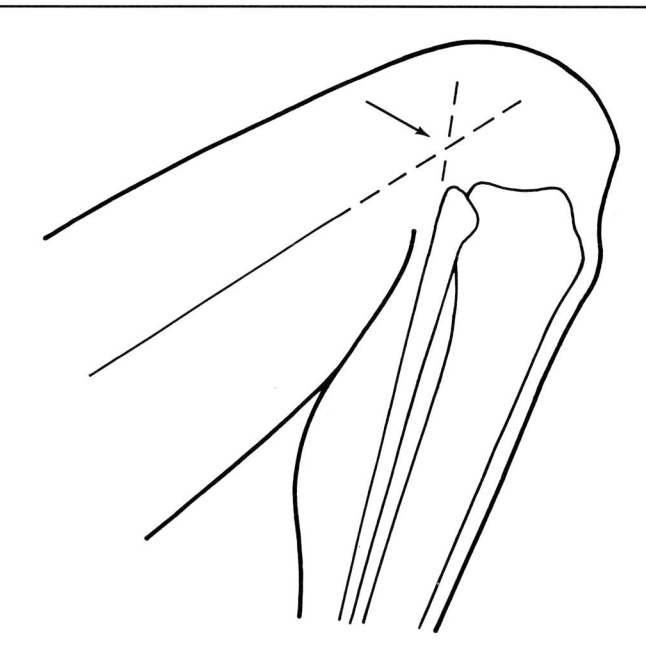

FIG. 3-27. Point of posterolateral entry where line drawn up from lateral intermuscular septum intersects with line drawn up from posterior aspect of fibula. Trocar and sharp cannula are placed, then directed slightly inferior and anterior to enter posterolateral compartment.

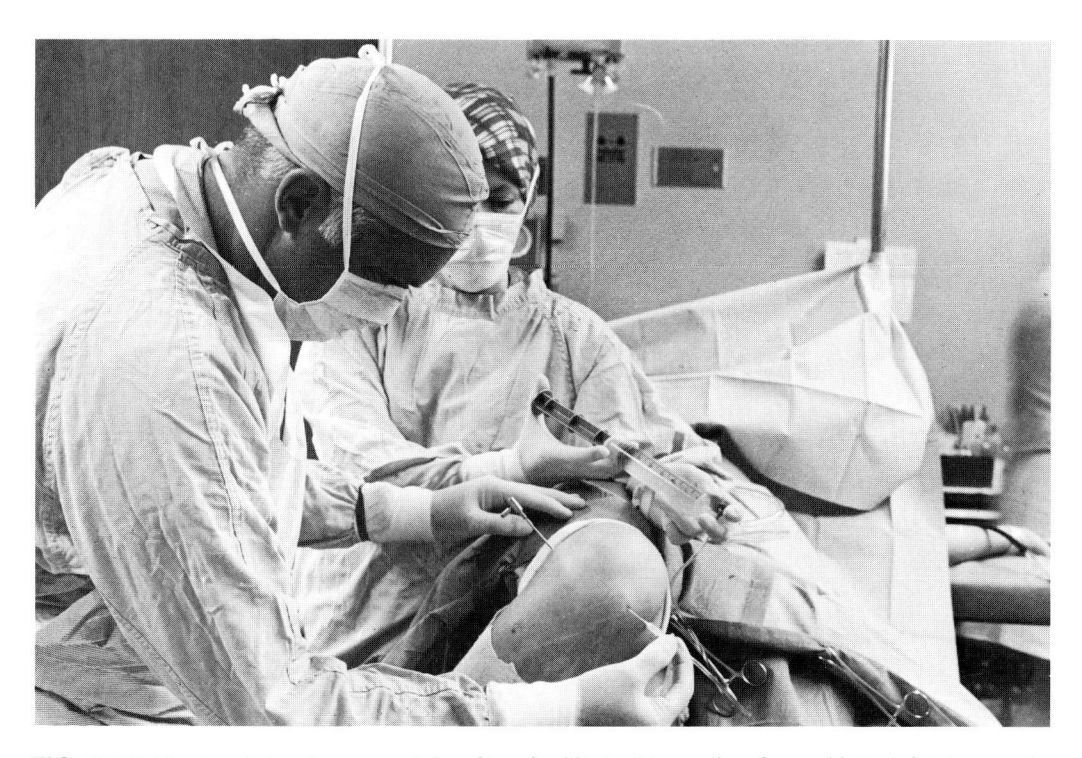

FIG. 3-28. Posterolateral approach is often facilitated by saline forced into joint to create maximal distension. Syringe from polyethylene catheter can be attached to No. 18 needle and placed through the previous anteromedial puncture site.

Basic arthroscopic techniques

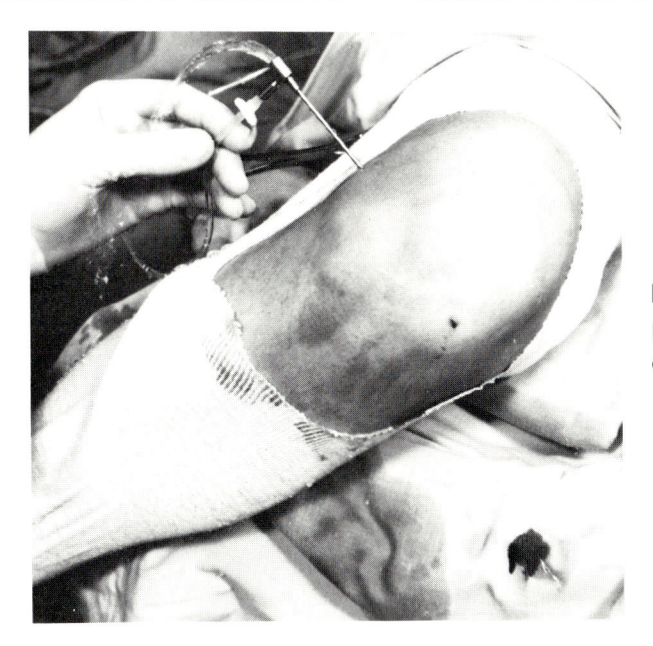

FIG. 3-29. Extrusion of saline from posterolateral puncture confirms entry.

Maximum distension of the joint may be compromised by minimal leakage from previous puncture wounds. The use of a small-diameter endoscope minimizes the leakage in multiple puncture techniques. When operative work is undertaken, a large inflow cannula is used. The cannula system eliminates the saline leakage, joint decompression, and lack of visualization. Further distension can be achieved by detaching the K-52 catheter from the cannula, attaching it to a No. 18 needle, placing it in the joint anteromedially (this area was anesthetized prior to initial puncture), and reinstilling saline (Fig. 3-28). Extrusion of fluid from the cannula again confirms entry (Fig. 3-29).

The internal landmark is the junction of the meniscus and the lateral femoral condyle. (See Fig. 7-4, *A* to *C*.) The contour is a little different here than on the medial side. Posterior loose bodies and posterior detached menisci are visible that cannot be seen from other approaches. It has been possible to enter the popliteus sheath in some cases, but in my opinion success was fortuitous. The popliteus sheath under the meniscus often houses loose bodies, which can be vacuumed out at this time. The popliteus sheath is best approached from the anterolateral inferior or superior side (Fig. 3-30).

FIG. 3-30. Popliteus tendon passing down sheath, seen from lateral approach. Photograph taken with rod-lens arthroscope.

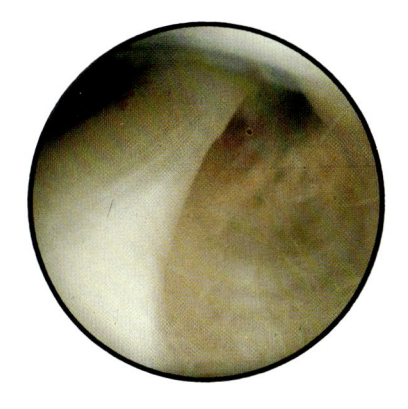

Diagnostic arthroscopy of the knee

Suprapatellar approach

Experience has shown that the suprapatellar approach is very important. The anteromedial view of the patella is often compromised by patient tightness under local anesthesia or by the scar tissue of previous surgery, even under general anesthesia. There are some patients who have a naturally tight patellar femoral articulation, which necessitates a suprapatellar approach. This is most easily performed with the patient's leg extended and the physician sitting medial to the knee while the assistant stabilizes the thigh to the outer side (Fig. 3-31). The point of entry is at the level of the superior margin of the patella and ¾ inch below the surface of the knee. The direction is perpendicular to the long axis of the leg and parallel to the floor. On entry it is possible to see the undersurface of the patella. (See Fig. 7-1, *A* and *B*.) Articular surface visualization is facilitated by manipulation of the patella. The intercondylar notch and the fat pad can be seen, as well as any loose bodies in the suprapatellar pouch.

A suprapatellar plica is more easily visualized from a superior view. It is also possible to see the other anatomic variations in the synovial lining, including the medial shelf.

In patients who have suspected subluxation or dislocation of the patella, a lateral suprapatellar inspection is indicated. The approach also facilitates inspection across the joint to a medial synovial plica, especially when incision or resection is being considered. The patient's leg is extended, and the physician and the assistant change places so that the physician is on the outer aspect of the knee. The puncture site and technique are similar to those of medial entry,

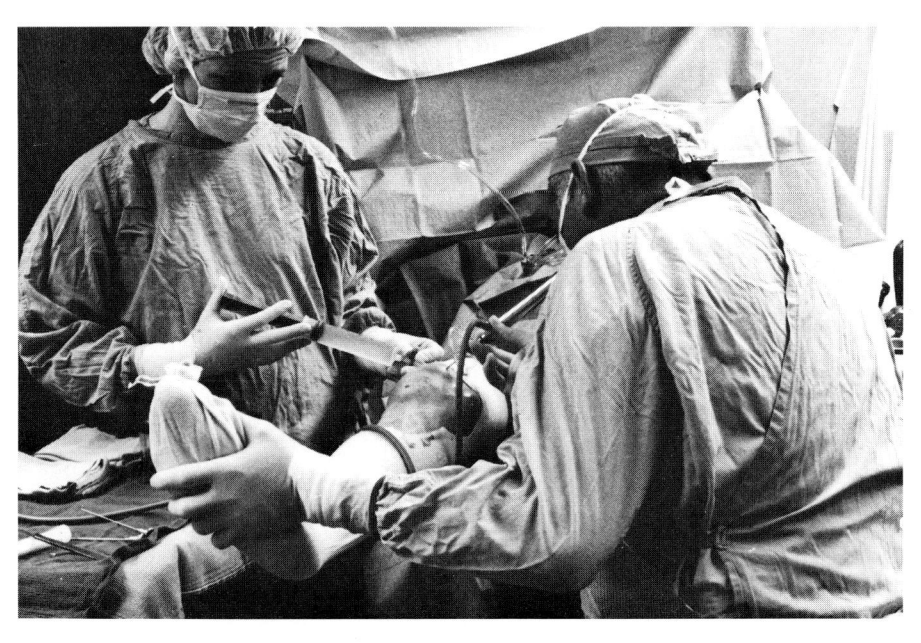

FIG. 3-31. Auxiliary suprapatellar inspection is commonly done from medial side at level of superior aspect of patella. If acute dislocation of patella is suspected, lateral inspection is indicated. This allows visualization down lateral sulcus for any potential loose bodies and also may allow defect in lateral femoral condyle to be seen.

Basic arthroscopic techniques

allowing visualization of the defect in the lateral femoral condyle. A loose body may be engulfed in the synovium along the lateral femoral condyle. (See Fig. 10-4, *B*.) Inspection down the popliteus sheath is possible by this approach (Fig. 3-30) and can facilitate the separate instrument puncture with triangulation to remove the loose body in this area.

Transpatellar tendon approach: Gillquist technique

Gillquist, Hagberg, and Oretorp[2] have advocated the transpatellar tendon approach for knee joint arthroscopy. Their approach starts 1 cm inferior to the tip of the apex of the patella and in the center portion of the patellar tendon. This approach has some universal value, and they have demonstrated an ability to view the suprapatellar pouch, both medial and lateral compartments, as well as entry into the posteromedial and posterolateral compartments in some cases using the single approach. They chose the large-diameter endoscope (4 mm) with a 30° incline view for the anterior chambers. As the endoscope makes an approach adjacent to the tibial spine into a posterior compartment, the endoscope is removed and the blunt trocar is placed in the cannula. These are then manipulated into the respective posterior compartment. At that juncture the 30° incline view is exchanged for a 70° incline-view endoscope, and viewing of the posterior compartment, the meniscal recesses, and the interior of the compartment walls is possible. These practitioners contend that a better inspection is made of the posterior cruciate ligament by this approach. Their approach also enables the surgeon to carry out arthroscopic surgery by a single viewing puncture. Fig. 3-32 shows the point of entry of the Gillquist approach. It is 1 cm inferior to the apex of the patella and in the center of the patellar tendon. There is good access above the fat pad.

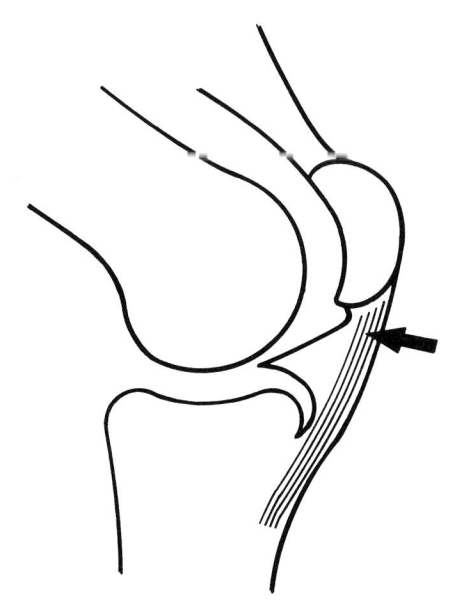

FIG. 3-32. Point of entry through the patellar tendon by Gillquist technique is 1 cm below patellar apex and above fat pad.

The disadvantages of this approach, from my experience, include a tender thickening in the patellar tendon for several months, especially if a larger diameter endoscope has been used. The disruption of the patellar tendinous fibers heals slowly and also with some palpable fibrosis. Some patients have found this unacceptable.

Modified Gillquist approach

The same total joint visualization is possible with a puncture site immediately adjacent to the patellar tendon, usually from the lateral direction. This prevents the disruption of the patellar tendinous fibers. This places the scope superior to the fat pad and gives surprisingly excellent access to the knee joint.

I have incorporated the Gillquist concept during inspection prior to arthroscopic surgery. Replacement of the endoscope with the blunt obturator may permit manipulation into the posteromedial space. The arthroscope is replaced for viewing. Most circumstances do not require the exchange to a 70° endoscope to view the posteromedial and posterolateral compartments. Viewing into the popliteus sheath is facilitated.

In some cases it is not possible to make this pass atraumatically, especially in a small person or a tight knee. Separate posteromedial and posterolateral punctures performed with a small scope may be necessary.

FOLLOW-UP

After an arthroscopic examination with local anesthesia, a simple compression bandage is applied to the puncture sites (Fig. 3-33). The patient is advised to remove this dressing the following day and to place adhesive bandages over the small wounds. Because patients frequently forget what they have been told in the operating room, the following week in the office their puncture wounds are inspected and the arthroscopic findings are reviewed (Fig. 3-34).

COMPLICATIONS

In two patients the saphenous vein was nicked with a No. 11 blade while making the posteromedial puncture. One patient bled for 3 days despite application of a compression dressing. The bleeding subsided spontaneously, and there was no further complication. The other patient underwent arthrotomy while under general anesthesia. Although the vein was ligated, there was no subsequent complication of phlebitis.

There has been no infection or unexplained synovitis as a result of arthroscopy. A few patients have developed synovial inflammation following open surgery, but neither anaerobic nor aerobic culture tests showed any positive results. There have been no wound infections following any arthroscopy in the past 7 years.

One patient who had a Waldius total-knee prosthesis with absorption adjacent to the cement line underwent arthroscopy, at which time it was determined that he had a preexistent low-grade infection. The hemarthrosis pro-

Basic arthroscopic techniques

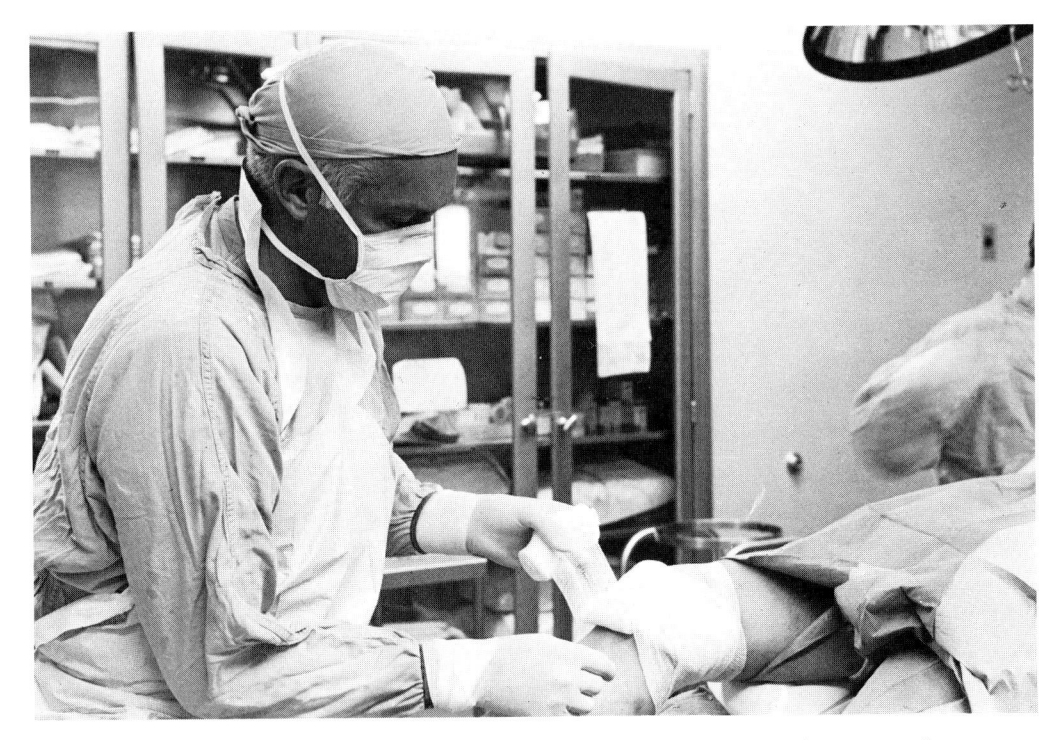

FIG. 3-33. After arthroscopic procedure, gauze bandages are placed over small puncture wounds, and sterile dressing compresses joint. Next day, patient may remove bandage and place small adhesive bandages over areas of entry.

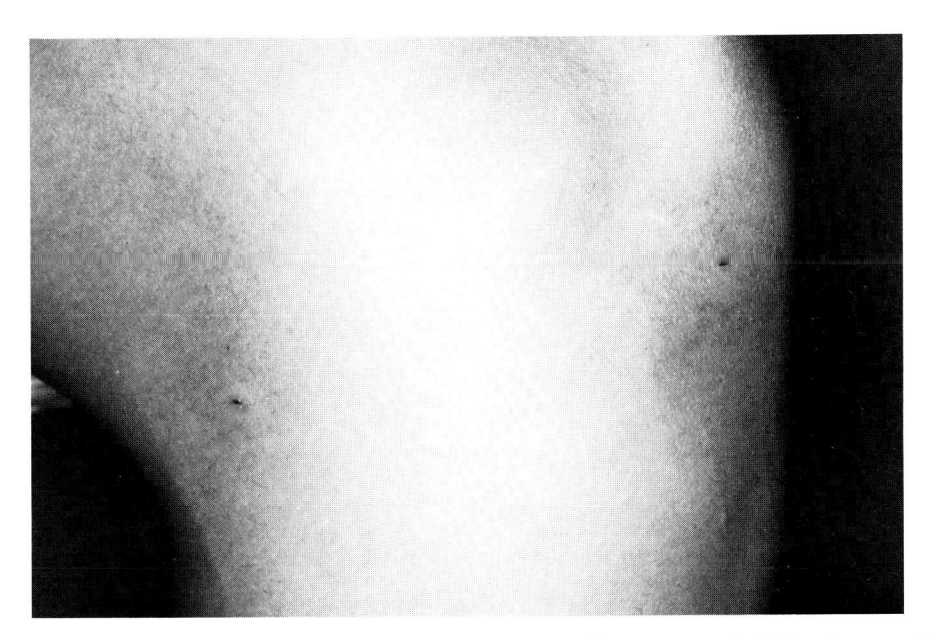

FIG. 3-34. Needlescope leaves small marks, seen here 1 week following multiple-puncture technique arthroscopy. Punctures are so small that no suture is required, and adhesive bandage is all that is indicated after second day. Surgery can be performed any day after arthroscopy without risk of infection.

duced during arthroscopy created a culture medium for the bacteria and subsequent drainage of the knee and removal of the prosthesis were necessary. However, we have performed arthroscopies on patients who had acutely infected knees, without any exacerbation of the condition or puncture site infection.

In one patient synovial fluid drained for 4 days after a loose body of 1-inch diameter was removed percutaneously from the posteromedial compartment with a Jaws modified pituitary rongeur during arthroscopy. No sutures were placed in the synovium or skin of this patient, in whom a skin incision of approximately 1 cm had been made. The problem cleared without sequelae.

One patient developed an infection following reconstructive surgery that was preceded by an arthroscopic examination. Another patient, with a loose, infected Waldius total-knee prosthesis, had this problem exacerbated following arthroscopy.

REFERENCES

1. Burman, M. S., Finkelstein, H., and Mayer, L.: Arthroscopy of the knee joint, J. Bone Joint Surg. **16**:255, 1934.
2. Gillquist, J., Hageberg, G., and Oretorp, N.: Arthroscopic examination of the posteromedial compartment of the knee joint, Int. Orthop. **3**(1):13-18, 1979.
3. Guten, G. N.: Methylene blue staining of articular cartilage during arthroscopy, Orthop. Rev. **6**:59, 1977.
4. Jackson, R. W., and Abe, I.: The role of arthroscopy in the management of disorders of the knee; an analysis of 200 consecutive examinations, J. Bone Joint Surg. **54**:310, 1972.
5. Jackson, R. W., and Dandy, D. J.: Arthroscopy of the knee, New York, 1976, Grune & Stratton, Inc.

Chapter 4

Anesthesia

Local anesthesia
    Technique
        Patient instruction
        Patient selection
        Patient monitoring
        Discussion
General anesthesia
    Technique
    Patient selection
Complications

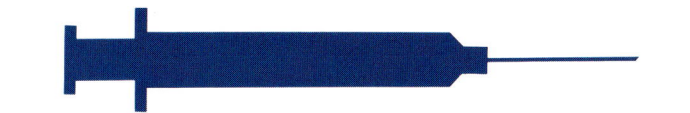

LOCAL ANESTHESIA

On October 30, 1972, I performed my first arthroscopy without having witnessed one. The lack of experience proved to be advantageous in developing the technique of knee joint arthroscopy with the patient under local anesthesia.

Mack Clayton[1] performed single-puncture inspection in rheumatoid patients in the late 1960s. Also, Boehler was reported to have used local anesthesia in some patients. Subsequently, McGinty and Mapza[4] and Pevey[5] reported on the use of local anesthesia. In the first patients, only 1% lidocaine was administered into the skin, subcutaneous tissue, and the synovium; no intra-articular tissue was anesthetized. Successful visualization of the anterior and

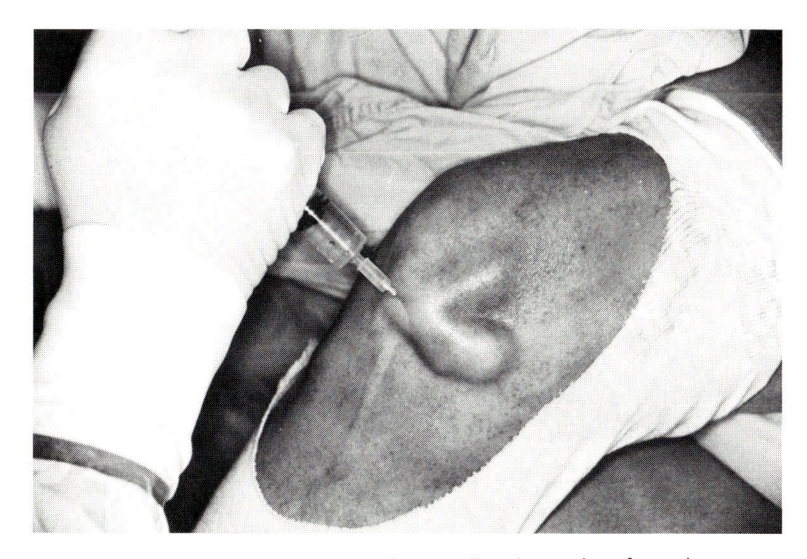

FIG. 4-1. Plain lidocaine, 1%, blocks infrapatellar branch of saphenous nerve. This decreases patient's proprioception and anxiety and increases comfort during procedure.

Diagnostic arthroscopy of the knee

superior compartments of the joint was accomplished. Subsequently it was realized that if the infrapatellar branch of the saphenous nerve were blocked, there was a decrease in the patient's sense of proprioception, and improved relaxation resulted (Fig. 4-1).

Initially a narcotic or sedative was given intravenously. Patients often became drowsy and occasionally nauseated, and they frequently vomited. The use of such medicine prolonged the outpatient stay in the recovery room. Also, patients were restricted from driving vehicles. Therefore this practice was stopped, and subsequent experience has shown it to be unnecessary.

Technique

After it has been established medically that arthroscopy is indicated, the patient is given the choice of having it performed under local anesthesia. Most patients readily accept this because of the simplicity and reduced risk of the procedure.

Plain lidocaine, 1%, is used. It has not been necessary to inject local anesthetic inside the joint cavity because an adequate infiltrative block of the infrapatellar fat pad and the infrapatellar branch of the saphenous nerve has sufficed for inspection of the anterior and superior compartments. For all sites, including posteromedial, posterolateral, and suprapatellar punctures, direct locally infiltrated 1% plain lidocaine is injected (Fig. 4-2). Normally 10 to 12 ml of lidocaine are used per puncture, but a higher dose is indicated in a sensitive person.

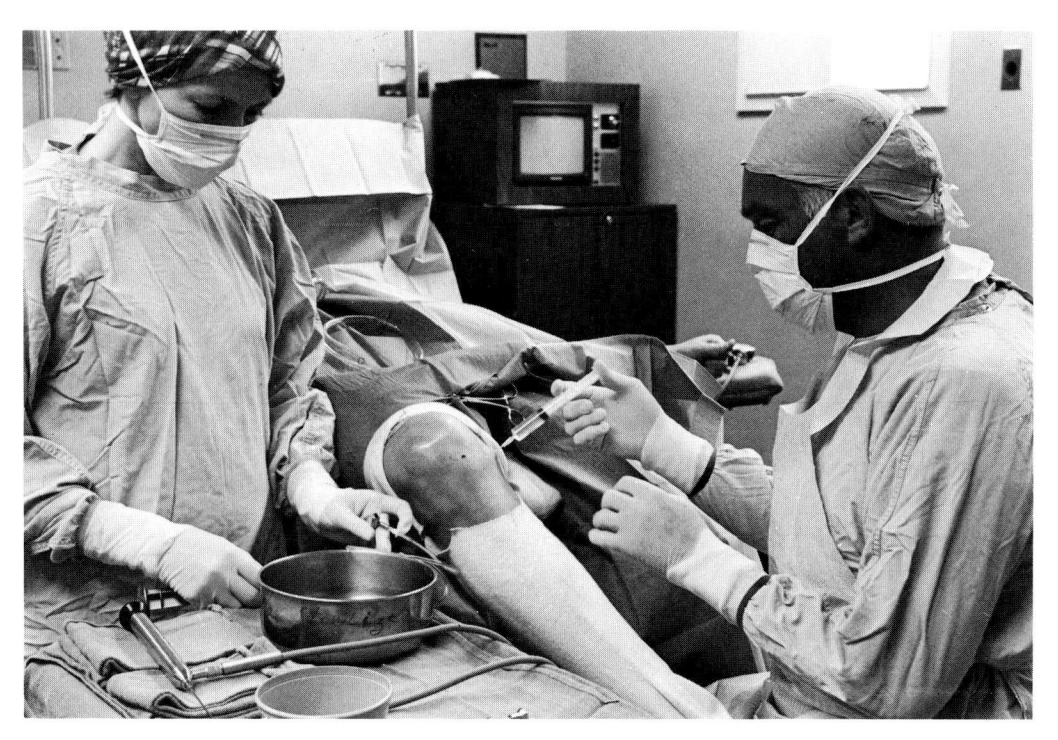

FIG. 4-2. Plain lidocaine, 1%, is injected directly into posteromedial compartment. Direct infiltration is also used in posterolateral approach.

It is essential that the patient not be in pain. A dialogue between the surgeon and the patient can prevent this; if there is any discomfort, the patient should speak up. If the cannula and trocar are in place when the discomfort occurs, remove the trocar, bend the K-52 catheter at the entry site, and place lidocaine through the cannula to that exact area (Fig. 4-3). This delivers the anesthetic better than does withdrawing the cannula or trying to pass a needle adjacent to the cannula to achieve adequate anesthesia in the area.

There are several other factors that facilitate arthroscopy when the patient is under local anesthesia. First and perhaps foremost is the security and confidence of the arthroscopist, whose attitude is readily perceived by the patient. Confidence transmitted to the patient will result in relaxation and decreased anxiety. Second, a gentle procedure carried out with dispatch (less than 15 minutes) is easily tolerated. Third, the patient's confidence and relaxation can be enhanced by word-of-mouth advertising by other patients who had successful arthroscopies.

Patient instruction

The physician should inform the patient of the nature of the arthroscopic procedure. One of the most valuable methods of allaying anxiety and fear is to give the patient a mimeographed instruction sheet about arthroscopy (see box on p. 64). First reading may create some anxiety, but at the time of the procedure the patient may find that it has reduced apprehension considerably. He will be pleased to find that the procedure is carried out as detailed.

After the procedure a dressing is applied. (See Fig. 3-34.) It is removed the following day, and adhesive bandages are placed over the multiple puncture wounds. If there is no indication for surgical intervention, the patient is exam-

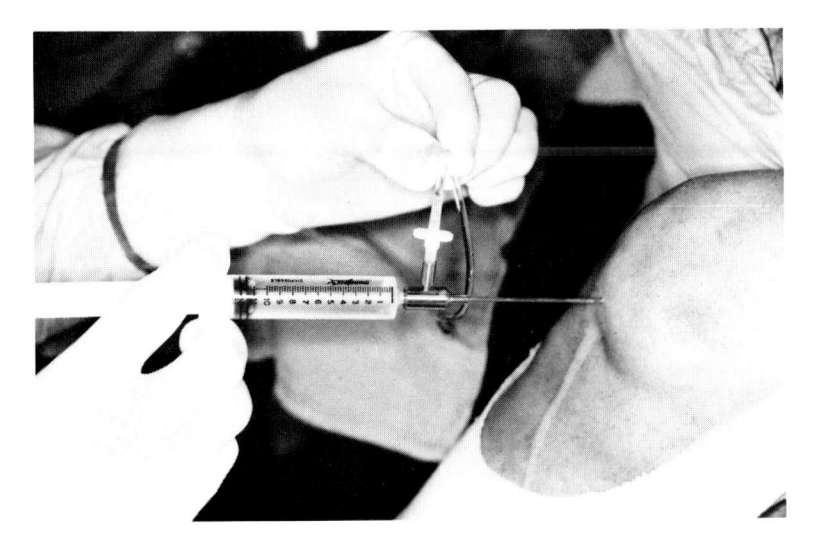

FIG. 4-3. If patient expresses some discomfort during insertion of scope, rather than withdraw cannula and reinsert needle, it is possible to pinch off K-52 catheter and infiltrate 1% plain lidocaine directly through cannula to tip, exact site where patient is having discomfort.

Diagnostic arthroscopy of the knee

> **Arthroscopy instructions**
>
> Arthroscopy (looking into a joint) is a relatively new procedure, now performed with a fiberoptic Needlescope of small diameter (2.2 mm). It takes about 10 minutes.
>
> Arthroscopy allows the physician to directly visualize almost every portion of the knee joint and provides an opportunity to improve diagnostic accuracy. The intended purpose is to prevent unnecessary surgery and permit earlier surgical intervention in those patients requiring an operation.
>
> The procedure is performed in the hospital outpatient operating room to provide ideal conditions. The procedure necessitates the use of a tourniquet (a tight tube) placed around your thigh to prevent any small amount of blood from obscuring the physician's vision. This tourniquet tightness is the most uncomfortable part of the procedure. If you remain relaxed and do not tighten up, the tourniquet will be more tolerable. Your leg is painted with a cool, brown antiseptic solution. Sterile sheets protect the area. Your knees will be allowed to bend so your legs hang down.
>
> You will have some discomfort with the "freezing" of the knee, which is similar to that done by a dentist. The medicine is 1% lidocaine and usually renders the knee painless. There may be a feeling of distension or occasional pressure without pain.
>
> There are complications to any procedure, and so it is with arthroscopy. There is less than 1% chance of complication. The known problems have been breakage of the fiberoptic scope, infection, allergy to the medicines used, and knee effusion (swelling). These are rare, and we take measures to prevent them.
>
> Now for your part:
> 1. You will be called by the hospital regarding your time of arrival.
> 2. Please shave your leg (groin to ankle) and shower prior to the test.
> 3. Bring a list of any known allergies to medicines and/or general medical problems for our information.
> 4. Anticipate 1 to 2 hours total time to get in and out of the hospital.
>
> Thank you.

ined approximately 1 week following the arthroscopic examination, and the arthroscopic findings are reviewed at that time. If the patient is scheduled for surgery, this review will be carried out the night prior to surgery. Surgery can safely be performed immediately, a day, or a week after Needlescope arthroscopy without an increased risk of infection.

I have performed these as early as 1 day and as late as 10 or more days after diagnostic arthroscopy for 7 years, with no patient developing infection of the small (2-mm) arthroscopic puncture wounds. In an occasional case contamination has required redraping and reprepping the patient, although with the Needlescope the eyepiece is at a safe distance from the surgeon's hand. When using an arthroscope in which the ocular lens is close to the hand, the chance of contamination is great, and it is safer to reprepare and redrape the patient prior to arthrotomy.

Patient selection for local anesthesia

The selection of patients for arthroscopic examination under local anesthesia is based on clinical judgment. If the patient has a diagnostic problem without clear-cut physical findings to support complaints, then arthroscopy is performed with a local anesthetic. Also, preoperative assessment is important in advising a patient who has had many previous surgeries. It affords an opportunity to discuss with the patient the arthroscopic findings, prospective surgery, and prognosis. Both the surgeon and the patient have increased confidence when a surgical procedure can be designed after direct observation of intra-articular findings.

Patients whose history and physical examination suggest a meniscal abnormality, but in whom positive findings are lacking, are also given a local anesthetic before arthroscopy. If physical examination is compromised because the patient has pain, diagnosis may be established by arthroscopy rather than by surgical exploration. This not only avoids the risks of general anesthesia but also eliminates unnecessary arthrotomy or meniscectomy. Misdiagnosis of patellar conditions (i.e., chondromalacia, dislocation, or subluxation) can be avoided. In some patients with condylar disease (e.g., osteochondritis dissecans), the status of the articular surface cannot be demonstrated on arthrogram or plain-film roentgenogram; arthroscopy can provide this information. Ligamentous injuries, both fresh and old, are amenable to arthroscopic examination. Synovial disease also lends itself to morphologic study by this technique.

Recent series have included a number of patients with medicolegal or Workmen's Compensation claims, who were seen for evaluation only. In the minds of the referring physicians these patients probably had no knee problem, and the consultation was to confirm that impression. Although we would like to think of arthroscopy as contributing in a positive way, examinations performed to rule out any existing abnormality allow the physician to confidently recommend conservative measures or return to work.

Patient monitoring

The arthroscopist can anticipate any sudden moves by the patient by being sensitive to his reactions. During the procedure with local anesthesia, the arthroscopist can monitor the patient's discomfort or anxiety by observing his breathing or deep sighing. The patient will tighten the Achilles tendon, which can be monitored easily by the surgeon, whose hand is on the patient's ankle. (See Fig. 3-10.) It should also be noted that when a patient under local anesthesia tightens the quadriceps muscle, the capsular tissues will be compressed, making it difficult to puncture the fascia. It is also possible to ascertain in certain cases the patient's relative pain threshold, which can be an important factor in clinical judgment.

Diagnostic arthroscopy of the knee

Discussion

When the technical principles previously outlined are carefully adhered to, it is possible to arthroscopically examine the entire knee joint with the patient under local anesthesia.

The value of local anesthesia cannot be overemphasized. With essentially no risk to the patient, a comprehensive evaluation of the diagnostic problem is possible, as are some therapeutic measures (e.g., removal of loose bodies). The patient's pain threshold and psychologic sensitivity to the knee problem can be evaluated during injection of the local anesthetic. Areas within the knee can be palpated to confirm the presence of an intra-articular abnormality.

As with any surgical procedure, there is no substitute for sound clinical judgment, knowledge of anatomy, preparation and organization, and perseverance in improving clinical skills through experience.

Tourniquet

The use of the tourniquet has been questioned. However, arthroscopy can be performed in 5 to 15 minutes, and the patient is able to tolerate the tightness on the thigh for this period of time. In fact, there is some anesthetic effect from ischemia. Inspection of the joint can be bloodless. At the end of the procedure the tourniquet is released, and the vascular characteristics of the synovium are documented.

Physician-patient relationship

Do not underestimate the effect of verbal and written explanation given to the patient to allay anxiety. An existing physician-patient relationship has proved to be important in establishing relaxation. Some of my more difficult patients have been those who were referred for arthroscopic examination only and with whom there was no opportunity to establish rapport.

Diagnostic value

Arthroscopy with local anesthetic was performed on patients in whom circumstantial evidence (i.e., history and physical examination, roentgenograms, and arthrogram) was not sufficient to warrant surgical exploration or on patients referred for evaluation only. Without arthroscopy, certain of these patients would have undergone empirical exploratory arthrotomy; others would have been treated conservatively. The matching of the right treatment to the right condition in this group of patients would have been a matter of chance. Arthroscopy under local anesthesia provided a method of reaching a correct diagnosis by direct evidence and hence of prescribing the appropriate treatment.

Clinical judgment

Some have suggested that arthroscopy serves as a substitute for sound clinical examination and judgment, and thus the traditional clinical skills of the physician are being neglected or diminished. On the contrary, the opportunity to combine direct inspection in the joint with clinical evaluation enhances one's skills as a clinician. It would be virtually impossible for one not to improve as a clinician while using this opportunity to correlate simple intra-articular viewing with preoperative evaluations.

GENERAL ANESTHESIA
Technique

The technique of arthroscopy is similar when performed with the patient under general anesthesia. Posteromedial and posterolateral inspections are still important in any patient in whom inspection from the anterior puncture shows normal findings because of the possibility of lesions not seen from other approaches.

The patient's position and preparation are the same as for arthrotomy. At the end of the arthroscopic procedure the equipment and tables are moved away, and separate Mayo stands and tables for the arthrotomy are positioned. A new water-impermeable drape is placed on the table.

Arthroscopy need not lengthen the duration of general anesthesia, but actually can shorten the procedure time. The inspection of the knee by arthroscopy is thorough; thus extensive surgical exploration and unnecessary arthrotomies are avoided. It is possible to make selective and rather limited incisions because of the knowledge of the intra-articular lesion gained by arthroscopy. Initially a time limit of 15 minutes for arthroscopy should be established, so as to not discourage the operating team. With experience arthroscopy is not a hindrance to the operating schedule but is of benefit to both the surgeon and the anesthesiologist.

The techniques for arthroscopy when combined with arthroscopic surgery are necessarily different and are described in Chapter 15.

Patient selection

Arthroscopy with general anesthesia is performed on patients who have not had a recent arthroscopy of the knee with local anesthetic but whose known clinical condition warrants surgical intervention.

A small percentage of patients who would be candidates for arthroscopy with local anesthetic for diagnostic purposes choose or are advised to have arthroscopy with general anesthetic because of personal or emotional reasons. This might include patients who have had multiple arthrotomies or because of subsequent painful injury to the knee. Only one of my patients experienced enough discomfort during the initial procedure with local anesthetic to request that the second be done with general anesthetic. Most patients, when given the choice, choose a local anesthetic if there is some certainty that an arthrotomy will *not* follow.

COMPLICATIONS

We have seen no complications from anesthetic in arthroscopy. No patients have shown sensitivity to 1% plain lidocaine, and none has developed pulmonary emboli or thrombophlebitis, even with an accompanying arthrotomy or arthroscopic surgery.

One out-of-town referral who requested outpatient diagnostic arthroscopy claimed a medical history of allergy to all "caines." The procedure was performed with a massive infiltration of 0.9% saline to distend the skin and deeper tissues. This was quite effective, and a single-puncture evaluation was performed. As a historical note, Fred C. Reynolds mentioned this method of anesthesia when I was a resident at Barnes Hospital in St. Louis.

It should be noted that patients 40 or more years of age who had accompanying arthrotomy were given postoperative low-dosage prophylactic warfarin sodium (Coumadin).

REFERENCES

1. Clayton, M. L.: Personal communication, 1979.
2. Johnson, L. L.: Arthroscopy of the knee using local anesthesia: a review of 400 patients, J. Bone Joint Surg. (Am.) **58**(5):736, 1976.
3. Johnson, L. L.: Diagnostic arthroscopy of the knee: the knee joint, Amsterdam, Excerpta Medica; New York, 1974, American Elsevier Publishing Co.
4. McGinty, J. B., and Mapza, R. A.: Evaluation of an out-patient procedure under local anesthesia, J. Bone Joint Surg. (Am.) **60**:787, 1978.
5. Pevey, J. K.: Out-patient arthroscopy of the knee under local anesthesia, Am. J. Sports Med. **6**(3):122, 1978.

Chapter 5

Diagnostic arthroscopy in clinical practice

Enhancement of clinical skills
Effect on patient management
Differential diagnosis
Arthroscopy versus arthrography
Effect on surgical design
Rehabilitation
Arthroscopy in joints other than the knee
Research
Review of diagnostic arthroscopy experience
    Choice of anesthetic
    Classification of patients
    Analysis
    Series I (1972 to 1975)
    Series II (1975 to 1976)
    Series III: general anesthesia (1975 to 1976)
    Series IV (1976 to 1978)
Patient management routine
Value of diagnostic arthroscopy
Learning arthroscopy

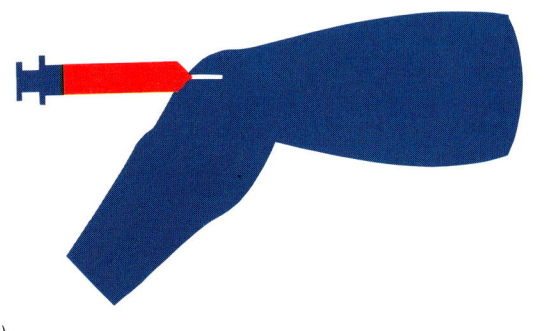

Arthroscopy has sparked the curiosity and interest of most orthopedists. Heretofore the technique with large-diameter endoscopes and general anesthetic, confining the inspection to the anterior portion of the knee joint, was not considered practical and thus was not embraced as part of routine management in orthopedics.

When the concept of arthroscopy was expanded to include the use of local anesthetic and inspection of posteromedial and posterolateral compartments, arthroscopy became a valuable necessity.

Still, some orthopedists vehemently reject the value of arthroscopy. It seems to challenge the competence and clinical abilities of some; others admit inability to technically perform the procedure with proficiency. This is in sharp contrast to the widespread acceptance by patients with knee problems who have come to understand the value of arthroscopy. Patients who realize that the interior of the joint can be inspected directly under local anesthesia will choose arthroscopy over an exploratory arthrotomy, regardless of the confidence they or the surgeon might have in the clinical evaluation.

Because proficiency in arthroscopy points up limitations of clinical diagnosis and lack of understanding of pathologic processes in patients with knee problems, orthopedists who have invested time, money, and energy in arthroscopy have been rewarded handsomely by improvement of diagnostic skills, understanding of pathologic findings, and general enjoyment of their practice. Those who have not expended the energy to become proficient in arthroscopy cannot make a valid criticism and simply do not know what they are missing.

ENHANCEMENT OF CLINICAL SKILLS

Interest in arthroscopy and its benefits does not negate the physician's desire to improve other clinical skills of physical examination, laboratory testing, or x-ray film interpretation. It provides further information with which to evaluate clinical judgment and diagnostic competence. A continued reshaping of clinical impressions is possible. For instance, during clinical review (documented later in this chapter) it is not unusual to find that either an additional significant diagnosis or one different from that made preoperatively was identified by arthroscopy. Also, in a few patients complete arthroscopic examination of the joint proves that no abnormality exists, although clinical, laboratory, or x-ray findings suggest one.

Certain conditions may be clinically suspected but confirmed by arthroscopy only. For example, subluxation of the patella can be a subtle condition. It can be overlooked clinically, but the specific lesion is seen arthroscopically in the lateral femoral condyle.

Correlation of clinical experience with arthroscopic findings increases the physician's confidence in caring for patients with knee problems, which certainly enhances the enjoyment of practice for the orthopedist/arthroscopist.

EFFECT ON PATIENT MANAGEMENT

A patient's symptoms, physical signs, and x-ray findings provide information on which the clinician may base one of three choices: conservative management (i.e., laboratory investigation, medication, or exercises); arthroscopic examination with local anesthetic for those patients in whom diagnosis is uncertain; or surgical intervention based on recognition of typical findings of an internal derangement or other surgically amenable abnormalities. Many patients will require arthroscopic evaluation if other attempts at diagnosis fail or they are unimproved after conservative treatment.

Over the past several years the management of acute knee injuries has evolved from a concept of "wait and see" to one of earlier definitive treatment. Evaluation of clinical instability or arthrographic evidence of intra-articular abnormalities is being substituted. The "wait and see" attitude really is "not seeing at all"; it is postponing treatment to a time when surgical repair might be compromised or the intra-articular injury may be permanent. This is compounded if the patient attempts to mobilize a knee with internal derangement.

Therefore arthroscopy has replaced the "wait and see" method with the "see" method. The aspiration of hemarthrosis, followed by roentgenography to rule out fracture and the subsequent application of a cast, is probably no longer generally accepted practice. Hemarthrosis is not considered a contraindication to arthroscopy. By the methods outlined in previous chapters, clear visualization can be achieved intra-articularly in the acutely injured knee. Thus there is little excuse for a delay in arthroscopy, resultant diagnosis, and treatment.

For example, a massive hemarthrosis may accompany a torn anterior cruciate ligament, a complete separation of a posteromedial meniscus, an acute dislocation of the patella, or condylar fracture. The only condition that can cause hemarthrosis and not require surgical intervention is an occasional contusion. The patient's acute pain may compromise the clinical examination, and in the presence of hemarthrosis the arthrogram loses its reliability. An arthroscopic examination provides an immediate definitive diagnosis. Appropriate early treatment is pursued with confidence.

Arthroscopy provides a means of differential diagnosis and direction in patient management. It allows a macroscopic inspection of the joint previously possible only by arthrotomy. Because fluid is instilled in the joint, the natural activities of flexion, extension, and rotation can be simulated during arthroscopic observation. This enhances recognition of various pathologic abnormalities. The subtle early degenerative changes not recognized grossly are readily apparent arthroscopically.

DIFFERENTIAL DIAGNOSIS

Many patients, when seen clinically, have symptoms suggesting intra-articular abnormalities but no positive physical, laboratory, or x-ray findings. They desire a definitive determination of the problem and some clear-cut direction for treatment. In the past such patients were advised to pursue conservative measures until the condition resolved through the natural course or worsened to such an extent that diagnosis was obvious. Even exploratory surgery may be acceptable to the patient if it is the only viable alternative to symptoms.

In contrast, arthroscopy provides a method of inspecting the interior of the joint completely to establish or rule out intra-articular abnormalities. The physician can then institute appropriate intervention or conservative measures based on this observation.

Arthroscopy provides understanding of management in vague diagnoses. Often patients have vague complaints referable to their knees but no sign of intra-articular abnormality. Typically, there is tenderness along the medial joint line, pain in the patellar area with some minimal patellar catching, or crepitus that is barely discernible. If symptoms are caused by chondromalacia of the patella, the physician can assure the patient that the natural history of this condition rarely produces serious consequences and that conservative isometric exercises and salicylates are indicated. If the chondromalacia is severe, then arthroscopic intra-articular shaving may be performed, often under the same local anesthetic. (See Chapter 17.) On the other hand, if a torn meniscus is injuring the articular cartilage, the treatment of choice is meniscectomy at an early date, before deterioration of the condylar surfaces results in permanent condylar injury.

A better understanding of the pathologic variations is possible when the arthroscopist correlates results of physical examination with intra-articular observations. Arthroscopic examination of the meniscal dynamics has shown that some menisci are more mobile than others. Certainly if there is no injury to the articular cartilage, the increased mobility of the meniscus need not be treated. However, if there is instability during high-level athletic performance, and if the patient understands the consequences, a meniscectomy might be indicated. Observations of "hypermobile meniscus" made arthroscopically have prevented unnecessary meniscectomy.

ARTHROSCOPY VERSUS ARTHROGRAPHY

Arthroscopy provides a diagnostic bridge between arthrography and subsequent surgical management. X-ray films provide only shadows for interpretation. At best, this is circumstantial evidence. The interpretation of lateral meniscal lesions by arthrography is difficult in the best of hands. Articular and synovial lesions usually are not recognized. A complete absence of the anterior cruciate ligament may be identified arthrographically but is also easily diagnosed on physical examination. Arthrography is compromised in the presence of hemarthroses, is of limited value if there are large loose bodies, and is of no value in discerning multiple small loose bodies. Arthrography provides limited information about synovial diseases or their morphologic characteristics.

Proponents of the use of arthrography and arthroscopy usually limit arthroscopic examination to the anterior compartments of the joint and use a large-diameter endoscope. Their judgment to continue using arthrography is clinically justified for the posterior aspects of the joint and menisci. Those areas can be documented arthrographically.

Certainly arthrography has been proved an excellent and reliable diagnostic means by those who regularly examine a large volume of patients. It should be continued accepted practice, especially in areas where there is no one skilled in arthroscopy.

I find the direct evidence provided by arthroscopy in all compartments of the joint preferable to the circumstantial findings of arthrography. At the present time I use arthrography for those patients who have juxta-articular cysts, to establish the extent of the mass prior to resection. Also, arthrography can be used if the physician feels that the arthroscopic examination had been compromised in some area or compartment of the joint.

EFFECT ON SURGICAL DESIGN

Arthroscopy provides additional information for the surgeon in designing and recommending a plan of treatment. It is not unusual that an anticipated surgical procedure is deemed unnecessary as a result of arthroscopy. With experience, interpretation of findings can rule out the need for exploratory arthrotomy or meniscectomy. In some situations arthroscopic findings greatly alter the anticipated surgical procedure or the location and extent of the incision necessary to perform the definitive treatment.

Arthroscopy can provide information important to maintaining a good physician-patient relationship in complex situations, such as when a second or third exploratory or reconstructive procedure is necessary. The presence or absence of articular degeneration affects the prognosis and is an important consideration when advising a patient who has had previous surgery and is anticipating another operation. The patient gains added confidence in the recommendation of surgery when he has a clear understanding of the anticipated results and the specific prognosis.

Arthroscopic evaluation may prove beneficial in patients with degenerative articular disease who are being considered for high tibial osteotomy or total-knee replacement. Standing x-ray examinations do not fully disclose the status of the articular cartilage or loose bodies in lateral compartments. Tibial osteotomy, which shifts weight bearing to a compartment with significant articular surface loss or meniscal derangement, should be avoided if possible. Patient selection and surgical results should improve treatment.

The arthroscopic surgical procedure may be combined with various conventional procedures. For example, arthroscopic inspection, meniscectomy, and compartment chondroplasty could give optimal intra-articular status of a joint immediately prior to high tibial osteotomy. Arthroscopic meniscectomy may precede capsular reconstruction for cruciate ligament instability and decrease the morbidity accompanying arthrotomy, thus limiting necessary repair and attendant scarring.

REHABILITATION

Rehabilitation is enhanced as a result of diagnostic arthroscopy. Significant abnormalities are known at the time of surgery, such as conditions in the posterior compartment, which if not recognized and treated properly would prolong or complicate the postoperative course. Loose bodies in the posterior compartment that are not visible anteriorly may be removed arthroscopically, thus preventing prolonged synovitis that would develop while this articular material was absorbed by the synovium. Virtually every recess of the knee joint can be examined and loose articular debris cleared.

Subtle lesions, such as horizontal cleft tears, can be seen with a small-diameter endoscope passing under the meniscus. In addition, posterior horn tears not visualized even from anterior arthrotomy can be seen by posterior arthroscopic examination. When these are observed prior to the initial surgery, they can be surgically managed, removing any potential cause of postoperative problems.

Arthroscopic surgery (Chapters 14 to 20) reduces the morbidity by virtue of the minimal puncture of the capsule. The rehabilitation is hastened as a result, especially in rheumatoid synovectomy. Enthusiasm for rapid return to competitive athletics must be tempered by the time necessary for internal tissue healing.

Patients who have recently undergone major reconstructive knee surgery and have a synovitis either accompanying or following surgery may benefit from arthroscopy and lavage.

After open meniscectomy an occasional patient will have recurring meniscal symptoms or persistent effusion. Prior to arthroscopy with local anesthetic these patients could only be encouraged to alternately rest and lift weight. Now if there is any unexplained morbidity 8 to 12 weeks after meniscectomy, a direct inspection should be considered. Although this may seem an oversell of arthroscopy, my observations have shown this not to be so. The procedure has shown tears of the meniscus in the opposite compartment not present at the time of the original surgery, presence of rather large loose bodies, and an occasional diffuse reactive synovitis. Also, three bucket-handle tears of the regenerated meniscus have been seen, one as late as 10 years after surgery.

The presence of loose bodies is the most common cause of effusion following meniscectomy. A preexisting articular injury may flake off more material. Arthroscopy can confirm this, and the material can be removed through the various arthroscopic cannulas. One of the most common causes of postoperative effusions and loose bodies is excessive progressive quadriceps exercise before healing of the surgical incision. Diffuse synovitis will respond to arthroscopic cleansing of fibrin, free synovial debris, and a single injection of cortisone. Removal will interrupt the naturally slow rehabilitative process. The patient will regain muscular strength faster and can resume activity sooner. When the inflammation and thickness about a joint are removed, the patient's confidence in arthroscopy is increased.

ARTHROSCOPY IN JOINTS OTHER THAN THE KNEE

It was only natural to apply the techniques learned in knee joint arthroscopy to other joints. Inspection and photographic documentation have been made in the temporomandibular, shoulder, elbow, wrist, finger, hip, and ankle joints. Early observations indicate these areas need as much attention as has been given to the knee. The result will be just as fruitful in patient care.

Surgical procedures, including intra-articular shaving, chondroplasty, and synovectomy, have been performed on the shoulder, elbow, and ankle joints. Diagnostic arthroscopy and arthroscopic surgery of joints other than the knee are covered in Part three.

RESEARCH

Investigational uses of arthroscopy are limitless now that it can be performed easily with the patient under local anesthesia. Naturally, patients are hesitant to agree to an exploratory arthrotomy for observation purposes. Some with osteochondritis dissecans, articular defects, or synovial abnormalities have agreed to direct arthroscopic observation.

The second-look arthroscopy has been the single most important means of establishing the results of arthroscopic surgery. (See Fig. 8-9.) Comparing the videotape recordings of the lesions, the entire procedure, and the subsequent follow-ups documents the healing of meniscal and articular cartilage. (See Chapters 17 and 18.) These evaluations have not only assisted in treatment of the patient but have also provided increased learning experience for the orthopedist. It has been possible to observe the natural history of osteochondritis dissecans. Direct evidence has been provided as to the extent to which the articular cartilage has loosened and the proper form of treatment. Healing articular defects are amenable to arthroscopic monitoring.

Observations and morphologic variations of synovial disease have been documented. The medical management of rheumatologic conditions can be monitored arthroscopically. Biopsy in synovial diseases is possible. Articular synovial debris can be submitted by cell block for investigational purposes. Articular changes in degenerative arthritis can be monitored. Arthroscopy may be beneficial in determining whether tibial osteotomy or articular resurfacing is necessary.

REVIEW OF DIAGNOSTIC ARTHROSCOPY EXPERIENCE

A review of a physician's clinical experience benefits not only that individual but also others who are performing the same procedure or caring for a similar pathologic condition.

The following review demonstrates some specific individual weaknesses in clinical judgment but provides continued conviction that arthroscopy is valuable.

In reviewing my arthroscopic series, several questions were asked: What insight was gained about clinical judgments? What erroneous tendencies were there prearthroscopically? Which conditions were frequently overdiagnosed or underdiagnosed? What effects did increased knowledge have on subsequent arthroscopic indications, methods, and techniques? What changes were made in subsequent patient treatment?

Three series, comprising almost 1,000 patients, were reviewed. *Series I* (October, 1972, to September, 1975) encompasses the first 400 patients (419 knees) treated under local anesthesia for whom comprehensive clinical records were complete. It should be noted that in a few of the early patients in this series arthroscopy was limited to the front of the knee joint. Most of the patients were examined after it was possible to inspect posteromedially. None of the patients had posterolateral inspections.

Series II (September, 1975, to September, 1976) includes 375 patients (384 knees) examined under local anesthesia. All had the benefit of the fully developed comprehensive arthroscopy of the knee; that is, the posteromedial and posterolateral compartments were examined even when anterior inspection showed normal findings. In Series II more patients than in the other series had medicolegal or Workmen's Compensation claims. Arthroscopic consultation was for the purpose of supporting the referring physician's clinical impressions that the knees were normal and to rule out the presence of occult lesions.

Series III (September, 1975, to September, 1976) includes 150 consecutive patients (162 knees) examined arthroscopically under general anesthesia immediately prior to an anticipated arthrotomy. All were patients from my private practice. A few had medicolegal or Workmen's Compensation claims.

Series IV (September, 1976, to September, 1979) includes 1,000 diagnostic arthroscopies. This group is similar to Series II and includes a large number of referral patients.

The arthroscopic surgical cases are summarized in Chapters 16 to 20.

Choice of anesthetic

Local anesthetic was used for those patients in whom the diagnosis was unconfirmed or the extent of injury or status of the disease process was unclear but arthrotomy was not anticipated. It was also used for those patients in whom the diagnosis seemed certain but for whom a general anesthetic for arthroscopy or arthrotomy was not indicated clinically because they had been referred for consultative arthroscopy only. These patients made up Series I, II, and IV.

General anesthetic was used for patients whose history, physical examination, or x-ray findings showed intra-articular lesions or internal derangement that necessitated arthrotomy. Arthroscopy was performed immediately prior to surgery. Series III comprised this group of patients.

Classification of patients

Patients were classified according to five diagnostic categories: meniscal lesions, patellar conditions, condylar disease, extrasynovial lesions, and synovial disease. A miscellaneous category included those patients who were undergoing arthroscopy for medicolegal or consultation purposes.

Patients who had typical symptoms referred to the medial joint line but no positive findings were classified as having a torn medial meniscus. If their symptoms were referred to the lateral joint line, they were placed in the torn lateral meniscus category. Those in the retained posterior meniscus category had had previous arthrotomies through a short anterior incision.

Patients were placed in the patellar or condylar disease categories if the typical history, physical examination, and x-ray evidence suggested those anatomic areas as the most likely sources of their symptoms.

In the extrasynovial disease category were those patients in whom ligamentous injuries, cystic changes, or juxta-articular bony abnormalities were anticipated. In the synovial disease category, patients, typical histories, and physical evidence suggested that symptoms were produced in the synovium.

Analysis

Findings of each arthroscopic examination were documented by narrative dictation. Drawings, cinephotography, and 35-mm slides are used to document unusual lesions. Virtually all surgical cases are recorded on television.

Presumptive, or prearthroscopic, diagnosis was compared with the actual arthroscopic findings. Diagnosis was considered correct if confirmed arthroscopically or an additional significant diagnosis was made; it was deemed incorrect if a different diagnosis or no diagnosis was made by arthroscopy. Critical analysis of prearthroscopic and postarthroscopic diagnoses provided information by which clinical impressions have been altered over the past several years.

With the prearthroscopic diagnosis in mind, it was determined on the basis of arthroscopic findings whether a lesion was surgically correctable, could be arthroscopically managed, or needed only conservative treatment.

Specific analyses of the four series, under each of the five disease categories, are considered in the following sections.

The reporting of experience in chronologic series provides a perspective on today's techniques and thoughts. Text concerning the first three series has been left unchanged from the first edition. An occasional comment has been added in light of my experience. Reexamining the reviews reminds us of the progression of the art of arthroscopy. It also prevents the delusion that what is known now has always been known. An open reappraisal of one's experience ensures continued progress toward better care for each patient. This method of review demonstrates, for one starting arthroscopy, the progression of skills and experience to be expected.

Series I (1972 to 1975)

Series I consisted of patients routinely seen in an active private practice. Very few had medicolegal or Workmen's Compensation claims or were referred for diagnostic or second-opinion purposes.

There were 259 male (64%) and 141 female (36%) patients, ranging in age from 8 to 61 years (median, 28 years). Right and left knees were equally represented.

Patients early in this series were examined only in the anterior compartments and the suprapatellar pouch. Subsequently the technique of posteromedial inspection was developed.

Meniscal disease

Initial review showed a considerable tendency prearthroscopically to overdiagnose torn medial menisci. They constituted almost half the prearthroscopic diagnoses. In part this reflects the frequency of this particular abnormality and the fact that symptoms in many knee conditions are clinically referable to the medial joint line.

Review of postoperative diagnoses showed that the diagnosis of a torn medial meniscus was correct in 24% of patients; a different diagnosis was confirmed in 40%; and no diagnosis was made in 24%, undoubtedly because posteromedial and posterolateral inspections were not carried out in Series I. Common different diagnoses were chondromalacia patellae, degenerative meniscal disease without a tear, or degenerative condylar disease. Eight patients in this group had a torn anterior cruciate ligament without a meniscal abnormality visible from the front. Findings in Series II and III, which included posterior inspection of all knees, suggest that posterior abnormalities in the presence of torn anterior cruciate ligaments were probably overlooked in Series I.

Clinical judgment was slightly better in diagnosis of a torn lateral meniscus in patients with symptoms but no clear positive physical or laboratory findings. Diagnosis was confirmed in nine patients (31%). Two patients had a tear of the lateral meniscus plus an old unrepairable tear of the anterior cruciate ligament. In 41% of the patients a different diagnosis was made, most commonly degeneration of the lateral meniscus or degeneration of the compartment with loose bodies. No diagnosis was made in 20% of patients. This figure is artificially high because no posterolateral punctures were made.

In 28 patients (29 knees), a prearthroscopic diagnosis of retained posterior horn was considered. These patients had had previous surgery carried out through a single short anterior incision. The retained posterior meniscus is commonplace after this type of meniscal arthrotomy, which, it is hoped, will be eliminated as a standard method of treatment. Suspected retained posterior horn was substantiated arthroscopically in over 90% of the patients. In only two patients was a different diagnosis made: one had a torn lateral meniscus, and the other had a dislocated patella. Arthroscopic findings in patients who have had meniscectomies carried out through a single anterior vertical arthrotomy convinced me of the necessity for removal of the entire meniscus through combined anterior and posterior incisions on the medial side.

The retained posterior horn is a clinical entity when the remaining meniscus is abnormal in shape, mobility, or tissue consistency. The arthroscopic techniques have eliminated the necessity for total meniscectomy, previously the only way to be certain of eliminating the posterior horn problem. With arthroscopic microsurgical methods the meniscal rim may be reshaped, resected, and redesigned so that it will not offend the joint. Currently all meniscectomies are less than total and have reshaped remaining posterior rims. These have proved asymptomatic on second-look arthroscopy. The diagnosis of a symptomatic retained posterior horn is only clearly determined under local anesthesia by palpation correlated with the sensation confirmed by the patient being examined.

Of all meniscal lesions, 38% were surgically correctable, 3% were arthroscopically managed, and 56% were conservatively managed; 3% were diagnosed only (miscellaneous cases). It is significant that more than half the patients with a torn medial meniscus required only conservative treatment.

In patients with a presumptive diagnosis of a torn lateral meniscus the arthroscopic examination identified a lesion that was surgically correctable in 37%; 62% were managed conservatively.

In presumptive diagnosis of reatned posterior horn, arthroscopic examination identified a surgically correctable lesion in 58% of the patients; 6% were treated arthroscopically and 34% were conservatively managed.

Of all patients undergoing arthroscopy for clinically suspected meniscal abnormalities with no positive findings, the majority required only conservative treatment, although a significant percentage still required surgical intervention. Arthroscopy provided a means of differentiating between these two groups of patients for determination of appropriate therapy.

In summary, more patients were categorized as having meniscal disease than actually had it. This was in part due to the presence of medial symptoms in a variety of abnormalities and to a predilection to assume that medial symptoms are meniscal in origin. Statistically, meniscal abnormalities make up the largest percentage of knee problems.

Few posterior inspections were carried out in this group; thus the number of "no diagnoses" was high.

Patellar conditions

In patients with knee problems, complaints are frequently localized to the area of the patella. An analysis of prearthroscopic impressions of patellar disease indicates that clinical judgment was correct most of the time; the diagnosis was substantiated in 21 of 37 knees examined. A combination of dislocation or subluxation of the patella and chondromalacia was the prevalent additional diagnosis. Occasionally loose bodies were identified even through the anterior puncture. Parapatellar synovitis was diagnosed in two young women with patellar pain and crepitus on flexion and extension and distal push of the patella against the femur. Clinical inspection showed no articular abnormality. A fringe of synovium about the patella was caught between the patella and the femur, producing the symptoms. Conservative measures were adequate for these patients and for most of those with chondromalacia of the patella.

Condylar disease

Patients with degenerative articular disease were examined for the purpose of evaluating the extent of disease or to determine whether a meniscal mechanical abnormality was the cause or aggravating condition. In a number of patients with osteochondritis dissecans, arthroscopy was performed to determine whether the articular surface was intact and to monitor healing in selected patients. Most young patients with osteochondritis dissecans had no loose articular fragments, and healing was accomplished with cast immobilization. Arthroscopic examination was carried out on a few patients with known loose bodies. Small bodies were removed through cannulas or with a pituitary forceps. Because of the technical problems involved in removal of larger loose bodies with a regular pituitary forceps, the reversed-tooth modified pituitary forceps was developed.

Prearthroscopic diagnoses were correct for all patients with condylar disease. Some additional significant diagnoses included degenerative or torn menisci, accompanying degenerative arthritis, and loose bodies. Loose bodies were invariably accompanied by a torn meniscus or degenerative arthritis.

In the condylar disease group most patients received conservative treatment, mainly because I was not adept at removing loose bodies with the arthroscope. Some loose bodies, however, were removed arthroscopically. The few surgically correctable lesions were in patients who underwent arthroscopy for a loose body or for drilling in osteochondritis dissecans. In four patients a degenerative torn meniscus that was promoting degeneration of articular cartilage was removed. Overall, 17% of condylar problems were surgically correctable, and 80% were conservatively managed.

Extrasynovial lesions

In those patients with extrasynovial abnormalities a torn tibial collateral ligament was the most common prearthroscopic diagnosis, followed by torn anterior cruciate ligaments.

The clinical impression was substantiated in virtually every patient. A significant number of patients with ligamentous injuries also had additional diagnoses. It was my impression at the time, before the posterior compartments were being inspected, that a patient could have an "isolated" tear of the anterior cruciate ligament. Posterior punctures revealed many meniscal tears and capsular hemorrhage accompanying "isolated tears." Also, some significant abnormalities accompanying the torn anterior cruciate ligaments were overlooked.

In 40% of patients with a torn tibial collateral ligament an additional diagnosis was made, most commonly of a torn medial meniscus. Five of these patients had no palpable defects in the tibial collateral ligament nor gross instability. This encouraged arthroscopic intervention in any patient with a partial tear of the tibial collateral ligament, to avoid mobilizing a patient with an unsuspected meniscal abnormality.

Forty-one percent of the patients in this group had surgically correctable lesions.

In patients with meniscal cysts arthroscopic examination rarely showed a bulge within or any degeneration of the meniscus. Subsequent resection of the cyst down to the meniscus was the best indication of the extent of meniscal destruction. If it was minimal, the meniscus was left in. Some patients developed tears with degeneration within 6 months; others have remained completely asymptomatic. These results do not give any clear-cut direction for the management of cystic changes of the menisci. However, the presence of a cystic meniscus with cystic degeneration down into the meniscal abnormality is an indication for meniscectomy.

I was interested in further analysis of the patients with postarthroscopic diagnosis of a torn cruciate ligament. There were 34 such patients in our series, 25 of whom had been clinically classified in other disease categories. In the group presumed to have a torn medial meniscus, 16 patients had torn anterior cruciate ligaments; in six it accompanied the torn lateral meniscus, and in ten it was an "isolated" lesion. In those patients thought to have a torn lateral meniscus, three had a torn cruciate ligament: two accompanied the tear and one was an "isolated" lesion. When a retained posterior meniscal horn was suspected, without physical evidence of a torn cruciate ligament, two such lesions existed. In the 18 patients with torn tibial collateral ligaments, four had an accompanying torn anterior cruciate ligament to some extent. It must be noted that in these patients with known torn tibial collateral ligaments, surgery was not considered because of the lack of a palpable defect or instability. In those 34 patients in whom a torn anterior cruciate ligament was the final diagnosis, surgery was recommended for 21; only one patient refused.

In those patients who underwent surgery, the repair of the anterior cruciate ligament was possible in only one. It was a fresh tear and technically amenable to repair. The others required a reconstructive procedure of some type because instability existed. This further emphasizes the importance of early diagnosis of acute hemorrhagic knees. Most of these patients were seen at a time when neither their original physician nor I recognized the magnitude of the abnormality.

Review of the anterior cruciate ligament tears shows that these can be occult lesions. Most are not diagnosed initially or suspected at the time of clinical examination in patients with diagnostic problems. The effusion or the patient's discomfort limits the physical examination. Experimental sectioning of the anterior cruciate ligament will not produce gross instability of the knee where there is an intact tibial collateral ligament and lateral capsular ligament.[1]

Synovial disease

In those patients with synovial disease, preoperative diagnosis was either known synovitis, on the basis of laboratory work, or differential diagnosis of common lesions. Two patients had a history of foreign bodies in the knee. Arthroscopic examination established the existence of a foreign body and articular cartilage scar in one patient. The other patient had no intra-articular foreign body. Most of the patients in this category had arthroscopy for diagnostic purposes, which proved valuable.

Summary

These were patients from my general orthopedic practice. Most were diagnostic cases before anticipated open surgery. In most I used anteromedial and posteromedial approaches. This accounted for the high percentage (24%) of "no diagnosis made." The retained posterior horn was identified with more certainty under local anesthesia and palpation.

The arthroscopic examination changed or corrected my clinical impression frequently, especially when I suspected a torn medial meniscus. Suspicion of chondromalacia was usually substantiated; most cases in my practice were mild and needed no treatment. Most incidences of degenerative arthritis were not severe enough for total-knee surgery and therefore were managed conservatively. The anterior cruciate ligament was torn more often than was suspected clinically, and the posteromedial inspection showed tears and capsular injury not seen from the "solo" anterior approach.

Series II (1975 to 1976)

Approximately half the patients in Series II were referred by other orthopedists for arthroscopic consultation. A large percentage of the referral patients were considered to have no abnormality, and the arthroscopy was performed to rule out a rare or occult abnormality that may not have been identified. A number of these patients had medicolegal or Workmen's Compensation claims.

Of the 375 patients in Series II, 243 were male and 132 were female. They ranged in age from 9 to 76 years. All were given local anesthetic. All knees were inspected posteromedially and posterolaterally, when indicated.

Meniscal disease

As in Series I, a high percentage of prearthroscopic diagnoses fell in the meniscal category. Statistical analysis of meniscal disease was similar in the Series II, although diagnostic abilities had improved with experience and inclusion of the posterior puncture to the routine examination. The apparent lack of statistical improvement was related to patient selection in Series II. Many believed to have no clinical abnormality were placed in the torn meniscus group by the referring physician, which accounts for no diagnosis being made in 30% of patients with a torn medial meniscus. With the addition of posterior compartment inspection, additional diagnoses were identified in 16% of patients and a different diagnosis was made in 23%. In the latter group, differential diagnosis was made between chondromalacia of the patella and meniscal abnormality with minimal positive findings. These patients were arbitrarily placed in the torn meniscus group preoperatively. Arthroscopy usually confirmed chondromalacia patellae.

In those referred patients in whom no abnormality was suspected on the basis of history or physical examination, the clinical impression was usually supported by arthroscopy. Many of these patients had emotional concerns or potential secondary gain. Had they been placed in a separate group, overall diagnositic accuracy would have improved statistically.

A torn medial meniscus was suspected in 115 patients. The diagnosis was confirmed in 36. Of these, an additional significant abnormality was diagnosed in 17 patients: degenerative arthritis in six, torn anterior cruciate in five, tear of the lateral meniscus in three, and torn anterior cruciate ligament and torn lateral meniscus in three.

A different diagnosis was established in 27 patients. Chondromalacia was present in 25. Degenerative arthritis was the second most common different diagnosis in the meniscal compartment, occurring in ten patients. An isolated torn anterior cruciate ligament was seen in four patients, and a torn lateral meniscus in two. Synovitis was seen in two patients, posterior cruciate ligament tear in one, subluxation of the patella in one, loose bodies in one, and a meniscal cyst in one.

Meniscal symptoms referable to the lateral joint line were seen in 45 patients. Of these, 16 had an isolated tear of the lateral meniscus. Three patients had an additional torn anterior cruciate ligament identified only at arthroscopy. A different diagnosis was established in 18 patients: degenerative meniscal or articular abnormality without a mechanical tear in seven; isolated anterior cruciate ligament tear, usually laying out in the lateral joint line and mimicking a torn meniscus in three; loose bodies in the posterolateral compartment in two; a torn anterior cruciate ligament and degenerative articular disease in one; and subluxation of the patella in one. Patellar tendon tear, chondromalacia, torn meniscus, and synovitis were each seen once. No diagnosis was made in eight patients, despite inspection of all compartments. This review shows that significant abnormalities, especially torn anterior cruciate ligaments, should be suspected when initial symptoms suggest meniscal disease.

It should be noted that posterior puncture revealed five torn lateral menisci that were not seen from the front and that four additional patients had loose bodies seen only in the posterior compartment.

A retained posterior horn was identified in 21 patients, 17 medially and four laterally. Thirteen of these patients had an additional diagnosis, most commonly degenerative arthritis or torn anterior cruciate ligament. It is significant that six of these patients had a posterior meniscal abnormality identified from the posterior puncture only. Some who had a retained posterior horn that was partially excised had a second old meniscal tear behind the line of resection. Four patients had loose bodies identified only by the posterior puncture.

In the group of patients prearthroscopically thought to have a torn meniscus, 23% had a significant abnormality found only by posteromedial and posterolateral puncture. Of torn medial menisci, 18% were identified by this route, as were 9% of loose bodies. Of those patients with a suspected retained meniscus following previous surgery, 48% had an abnormality identified only by the posteromedial and posterolateral puncture of a meniscal tear.

Review of the meniscal group showed again the surprising number of additional abnormalities identified only arthroscopically, in particular by the posterior inspection. I believe this points to the value of arthroscopy, rather than to lack of clinical expertise.

Patellar conditions

Analysis of patellar abnormalities in this series was similar to Series I, with some differences. Four patients had experienced a direct blow to the patella, which injured the articular surface. Some patients with bipartite patellas that showed no fragmentation at the junction had articular abnormalities different from the original observations. After inspection of several patients with bipartite patellas, it was learned that about half had symptomatic separations very much like a nonunion with articular irregularities at the junction.

The clinical impression was substantiated by the arthroscopic examination in most of the patients with patellar disease. Additional diagnoses included chondromalacia, loose bodies, and subluxations. Most patients with dislocation or subluxation also had loose bodies or chondromalacia. Three patients in whom patellar abnormality was the primary diagnosis also had a torn meniscus. One patient had a torn anterior cruciate ligament accompanying a dislocation. Most loose bodies were from the lateral femoral condyle and rested in the lateral sulcus or in the posterolateral compartment. Most were managed arthroscopically.

The main advantage of arthroscopic examination of patients with patellar problems is that surgery or a rehabilitative regimen can be specifically designed

Condylar disease

The prearthroscopic diagnosis of condylar disease was substantiated in virtually every patient. The additional diagnosis of loose bodies or degenerative changes accompanied the primary diagnosis, and an additional torn meniscus or retained posterior horn was seen in two patients. A different diagnosis was made in two patients: one had loose bodies from osteochondromatosis; the other had severe synovitis with catching and popping in the joint mimicking loose bodies and degenerative changes.

Arthroscopy in condylar diseases can establish the extent of the articular erosion, determine whether there is loss all the way down to raw bone, necessitating surgical articular resurfacing, or determine whether the underlying cause of articular injury is a mechanically torn meniscus that should be surgically removed. Additionally, diffuse degenerative change with loose bodies can be managed arthroscopically, followed by anti-inflammatory medication and isometric quadriceps exercises. This regimen has rendered many patients virtually asymptomatic who otherwise might have been considered for joint resurfacing or total-knee replacement.

Extrasynovial lesions

Forty-eight patients had extrasynovial lesions, arthroscopically confirmed in most.

A significant number of additional diagnoses were made. Most commonly, a torn anterior cruciate ligament was accompanied by a torn medial meniscus. It should be noted that a torn meniscus was suspected, but the primary abnormality was diagnosed as a torn anterior cruciate ligament with minimal instability. One patient had an acute dislocation of the patella as well.

In patients with old ligamentous instability, whether an isolated cruciate ligament tear or rotary instability, concomitant degenerative arthritis, torn meniscus, or loose body was virtually universal. In patients who had previous arthrotomies and an old tear of the anterior cruciate ligament, the most common accompanying abnormality was a retained posterior horn, with degenerative arthritis and loose bodies. Four patients with an old tear of the anterior cruciate ligament had an unidentified torn meniscus. Identification of these additional abnormalities assisted in planning reconstructive surgery and advising patients of the expected prognosis.

In patients who had acute injuries to the knee, the diagnosis of a torn tibial collateral or cruciate ligament was usually correct. These were generally accompanied by a torn meniscus, either medially or laterally.

Torn tibial collateral ligaments were accompanied by tenderness without gross instability or a palpable defect. This was substantiated arthroscopically in eight of 11 patients. One had only a torn meniscus; another had a partial tear of the anterior cruciate ligament that was not identified clinically. A third patient had degenerative arthritis in the medial compartment, which produced acute pain in the area of the tibial collateral ligament.

Torn anterior cruciate ligaments were commonly accompanied by a torn meniscus, usually laterally. The value of arthroscopy in acute ligamentous injury is identification of those patients for whom surgical intervention is indicated. It was learned from posterior puncture that acute anterior cruciate ligament injury is not isolated; it is always accompanied by hemorrhagic changes in either the posteromedial or posterolateral capsule and either a torn meniscus or a loose body.

In all, 49 patients (16%) had a postarthroscopic diagnosis of torn anterior cruciate ligament. Of these patients, 24 were thought to have meniscal abnormalities as the primary diagnosis; patellar disease was suspected in one; and 34 had been classified as having an extrasynovial or ligamentous lesion.

Seven patients had a tear or attenuation in the anterior cruciate ligament; all had hemorrhage. Most patients with a torn anterior cruciate ligament had an associated abnormality, the most common being a meniscal tear in 37% and degenerative arthritis in 22%.

Diagnostic arthroscopy in clinical practice

Of continued concern were eight patients who had had a previous meniscectomy through a short anterior incision in the presence of a torn anterior cruciate ligament. They remained symptomatic, with either a large meniscus that was catching and popping in the posterior compartment or degenerative arthritis with loose bodies. It was common to find a subtotal meniscectomy with an existing old tear of the posterior horn behind the line of meniscal resection. (See Fig. 7-6, *H*.)

Two patients had a torn anterior cruciate ligament accompanying an acute dislocation of the patella. These were not recognizable clinically because the patients' pain limited the physical examination.

Synovial disease

In a number of patients only primary synovial disease was suspected. However, some had acute inflammatory degenerative arthritis with loose bodies causing a synovial reaction, and others had intermittent joint pain with swelling not established by arthroscopic examination. Other abnormalities observed include gout, pseudogout, pigmented villa nodular synovitis, and osteochondromatosis. Osteochondromatosis was managed in three patients without synovectomy by vacuuming loose bodies from the joint; they have remained asymptomatic for over a year.

Arthroscopy is of benefit in synovial diseases for establishing the conditions morphologically and providing access for biopsy. Appropriate medical and surgical recommendations can then be made.

Summary

At this point I was improving technically, especially with both posterior punctures added to the routine. Many of these patients were referrals for diagnostic purposes and returned to their orthopedists for definitive treatment. Arthroscopy still identified an additional or different diagnosis than was suspected clinically, especially in the medial meniscal groups. By now I recognized the lesion of subluxation patellae on the lateral femoral condyle. Associated surgical injuries with a patellar dislocation were not uncommon, a further reason for arthroscopic examinations. The value of arthrotomy in condylar disease was assessment for high tibial osteotomy or total-knee replacement.

Subsequent arthroscopic surgical experience, plus follow-up inspection, has modified evaluation of a retained posterior horn. It seems that the mere presence of a regrown or retained posterior horn is not what produces clinical symptoms. If the posterior horn has abnormal tissue (e.g., ganglion cyst) or abnormal mobility, it produces symptoms. This often may be determined as the offending lesion by direct palpation under local anesthesia. The presence of a retained posterior horn mass may be associated with overlooked subtle instability (lateral pivot shift) and yet incriminated as the sole cause of the patient's problems. (See Chapter 16.)

Morphologic identification of various synovial conditions was now possible.

Series III: general anesthesia (1975 to 1976)

Patients in Series III had *not* had recent arthroscopy; however, on the basis of history, physical examination, and x-ray findings surgical exploration of the knee was warranted. All patients were given general anesthetic, and arthroscopy was carried out immediately prior to arthrotomy.

All patients in Series III were from my private practice. Only a few had medicolegal or Workmen's Compensation claims. Of the 150 patients, 122 were male and 28 were female. Their median age was 28 years.

Twelve patients had bilateral conditions, either a meniscal abnormality in the opposite compartment or bilateral patellar conditions; a few patients had bilateral degenerative disease or osteochondritis dissecans.

The preoperative diagnosis was substantiated in 54% of the patients, and an additional significant abnormality was identified in 22%. Clinical diagnosis was incorrect in 20%, and in 4% no abnormality was found within the joint, despite anterior, posteromedial, and posterolateral inspection and suprapatellar puncture.

Meniscal disease

Meniscal abnormalities most often misdiagnosed were an accompanying tear or an isolated tear of the meniscus in an opposite compartment. Some patients had loose bodies that mimicked a torn meniscus, and in three instances an acute dislocation of the patella with marked knee swelling was mistaken for an acute meniscal lesion.

Patellar conditions

In the patellar group it was more common that a presumptive diagnosis was substantiated arthroscopically and surgically. In those patients with dislocations of the patella, one had a tear of the posterolateral meniscus identified only through that arthroscopic approach, and two patients had additional loose bodies. One patient was thought to have a ruptured patellar tendon because of inability to extend the knee. The tendon was normal, but there was acute synovitis of the joint of a rheumatologic type.

Condylar disease

Suspected condylar disease was usually substantiated by arthroscopy. A few patients in this group had additional loose bodies.

Fifteen patients were treated arthroscopically, usually for loose bodies that mimicked some other condition. The loose bodies were removed either by vacuuming or with the Jaws modified pituitary rongeur under arthroscopic control.

Extrasynovial lesions

Patients thought to have extrasynovial lesions, torn ligaments, or old instability of the joint most commonly had an unsuspected meniscal tear. In a few patients with massive hemarthrosis with mild instability, torn cruciate ligaments were clinically diagnosed on the basis of a twisting injury, an acute pop in the knee, and massive hemarthrosis. Arthroscopic inspection showed that these patients had a torn meniscus.

Patients with ligament injuries often have an additional torn meniscus. An isolated meniscal tear or an acute dislocation can mimic a ligament injury.

Synovial disease

Prior to synovectomy in one patient with rheumatoid changes in the knee, arthroscopy was carried out to substantiate synovitis and to rule out joint thickening as the basis of capsular thickening.

Summary

This was a group of my patients who I thought needed open surgery. The arthroscopy immediately preceded the anticipated arthrotomy. Additional and different diagnoses again were common. The arthroscopic inspection changed or prevented an unnecessary arthrotomy. Unsuspected lesions could be discovered and the surgical approach changed to manage all the intra-articular lesions. Four percent did not require the surgery I had anticipated. In spite of increased interest in knee problems and improving skills in arthroscopy, this technique is still altering my clinical impressions and surgical approaches. Simple arthroscopic surgical techniques were sufficient treatment in 10% of this group.

Series IV (1976 to 1978)

This series includes 1,000 patients that had diagnostic arthroscopy performed between September, 1976, and August, 1978 (Table 1). The procedures were performed with a Needlescope and by the multiple puncture technique outlined in this text.

The average age of the men was 31 years, and the women averaged 30 years. The youngest patient was 10 and the oldest 79. The right and left knees were involved almost equally.

This series was initiated after 5 years of arthroscopic experience with the knee joint; actually, the practice was almost totally limited to the knee joint. The clinical diagnoses were based on customary evaluations, including plain film x-ray examination. The patients were categorized according to their pre-arthroscopic diagnosis.

TABLE 1. Diagnostic arthroscopy patients (1976 to 1978)

Problem area	1976 to 1977	1977 to 1978	Total
Normals (6%)	30	33	63
Meniscus (44%)	285	206	441
Patellar (23%)	82	151	233
Condylar (11%)	59	51	110
Extrasynovial (8%)	42	42	84
Synovial (7%)	30	39	69
TOTAL	478	522	1,000

Normal knees

There was a prearthroscopic diagnosis made of normal knees in 63 patients. Following the arthroscopy it was confirmed in 81%. The most common other diagnosis was chondromalacia of the patella or a torn cartilage. One patient had discoid lateral meniscus, another had a subluxed patella, and one had loose bodies.

Meniscal group

Torn medial meniscus was the prearthroscopic clinical diagnosis in 229 patients. My arthroscopy confirmed this in 35%. In 22% there was a torn medial meniscus, but an additional and surprising significant finding was that in 42% of patients there was a completely different diagnosis than the prearthroscopic diagnosis of a torn medial meniscus.

When a torn meniscus was diagnosed, there was a 25% chance of arthritic change seen by arthroscopy before any surgery had been performed. This is significant in evaluating the effects of meniscectomy, whether open or by arthroscopic means, in any series concerning the results of the treatment of a torn meniscus. When I made a clinical diagnosis of a torn medial meniscus, the lateral meniscus was torn in 5% of the patients. Of this group 10% revealed no such condition on comprehensive arthroscopic examination. There was an 11% chance of chondromalacia mimicking a torn medial meniscus. A torn anterior cruciate ligament accompanied the torn medial meniscus in 3% and mimicked the torn meniscus in 4%.

Torn lateral meniscus

There were 89 cases in which the prearthroscopic clinical impression was a torn lateral meniscus (72%). That impression was confirmed in 34% of patients. In an additional 37% a concomitant significant abnormality was identified. The diagnosis of a torn lateral meniscus prearthroscopically was wrong in 28% of the patients. When prearthroscopic impression was a torn lateral meniscus, it was correct in 72% of patients. The common additional diagnoses were a torn anterior cruciate ligament in 16% and degenerative arthritis in 8%.

A common problem mimicking a torn lateral meniscus was a degenerative torn knee with a torn anterior cruciate ligament and no torn meniscus. The torn anterior cruciate ligament was present in 22% of the 89 patients with preoperative impression of a torn lateral meniscus. About 7% of patients in this group had no positive arthroscopic findings or were considered normal.

Postoperative evaluations

There were 56 patients who had a previous medial meniscectomy by open methods and who were having postoperative arthroscopic evaluation because of symptoms. Of these, 26% had a palpable symptomatic posterior horn remnant that was either abnormal in mobility, shape, or tissue. This was determined under local anesthesia and correlated with the patient's symptoms by palpation.

Twenty-one percent of these patients had a torn anterior cruciate ligament; 50% had degenerative arthritis; 14% had a torn lateral meniscus that was found by arthroscopy after they had already had the medial meniscectomy. Therefore the common reasons for a repeat arthroscopic examination following open medial meniscectomy were inadequate resection of the meniscus, the presence of a torn anterior cruciate ligament, or an unobserved torn lateral meniscus.

It is of special significance that, after the medial meniscectomy with problems, it was found that 50% of these patients had degenerative arthritis. Compare this with the 25% with a torn medial meniscus who had degenerative change prior to the meniscectomy.

Eighteen patients had a previous open lateral meniscectomy with symptoms significant enough that a repeat arthroscopic examination was considered. About 77% of the patients had degenerative arthritis producing the symptoms. Two patients had a torn medial meniscus, which had either been overlooked or had occurred since their lateral meniscectomy. Nine patients had a postoperative medial and lateral meniscectomy. Seven of the nine had degenerative arthritis; three had a torn anterior cruciate ligament.

In summary, the postoperative evaluations were necessary following the meniscectomy for degenerative arthritis. Joint instability was related to a torn anterior cruciate ligament and a possible overlooked torn meniscus in the opposite compartment.

Patellar diseases

There were 148 patients who had a prearthroscopic impression of chondromalacia of the patella. This diagnosis was confirmed in 50%. An additional 34% had chondromalacia as well as an additional diagnosis; and in only 15% was there a different diagnosis. Of the additional diagnoses, the most common were degenerative arthritis (35%) and loose bodies (35%). Where the prearthroscopic diagnosis was chondromalacia of the patella, it was correct 85% of the time.

There were 22 patients with a different diagnosis than the prearthroscopic assumption of chondromalacia. There were six patients in whom there was no diagnosis made, all of whom had a medial shelf or plica, and three of whom had a torn meniscus. In prearthroscopic diagnosis, chondromalacia of the patella was most often correct. The presence of degenerative arthritis opposite on the femoral side in one of the compartments should not be overlooked, and the management of loose bodies should be performed by vacuuming at the time of diagnostic arthroscopy. Further discussion of the treatment of chondromalacia is found in Chapter 17.

Dislocation and subluxation of the patella

There were 25 patients who had a prearthroscopic diagnosis of dislocation of the patella. It was significant that there was an additional abnormality in 80% of the patients. Most commonly it was a loose body or injury to the articular surface or a defect on the lateral femoral condyle with degenerative arthritis. In one patient there was a torn cruciate ligament and a significant medial capsule hemorrhage that mimicked the dislocation.

There were 35 patients who had a subluxation of the patella. When that was a clinical impression, it was correct 94% of the time. Only 30% had an isolated subluxation with no additional findings. In 64% there was an additional finding, most common of which was chondromalacia of the patella. In only three patients, or 6%, was there a different diagnosis. One was chondromalacia without subluxation, and the other two had a torn meniscus. It is important to note that two patients with subluxation and chondromalacia also had a lateral plica, which may well have been scarred tissue from the subluxation.

Other patients in the group had prearthroscopic, postpatellectomy, or post–Hauser procedure diagnosis of fracture, and all had articular abnormalities of the patella that were amenable to intra-articular shaving.

Chondral defects

There were 48 patients in whom arthroscopy confirmed diffuse degenerative arthritis of the knee. This was usually accompanied by degeneration of the meniscus. There were 29 patients in whom degenerative arthritis affected only the medial compartment, including degenerative changes of the meniscus. The changes were most often associated with loose bodies and chondromalacia. Many of the patients had had a previous meniscectomy. There were a number of cases of osteochondritis dissecans, loose bodies, previous fractures, and osteonecrosis. The diagnosis was virtually correct in every case in which the prearthroscopic impression was degenerative arthritis.

Extrasynovial lesions

There were 138 patients from 1,000 total whose anterior cruciate ligament was a major diagnostic problem. This constituted 13% of the patients undergoing arthroscopy for diagnostic purposes.

It was determined by multiple puncture technique that 10% of the patients had only an isolated tear in the anterior cruciate ligament. There may have been some small capsular hemorrhage, but no additional ligamentous, patellar, condylar, or meniscal injury. When the anterior cruciate ligament was torn, the patient had a 50% chance of also having degenerative arthritis.

A torn meniscus frequently accompanies a torn anterior cruciate ligament. In this series 39% of the patients had a torn meniscus. About 34% of the patients had a previous meniscectomy. Therefore, when the patient underwent arthroscopy for diagnostic purposes and the arthroscopy demonstrated that there was a torn anterior cruciate ligament, the chance of having had previous surgery or an existing torn meniscus was 73%.

When all cases were reviewed, there was either a torn meniscus or a previous meniscectomy on the medial side in 62%; the lateral side had a torn meniscus or one previously removed in 25%; and 22% of the patients had either both menisci torn or previously removed.

It should be noted that 6% of the patients with a torn anterior cruciate ligament had a previous medial meniscectomy with degenerative arthritis and still had persistent problems because the arthroscopy showed a torn lateral meniscus. This probably was overlooked at the time of previous open surgeries.

Synovial conditions

There were 69 patients with prearthroscopic assumption of a synovial condition. The most common was a contusion of the synovium (37%). Various other rheumatoid and synovial conditions were diagnosed, including four cases of medial shelf, three of suprapatellar plica, and one synovial tag and capsular rent following a puncture wound from arthroscopic surgery. One patient had a torn anterior cruciate ligament that was undiagnosed clinically, and there were several cases of nonspecific synovitis that were serologically negative.

In summary, the review of these cases shows the continued necessity in my practice for arthroscopic surgery because of the additional significant abnormalities that accompany my prearthroscopic diagnosis. In addition, there was a significant number of different diagnoses present.

Additional diagnosis

The medial meniscal group was most notable, having additional diagnoses in 22%. These were accompanying degenerative arthritis, torn lateral meniscus, and torn anterior cruciate ligament. The torn lateral meniscus had an additional diagnostic incidence of 37%, which was most commonly a torn anterior cruciate ligament or degenerative arthritis. In the postoperative evaluation the additional presence of a torn anterior cruciate ligament and degenerative arthritis or an opposite torn meniscus was of special significance.

In chondromalacia of the patella an additional diagnosis of loose bodies and degenerative arthritis in the joint certainly could affect the prognosis and/or the treatment. The additional presence of loose bodies and articular injuries, dislocations, and subluxations that needed diagnosis and treatment was certainly an indication for arthroscopy in those situations.

In degenerative arthritis the additional diagnoses were not as significant as in the other groups. When a torn anterior cruciate ligament was present, it was manifested by instability. Only 1% were isolated cases. Of those patients, 99% had either degenerative arthritis or a torn meniscus necessitating diagnosis and treatment. Additional diagnoses were not common in the synovitis group.

Different diagnosis

The most striking incidence of different diagnosis was in the medial meniscal prearthroscopic group; 42% of the patients had a diagnosis different from torn medial meniscus. In 10% there was no diagnosis made, whereas 14% had chondromalacia mimicking a torn meniscus, and 4% had a torn anterior cruciate ligament alone, without meniscal change. About 28% of the patients with a torn lateral meniscus had a different diagnosis. Degenerative arthritis and a torn cruciate ligament most often mimic the torn lateral meniscus. Of those patients, 7% were normal. The postoperative evaluations showed very few different diagnoses other than the possibility of a torn opposite meniscus in several instances. Chondromalacia of the patella was rarely diagnosed differently. Six patients had no diagnosis made, six had a medial shelf, and three had a torn meniscus. Different diagnoses for subluxation of the patella included two patients who had a torn meniscus and one with chondromalacia. When I suspected a dislocation of the patella, only one patient had a torn anterior cruciate ligament and some medial capsular hemorrhage that mimicked the dislocation of the patella when it was diagnosed arthroscopically.

There were few different diagnoses when degenerative arthritis was suspected.

The group of patients with synovitis rarely showed a different diagnosis other than the synovial condition. Occasionally there were patients who thought they had synovitis because of a history of effusion and swelling of the joint; but biopsy showed a normal knee.

Summary

A review of the 1,000 patients included in my 5-year study of arthroscopy and problems of the knee continues to demonstrate that ultimate diagnostic accuracy is improved by arthroscopy, as are the prognostic expectations that the patient can be informed of. The arthroscopy dictates whether an operation is necessary, how it should be done, and what route should be taken, and it affords an opportunity to limit the number and size of incisions.

After 5 years of interest and arthroscopic experience, a question certainly could be asked: why is my clinical impression still erroneous in a rather significant number of patients with a torn medial meniscus (42%), torn lateral meniscus (28%), and chondromalacia (15%)? I want to believe the answer is that arthroscopy is the best possible opportunity to make an accurate diagnosis. In addition, arthroscopy has significantly improved my awareness of clinical and concomitant conditions as I reviewed other cases; still, there are surprises. Therefore I have come to the same conclusion I reached before, that is, no matter how good my clinical judgment is or has been, there is still a need for the benefit of arthroscopy in arriving at an accurate diagnosis from which to make a therapeutic recommendation.

PATIENT MANAGEMENT ROUTINE

The effectiveness of a practicing surgeon is not based solely on a technical ability to perform an operation. Personal and office staff competence, as well as hospital organization, is essential, affecting the patient's surgical treatment and the operation itself. The following brief description outlines the general management of patients seeking consultation in my office.

There are two groups of patients who call for treatment and/or opinions. First is the referral patient from another orthopedic surgeon. The patient may only request a second opinion. Either the patient or the physician might request that the case be taken over by the arthroscopist. Currently, work-ups have been carried out on most patients before they report for arthroscopic surgical procedures. It is necessary to rely on the work-up of the referring orthopedic surgeon and the accompanying medical reports and x-ray films in determining the feasibility for the specific service being requested.

The second type of patient is from one's own general orthopedic practice with a knee, shoulder, elbow, or other joint problem.

The standard clinical examination and x-ray and laboratory evaluations are performed. These patients are then categorized.

I decide whether this is arthroscopy for diagnosis only or for treatment. The patient may request diagnosis only and then to be included in the problem review before any surgery is performed. This is often the case prior to any major reconstructive surgery, whether it be ligamentous or high tibial osteotomy and joint replacement. Many patients are now aware of the possibilities of arthroscopic surgery. At the original visit the decision can be made to perform the indicated transcutaneous surgical procedures.

A decision is then made concerning whether to use local or general anesthesia. Usually diagnostic arthroscopies are performed under local anesthesia. Occasionally an anticipated simple surgical procedure, for conditions such as loose bodies or plica or for intra-articular shaving of the patella, can be performed under local anesthesia as well. The other types of surgical procedures require general anesthesia. Occasionally a patient will request general anesthesia for personal or emotional reasons. The surgeon, after evaluating the patient, may advise a general anesthetic to ensure the success and adequate view of the arthroscopy.

The most important dimension is the ability to palpate different structures within the knee and determine, with the patient's cooperation and assistance, what is producing their symptoms. This is especially so in cases of medial shelf disease. That diagnosis is best confirmed under local anesthesia; the knee can be sectioned at the same time. If further diagnosis indicates additional treatment in the knee and a general anesthetic is required, the patient can be more completely anesthetized after examination under local anesthesia.

Many outpatients were given local anesthetics, especially in Series IV, for research purposes or for second-look arthroscopies.

A decision is then made on whether the patient should be admitted to the hospital or be cared for as an outpatient. Ingham Medical Center in Lansing, Michigan, has gradually responded to the increased need for outpatient care and has provided the physical facilities to manage same-day surgery. Other arthroscopic surgeons use surgical centers for this type of work. The advantage of working in a general hospital is that many patients require medical work-ups or internal medical or cardiac monitoring during their hospital stay. In addition, because the surgeon is not limited to arthroscopic surgery only, the use of a general hospital facility is important.

The patients who are selected for outpatient local diagnostic arthroscopies have approximately a 30% chance of an intra-articular abnormality that later requires surgery. Of course, if we could tell which 30% that was, we would not have to use this diagnostic method.

Open surgery was contemplated in Series III for 158 knees; the proposed surgery was carried out in 62% of the patients. Arthroscopy immediately preceding the surgery altered the exposure or design in 20%. Many of these patients had a tear of the opposite meniscus, some with no abnormality on the side of the referred pain other than the anticipated lesion. More important, 10% of patients were treated just by arthroscopy. This was usually removal of loose bodies not requiring surgical intervention. Heretofore, in Series IV, these patients would have required an arthrotomy.

Eight percent of the patients did not require surgery or arthroscopic management. It is significant that 4% of the patients, or six in whom a torn meniscus was expected, had no abnormality at all in spite of a multiple-puncture inspection. On three occasions a torn medial meniscus was diagnosed clinically, but the arthroscopy prior to arthrotomy established a dislocation of the patella as the cause. On four occasions a torn lateral meniscus was misdiagnosed as a torn medial meniscus. One patient had a torn meniscus and an additional medial meniscal tear that required surgery.

Certainly, when one is considering open surgery, the arthroscopy can reduce the surgical exposure necessary, determine the exact area of the lesion, and eliminate unnecessary exploratory arthrotomy.

Furthermore, when 21 patients with ligamentous instability were examined under general anesthesia, eight showed a medial compartment instability with an unsuspected torn lateral meniscus. Most commonly this was examined only by the posterolateral puncture. Again, arthroscopy altered the open surgical design.

The significance is not so much that there was a clinical diagnostic error in 18% of these patients, but rather that they did not undergo unnecessary arthrotomy and/or surgery. There are unsuspected findings at the time of arthroscopy, prior to surgery, that can condition the prognosis. A partial tear of the anterior cruciate ligament, even with a small portion catching in the lateral compartment, is not amenable to repair. Also, there can be articular cartilage injury necessitating chondroplasty that was not suggested even on preoperative x-ray films.

The comprehensive examination also demonstrates the importance of visualization into the posterior compartment. A separate review by David Shneider of our combined cases showed that when there was a torn anterior cruciate ligament demonstrated on x-ray examination, there was a 70% chance of a torn meniscus. Also, when this examination was performed with the small-diameter scope and under local anesthesia, 36% of the medial meniscus tears were not visualized from the anterior puncture alone (despite the good access to the posterior horn from anterior). Thirty-two percent of the torn lateral menisci were not visualized from the anterior inspection. Therefore the emphasis is on adequate posterior visualization, whether achieved by the separate posteromedial and lateral punctures as outlined before, or by the Gillquist method. The important fact is that the posterior compartment must be visualized. Twenty-eight percent of patients in Series II had their significant pathologic abnormality visualized only by that posterior puncture.

Arthroscopic observations of meniscal degeneration have improved understanding of meniscal conditions. The recognition that fringe tears can mimic a complete tear explains the negative findings of exploratory surgery in the past. Fringe tears can produce a positive McMurray sign; yet, when the knee is opened, cleaned, and dried, the lesion is not visible to the naked eye. In the past, unnecessary meniscectomies have been performed to alleviate symptoms. However, the fringe tear will cleanse itself, and the signs and symptoms will disappear. (See Chapter 8.)

VALUE OF DIAGNOSTIC ARTHROSCOPY

Diagnostic arthroscopy has had and continues to have a major impact on my clinical practice. This simple, efficient, practical diagnostic method has enhanced clinical skills and improved patient care. Arthroscopy has provided information that both dictated and contraindicated surgical intervention. No unnecessary incisions have been made. Simple procedures have been performed arthroscopically, thus avoiding arthrotomy. Patients have enjoyed a smoother rehabilitative process. At the same time, general understanding of meniscal degeneration and healing, articular cartilage healing, and synovial morphologic patterns has increased. I expect that others, regardless of clinical proficiency, would find similar benefits from inclusion of diagnostic arthroscopy in their practice routine.

LEARNING ARTHROSCOPY

The following is offered as a method of becoming proficient in arthroscopy.

Short of individual instruction, which is difficult in arthroscopy, instructional courses, reading materials, and audiovisual programs can be helpful. Nothing supersedes personal experience; the use of clinical models has limited value. The neophyte arthroscopist should obtain an above-the-knee amputation specimen and freeze it until there is free time to explore the joint. A constricting tie around the thigh above the suprapatellar pouch will prevent leakage of saline. The amputation specimen femur may be clamped in a vise and draped as for surgery. The complete surgical setup, including an assistant, will better prepare the potential arthroscopist for the procedure. After extensive viewing, the joint may be opened for the gross correlation of findings. Because a cadaver is not supple and does not maintain distension well, arthroscopic viewing is difficult, but it could be a second choice. This laboratory experience should precede one's surgical attempts.

The first clinical arthroscopies should be performed under general anesthesia on patients for whom the surgeon anticipates arthrotomy. The arthroscopy should be limited to 15 minutes, whether any viewing is accomplished or not. Prolonged viewing will bore the anesthesiologist and enrage the surgeons who are planning to follow you in the operating room suite. Both arthroscopy and the arthroscopist will acquire a bad reputation because of the inconvenience produced. With experience, the neophyte arthroscopist will become skilled enough to perform the complete arthroscopy in the allotted time. If no diagnosis is arrived at arthroscopically, one should proceed on the basis of clinical judgment. As the surgeon becomes more confident in his abilities, arthroscopy will influence decisions and even contradict preoperative clinical impressions. The contribution of arthroscopy to care of patients will be appreciated.

After technical confidence has been achieved, arthroscopy may be performed with the patient under local anesthesia. It is best to select a confident and relaxed patient. The surgeon should also be confident and relaxed. The techniques are the same. The posteromedial approach will be easier to master than the posterolateral routine. With perseverance, most orthopedists will become competent in diagnostic arthroscopy.

REFERENCE

1. Johnson, L. L.: Lateral capsular ligament complex: anatomical and surgical considerations, Am. J. Sports Med. **7**(3):156, 1979.

Chapter 6

Documentation

Dictated narrative
Chart documentation
Still photography
    Camera and adapter
    Film
Movie photography
Television

Immediate documentation following arthroscopy is essential. Experience has shown that time lapse between the end of the procedure and documentation of findings (i.e., for performance of another arthroscopic examination) results in greatly diminished recall. Therefore a dictated narrative should be made immediately following the procedure—before phone calls, patient discharge, or extraneous conversation.

DICTATED NARRATIVE

The narrative entered on the outpatient report should include a brief history and results of physical examination of the patient (Fig. 6-1). Prearthroscopic diagnosis and postarthroscopic findings are documented. The procedure is always recorded in a routine manner, regardless of how it was technically accomplished.

Findings in the patella and suprapatellar pouch are recorded first because this area is usually examined first. However, in patients with tight, fat, or scarred knees complete inspection under the patella is not possible from the initial anteromedial puncture, and the area must be inspected later in the procedure by suprapatellar puncture. Findings are still recorded first.

The next paragraph should describe the anterolateral compartment, its meniscal substance, and its articular surface in the tangential view.

Findings in the intercondylar notch are described next in a separate paragraph, including status of the fat pad, size, fibrosis, and ecchymosis, as well as inspection of the anterior cruciate ligament and the presence of loose bodies.

Documentation of the anteromedial compartment should include findings on the articular surface and in the meniscal substance, extent of examination, any limitations due to mechanical tightness inherent in the knee, and technical problems.

Findings in the posteromedial compartment include those of the articular surface and the meniscus, as well as the presence of loose bodies or synovitis and the status of the posterior cruciate ligament. This compartment is not

Example of dictated narrative

The patient is a 28-year-old white man who has had previous medial and lateral meniscectomies, with attenuation of the anterior cruciate ligament. He has catching and pain on the outer aspect of the right knee in spite of lateral meniscectomy. Arthrography does not show any specific abnormality at this time.

Physical examination shows a stable patella and a relatively stable knee, with only minimal evidence of anterior cruciate laxity. There is some crepitus over the lateral joint line in the lateral femoral condyle, but no acute tenderness, no heat, no effusion.

CLINICAL DIAGNOSIS. Status postoperative medial and lateral meniscectomies, right knee: partial tear in anterior cruciate ligament. No instability.

PREOPERATIVE DIAGNOSIS. Status postoperative medial and lateral meniscectomies: partial tear in anterior cruciate ligament.

POSTOPERATIVE DIAGNOSIS
1. Posterior horn in lateral meniscus
2. Degenerative arthritis, moderately severe, in lateral femoral condyle
3. Status postoperative medial meniscectomy
4. Attenuated anterior cruciate ligament

PROCEDURE. The patient was placed on a table. A tourniquet was placed high on the right thigh. The entire right knee was prepared with Betadine and sterile draped so as to expose the area.

Plain lidocaine 1% was injected into the infrapatellar fat pad and the infrapatellar branch of the saphenous nerve. A sharp and then a blunt trocar were placed in the joint, and the joint was distended with saline.

The undersurface of the patella was seen and found to be smooth. There is mild synovitis of the joint. Minimal stardusting was vacuumed out of the joint.

The lateral compartment shows diffuse degenerative articular changes, chunky and fibrillar in nature.

The lateral meniscus shows rather prominent size near the area of the posterior horn and some tibial condylar fibrillation.

The intercondylar notch shows an attenuated anterior cruciate ligament.

The medial compartment shows a small regenerated meniscus and no articular injury.

A separate posteromedial puncture shows only a minimal remnant of the posterior meniscus, with no separation.

A separate posterolateral puncture shows a rather large posterior lateral meniscus. The meniscus was palpated and popped back and forth. The patient feels that this duplicates his symptoms of instability in the lateral joint line.

The fluid and equipment were removed. A sterile dressing was applied, and the patient was taken to the recovery room in good condition.

RECOMMENDATIONS. I would recommend arthrotomy through a transverse skin incision after the fashion of Bruser, with the patient in a cross-legged position. The posterior horn of the lateral meniscus should be removed. Some shaving of the lateral femoral condyle might be in order. The patient should be told that the prognosis is not good because of the presence of degenerative lateral compartment disease.

inspected if anteromedial findings indicate that surgical exploration will be performed in this area.

Recorded findings of the posterolateral compartment include the status of the meniscus and articular surface of the posterior femoral condyle. Occasionally it is possible to describe the popliteus tendon and its sheath, as well as the presence of loose bodies.

Any technical problems are documented, as is the completeness of the examination. Occasionally there are limitations to areas inspected, which should be noted as due to technical inability, scar tissue, obesity, or lack of cooperation of the patient.

The last paragraph includes recommendations concerning whether the patient was referred only for consultation or is going to be treated by you.

Very often there is an interval between the arthroscopy and evaluation and the time of surgery, so some details can be forgotten. It is especially important to record not only the findings but also the recommendations for a surgical plan.

CHART DOCUMENTATION

When the patient record is dictated, the postarthroscopic diagnosis and date are written on the patient's office chart in case the dictation is lost. For those patients undergoing diagnostic arthroscopy for another orthopedic surgeon, I fill out a worksheet (Fig. 6-1). The top copy is placed in an envelope and accompanies the patient on the return visit to the referring physician. Often the typewritten record is not available at the time of the arrival of the patient at the referring physician's office. This method provides that physician with the necessary information to have an intelligent discussion with the patient. The undersheet is a copy of NCR paper and becomes a part of our permanent record.

Diagrams, charts, and drawings can be helpful, especially early in arthroscopic experience; familiarity with arthroscopic descriptions diminishes the need for diagrams. The diagram shown in Fig. 6-2 serves for both right and left knees. A more definitive illustration of findings can be added, including those from the posteromedial and posterolateral compartments.

STILL PHOTOGRAPHY

There is a universal desire by those embarking on arthroscopy to produce photographic documentation. Even a hazy, poorly illuminated, artistically and photographically uninteresting slide will excite the novice arthroscopist. A slide of a lesion may be of interest to the arthroscopist and the patient, but with the passage of time it will bring only a ho-hum reaction from even the arthroscopist.

Slide photography has some limitations because of the number of frames on any given roll of film. By the time the film has been developed, much about the patient and the arthroscopy has been forgotten. Unless one is compulsive about record keeping (i.e., identifying film as to the exact patient, compartments, and findings), there frequently will be many slides of little recognizable

Diagnostic arthroscopy of the knee

```
                ARTHROSCOPY:  DICTATED REPORT TO FOLLOW

Name                                    Office #           Date

Referring Doctor                        Age       Race         Sex

R    L    Hip     Knee    Ankle    Shoulder    Elbow    Wrist    Finger

Onset:         How:                When:           Where:

COMPLAINTS     SITE      PHYSICAL EXAM                      XRAY
Pain           Antero    Normal              Warm           Normal
Crepitus                 Obese               Patellar       Narrowing
Catching       Medial    ROM_____             Pain           Osteochondritis
Locking                  Incision            Crepitus       Patellar defect
Swelling       Lateral   Instability         Instability    Loose Body
Heat                     Tibia Vara          Dislocation    Calcification
Instability    Postero   Genu Valgus         Pain w/ Push   Fracture
Giving Out               Tender              Pain w/ contr. ARTHROGRAM
Popping        Patellar  Swollen
Numbness                 Positive McMurray

Surgery:_____

Anesthesia:  Local  General  Spinal  IV Regional  Apprehensive  Relaxed

Pre Op DX

Post Op DX

Findings:
Patella

Suprapatellar Pouch

A-L

ICN

A-M

P-M

P-L

Alternate
Puncture

Therapeutic:  Loose Bodies    Lavage    Forceps Removal    Section Plica    Biopsy
              Intra Articular Shaving    Patella    Condyles    Menisectomy
Recommendations:
                                               Lanny L. Johnson, M.D.
```

FIG. 6-1. Worksheet is filled out with ballpoint pen and taken by patient undergoing diagnostic arthroscopy back to referring physician. This is NCR paper, which provides copy for our records.

value. Also, with hundreds of slides, many will be duplications. Some of these problems have been overcome by the Olympus OM system with a Data Back II (see Fig. 6-4), which places a selected number and letter on the photograph. (See Fig. 6-5, *B.*) The date on the photograph is useful later. Slide photography is not a practical recording method except for rare cases, medicolegal claims, or for establishing a slide file for teaching purposes.

Documentation

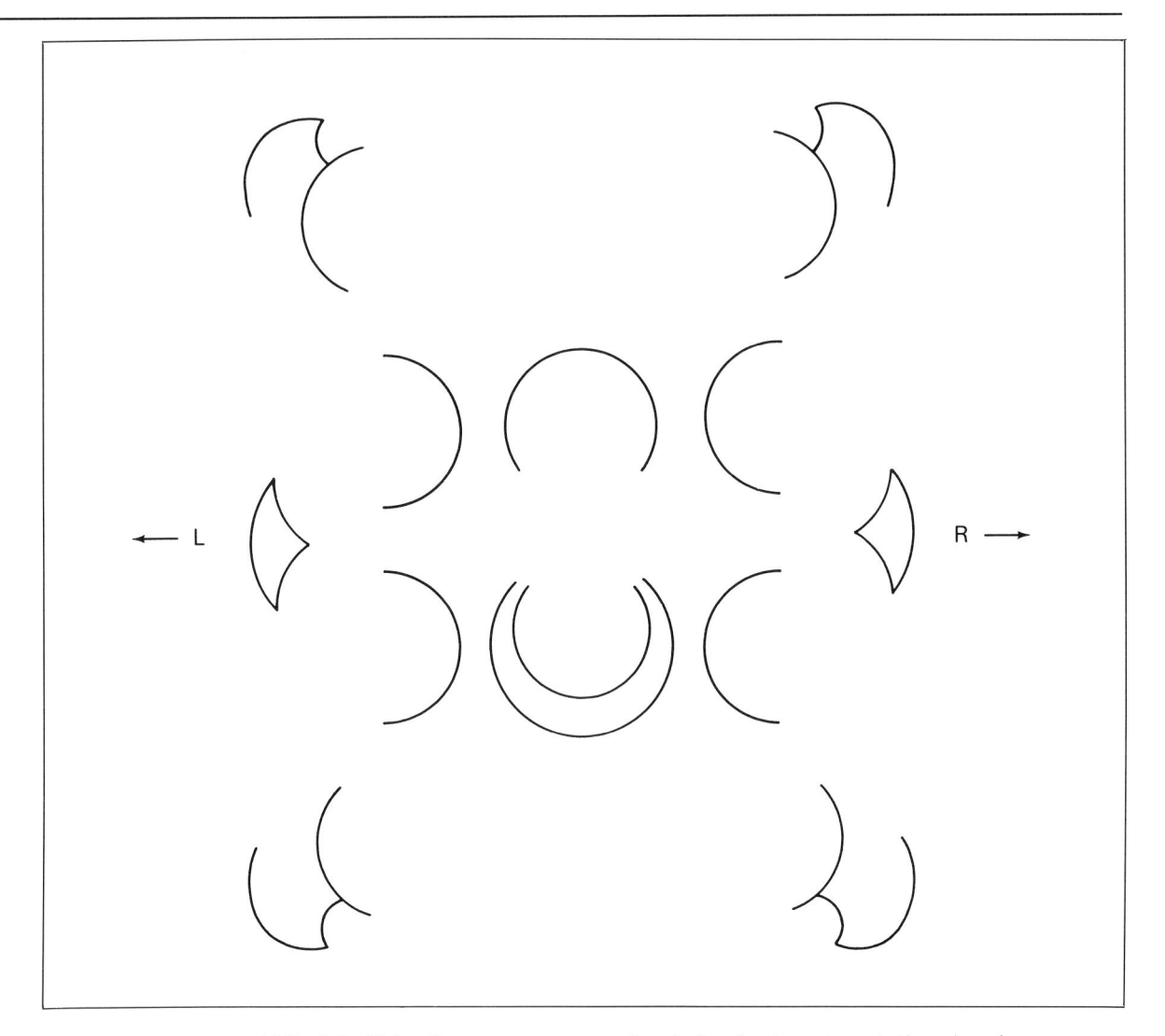

FIG. 6-2. This diagram serves as basis for further descriptive drawings.

Photography is a function of light that produces an image on photographic film. In arthroscopy the variables are the amount of light that can be thrown on an object, the amount absorbed by the object, and the amount of light that can come back through the lens of the endoscope. It is axiomatic that the smaller the diameter of the endoscope, the smaller the amount of light that can be thrown on the object. The smaller the diameter of the arthroscopic lens, the smaller the amount of light that can be transmitted to the film. Therefore the smaller endoscopes have less photographic capacity. The quality varies with the amount of light thrown on the subject. An excellent photograph is less likely with the 1.7-mm diameter Needlescope than with an endoscope of 5 to 6.5 mm diameter.

Other variables include the transmission of light along fiberglass bundles. If there is breakage of the fiber bundles, which occurs over a period of time, or corrosion over the end of the bundles, there will be diminution of light transmission. (See Chapter 2.)

Diagnostic arthroscopy of the knee

Most available illuminators provide ample light for viewing with any endoscope. The quality of the illuminator is more critical with the smaller diameter endoscopes and fiberoptic bundle mass. The more powerful output will throw more light on an object; hence viewing will be clearer. It is my opinion that the serious arthroscopist will require a Dyonics Model 500 Illuminator or a Storz xenon light source for optimal viewing and photography. The Sylvania Colorarc 300/16 lamp is used with the Dyonics Model 500 Illuminator.

It should be noted that light bulbs lose power with time. Before they burn out, light can be diminished to a rather significant degree. The effective light can be greatly compromised for documentation yet not recognized on direct viewing. Thus, for excellent photographic work and bright video images, frequent bulb inspections and replacements are essential.

Camera and adapter

I first used the 35-mm Olympus Pen F single-lens reflex camera with a single-lens arthroscopic adapter (Fig. 6-3). This type of adapter is short and therefore shortens the lever arm on the arthroscope. The single lens produces the brightest, sharpest image. Also, the thumb screw provides a secure attachment to the arthroscope. The half frame feature produces double the slides per roll with less film border around the arthroscopic image. (See Fig. 6-5, *A*.)

Currently, I favor the 35-mm Olympus OM-2 single-lens reflex camera for endoscopy (Fig. 6-4, *A*). Clear viewing through the F-9 screen is the choice for endoscopic work. In fact, one should choose a camera system that provides a clear endoscopic viewing screen to replace the conventional ground glass. These are available for Nikon-F, Olympus Pen F, and OM systems as well as for the Canon F-1.

The OM system provides the power winder (three shots per second) and the Data Back (Fig. 6-4, *B*). The winder facilitates the taking of serial photo-

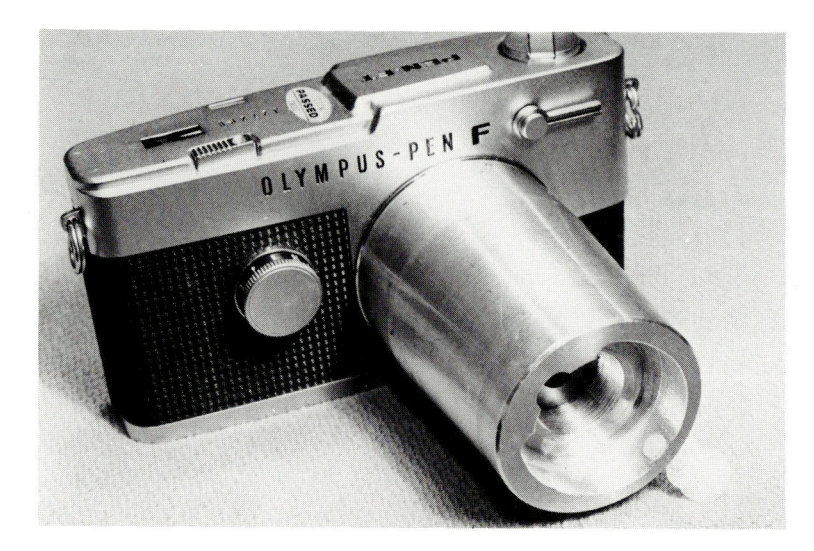

FIG. 6-3. Universal lens attachment permits freedom of motion for photographic purposes.

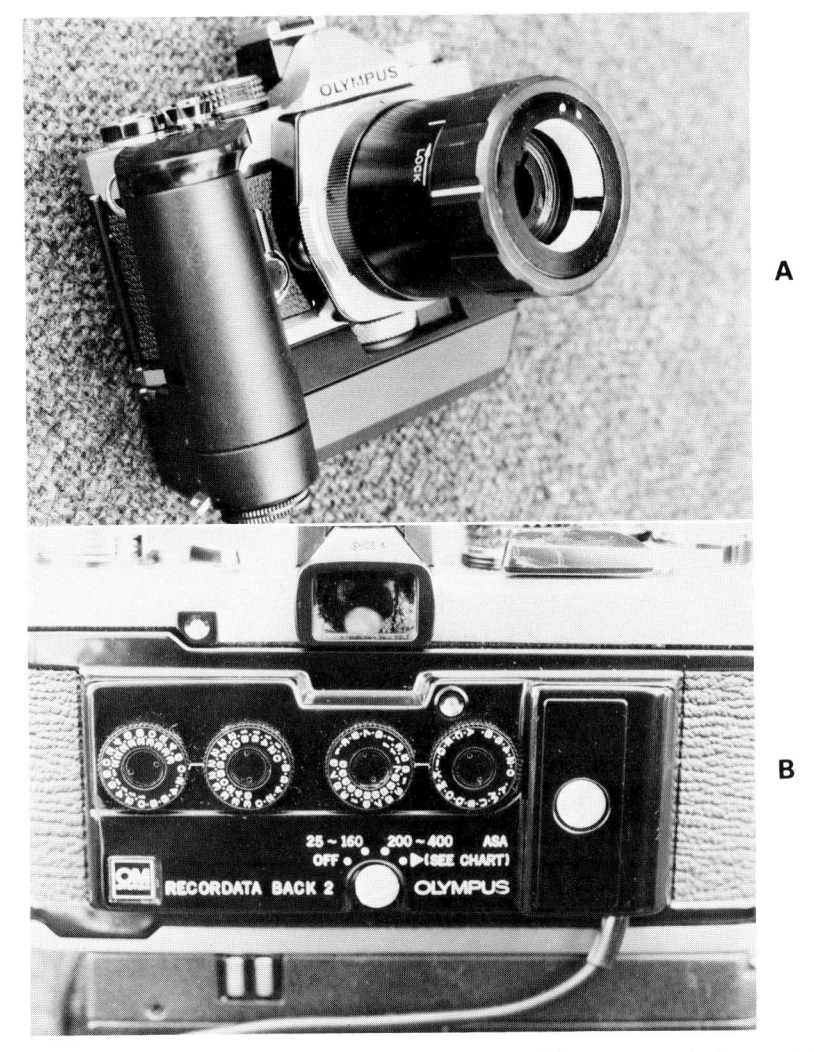

FIG. 6-4. A, Olympus OM-2 35-mm camera system with power winder and Dyonics deluxe arthroscopic attachment. **B,** Data Back recorder for Olympus system.

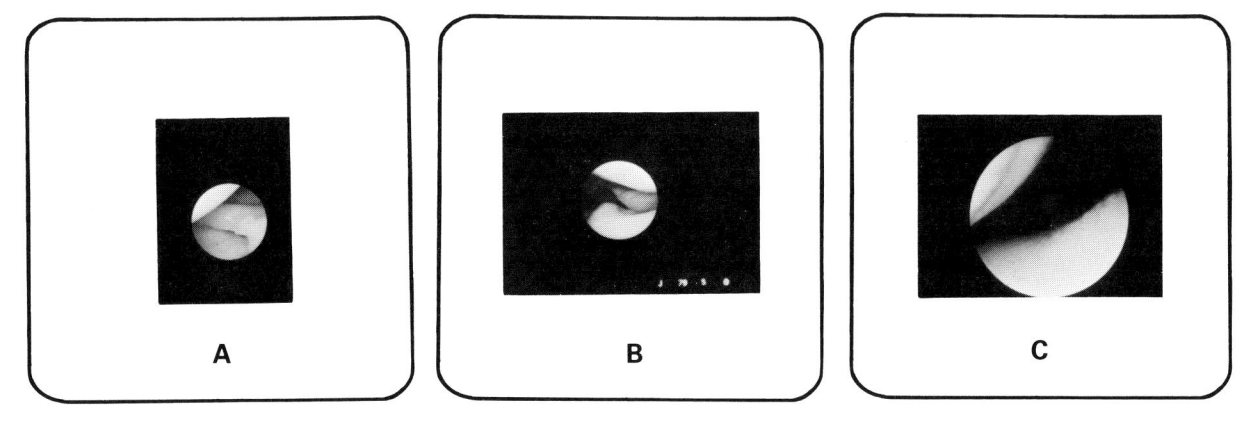

FIG. 6-5. A, Pen F half-frame slide of a femoral condyle and the meniscus. **B,** Olympus OM-2 system with Data Back recording photograph of patellofemoral joint. **C,** Available light photograph of the patellofemoral joint taken through a 135-mm lens with a Nikon camera and a simple pinch-type arthroscopic attachment. Notice the increased diminution of light plus optical clarity.

Diagnostic arthroscopy of the knee

graphs during surgical procedures without the necessity of manipulating a lever. There has been no need for an automatic winder (five shots per second). The data back places letters and/or numbers on the film so that dates or diagnostic codes can be imprinted (Fig. 6-5, *B*).

A deluxe camera adapter with a simple, secure twist-locking mechanism has been developed by Dyonics. (See Fig. 6-4, *A*.) Some physicians favor a pinch adapter attached to a conventional lens system. This produces a larger image on the film but less clarity and brightness because of the multiple lens surfaces the image must traverse (Fig. 6-5, *C*). In addition, the pinch-type adapters frequently and easily disengage.

Film

I originally used Kodak Ektachrome ASA-64 film, the Dyonics Model 400 Illuminator, and shutter speeds in the range of $1/8$ to $1/30$ second. When the slides were edited correctly and enough of the bright femoral condyle and meniscus was included, the image could be documented. Photography improved with adoption of a light source in the 550-K range, the Dyonics Model 500 Fiberoptic Illuminator (see Fig. 2-5), which provided increased photo-

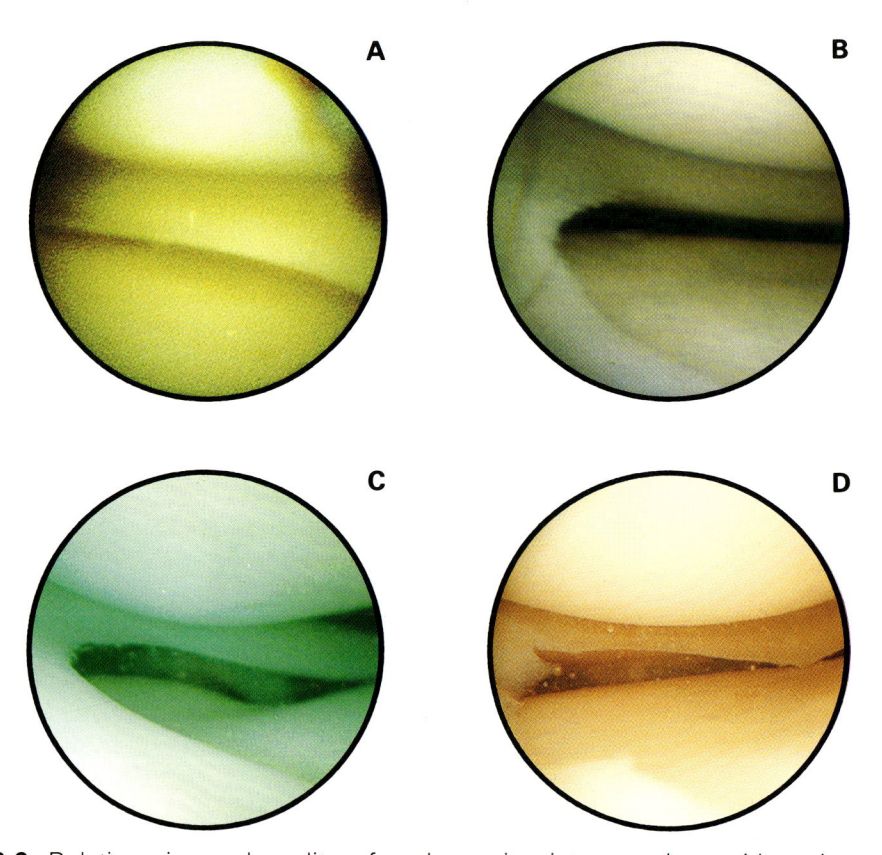

FIG. 6-6. Relative size and quality of endoscopic pictures taken with various endoscopes. **A,** Original Needlescope with available light. **B,** Model III Needlescope with flash generator. **C,** Dyonics rod lens with flash generator. Methylene blue is used as contrast medium. **D,** Endoscopic view taken with Storz rod-lens scope with flash generator.

graphic capacity even in dimly lit areas on slides. I switched to the high-speed Ektachrome ASA-160 film, which can be pushed to an ASA of 1,000 during processing (Fig. 6-6, *A*), thus improving documentation of darkened recesses of the knee.

I currently use a new Ektachrome ASA-400 film for slide photography. This is readily available, produces an especially clear image with the rod-lens system and available light, and is locally processed on a 24-hour basis. The present system of the Model 500 Illuminator, a 5-mm diameter light cable, and the new Ektachrome ASA-400 film provides a simpler method and produces documents of the same quality as the flash generator. I use speeds of $1/30$ second for the intercondylar area and $1/15$ to $1/8$ second in the suprapatellar pouch. Extremely bright areas off the femoral condyle and cases of osteochondritis dissecans will probably require $1/60$- to $1/125$-second exposure. We have not used through-the-lens metering.

The Dyonics Model III Needlescope produces a good photograph with a Storz flash generator and Kodachrome ASA-64 film. This model has a wide angle of view, compared with that of the Needlescope Model II (Fig. 6-6, *B*). With the small-diameter arthroscopes, consistently good black-and-white reprints can be produced with Kodak 2475 recording film exposed at $1/15$ second and with standard processing. This is even possible using the 2.2-mm Needlescope and the Dyonics Model 450 Illuminator. Although black and white photographs made with regular stock film can be used, there is some graininess and they do not have the definition of color prints.

Consistently good films can be made with either the Dyonics rod-lens scope or the Storz-Hopkins rod-lens system. The Dyonics rod-lens system (Fig. 6-6, *C*) provides a wide-angle view of the entire meniscus and the femoral condyle. Methylene blue was placed in this joint for contrast. The Storz 4-mm endoscope (Fig. 6-6, *D*) provides a slightly wider view. The light source used

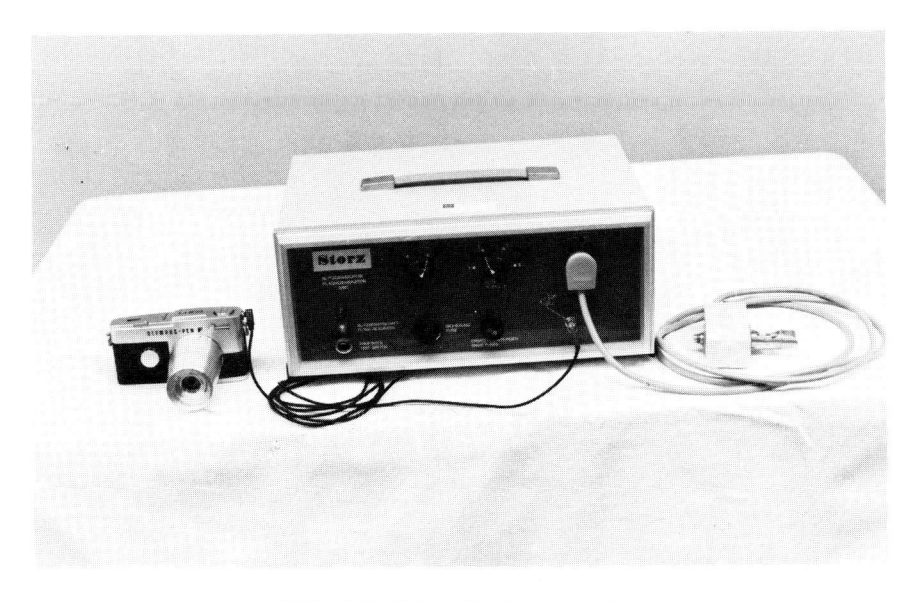

FIG. 6-7. Storz flash generator.

was the Storz flash generator; the film was Kodachrome ASA-64. A yellowish photograph is typical because of the light balance with the endoscope and film and does not represent pathologic abnormality. For photographic purposes the rod lens has less stigmatism and color aberration. This is not necessarily apparent with direct viewing but can be seen by comparison of photographs.

In the past, the best photographic slide documents that I have seen have been made with the Storz flash generator, which produces abundant light for excellent photography and has the advantage of a flash unit attached to the endoscope. Flash units that have their origin within the light box lose a considerable amount of potential light. A percentage of the effective light is lost for every foot it travels down a fiberoptic cable. Most light cables are 6 feet long. Therefore, if the flash unit is within the box, 48% of the potential light is lost. In addition, 30% of the light is lost at each interphase. These high light losses are reduced by the Storz flash generator because the source is attached directly to the endoscope (Fig. 6-7). The use of Ektachrome ASA-400 film and available light has eliminated the necessity for the flash generator system.

MOVIE PHOTOGRAPHY

Movie photography has a definitive advantage in that the entire arthroscopic examination is duplicated on film (Fig. 6-8).

Composition not possible with still photography is most effective, and observation of the flow of fluid and the motion of the intra-articular tissues (i.e., synovium, menisci, or loose bodies) is valuable. This method of documentation is somewhat impractical, however, because of the high cost of the film and the expense and weight of the equipment.

Good photography was achieved with the 8-mm Beaulieu direct-viewing, motor-driven, Super 8 camera with Ektachrome 7241 high-speed single-perforated film. However, because this film did not lock solidly during exposure, I switched to a 16-mm Beaulieu camera with 7241 double-perforated film (Fig. 6-9). This also allows flexibility in editing for both right and left knees during the final production of a finished film.

It was necessary to use the Dyonics Model 500 Fiberoptic 500-K Illuminator to achieve enough light. With an additional light source (i.e., a light wand), it is possible to photograph with the 1.7-mm scope. Adequate photography can be accomplished using the 2.2-mm diameter scope with the light provided within its cannula. Because areas in the distant range are rather dark, a circumferential halo light was devised, which increases the light by sixteen times, producing an excellent image.

Cinephotography with the Storz 3.5- and 5-mm endoscopes produces sharp, clear, well-illuminated photographs. I have used the Dyonics rod-lens system with similar photographic results.

Although the Dyonics rod-lens system has a slightly narrower field of view, it focuses closer to the object than does the Storz 5-mm endoscope. The choice between them is a matter of the user's preference.

Recently I have favored the Beaulieu Super 8 (Fig. 6-10) over the Fuji XL-1000 Single-8 camera. The camera has many excellent features for use

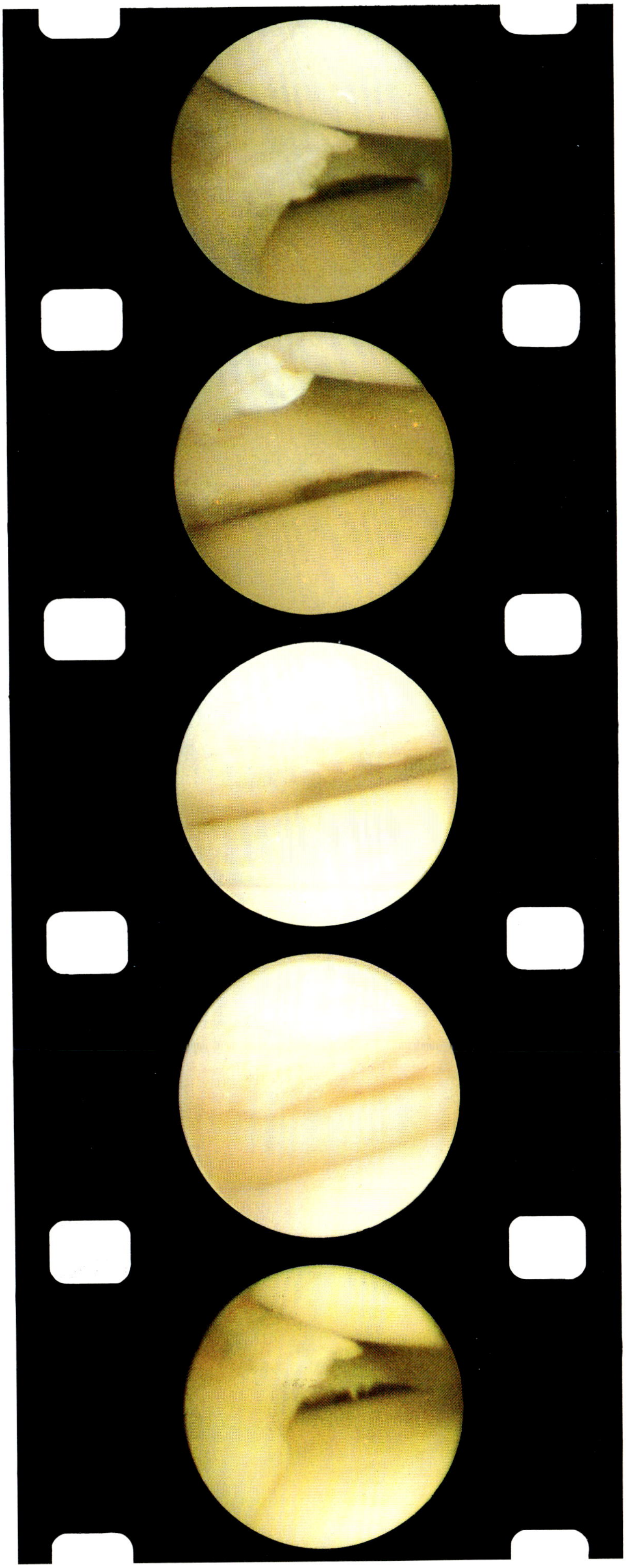

FIG. 6-8. Cinephotography provides best method of documenting endoscopic views with 2.2-mm Needlescope.

A Lateral femoral condyle is superior, and meniscus with irregularity along its inner border is to left.
B Deeper, posterior horn of meniscus comes into view.
C Needlescope, 2.2-mm diameter, under meniscus.
D Further penetration of endoscope shows horizontal cleft tear in undersurface of meniscus.
E Retraction of endoscope shows elevated inner border of meniscus. Tear was identified only by proceeding under meniscus with small-diameter endoscope. Dynamics of pistoning are well illustrated.

Diagnostic arthroscopy of the knee

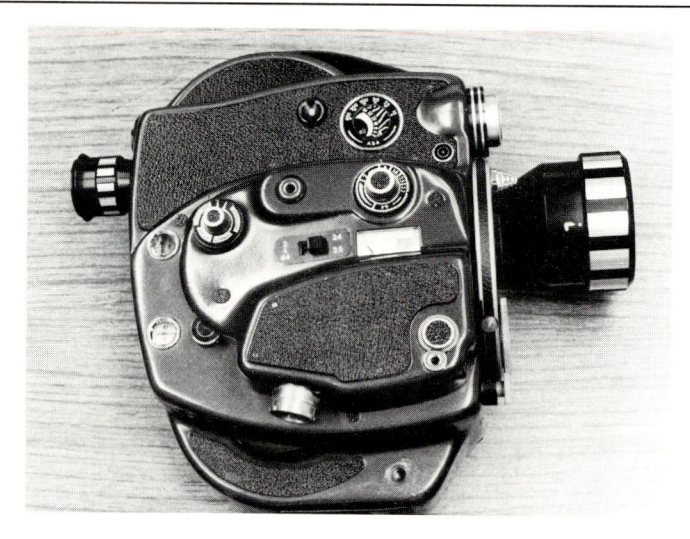

FIG. 6-9. Beaulieu 16-mm movie camera with Dyonics lens mount.

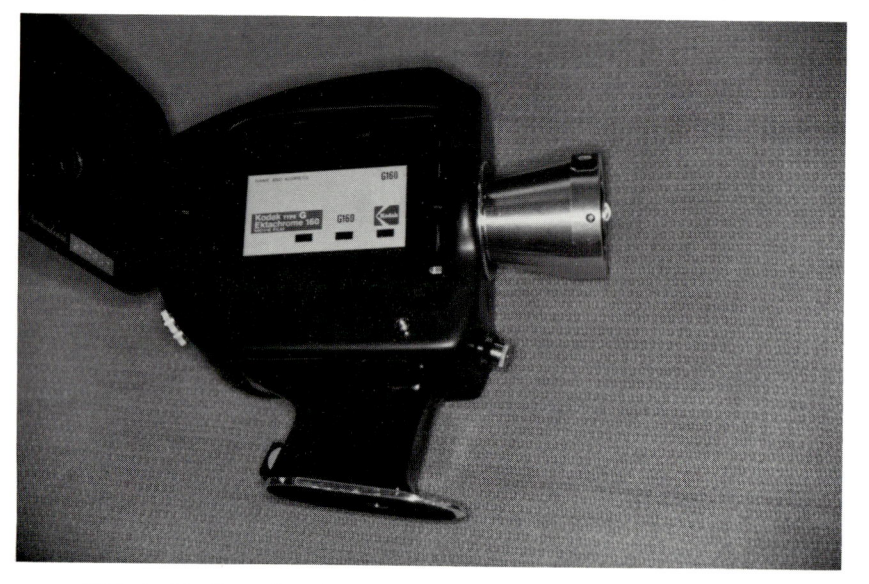

FIG. 6-10. Beaulieu Super 8 camera with cassette loading.

outside arthroscopy. Its main advantage is the ability to use available Kodak Super 8 cassettes. After processing they are excellent for record keeping. They may be viewed on Super 8 viewing devices or projector equipment that many arthroscopists already have for home movie systems. For professional reproduction the film would have to be changed to 16 mm for inclusion in a presentation.

TELEVISION

Modern videotape equipment makes it possible to document endoscopy with television cassettes.[1,2] Because there is no wait for film to be developed, what was observed through the endoscope can be reviewed immediately. Adequacy of the arthroscopic examination can be confirmed, or, if a part of it was

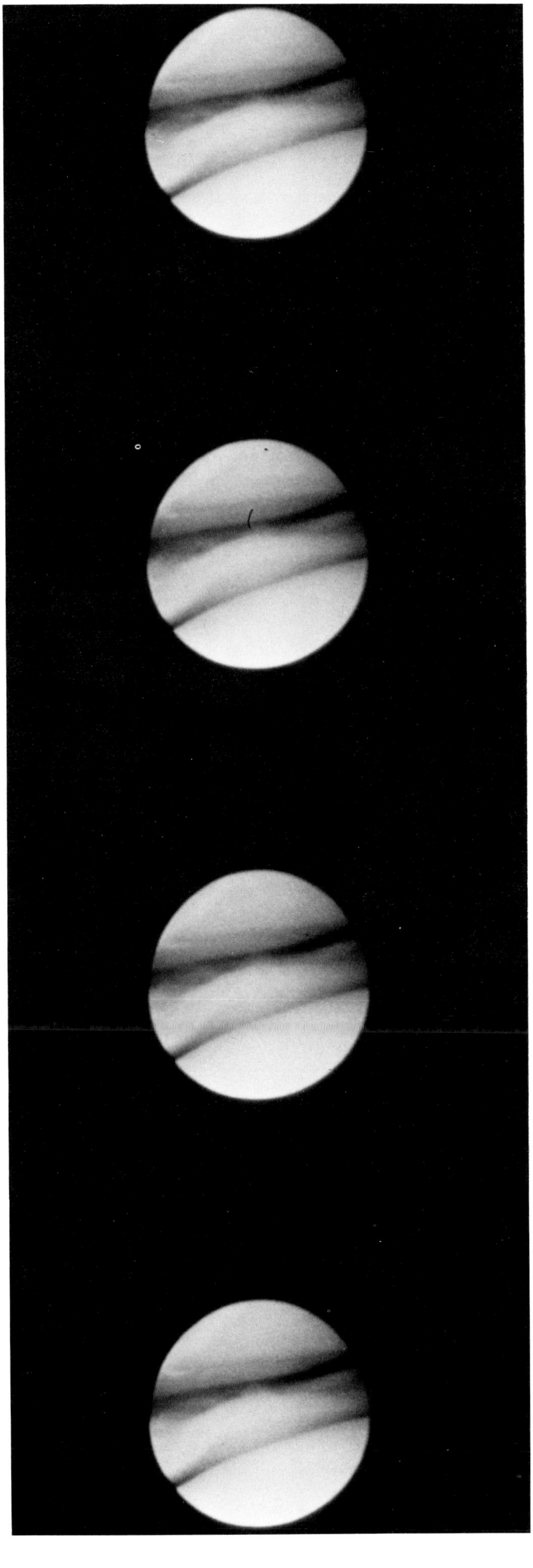

FIG. 6-11. Videotape transferred from movie film. Reproduction can be either black and white or color. It is costly.

Diagnostic arthroscopy of the knee

not satisfactory, it can be repeated right away. Some findings can be observed on the television screen that are not seen by direct vision.

For the past 2 years I have performed arthroscopic surgery with direct viewing from a television monitor. A simultaneous recording was made of every endoscopic surgical procedure. The video cassettes are stored in my office library. Jackson reported on a hospital making this same investment in video equipment and record keeping.[1]

With this video technique the surgeon has an excellent and comfortable body position. Both hands are free during endoscopic surgery. (See Chapter 20.) In addition, others may view at the same time. This enhances the operating room morale, provides immediate visualization for the instruction of other surgeons, and establishes a permanent record for comparison studies in research. Furthermore, materals can be edited for teaching seminars. I have not found any teaching value in having a student handle the television camera. It increases the weight of the instruments in the student's hands and produces one more item to think about.

As the number or volume of arthroscopic cases performed and recorded has grown and the need for research and documentation increased, a video editing system was added to my library. A video editing system and a film library are added conveniences for rapid viewing and reviewing of cases as well as compilation of teaching material.

Videotape can be converted to 16-mm movie film (Fig. 6-11). This is expensive ($64 per minute) but is a way of changing one principal means of documentation to another medium, including editing for movies and slide presentations.

The Medic III television system consists of a free-standing movable cabinet with locking doors in both front and rear. The monitor mount is capable of 350° rotation without destroying or entangling the cables. It has an adequate storage area below for tapes and accessories. Sliding shelves provide easy access to both the camera and the videotape recording equipment. A formica surface ensures the continued handsome appearance of the cabinet (Fig. 6-12). Also, the video monitor is at the eye level of the surgeon. Wall-mounted televisions or those placed on low carts are cumbersome.

The system has three basic pieces of equipment: color camera, a cassette videotape recorder, and a color monitor.

The Hitachi 9017 camera is a single-tube color camera with a remote-control unit and 15 feet of interconnecting cable. The camera head weighs less than 4 pounds. It is supplied with a 25-mm lens with a 16-mm C-mount for clinical documentation other than arthroscopy. There are 250 television lines and horizontal resolution, as well as a built-in color-bar generator for precision setup. The Hitachi 9017 illumination system has been of relatively low cost and high quality. The potential buyer should know that the cost of medical video systems is not necessarily commensurate with their quality; frankly, the opposite seems to be so. Investigate thoroughly and discuss options with a local video consultant. The Hitachi GP-5 system is an economical, good quality system.

Documentation

The color videotape recorder uses ¾-inch cassettes. It has a positive freeze-frame control. A built-in headphone jack provides for personal or private review of the material, as well as for sound dubbing. There is a remote control unit with 15 feet of cable, so the circulating nurse can manage the system.

The color monitor, a 12-inch in-line Trinitron Plus picture tube, is capable of standard telecast and closed-circuit television signals. It has an automatic color switch and automatic fine tuning.

A suspension system has been designed using the Storz articulating optical attachment (Fig. 6-13). This provides ease of movement and a sterile field.

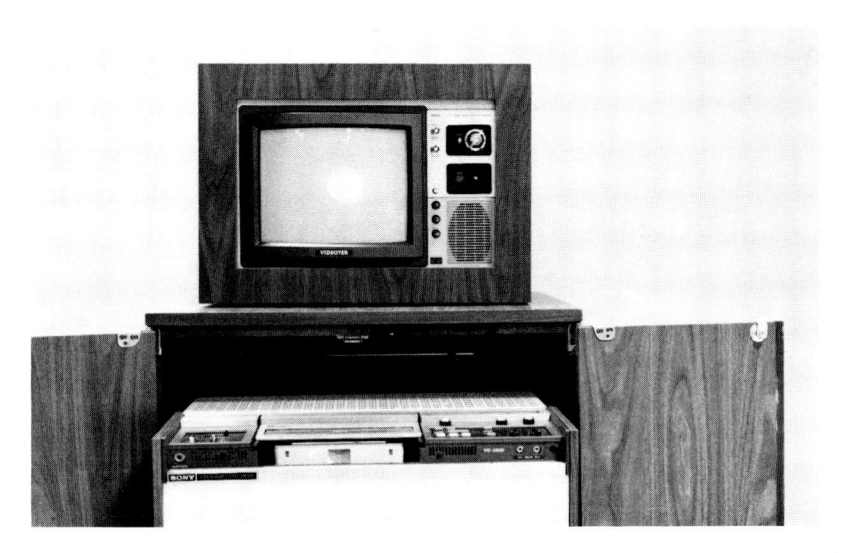

FIG. 6-12. Videotape has proved to be excellent means of recording endoscopic abnormalities. (Equipment assembled by R. P. Hermes Co., Detroit.)

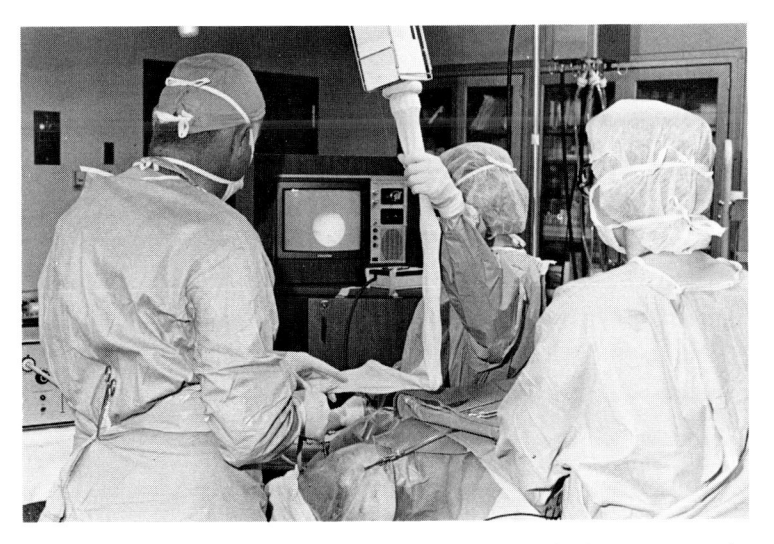

FIG. 6-13. Operative setup with Storz articulated device in between arthroscope and Hitachi camera suspended from bracket on operating table light. Viewing from video monitor is possible during this surgical procedure.

It couples nicely from the endoscope to the video monitor with a Dyonics C-mount adapter. There are other balance types of supports for television cameras, but their bulk and lack of mobility are drawbacks.

REFERENCES

1. Jackson, D. W.: Video arthroscopy: a permanent medical record, Am. J. Sports Med. **6**(5):213, 1978.
2. McGinty, J. A.: Closed circuit television in arthroscopy, Int. Rev. Rheumatol., special edition devoted to arthroscopy, pp. 45-49, 1976.

Chapter 7

Arthroscopic anatomy

Normal arthroscopic anatomy
Anatomic compartments: technique and pathology
    Anterolateral compartment
    Intercondylar notch
    Anteromedial compartment
    Posteromedial compartment
    Posterolateral compartment
Modified Gillquist technique
    Suprapatellar pouch
    Medial compartment
    Posteromedial compartment
    Intercondylar notch
    Lateral compartment
    Posterolateral compartment

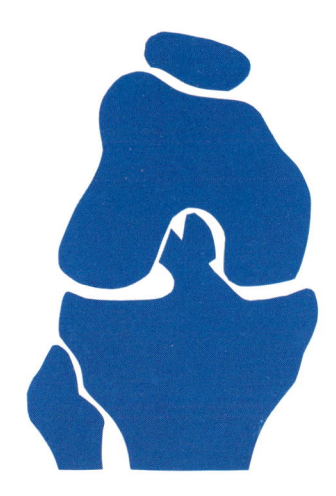

NORMAL ARTHROSCOPIC ANATOMY

A recognition of the normal anatomy and its variants is essential to any pathologic interpretation. The opportunity to perform arthroscopy on patients as young as 3 years of age and as old as 70 has allowed an understanding of the normal anatomy for any given age and an appreciation of normal degenerative changes. The following description and illustrations will help to establish a basis from which change can be recognized.

In the knee joint of a person under the age of 15 years the meniscus is thin in the anteroposterior and vertical dimensions. There is a very sharp inner margin without degenerative changes. The meniscus lies flat and very close to the tibial condyle. Even when valgus strain is applied to the knee, the meniscus elevates only slightly off the condyle. There is a smooth transition from the meniscus to the synovium.

Views of the meniscus from the posteromedial and posterolateral compartments show a clean junction with the articular cartilage. There is no pileup of synovium at the posterior slope of the meniscus, and the contour is smooth, with no irregularities. The meniscus fits firmly against the condylar surfaces.

Articular cartilage in preadolescents is absolutely smooth, usually white, and has no areas of roughening.

In teenage girls the patellar surface is normally smooth, but there may be shaggy synovial fronds hanging about the patella. Often these become symptomatic if they are caught between the patella and the femoral condyle. Synovial fronds can become hemorrhagic, mimicking chondromalacia patellae. In many young girls patellar pain and positive findings of patellar crepitus are not due to articular surface changes but to catching of the peripatellar synovium (Fig. 7-1, *B*).

Diagnostic arthroscopy of the knee

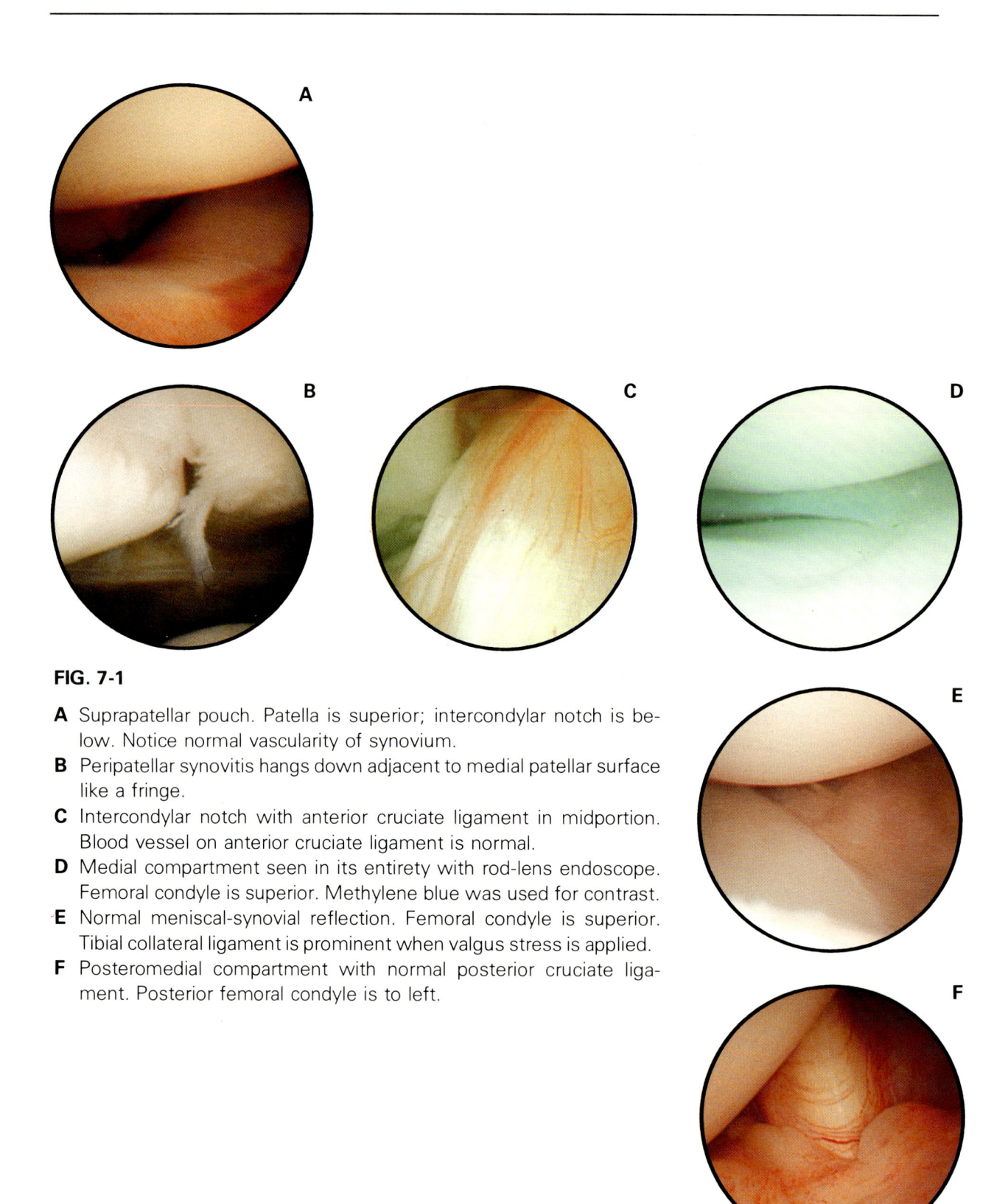

FIG. 7-1

A Suprapatellar pouch. Patella is superior; intercondylar notch is below. Notice normal vascularity of synovium.
B Peripatellar synovitis hangs down adjacent to medial patellar surface like a fringe.
C Intercondylar notch with anterior cruciate ligament in midportion. Blood vessel on anterior cruciate ligament is normal.
D Medial compartment seen in its entirety with rod-lens endoscope. Femoral condyle is superior. Methylene blue was used for contrast.
E Normal meniscal-synovial reflection. Femoral condyle is superior. Tibial collateral ligament is prominent when valgus stress is applied.
F Posteromedial compartment with normal posterior cruciate ligament. Posterior femoral condyle is to left.

114

The ligamentous tissue is easily identified. Frequently a well-formed blood vessel is seen running the length of the synovium on the cruciate ligament (Fig. 7-1, C). With a drawer test it is easy to discern minimal normal laxity in that ligament. With anterior displacement of the tibia on the femur there is minimal motion and rapid tightening of the anterior cruciate ligament. It also is apparent that there is a twisting and untwisting of the anterior cruciate fibers during tightening and relaxation, very much as if they were constructed like cable. Because there is generally no overlying fat, the cable appearance of the anterior cruciate ligament is seen beneath the synovium.

The tibial collateral ligament has a prominence immediately subsynovial, adjacent to the meniscus and in the slot medial to the medial femoral condyle. It is possible with valgus strain on the knee to bring this ligament into relief to demonstrate its integrity (Fig. 7-1, E).

The posterior cruciate ligament can be seen easily in posteromedial inspection as it courses from the posterior aspect of the tibia up into the intercondylar notch (Fig. 7-1, F).

The popliteus tendon can be seen in three different areas. From an anteromedial approach, it is visible under the lateral meniscus, where it courses through the area devoid of coronary ligament (Fig. 7-2, B). Its attachment is seen from an anterolateral approach down the sulcus lateral to the femoral condyle (Fig. 7-2, C). The most complete inspection of the popliteus tendon is carried out from the posterolateral or anterolateral approach. It is often possible to pick up the course of that tendon and follow down its sheath as it courses posterior and inferior to the meniscus (Fig. 7-2, D). The tendon has a silvery appearance in a young person, and crosshatching of collagen bundles is often apparent.

The synovium is flat, with only a rare villous formation. Normally, only a fine pattern of vascularity is observed (Fig. 7-2, E). Synovial folds are common in the suprapatellar pouch and along the medial wall of the joint connecting to the fat pad.

During adolescence the meniscus begins to degenerate. The first sign is translucency of its inner border; otherwise, there are no significant findings that could be considered normal. It should be noted that those individuals who are involved in vigorous athletic endeavors will have earlier degenerative meniscal changes, possibly including early fringe fragmentation. If there has been some significant injury, fragmentation of the meniscus or injury to the articular surfaces may result. (See Fig. 8-1.)

In the third decade of life, fringe degeneration of the meniscus, including fringe tags, is common. Normally, the brilliant white cartilage seen in the young knee starts to take on a yellow hue. The synovium is more villous and a bit more vascular.

Over the subsequent decades it is common for degenerative changes of the meniscus to increase. The meniscus may develop yellow streaks. Thickened areas in the meniscus make its surfaces smooth and rounded. It increases in girth. Posteromedial and posterolateral punctures show the meniscus to have convoluted rather than smooth surfaces.

Diagnostic arthroscopy of the knee

NORMAL ANATOMY

FIG. 7-2

A Anterolateral compartment. Entire lateral meniscus, with femoral condyle superior. Methylene blue used in joint for contrast.

B By pistoning toward posterolateral corner of lateral compartment, popliteus tendon can be seen under meniscus. No coronary ligament in area, and popliteus tendon is seen beyond notch in tibial surface.

C Anterolateral approach down sulcus, above popliteus tendon. Lateral femoral condyle is to right. Opening seen beyond is into posterolateral compartment. Popliteus tendon inferior, between 5 and 6 o'clock.

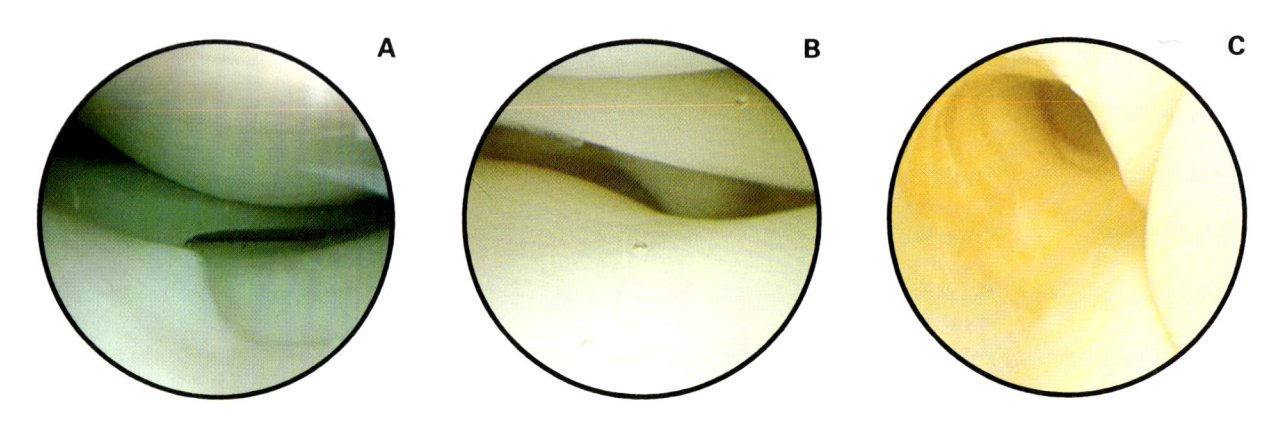

D Posterolateral compartment. Popliteus tendon crossing obliquely, going down its sheath beneath and posterior to meniscus. Femoral condyle superior. Methylene blue utilized for contrast. It is possible to pass small-diameter endoscope down popliteus sheath to vacuum out loose bodies, if they exist.

E Posterolateral approach. Normal femoral-condylar-meniscal junction. Meniscus has no tears. Normal synovial vascularity on posterior wall. No loose bodies.

F Saline is rapidly absorbed by normal synovium and looks like glistening silver balls.

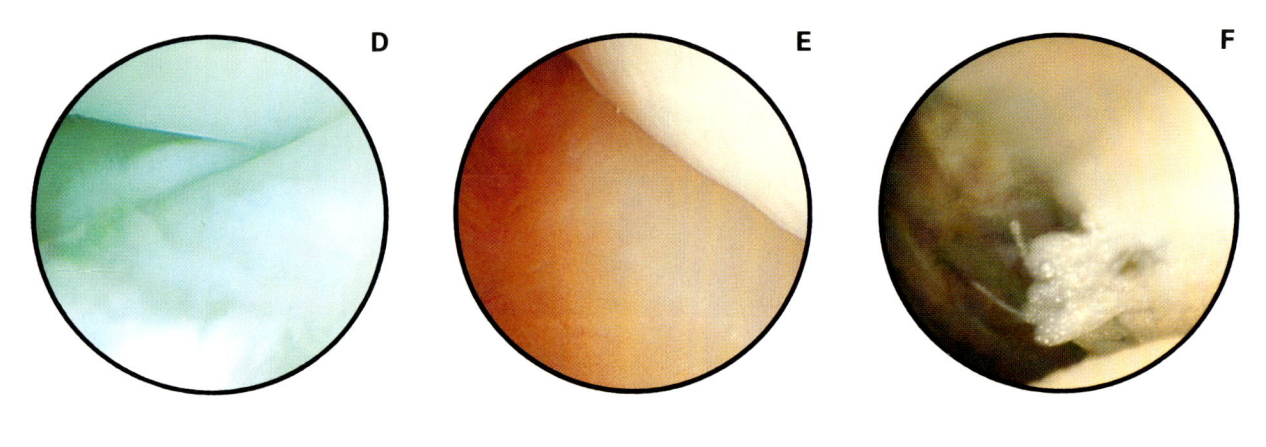

The articular surfaces lose their brilliance and sharp edges. The first sign of degenerative change is a smooth cobblestoning, which can advance to complete loss of articular surface and the uncovering of yellow bone. (See Chapter 8). The normal degenerative process can include development of osteophytes. The synovium becomes considerably more villous and proliferative, especially in the posteromedial and posterolateral compartments. Projections are seen coming off the posteromedial and posterolateral synovial reflections of the meniscus as well as the fat pad.

There is a time at which the normal degenerative changes in the knee take on clinical importance. Histologic sectioning of torn menisci, even in young people, indicates that there has been prior degenerative meniscal change. It is apparent that a virgin meniscus does not tear, except perhaps off of the synovial attachment, in a young person. Severe degenerative meniscal changes are usually accompanied by instability and mechanical malalignment (i.e., tibia vara).

With the instillation of saline it is not uncommon for a localized area of synovial fluid to appear syrupy (as one might see if sugar were dropped into a glass of water). This is normal. Otherwise, there should be no particles, or stardusting, in the synovial fluid. (See Chapter 8.) It is not uncommon for the saline to be rapidly engulfed by the synovium, where it appears as glistening little silver balls inside the synovial villi (Fig. 7-2, F).

ANATOMIC COMPARTMENTS: TECHNIQUE AND PATHOLOGY

The technique outlined in Chapter 3 illustrates the mechanics of entering the individual anatomic compartments of the knee. The arthroscopic views of each compartment are unique. For instance, the medial meniscus in a normal knee lies closer to the tibial condyle, even with valgus stress, than would the lateral meniscus with varus stress. The lateral meniscus tends to ride up off the tibia in a normal knee. Anatomic landmarks are seen in specific compartments. The posterior cruciate ligament is best seen from the posteromedial puncture (Fig. 7-1, F); the origin of the popliteus tendon is seen from an anterolateral approach, and through a posterolateral approach it can be seen coursing back behind the meniscus; the anterior cruciate ligament is seen only from the intercondylar view (Fig. 7-1, B).

Some pathologic abnormalities are unique to a particular anatomic compartment. Compression fracture or articular defect of an acute dislocation of the patella is seen in the anterolateral compartment, at a site one meniscus breadth superior and lateral to the meniscal-synovial reflection. (See Fig. 7-3.) It has been noted that most loose bodies collect in the posterolateral compartment as a result of gravity because when a person sits, the thigh is normally in slight external rotation.

Each of the following sections illustrates an anatomic compartment. Technique is demonstrated, and the role of each member of the arthroscopic team in achieving visualization of that compartment is outlined. The facing pages show normal anatomic structures visualized in the area, as well as illustrations of pathologic abnormalities that are unique to the respective compartment.

Anterolateral compartment

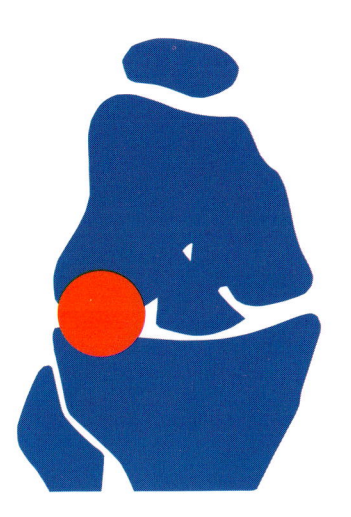

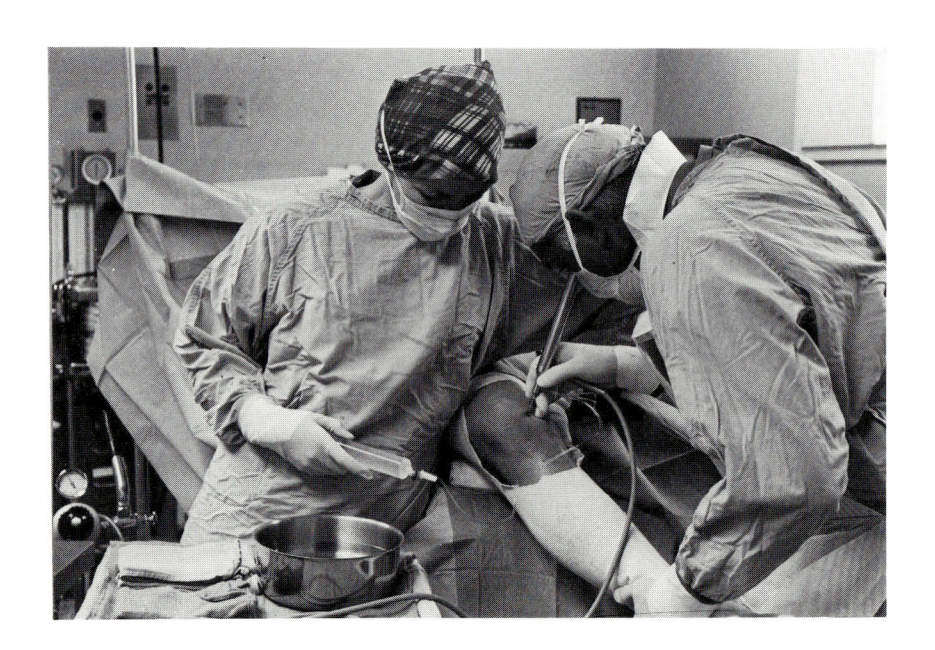

Patient	The patient is supine on the table, with his legs hanging free over the end.
Assistant	The assistant stands next to the patient's thigh and supports the inner distal femur with her hand.
Physician	The physician stands. With his free hand he applies varus stress to the knee, which, when coupled with approximately 15° flexion of the knee, usually opens the joint to maximum. To view a defect in the lateral femoral condyle, maximal distension, which pushes the synovium off the condyle, may be necessary. The physician may move to the lateral side of the patient's leg and apply varus strain with his hip and body. This frees both hands for inspection and cleansing.

Arthroscopic anatomy

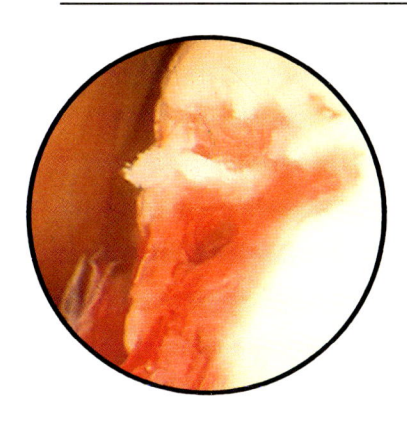

MULTIPLE PUNCTURE TECHNIQUE

FIG. 7-3

A Tangential view of lateral femoral condyle shows acute dislocation of patella. There also may be depression with roughening in subluxation of patella. Normal knee may have minimal depression without roughened articular surface. Loss of articular surface may accompany acute dislocations.

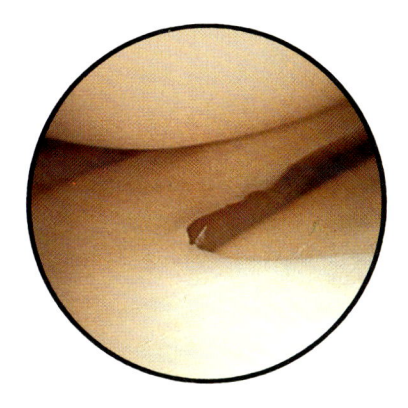

B Entire lateral meniscus. Femoral condyle is superior. Meniscus has sharp normal margins. Lateral meniscus elevates off tibial condyle with varus stress slightly more than medial meniscus would with valgus stress.

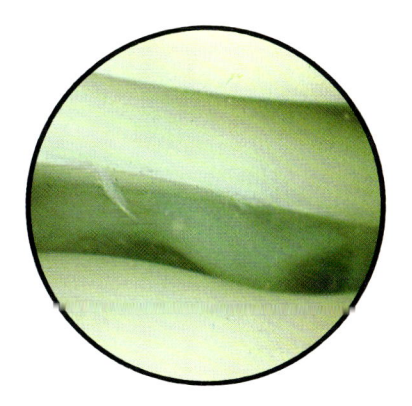

C Methylene blue in joint for contrast. View under lateral meniscus to area where popliteus tendon crosses posterolaterally. Area is devoid of coronary ligament. Tendon has lighter color of reflection than does meniscus, which assists in identification.

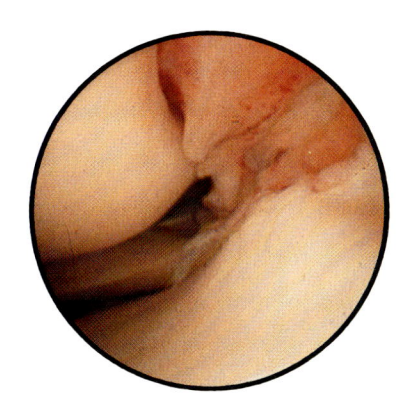

D Lateral compartment is first viewed adjacent to tibial spine. Landmark for orientation is junction between femoral condyle and tibial spine. Penetration brings posterior horn of lateral meniscus into view. Hemorrhage is seen in intercondylar notch.

Diagnostic arthroscopy of the knee

Intercondylar notch

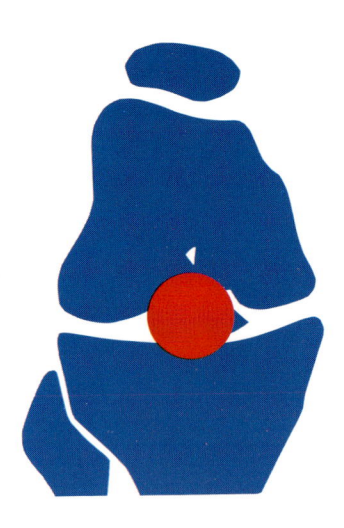

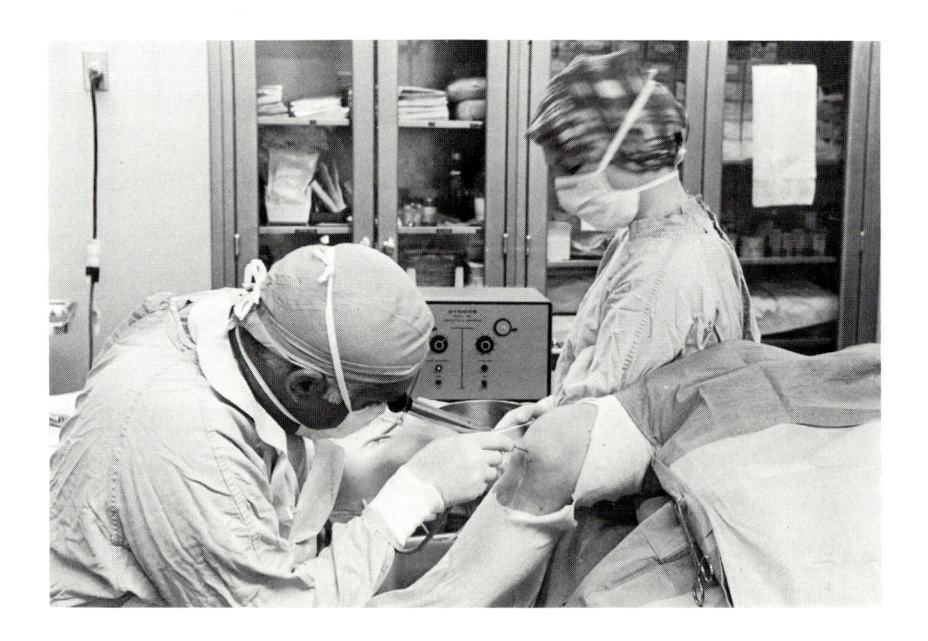

Patient	The patient is supine, with his legs hanging free over the edge of the table.
Assistant	The assistant stands next to the patient, stabilizing the distal thigh with her elbow or body.
Physician	The physician sits with the patient's foot in his lap at between 45° and 90° flexion. It is possible to visualize the notch and perform a drawer test to document the integrity of the anterior cruciate ligament.

Arthroscopic anatomy

MULTIPLE PUNCTURE TECHNIQUE

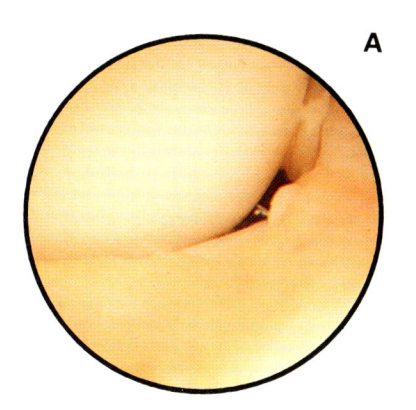

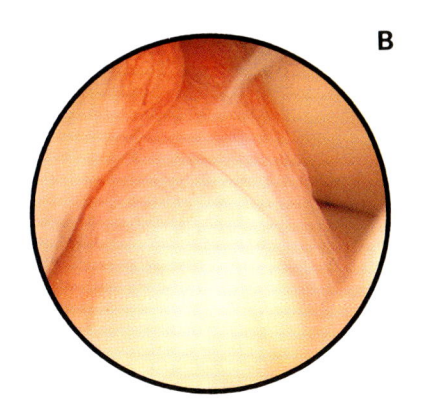

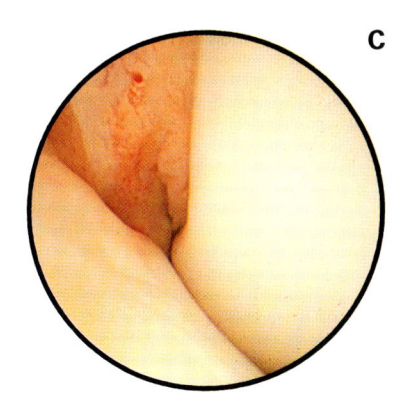

FIG. 7-4

A Junction of lateral femoral condyle and intercondylar notch is anatomic landmark.
B Anterior cruciate ligament with some increased vascularity but no tear. Medial approach reduces fat pad interference.
C Junction of medial femoral condyle and intercondylar notch. Notice synovial vascularity in foreground. Extreme anterior horn of meniscus seen in this area.
D Bucket-handle tear on lateral side of notch. Considerable synovitis and partial disruption of anterior cruciate ligament.
E Loose bodies in intercondylar notch can be removed with Jaws modified pituitary forceps while patient is under local anesthesia.
F Tear of anterior cruciate ligament, with massive disruption and hemorrhage. Direct preoperative evaluation of cruciate ligament provides evidence as to its integrity and repairability.
G Posterior cruciate ligament may be seen from anterior approach in this patient (whose anterior cruciate ligament is partially absent). It courses from 2 to 7 o'clock.

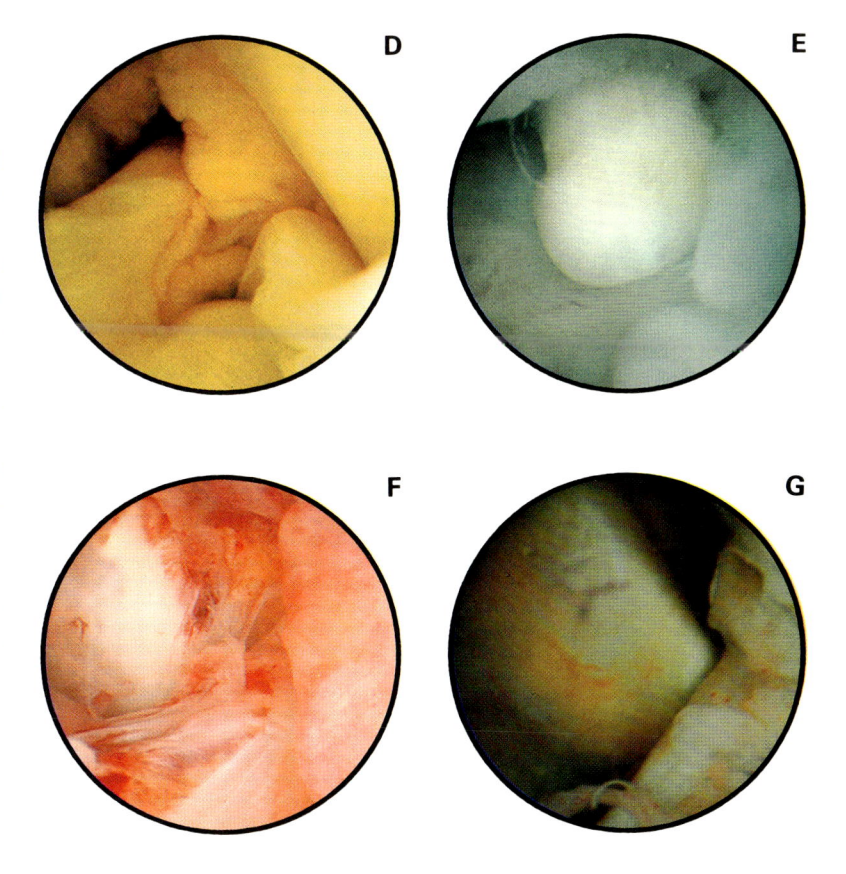

Diagnostic arthroscopy of the knee

Anteromedial compartment

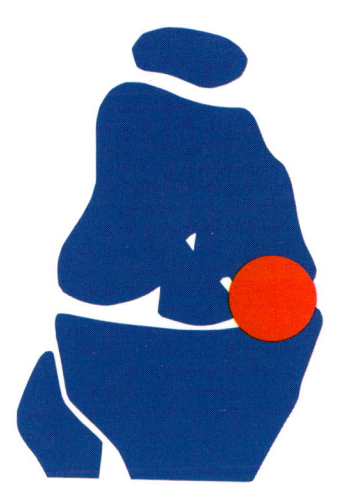

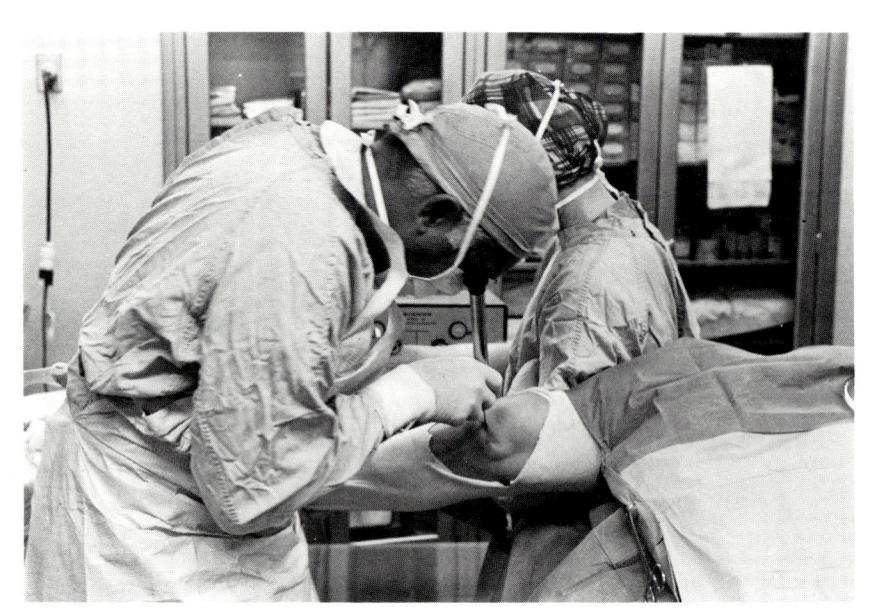

Patient	The patient is supine on the table, with his legs hanging free.
Assistant	The assistant stands to the patient's side and supports the distal femur with her elbow.
Physician	The physician stands and applies a valgus stress with his free hand. It may be necessary to flex and extend the patient's leg and rotate it internally and externally to complete the composite viewing of the medial compartment.

    The original direction of entry is 30° laterally. However, redirection of the endoscope in a patient with scar or fat tissue may be necessary. Redirection should *not* be considered a lack of ability but a matter of appropriate technique. It is done by removing the endoscope and reinserting the blunt trocar. The cannula and trocar are retracted into the subcutaneous tissue. The capsule is repunctured toward the medial compartment.

Arthroscopic anatomy

MULTIPLE PUNCTURE TECHNIQUE

FIG. 7-5

A Entire anteromedial compartment, with meniscus below femoral condyle.

B With valgus strain on knee, meniscus raises up in serpentine fashion. This amount of elevation is normal in mobile knee joint. To move under meniscus, it is important that meniscus be elevated in this manner. Scope is then placed under an elevated area. Valgus stress is reduced for viewing under meniscus.

C With methylene blue in medial compartment, most extreme anterior portion of horn of meniscus is seen at synovial reflection.

D Endoscope pistoned forward to visualize anterior portion of posterior horn.

E Normal posterior horn and posterior compartment beyond.

F Tear of notch attachment of medial meniscus.

G Same bucket-handle tear in notch. Frequently this is difficult for the uninitiated arthroscopist to diagnose because meniscus mechanically interferes with penetration of joint.

H Remaining rim of meniscus in bucket-handle tear. Notice abnormal size and contour. Small meniscus indicates bucket-handle tear.

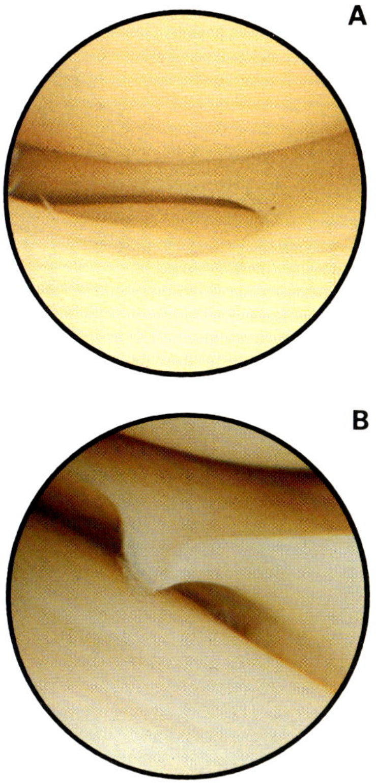

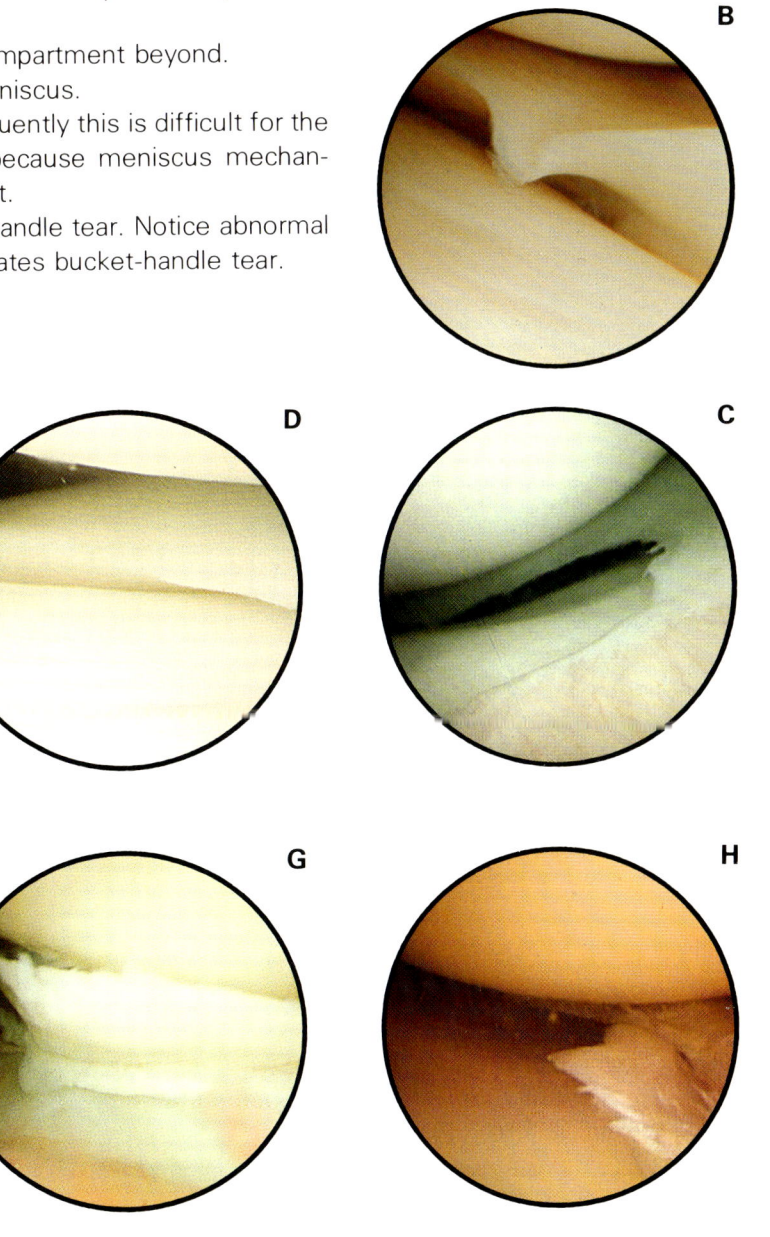

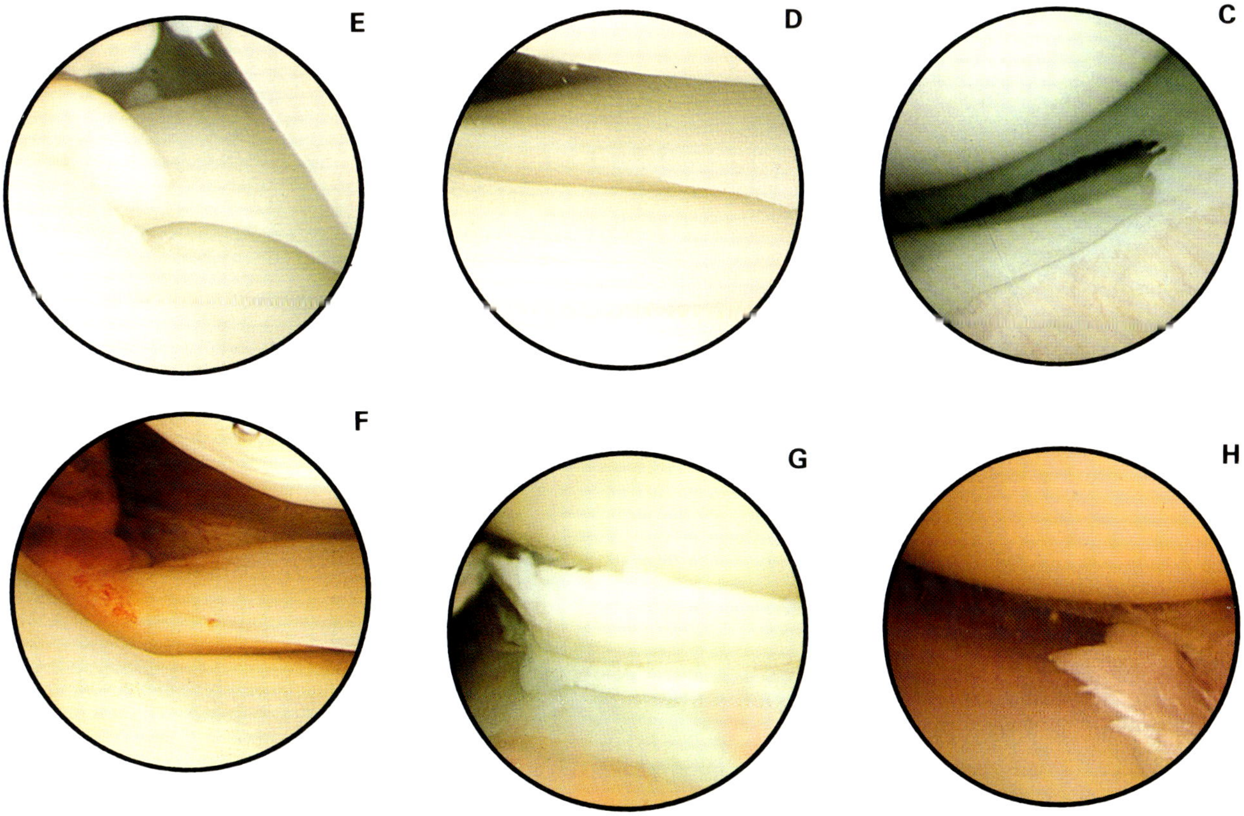

123

Diagnostic arthroscopy of the knee

Posteromedial compartment

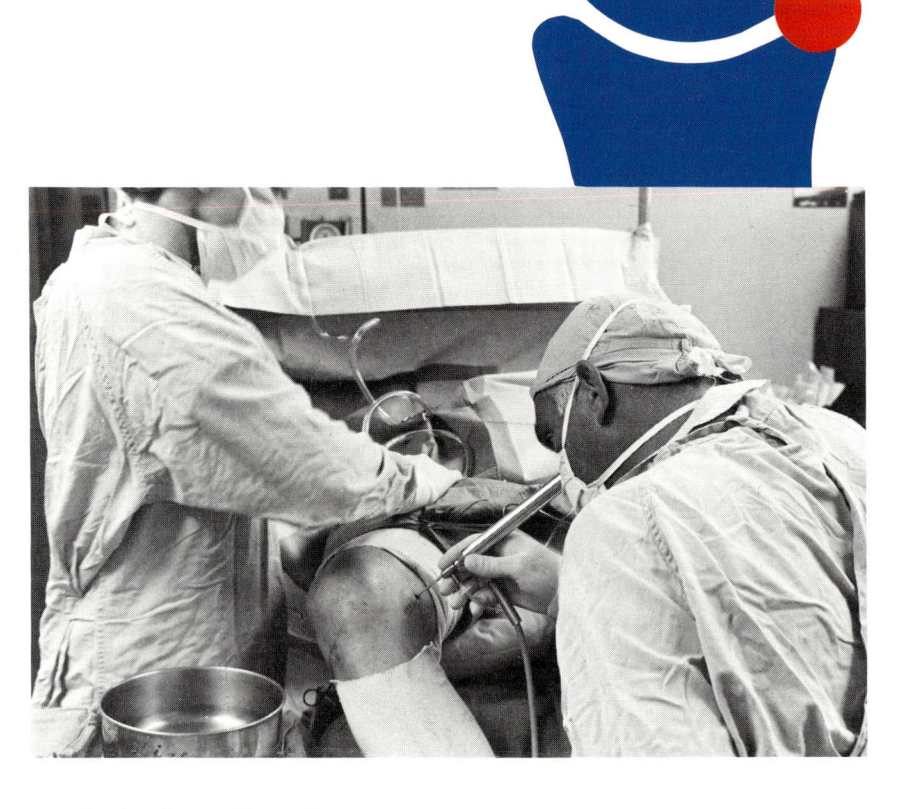

Patient	The patient's thigh is allowed to roll into external rotation. The knee is flexed approximately 90°.
Assistant	The assistant stabilizes the distal femur.
Physician	The physician sits with the patient's foot in his lap. Arthroscopic approach is made from the posteromedial corner.

Maximal distension of the joint is essential to entry of the posteromedial compartment. Entry is posterior to the condyle and superior to the meniscus. Inspection of the compartment proceeds from the landmark junction of the femoral condyle and the meniscus. The posterior cruciate ligament and the posterior horn of the medial meniscus can be visualized. In some patients, internal rotation of the tibia on the femur allows the meniscus to drop off the medial femoral condyle, making it possible to see vertical tears or abnormalities that would not be visible when the meniscus is resting against the femur. Retained posterior horns may be evaluated in this area.

Arthroscopic anatomy

MULTIPLE PUNCTURE TECHNIQUE

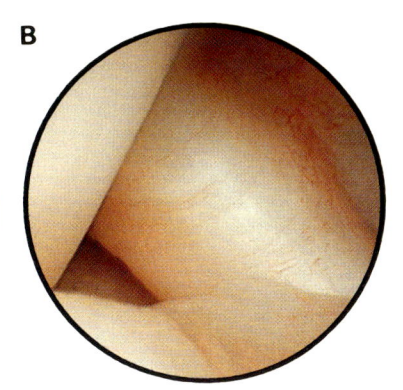

FIG. 7-6

A Posterior cruciate ligament seen just beyond junction of meniscus and femoral condyle.
B Close-up of normal posterior cruciate ligament in posteromedial compartment.
C Old separation of medial meniscus off posterior horn, not visible from front. No hemorrhage seen.
D Pistoning into cleft shows posterior tibial condyle deep in cleft.
E Subacute posterior horn tear of medial meniscus.
F Acute posteromedial horn tear of meniscus, with hemorrhage in posterior capsule.
G Internal rotation of tibia on femur drops meniscus away from femur. Occult tears may be seen. Fronds of old anterior cruciate ligament tear were catching in joint.
H Retained posterior horn after anterovertical arthrotomy and removal of meniscus. There was second tear posterior to removed portion of meniscus. Retained posterior horn was torn off its attachments, necessitating resection to reduce symptoms. Probably was an original untreated lesion.

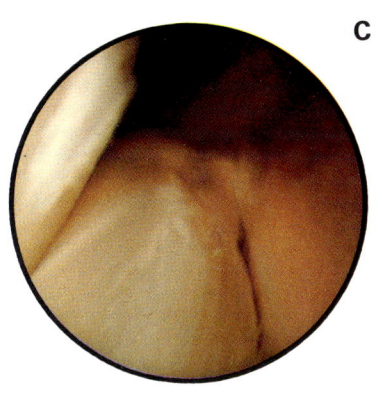

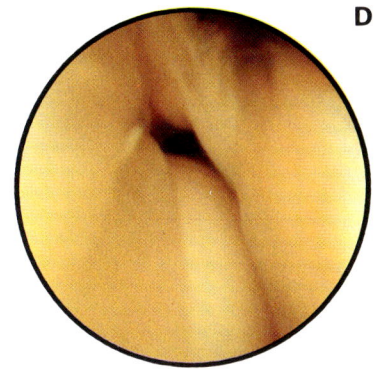

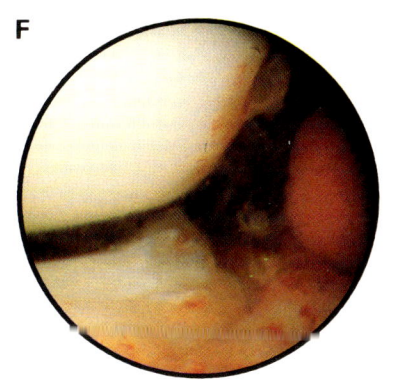

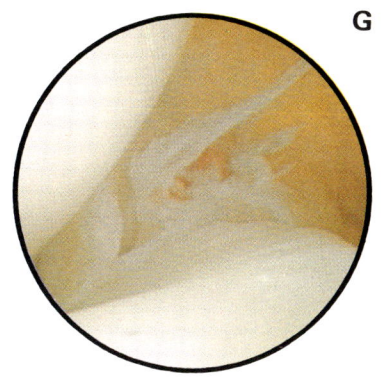

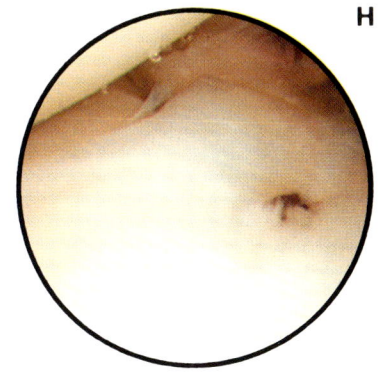

125

Diagnostic arthroscopy of the knee

Posterolateral compartment

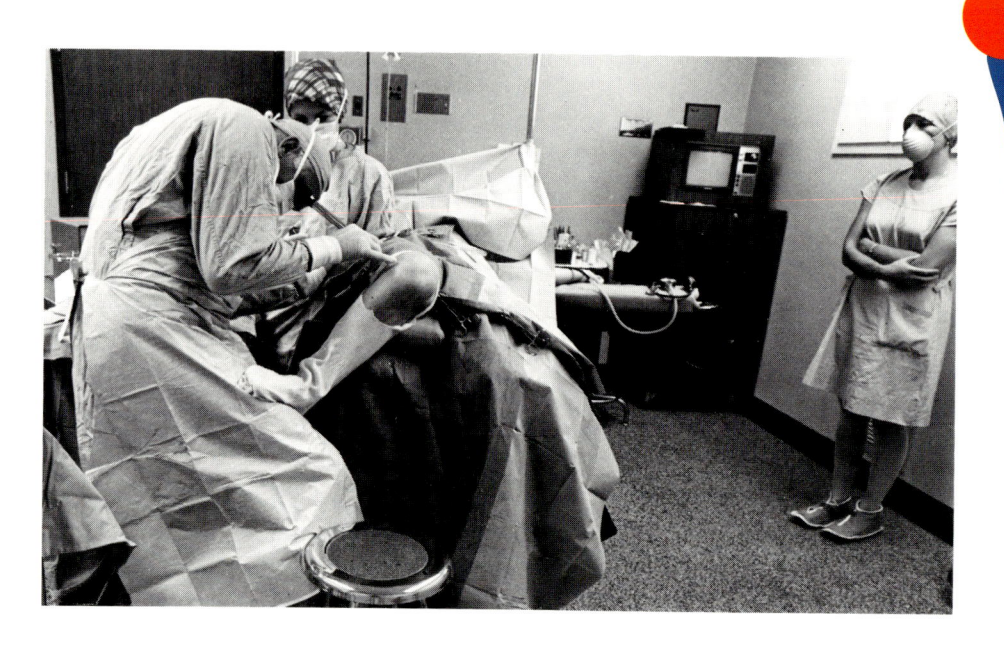

Patient The patient is rolled slightly to the side of the uninvolved extremity. The knee is brought up into flexion of approximately 100°.

Assistant The assistant is superior to the patient's side.

Physician The physician stands next to the patient, with his foot on a stool rung and the patient's foot supported on his thigh.

The puncture is made at a point where a line drawn along the intermuscular septum intersects with a line drawn from the posterior aspect of the fibula. The endoscope is directed slightly anteroinferiorly to enter the posterolateral compartment. The junction between the meniscus and the articular surface can be visualized. Often the popliteus tendon is seen as it enters the sheath posterolateral to the meniscus. Posterior horn tears not visible anteriorly are frequently identified, as is hemorrhagic fragment of the anterior cruciate ligament. Loose bodies collect in the posterolateral compartment. There may be isolated tears of the anterior cruciate ligament without any tear of the menisci. Invariably hemorrhage is seen within the posteromedial or posterolateral compartment, indicating an injury that cannot be documented clinically or arthroscopically from anterior puncture only. This approach has not been necessary with the exposure provided from an anterior direction under general anesthesia and the thigh held by the Surgical Assistant.

Arthroscopic anatomy

MULTIPLE PUNCTURE TECHNIQUE

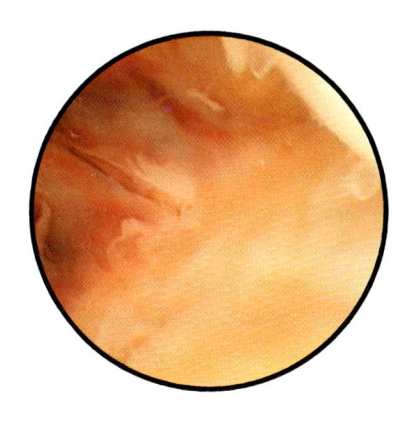

FIG. 7-7

A Torn menisci not visible anteriorly are often seen in posterolateral compartment, especially in patients with torn ligamentous structures. If knee opened medially only, posterolateral tear of meniscus probably would be missed. Arthroscopic inspection allows design of surgical approach. Area cannot be visualized anteriorly even with small-diameter endoscope because mass of meniscus blocks view.

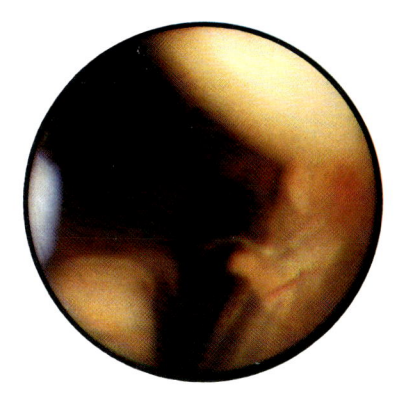

B Complete cleft in posterolateral meniscus.

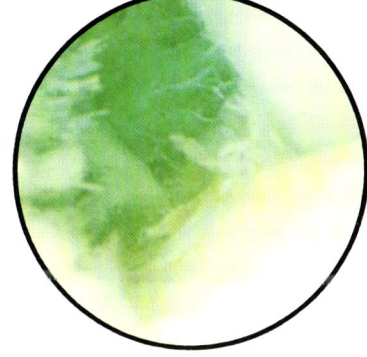

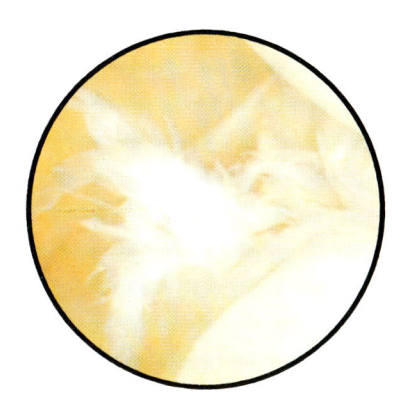

C Posterolateral compartment collects many loose bodies and provokes rather marked degenerative synovitis. Methylene blue in joint for contrast.

D Posterolateral puncture has been especially important in diagnosing anterior cruciate ligament injuries. Loose fragments of anterior cruciate tissue can be seen.

Diagnostic arthroscopy of the knee

MODIFIED GILLQUIST TECHNIQUE

The Gillquist method* of arthroscopic technique demands a transpatellar tendon approach and a single puncture inspection. Access to the posterior compartments is via the intercondylar notch and adjacent to the tibial spine (Fig. 7-8, A). The single puncture and intercondylar approach to the posterior compartments can be modified without the obvious potential injury to the patellar tendon. When a general anesthetic is administered, a 4-mm rod-lens arthroscope placed lateral to and opposite the tip of the patella can visualize all these areas if the thigh is firmly secured. The transpatellar puncture advocated by Gillquist is not performed because many of my patients complained of pain and thickness in the patellar tendon for several months after the transpatellar tendon approach.

This method functions well in the arthroscopic surgical setup (Fig. 7-8, B).

---

*Gillquist, J., Hagberg, G., and Oretorp, N.: Arthroscopic examination of the posterior compartment of the knee, Int. Orthop. (SICOT) **3**:13, 1979.

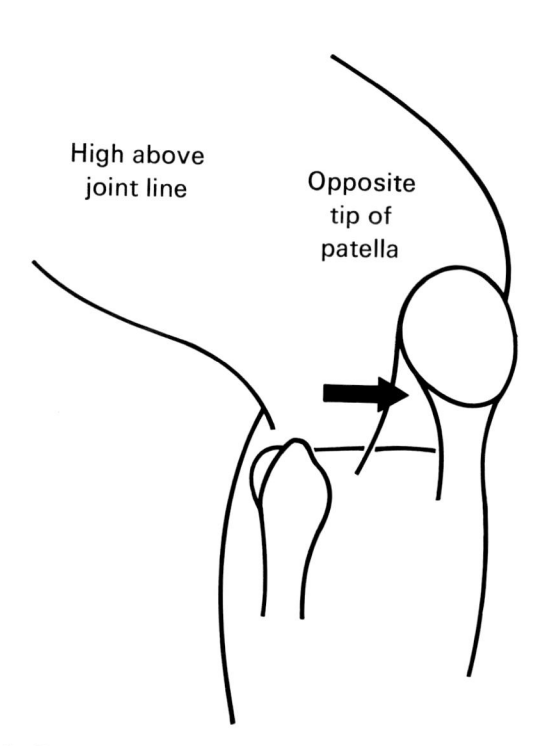

FIG. 7-8. A, Puncture placement for modified Gillquist technique.

Arthroscopic anatomy

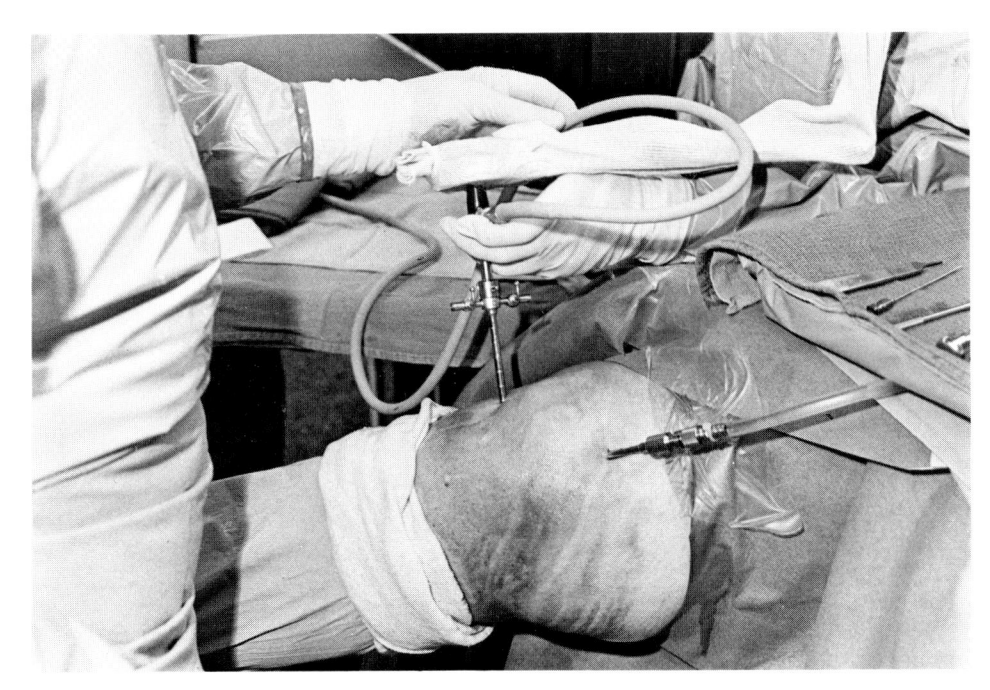

FIG 7-8, cont'd. B, Ideal placement site is higher than was previously thought to be correct. It is lateral and opposite the distal pole of the patella. Notice the inflow cannula site medial and superior to the patella.

Diagnostic arthroscopy of the knee

Suprapatellar pouch

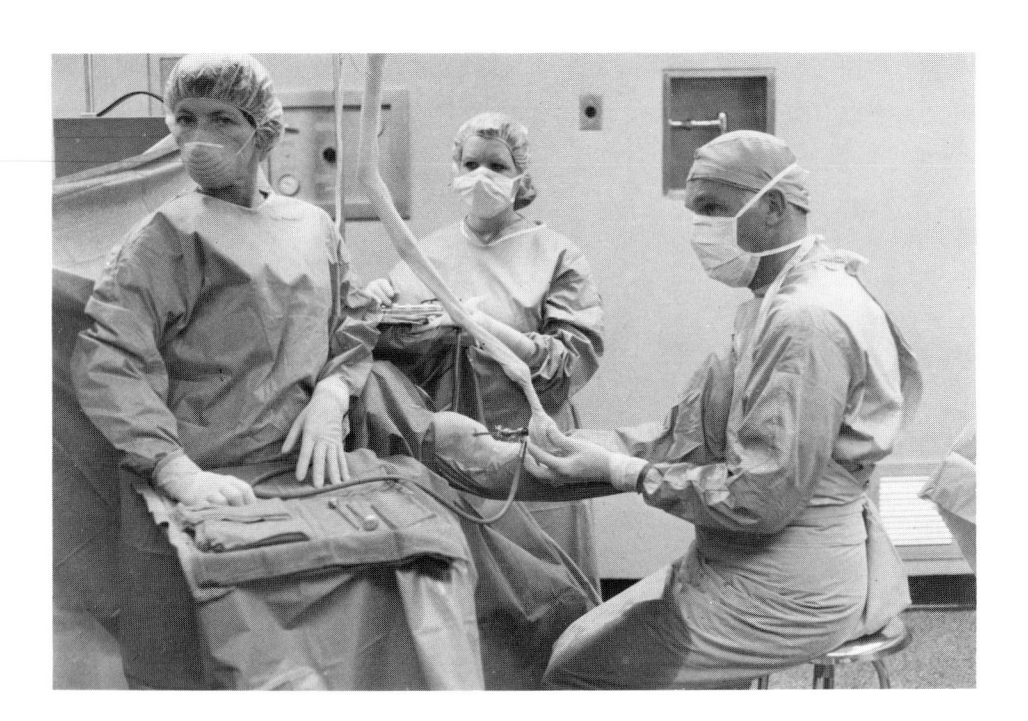

Patient	The patient is in the supine position with the thigh secured in the Surgical Assistant.
Knee	The knee is extended and hyperextended, even to flexion, to inspect tracking.
Assistant	The assistant is lateral to the thigh, assisting with the arthroscope and the articulating viewing device.
Physician	The physician sits with the patient's sterile foot against the chest.
Arthroscope	A lateral placement is preferred, opposite the apex of the patella.

Arthroscopic anatomy

MODIFIED GILLQUIST TECHNIQUE

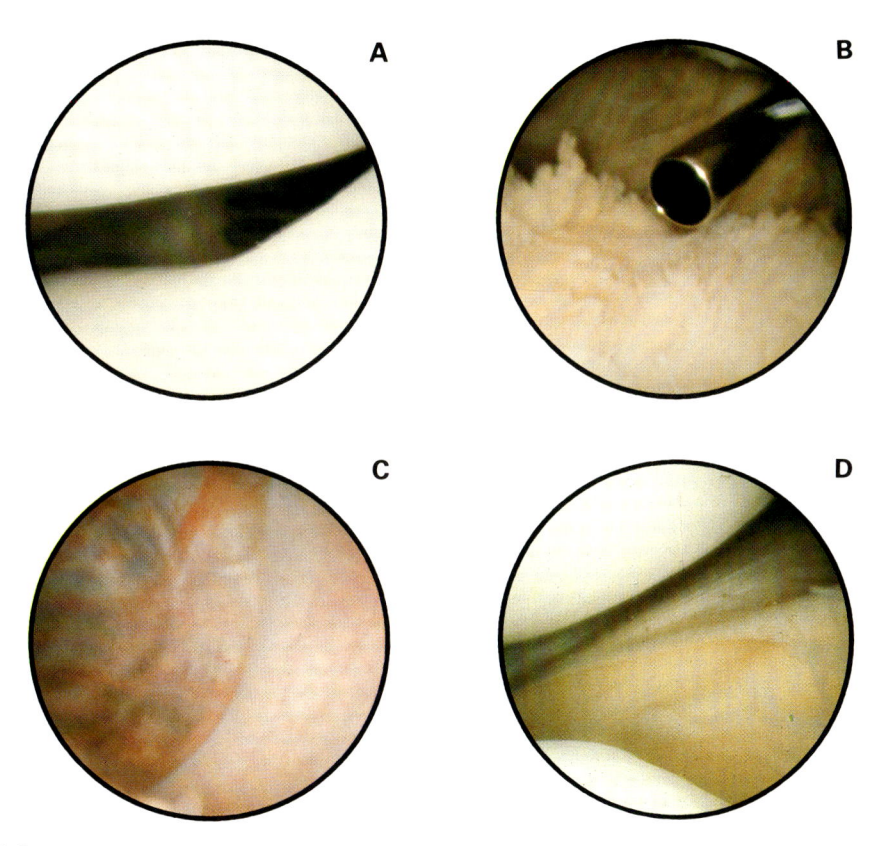

FIG. 7-9

A Patellofemoral joint is viewed from anterolateral peripatellar approach. Leg is in extension.
B Arthroscopic view shows inflow cannula, from superior and medial, and adjacent synovium.
C Further penetration into the suprapatellar pouch shows suprapatellar plica, a common anatomic finding.
D Move toward medial compartment shows patella above, medial femoral condyle below, and small medial shelf fold, or plica, between the two structures. Leg is in maximally extended position.

Medial compartment

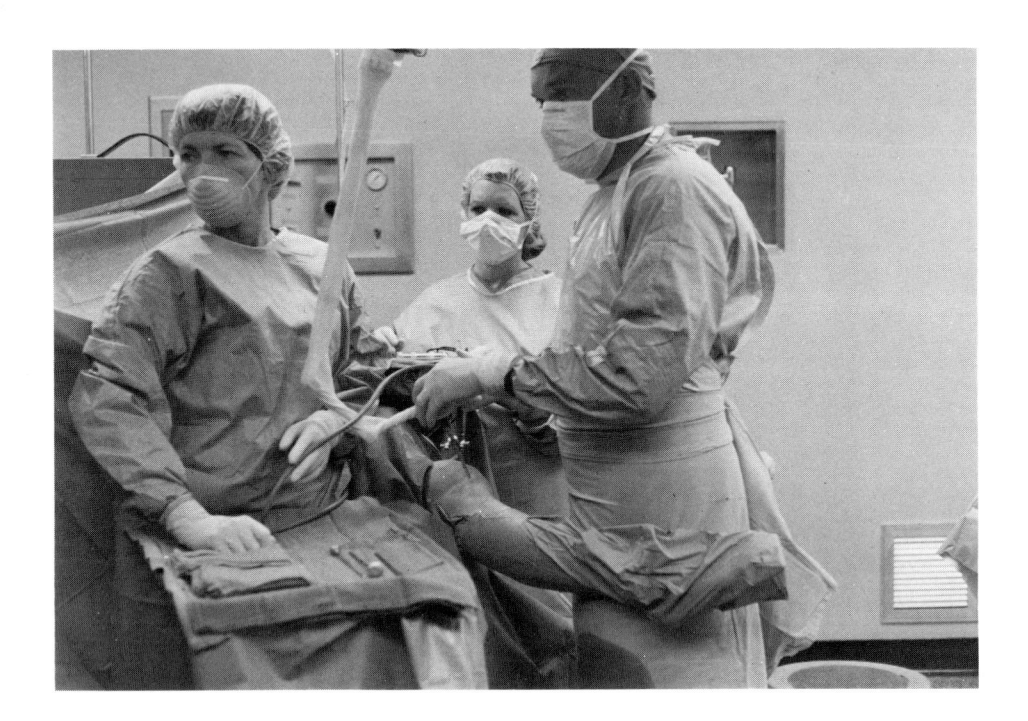

Patient	The patient is supine.
Knee	The knee is in 15° flexion with valgus stress and external rotation.
Assistant	The assistant is lateral to the patient's thigh.
Physician	The physician assumes a position at the inner aspect of the patient's leg and applies a valgus stress with the hip. Rotation of the leg at the knee joint may be controlled by the physician's hand on the foot or ankle.
Arthroscope	The arthroscope is in the lateral position.

MODIFIED GILLQUIST TECHNIQUE

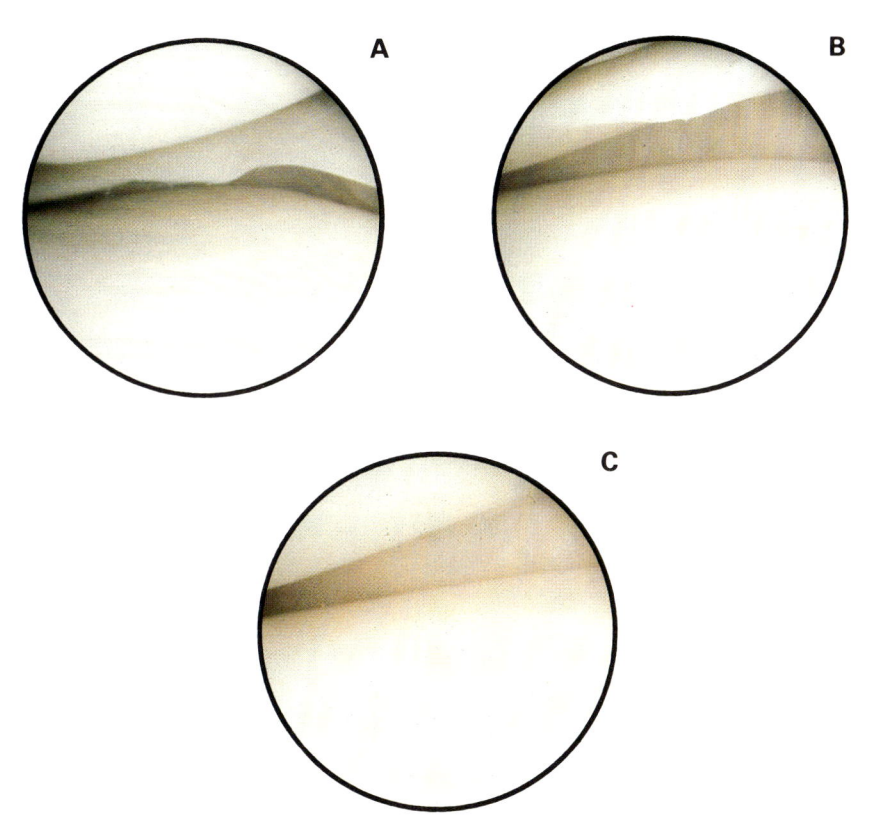

FIG. 7-10

A Femoral condyle is above, meniscus is in midfield, and tibial plateau surface is below.
B Knee is brought into valgus strain and external rotation, and arthroscope starts to move under meniscus. This is only possible with small-diameter scope and under local anesthesia. Thigh secured in Surgical Assistant device permits this maneuver with large-diameter scope and patient under general anesthesia.
C Meniscus is superior and coronary ligament in photographic midfield is immediately above tibial plateau.

Diagnostic arthroscopy of the knee

Posteromedial compartment

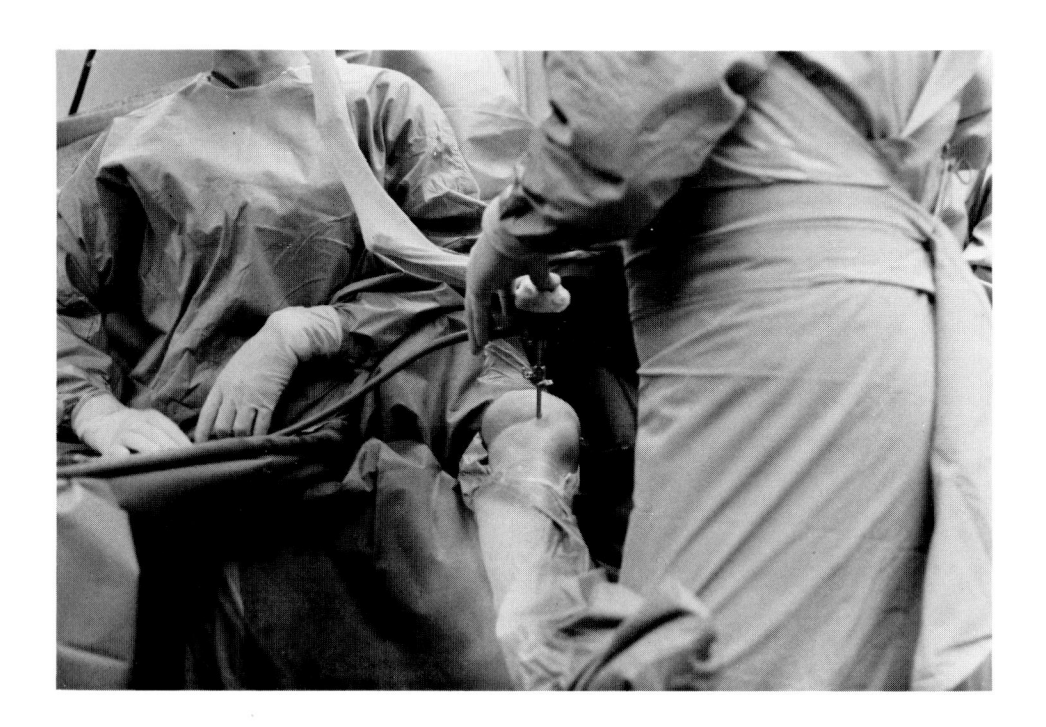

Patient	The patient is supine.
Knee	The knee is in 15° flexion and valgus strain.
Assistant	The assistant is lateral to the patient's thigh.
Physician	The physician views the posterior horn of the medial meniscus at its attachment near the tibial spine. From that point, entry is possible in most patients under direct vision into the posterior medial compartment. This route passes by the posterior cruciate ligament to the lateral side and the medial femoral condyle to the medial side. Rotation of the 30° inclined arthroscope to the medial side with knee flexion to 45° shows the entire compartment. A 70° inclined arthroscope has not been necessary, as Gillquist suggests. This may be due to the more lateral entry point. In some patients the arthroscope may be replaced by a blunt obturator and the posterior entry accomplished by manipulation. The arthroscope is replaced for viewing. In some small or arthritic patients this maneuver may not be possible, and a separate transcutaneous posteromedial puncture is necessary.
Arthroscope	The arthroscope is a 30° inclined rod lens, occasionally at a 70° inclined view.

Arthroscopic anatomy

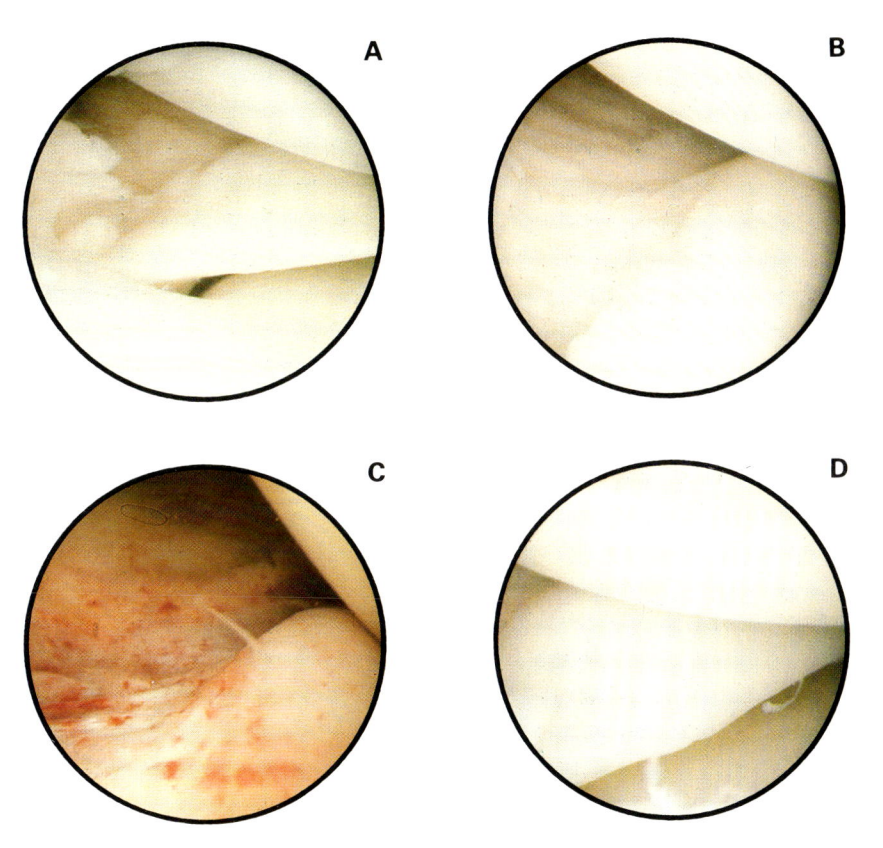

MODIFIED GILLQUIST TECHNIQUE

FIG. 7-11

A First move toward posteromedial compartment is to visualize extreme posterior horn attachment of medial meniscus. Telescope can be exchanged for blunt trocar, and blunt trocar and cannula can be manipulated into posterior compartment.

B Telescope is exchanged for cannula. Femoral condyle is above, meniscus is inferior and to right, and posterior capsule is left. Visualization is through space between medial femoral condyle and tibial spine.

C With 70° endoscope extreme medial wall of posterior medial compartment is seen. There are small areas of synovial hemorrhage due to trauma in this patient.

D On retraction of arthroscope, posterior horn of meniscus comes into view. Femoral condyle is above.

Diagnostic arthroscopy of the knee

Intercondylar notch

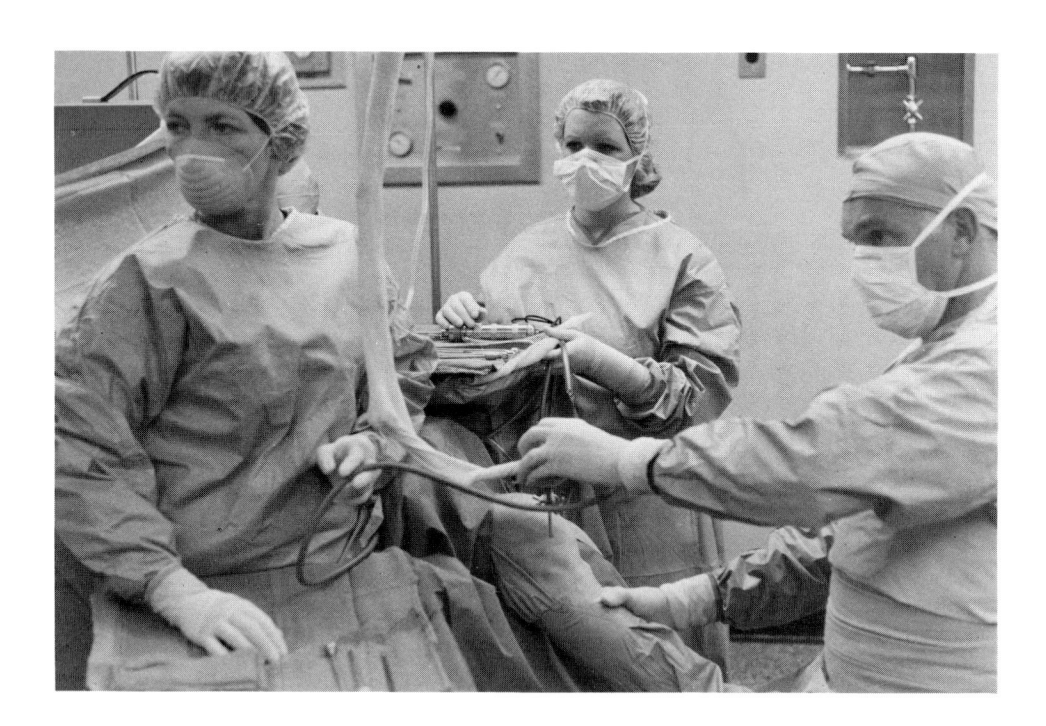

Patient	The patient is supine.
Knee	The knee is in 90° flexion with the foot resting in the surgeon's lap.
Assistant	The assistant is lateral to the patient's thigh.
Physician	The physician is seated. A drawer sign may be observed with manipulation of the tibia forward.
Arthroscope	The arthroscope is retracted and the inclined view turned toward the intercondylar notch. This prevents tangling with the membranous (alar) ligament.

MODIFIED GILLQUIST TECHNIQUE

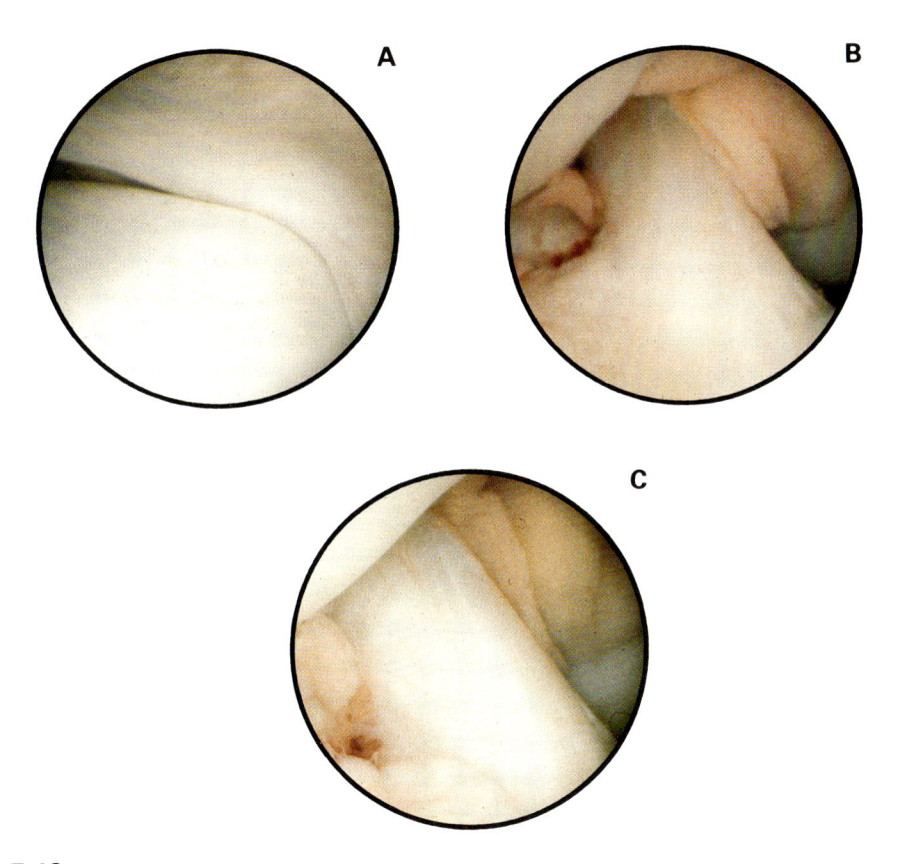

FIG. 7-12

A Arthroscope is retracted with leg in maximal distension. It is possible to see most extreme anterior horn of medial meniscus. Distension moves meniscus from normal position to over condyle. This is normal mobility on the meniscus anterior horn.

B Anterior cruciate ligament is in midfield and posterior cruciate ligament is immediately to left with fat and synovium covering it. This is relaxed position.

C Drawer sign is noted after stretching cruciate ligament and moving tibia forward. Dynamics of knee can be studied in this manner.

Diagnostic arthroscopy of the knee

Lateral compartment

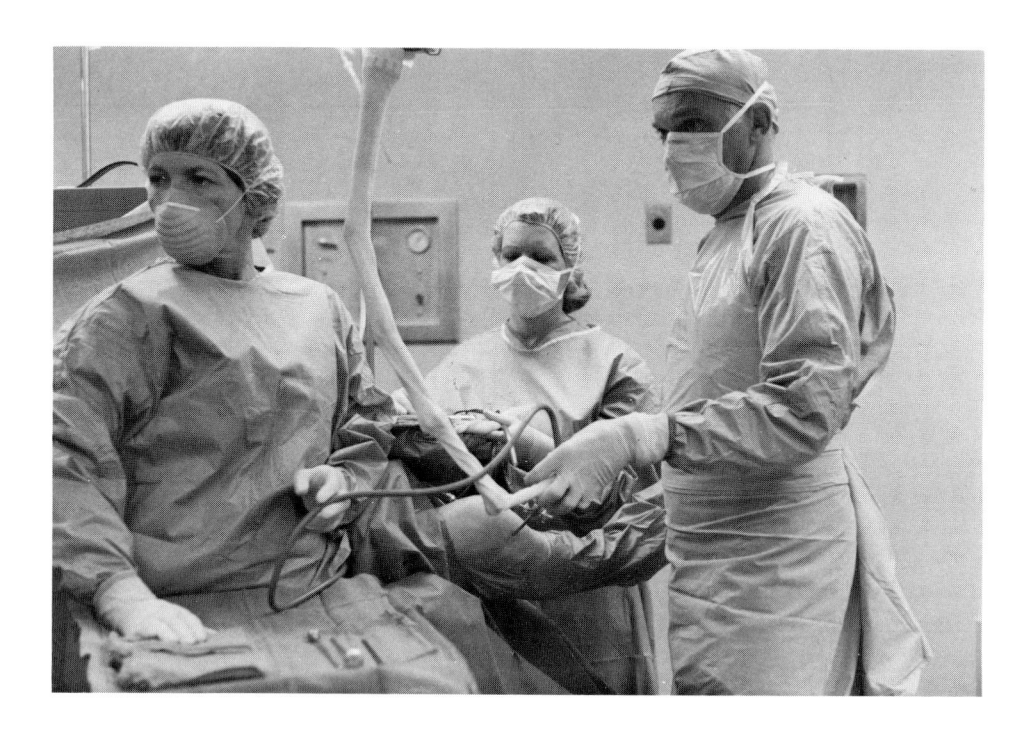

Patient	The patient is supine.
Knee	The knee is in varus strain with flexion up to 90°.
Assistant	The assistant is lateral to the patient's thigh.
Physician	The physician assumes a position lateral to the leg. A varus force is applied to the patient's leg with the physician's hip or thigh. As flexion is applied, the thigh tends to go into external rotation. This is controlled with the physician's hand on the patient's foot or ankle. The posterolateral compartment, especially the area above the meniscus adjacent to the popliteus tendon, is best exposed with the knee in 90° flexion, internal tibial rotation. At this point the ankle is actually pushed toward the ceiling. This is similar to the familiar "figure 4" position to expose the lateral meniscus by open methods. If the patient has a torn anterior cruciate ligament, then external rotation of the tibia is often necessary to keep the joint space open. This has eliminated the necessity of the more technically difficult transcutaneous posterolateral approach. An additional move can be made lateral to the condyle, into the lateral sulcus, and down the popliteus tendon sheath.

MODIFIED GILLQUIST TECHNIQUE

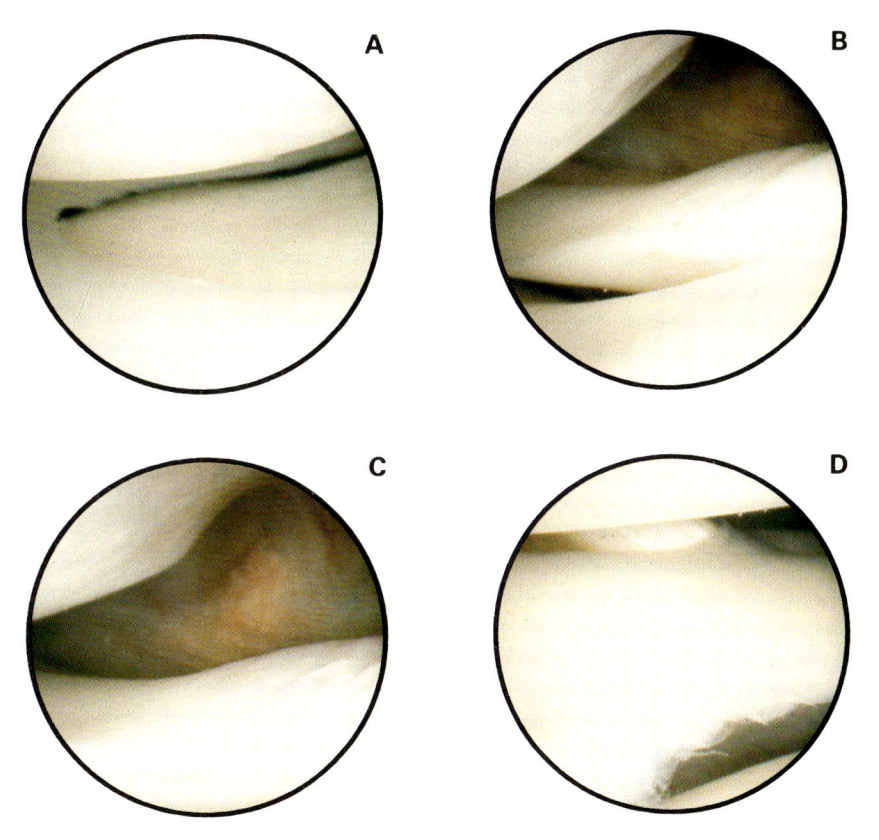

FIG. 7-13

A Overview of lateral compartment shows femoral condyle above and anterior horn of medial meniscus in foreground.

B With penetration of arthroscope, extreme posterior horn attachment of lateral meniscus in midfield is seen. Lateral femoral condyle is superior and to left.

C Through manipulation arthroscope passes on superior side of the meniscus below and femoral condyle above. It is possible with rotation and angulation to view over lateral meniscus and into posterior sulcus.

D With retraction and lateral movement of arthroscope, femoral condyle is above and meniscus is in midfield. Popliteus tendon can be seen between meniscus and femoral condyle. The leg is almost in a "figure of 4" position.

Diagnostic arthroscopy of the knee

Posterolateral compartment

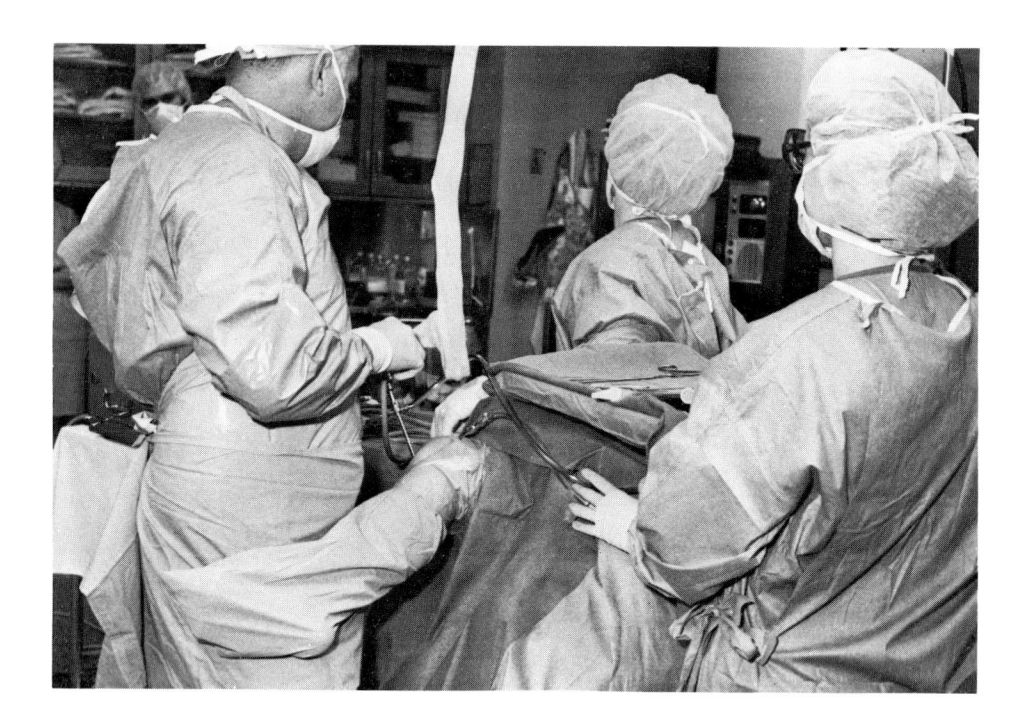

Patient	The patient is supine.
Knee	The knee is in varus strain with flexion up to 90°.
Assistant	The assistant is lateral to the patient's thigh.
Physician	The physician reduces the varus strain to allow distension of the capsule over the lateral sulcus. The horizon of the condyle is followed with the arthroscope to the popliteus tendon, and penetration is superior into the lateral sulcus.

Arthroscopic anatomy

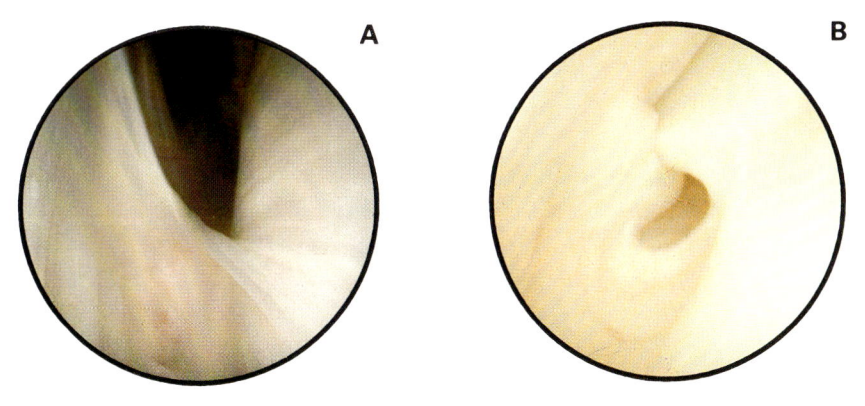

MODIFIED GILLQUIST TECHNIQUE

FIG. 7-14

A Superior view in lateral sulcus shows normal fold of synovium, which could be considered a plica. It is a normal variant and never seems to be symptomatic.
B Further penetration with arthroscope from lateral position permits passage down popliteus sheath. Opening of the sheath is in center.

Chapter 8

Pathology

Pathologic arthroscopic findings of the meniscus
Meniscus in service of the articular cartilage
Condylar disease
Osteochondritis dissecans
Articular disease
Ligamentous injury
Capsular tissue
Synovial disease
Healing of intra-articular tissues
Articular cartilage healing

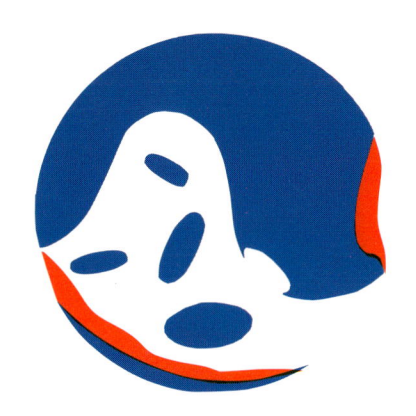

PATHOLOGIC ARTHROSCOPIC FINDINGS OF THE MENISCUS

The degenerative changes in menisci are mentioned in Chapter 7. The stage at which these become pathologic must be determined by interpretation of the patient's symptoms. Some patients have diffuse meniscal degeneration that is of little clinical significance because it is due to the aging process. Radiographically, juxtacortical increased densities may be apparent. Other patients have degenerative meniscal disease with large fragmentation or tears, which accelerate the degenerative process within a compartment.

Pathologic inspection of a cross section of menisci shows degenerative changes within the meniscal substance and a cleft separation between collagen fibers[2] (Fig. 8-1). A virgin meniscus rarely tears in its substance, except with cruciate ligament injury. However, it is possible for it to tear off of its synovial attachment (see Fig. 9-2, *A* and *B*) without there being degenerative changes within the meniscal substance itself.

Arthroscopically the earliest sign of degeneration of a meniscus is that the inner border loses its opaque nature and becomes translucent (Fig. 8-1, *A*). Arthroscopically it appears as though one is looking through ground glass.

This inner border can fragment and produce irregularities known as fringe tags (Figs. 8-1, *B*, and 8-2, *A*). These are asymptomatic. The small pieces that fragment out are cleaned by the synovial fluid and absorbed in the synovium.

A translucent inner border may separate from the body of the meniscus and appear as a fringe tear (Figs. 8-1, *C*, and 8-2, *B*). This particular lesion can mimic catching in or popping of the joint, often associated with a torn meniscus. In addition, it can produce a positive McMurray sign. Such a lesion is very difficult to identify during conventional surgery because the knee has been dried. Magnification by arthroscopy and floating of the fringe tag in a fluid medium are advantageous in identification. Many patients with positive physical findings of a torn meniscus but no lesion confirmed at surgery have been given meniscectomies "anyhow." They probably had fringe-type lesions. Obviously the symptoms are eliminated by total meniscectomy. However, these lesions need no surgical treatment; they are absorbed by the synovium, and the patient becomes asymptomatic.

Further evidence of degeneration is a cleft tear (Figs. 8-1, D, and 8-2, C). This may be a parrot-beak separation or a complete separation of the meniscus through its substance, forming a bucket-handle tear. This is the manifestation of deep interstitial fragmentation that has completely given way to stress. These interstitial defects can be palpated with a probe even before there is a separation of the meniscal surface.

A few patients examined arthroscopically for positive meniscal symptoms, including instability, have had normal findings. On repeat examination because of persistent symptoms for 4 to 6 months, a torn meniscus became apparent. There probably was a cleft tear deep to the meniscal surface or skin, which was not seen by the arthroscopist because it had not broken through the skin; yet fragmentation deep in the meniscus produced symptoms. Arthroscopy with local anesthetic allows repeat examination of these patients with ease and low risk. Therefore I believe that meniscectomy should not be performed in the absence of definitive arthroscopic evidence.

Meniscus injury can occur without resulting in a complete tear. In recent years I have observed deformation of the meniscus, that is, by a tearing ligamentous injury or even compressive forces, through which the meniscus can be injured internally, resulting in the deformation of its substance from the normal clean-cut triangular appearance. Or there can be deformation at its

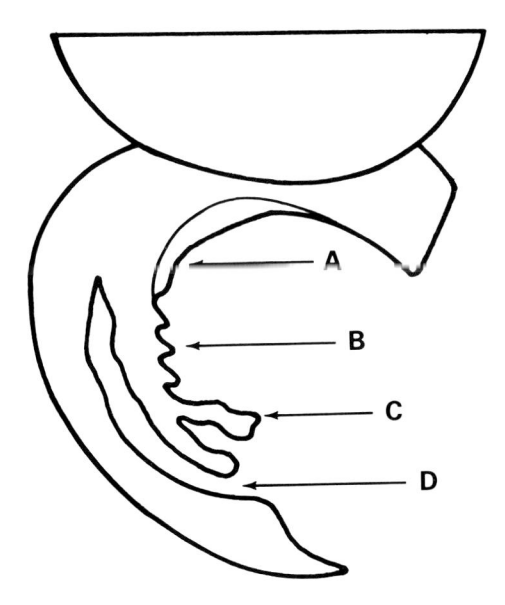

FIG. 8-1. *A,* Translucent inner border is first sign of degeneration of meniscus. *B,* Fringe tags occur when some translucent area sloughs off. *C,* Fringe tags or elevations of translucent inner degeneration may catch in joint and mimic positive McMurray sign. *D,* Cleft tears or complete tears within meniscus can occur when collagen bundles completely separate.

Diagnostic arthroscopy of the knee

FIG. 8-2

A Fringe tags.

B Fringe tear.

C Cleft tear.

D Diffuse degeneration.

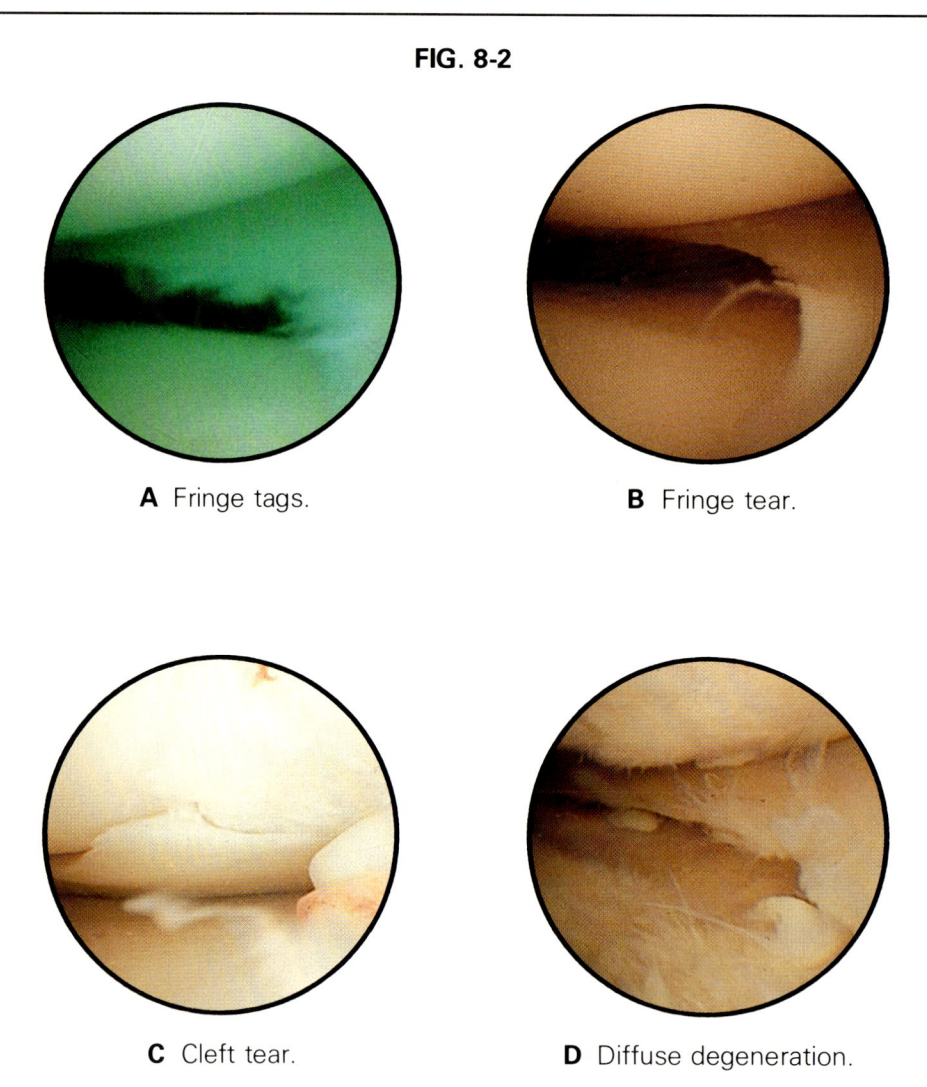

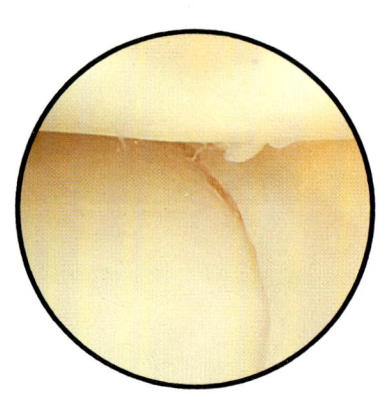

E Regenerated meniscus after total meniscectomy.

attachment. This lesion, of itself, does not require any surgical treatment, unless there is evidence of previous injury and/or disease. In an occasional patient it could be pain producing, which can be determined best by arthroscopy under local anesthesia. In a rare instance meniscectomy might be necessary.

Some patients have complete degenerative meniscal disease with large fragmentation tears that accelerate the degenerative process within the compartment (Fig. 8-2, *D*). This particular type of degeneration can be interrupted by arthroscopic meniscectomy. Even in the presence of substantial compartment loss, the knee can be improved.

Gross disruption of the meniscus affecting the articular surface is also an indication for meniscectomy.

There is another circumstance of diffuse degenerative meniscal and compartment disease without a specific mechanical meniscal lesion. This type of patient does not benefit from open surgery or extensive meniscal removal, since the degenerative changes are not being produced by the meniscus, but are general and diffuse. The absence of the meniscus will frequently lead to progression of degeneration in that compartment.

Arthroscopic observation of degenerative meniscal disease has added to our understanding of the management of meniscal abnormalities.

MENISCUS IN SERVICE OF THE ARTICULAR CARTILAGE

The importance of the meniscus has been well established;[1] it is in service of the articular cartilage. Some peripheral detachment or hypermobility of the meniscus is not an indication for removal unless the meniscus tear, degeneration, or motion is doing a disservice to the adjacent articular cartilage. Symptoms that interfere with the patient's job or life style may also justify meniscectomy in a chronic peripherally detached meniscus in the absence of articular cartilage injury. However, unless the meniscus is violating the articular cartilage as demonstrated arthroscopically, the patient is best off without meniscectomy if the symptoms are tolerable.

The ease and safety of arthroscopy with local anesthetic allows monitoring by repeat examination. The effects of the meniscus on the articular cartilage can be monitored before permanent articular cartilage changes are manifest by roentgenographic changes.

CONDYLAR DISEASE

Arthroscopy provides a method of study of condylar disease and its treatment in patients with articular cartilage defects. (See Fig. 11-3, *D*.) Such defects may be traumatically or surgically produced. I have followed up on patients who have had drilling procedures on fragmented and fissured patellar surfaces and have observed curettage and drilling procedures on the femoral condyle. Articular defects of up to 2 cm in diameter will generally heal with vascular fibrous tissue in 6 weeks; by 12 weeks there will be a complete fibrocartilage replacement devoid of a vascular base, and the patient may commence increased physical activity. Arthroscopy provides direct vascular monitoring of the tissue healing.

Diagnostic arthroscopy of the knee

FIG. 8-3. Arthroscopic view of 9-week-old articular defect that was curetted down to bone. Redness and vascularity have been seen to last from 3 to 6 months, depending on size of lesion.

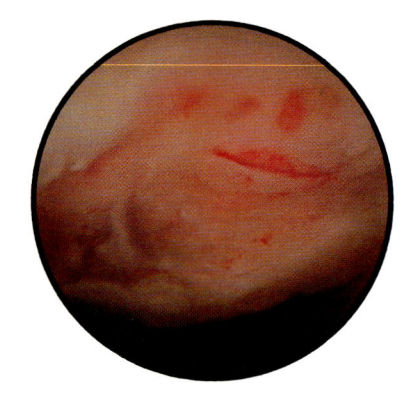

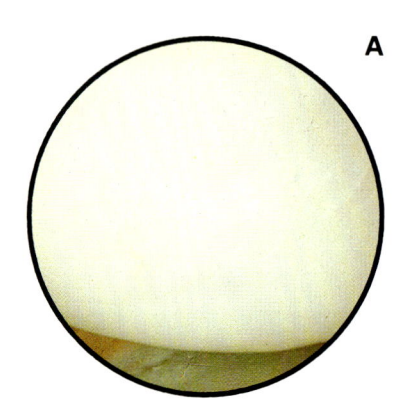

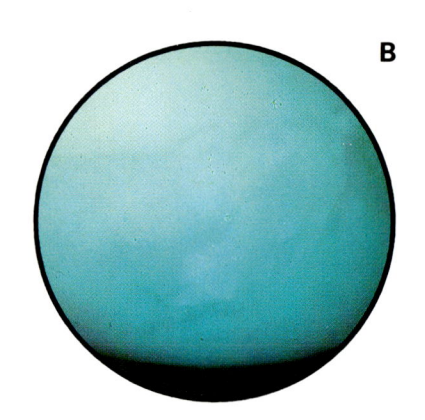

FIG. 8-4

A Arthroscopic photograph taken of smooth articular surface 1 year following open debridement down to bleeding bone. Notice the smooth surface.

B Same lesion with instillation of methylene blue shows slight roughening and incongruity of regenerated articular surface. Compare this healed lesion at 1 year with 9-week-old lesion in Fig. 8-3.

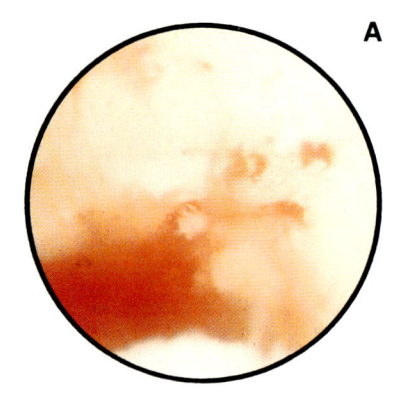

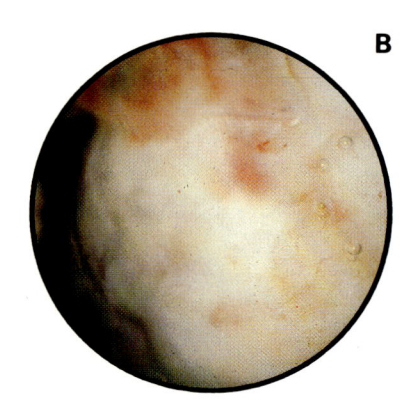

FIG. 8-5

A Acute drilling of osteochondritic lesion, transcutaneously and through intact articular cartilage, shows immediate backflow of blood when tourniquet is released.

B At 6 to 9 weeks following the multiple drilling there is still small punctate evidence of the vascularity in each drill hole, but palpation shows osteochondritic lesion to be secure.

In larger defects of up to 5 cm in diameter (Fig. 8-3), it takes as long as 6 to 12 months to obtain articular healing sufficient to bear weight. Following and monitoring these defects with arthroscopy under local anesthetic shows that the active healing as visualized arthroscopically correlates well with the clinical signs of decreased heat and inflammation (Fig. 8-4).

Drilling the articular bed will bring a blood supply into the area through the small drill holes. At 6 weeks the repeat arthroscopic examination shows each drill hole to have a vascular base, indicated by the redness at each drill site (Fig. 8-5).

Articular lesions near a synovial reflection will heal from the pannus covering. Also, the follow-up studies of patellar shaving show articular fibrous reactive tissue healing by 2 months without drilling down to bone.

OSTEOCHONDRITIS DISSECANS

Osteochondritis dissecans can be followed clinically in conjunction with arthroscopy with local anesthetic. In osteochondritis dissecans there is no correlation between symptoms and separation of the articular surfaces. The unseparated lesion can be monitored while treating with cast immobilization. Most defects heal in 6 months. The examination is enhanced by instillation of methylene blue for contrast. (See Fig. 8-4, *B*.)

When drill holes are made in an articular surface, as in a case of intact osteochondritis dissecans, there will be a small "shoestring" type of fibrous tissue protruding from each drill hole. This has been seen as late as 3 months after surgery. I presume that they eventually cleanse themselves. Surgical treatment of osteochondritis dissecans is discussed in Chapter 15.

ARTICULAR DISEASE

It is not unusual to observe articular injury or degeneration from articular disease arthroscopically prior to surgery. Articular disease worsens prognosis. Defects, in the compartment opposite that with the major suspected pathologic abnormality, have been seen which would probably have gone unnoticed in the absence of arthroscopy or with a unicompartmental arthrotomy. These defects have been curetted or debrided of articular cartilage or drilled to vascular bone prior to the Intra-articular Shaver methods.

Fissuring articular clefts often accompany patellar dislocations. Rather than shaving these patellar clefts, multiple 1-mm holes are drilled in each cleft. Repeat arthroscopic inspection at 4 months shows sealing over of these clefts, and the patient becomes relatively asymptomatic. It may be possible to manage selected articular disease without complete debridement or shaving, which often does not provide the best long-term results.

More recently I have used the Intra-articular Shaver for debridement in conjunction with the arthroscopic management of this particular entity. (See Chapter 18.)

Diagnostic arthroscopy of the knee

LIGAMENTOUS INJURY

A number of patients have had intraligamentous hemorrhage that would have gone unnoticed without arthroscopy. This is commonly seen with rotation injury to the knee and hemarthrosis. Arthroscopic examination shows no separation of either menisci. There is a so-called isolated anterior cruciate tear without disruption of the synovium. (See Fig. 12-1, A.) It may be hemorrhagic throughout its entirety, indicating the tear. Blood may disseminate through the adjacent subsynovial tissues in the intercondylar notch or into the fat pad. It should be noted that the so-called isolated anterior cruciate injuries universally show at least posteromedial and posterolateral capsular hemorrhage in the absence of posterior meniscal tears, but not to the extent that surgical repair is indicated. An isolated anterior cruciate injury is really a gross determination and does not reflect the diffuse disruption within the capsular tissues. Initially the knee may appear stable but may become lax with time.

I also have observed patients with minimal anterior cruciate injury, as seen arthroscopically and not detected clinically, progress within 3 years to marked rotational instability in the complete absence of the anterior cruciate structure (also seen arthroscopically). The apparent structure of the anterior cruciate ligament does not indicate its mechanical status. Performance of a drawer sign at the time of arthroscopy can be of some assistance in evaluating the integrity of that ligament.

The posterior cruciate ligament is equally vulnerable to minor injuries that often go unnoticed because the arthroscopy is performed through a single anterolateral portal. The posterior medial approach gives a much better view of the posterior cruciate ligament, and, as mentioned before, this compartment should be a part of every arthroscopic routine. The gross instability of the posterior cruciate ligament is often obvious clinically, but the status of the meniscus and the posterior medial compartment can be evaluated prior to any reconstructive surgery.

Some tears of the tibial collateral ligament are seen only intra-articularly. The patient has tenderness in the area but no palpable defect in the ligament. There is a synovial separation above the meniscus or hemorrhagic changes such that the tibial collateral ligament can be visualized from inside the joint. Tears and stretches of the popliteal tendon have been seen with hemorrhagic changes, but they do not require surgical repair.

CAPSULAR TISSUE

In patients with previous capsular injury and scar, the cannula and trocar meet more resistance during capsular penetration. It is a well-known principle of hand surgery that scar about the small joints and gliding tissues of the hand can be an impairment to function. The same is so of the knee joint but has not been given the same emphasis.

Furthermore, people who have had multiple surgical procedures have capsular fibrosis and constriction that does not permit mobility or distension of the joint. The most traumatic production of fibrosis follows a total-knee replace-

Pathology

ment. Arthroscopy shows the total knee virtually encased within the capsular structures (Fig. 8-6).

Scar is a result of every injury. Arthrotomy produces not only capsular scar, but intra-articular adhesions as well (Fig. 8-7). We have even seen intra-articular fibrosis bands protruding from the joint following arthroscopic lateral release. They have often been observed in patients who have had patellectomy and open synovectomy.

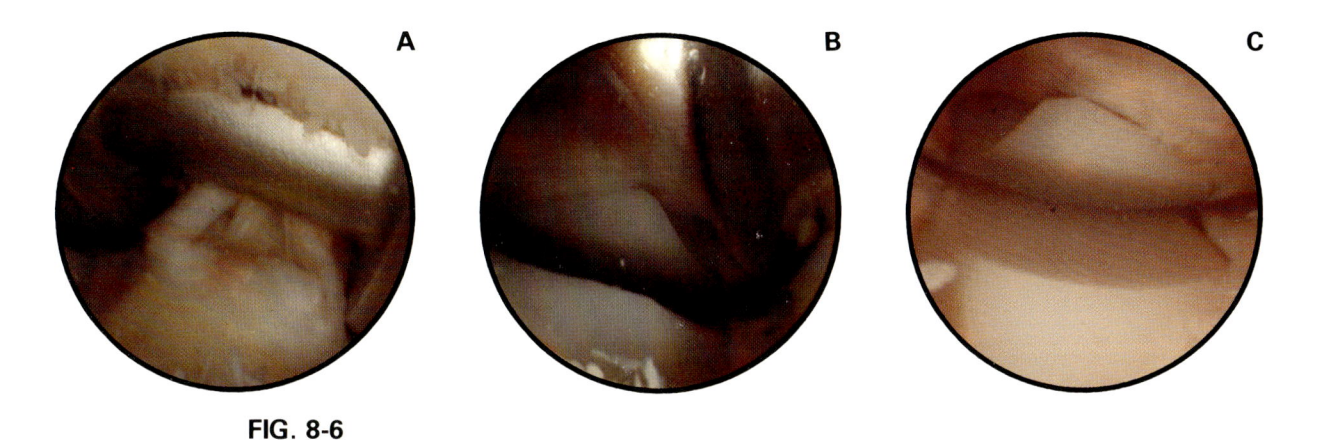

FIG. 8-6

A Arthroscopic view of geometric total knee showing transverse bar and tibial spine below.
B Arthroscopic view of geometric total knee with femoral condyle above and tibial plateau below.
C View of the opposite condyle showing femoral metallic component above and tibial polyethylene component below.

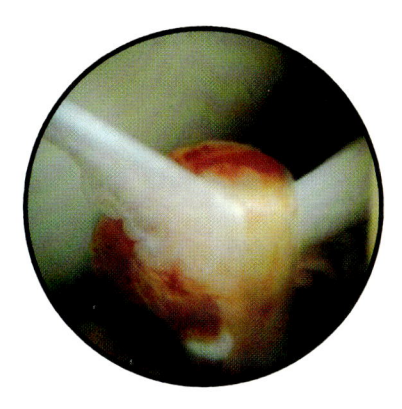

FIG. 8-7. Early fibrous adhesion approximately 6 weeks following open arthrotomy. Maturation occurs at approximately 3 to 6 months, with fibrosis replacing vascularity.

Diagnostic arthroscopy of the knee

FIG. 8-8

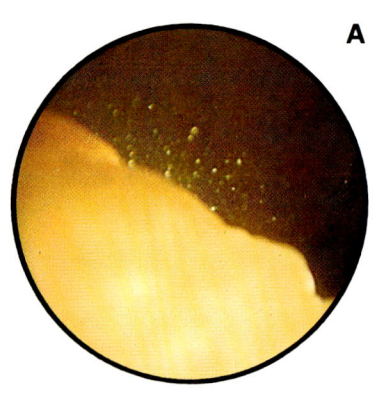

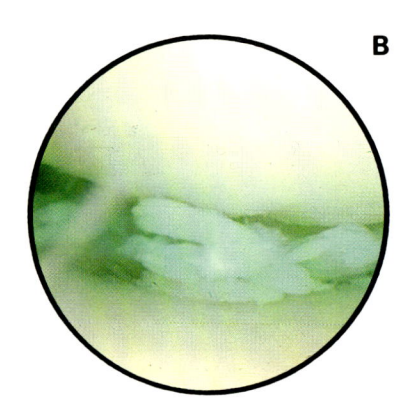

A Stardusting. Loose synovial and articular fragments seen in suprapatellar pouch with transillumination.

B Multiple loose bodies between tibia and femur in medial compartment. Methylene blue enhances visualization.

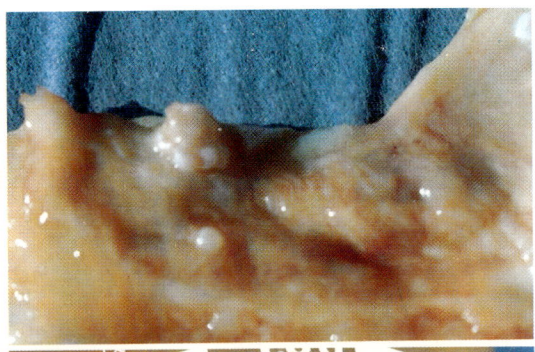

C Articular cartilage is engulfed by synovium if not removed from joint. May produce thickened synovium and capsule.

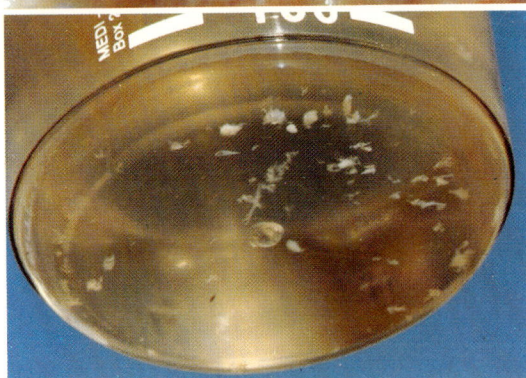

D Loose bodies vacuumed from joint through cannula.

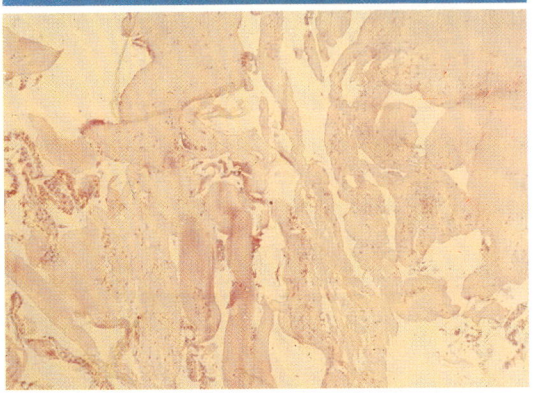

E Photomicrograph of synovial fluid cell block, including articular cartilage of synovial debris.

SYNOVIAL DISEASE

Synovial characteristics of aging are a response to gradual articular degenerative process. Small flakes of articular cartilage appear arthroscopically as stardust (Fig. 8-8, *A*), producing diffuse villous synovitis. Large loose bodies are easily seen (Fig. 8-8, *B*). Substantial synovial morphologic alterations occur in degenerative changes with loose articular pieces. The synovium eventually engulfs the articular cartilage (Fig. 8-8, *C*), but it may be removed through the arthroscopic cannula (Fig. 8-8, *D*). Because a synovial fluid cell block allows diagnosis of intra-articular tissue disease, biopsy is not required (Fig. 8-8, *E*). Lavage reduces the synovial reaction of edema, fibrosis, and capsular thickening. Synovial characteristics in various diseases are elaborated on in Chapter 13.

HEALING OF INTRA-ARTICULAR TISSUES

The method of meniscal healing is dependent on the extent of the injury and/or excision of meniscal tissue. If the meniscus has been completely disrupted from its synovial attachment or is removed surgically at that same level, then a rim of fibrosed tissue will regenerate from the synovium lining and its vascular bed (Fig. 8-9).

Scapinelli[3] reported studies on knee joint vascularity by injection methods. Review of his plates indicates a vascularity permeating the meniscus at a level heretofore not generally recognized. In some instances the injection dye came as much as two thirds into the area of the visible meniscal tissue. Immediately following subtotal arthroscopic meniscectomy the tourniquet is released and there is a surprising inflow of vascularity in the area of the meniscus (Fig. 8-10). The vascularity decreases with age. Subsequent arthroscopic inspections have demonstrated hemorrhage, fibrosis, and a regenerated meniscus on the basis of this vascularity. The question may be raised: Why does a meniscus not heal itself when it tears in an area of vascularity, for example, two thirds of the way back into visible meniscal tissue? The problem is that the detached peripheral tissue is somewhat devoid of vascularity. Once torn, it is abnormally mobile and never has a chance to reunite with its base. Of course, peripheral torn menisci at the level of the synovium can reunite in young people, although they might continue to produce symptoms.

The third way in which I have observed meniscal tissue healing is if the resected area was superficial even to the potential blood supply (Fig. 8-11). This shows the regrown tissue 2 months following total arthroscopic meniscectomy of the area not down to blood supply. A biopsy taken at this time of the regrown meniscus shows a fibrocartilaginous tongue of added-on meniscal tissue. High-powered examination shows this to be a fibrocartilage. Presumably it was either produced from the meniscus itself or was the result of blood clot adhering to the surgically roughened meniscus surface. It is a reactive fibrosis.

Diagnostic arthroscopy of the knee

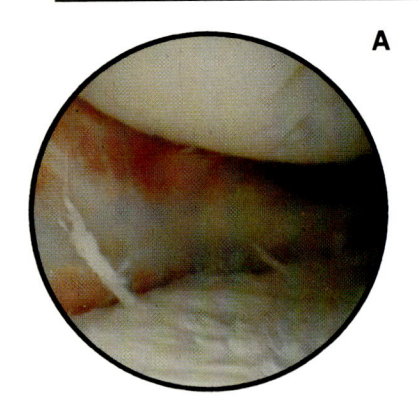

FIG. 8-9

A Arthroscopic view of arthroscopic total meniscectomy 3 months after surgery. Notice synovial contribution to small regenerated meniscus and mild degenerative arthritis in tibial plateau.

B Ten years after open total meniscectomy. Notice smooth articular cartilage and small regenerated rim from capsular and synovial contribution.

C Experimental lesion produced in dog meniscus showing synovial contribution filling defect at 2 weeks.

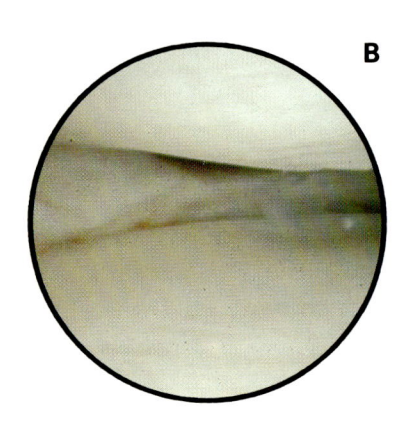

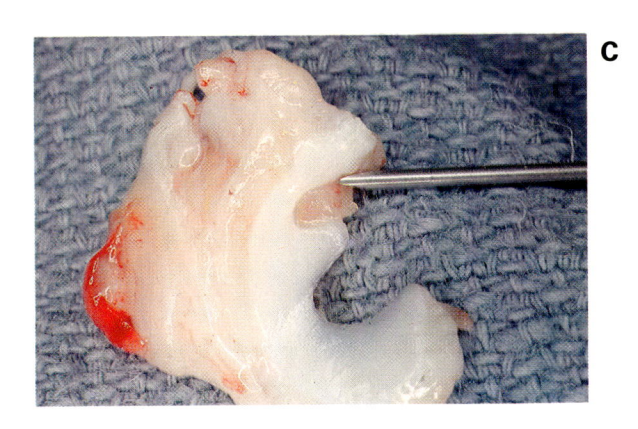

D Arthroscopic view of lateral compartment and popliteus tendon shows a regenerated meniscus 2½ months after virtually complete arthroscopic meniscectomy.

E Arthroscopic view taken of regenerated meniscal rim 3 months following total meniscal removal. Tourniquet is elevated.

F Arthroscopic view of patient in **E** but with tourniquet released. At 3 months there is still considerable vascular contribution to regrown fibrous tissue.

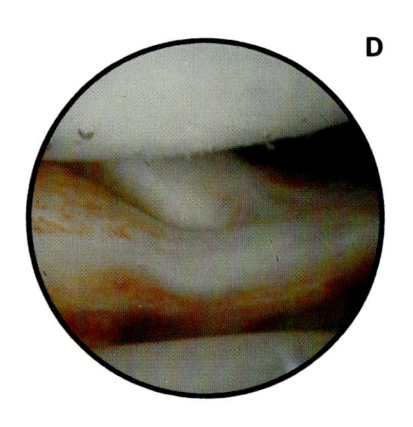

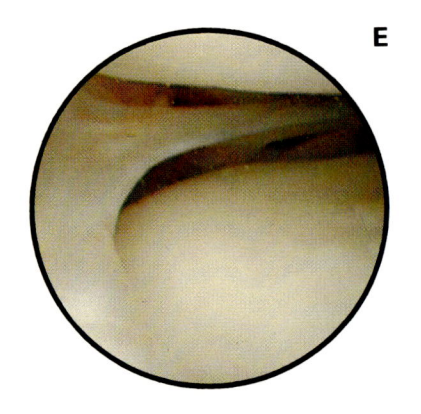

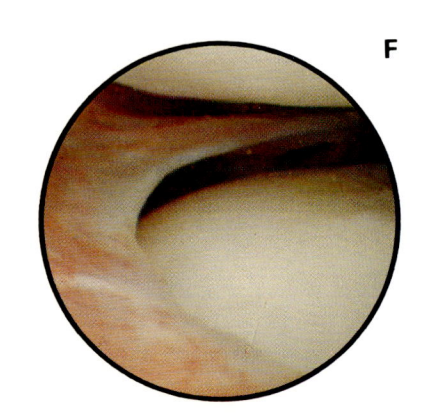

Pathology

FIG. 8-10

A Arthroscopic view taken at the completion of subtotal or selective arthroscopic meniscectomy. Tourniquet just released.
B After tourniquet release. Notice vascularity coming into meniscus in area heretofore not recognized.

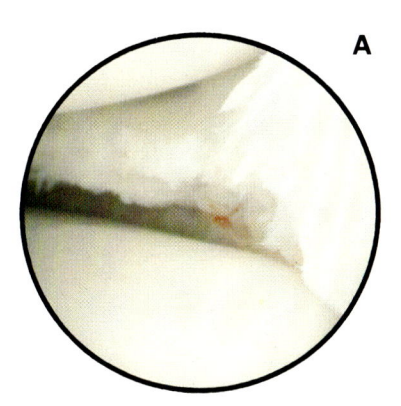

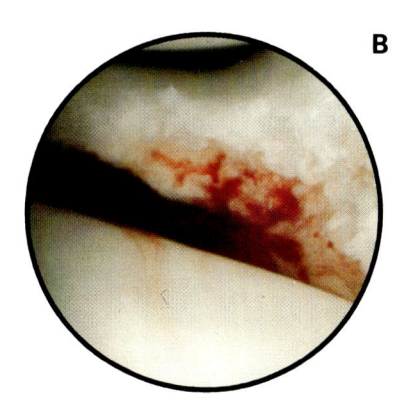

FIG. 8-11

A Arthroscopic view taken 2 months following subtotal or selective arthroscopic meniscectomy. Notice bridge of regrown tissue added to medial meniscus.
B Tissue biopsied under direct vision.
C High-powered photomicrograph of same tissue showing fibrocartilaginous tissue added onto meniscus.

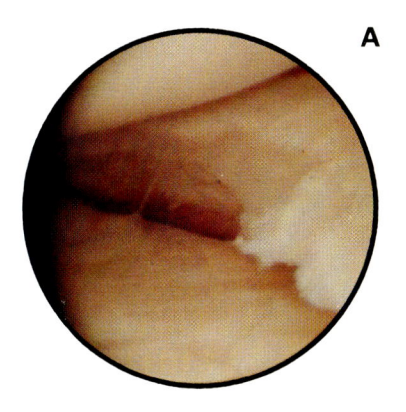

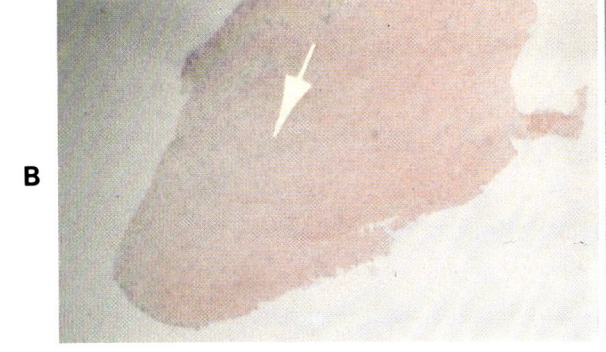

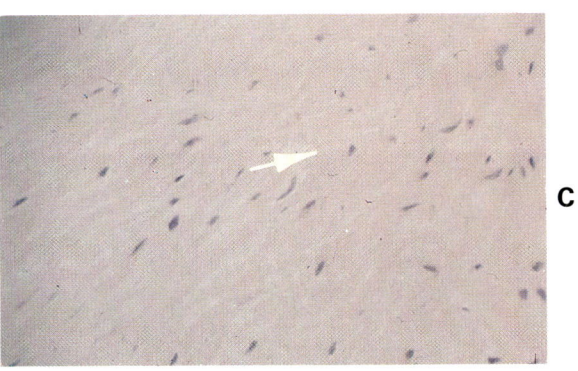

Diagnostic arthroscopy of the knee

ARTICULAR CARTILAGE HEALING

An acute traumatic injury to the patellar articular cartilage may be down to and including bony tissue (Fig. 8-12). On the condylar surface 1 week after injury there will be a fibrous tissue clot covering the surface (Fig. 8-13, A). This does not fill in the articular defect but just covers the base. When an articular defect is created surgically down to bone, either by drilling or curettage, it follows the same course as the natural history of an acute injury (Fig. 8-13, B). There will be a fibrous bed of vascularized tissue seen as much as 12 weeks later, especially in the larger defects (Fig. 8-13, C). Depending on the size of the defect (the smaller defects healing in a shorter period of time), the articular surface will fill in with a more mature fibrous tissue. By the end of 1 year there can be complete maturation (Fig. 8-14). Arthroscopy under local anesthesia has proved viable in monitoring the healing of the defects. There is an exact correlation between the arthroscopic view in the absence of inflammatory and healing processes and the clinical resolution of symptoms.

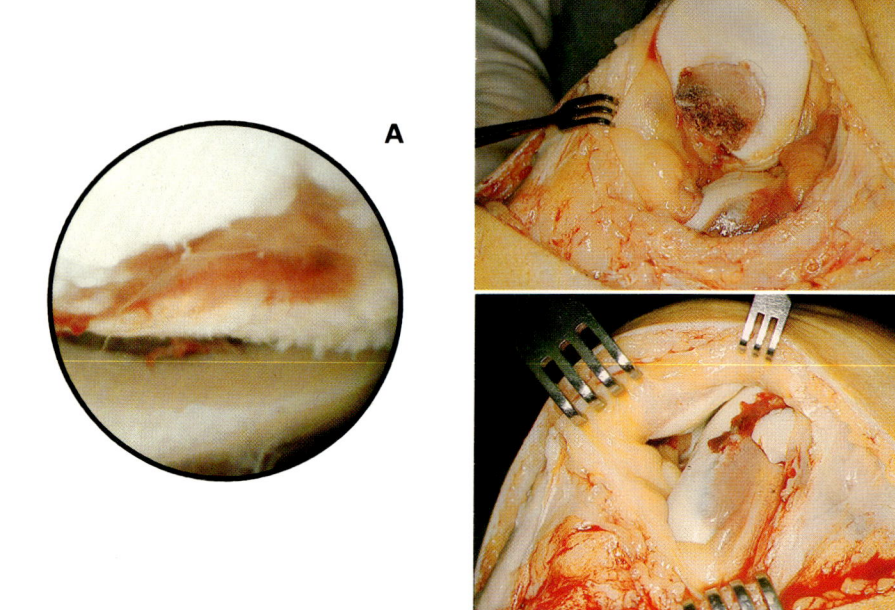

FIG. 8-12

A Arthroscopic view of area avulsed from femoral condyle 7 days before. Notice early fibrous bed.
B Gross anatomic view of patella 1 week following acute dislocation. Notice fibrous clot filling base of defect that had been avulsed down to bone.
C Lateral view of same patient showing avulsed portion of patella healed down to synovial overgrowth in lateral femoral condyle 1 week following injury.

154

Pathology

FIG. 8-13

A Articular defect of medial femoral condyle immediately after injury. Defect was full-thickness loss of articular cartilage, and blood supply was only evident by suction and decompression of joint in this area.

B Tibial plateau with 2-mm area curetted out of sclerotic bone. Suction and decompression demonstrate vascularity less than 1 mm adjacent to surface.

C Arthroscopic view approximately 12 weeks after surgery of large defect showing fibrous tissue. Healing in maturation on this size lesion would take approximately 3 months.

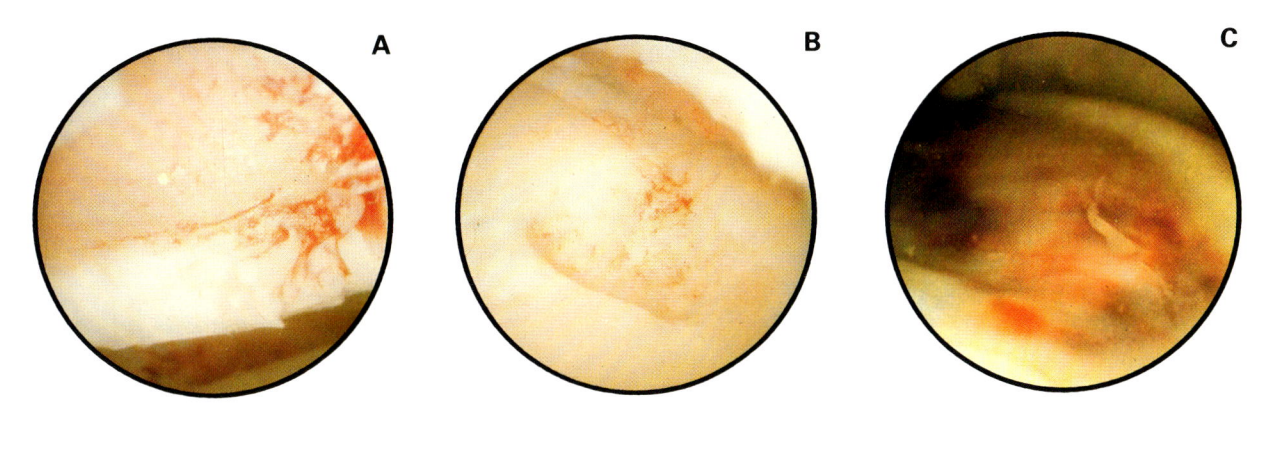

FIG. 8-14

A Arthroscopic view of an acute articular avulsion down to, but not including, bony surface 1 day after injury.

B Eight months following acute articular injury not involving bone, similar to that in **A**. This patient underwent intra-articular shave debridement of area. Notice resurfacing of even bone in patient under 30 years of age.

C Several months following acute articular injury down to, but not including, bony surface, ragged edge and progressive degenerative change are seen without resurfacing of bony defect in older patient.

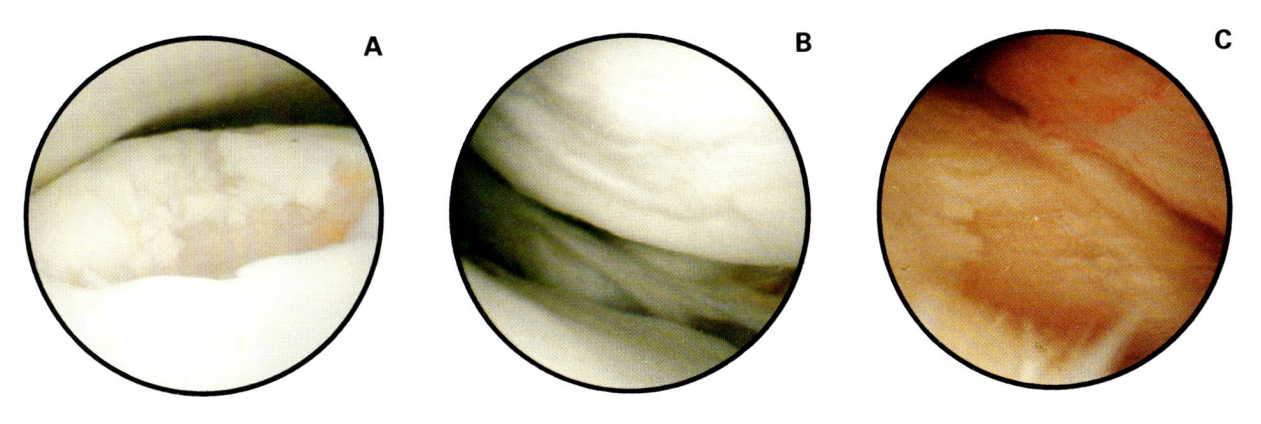

Diagnostic arthroscopy of the knee

In some acute articular injuries the articular cartilage will be denuded but not include a bony fragment. There will be either no bleeding or a microscopic amount of bleeding seen only by arthroscopy (Fig. 8-14, *A*). Untreated, these lesions progress with degenerative changes around their edges with continued flaking off of articular cartilage and only rarely fill in the base with fibrocartilage (Fig. 8-14, *C*). When this acute type of injury is managed arthroscopically by transcutaneous intra-articular shaving, I have reduced the morbidity by removing the debris and potential debris, and I have observed, as early as 1 month later, fibrocartilaginous healing across the defect (Fig. 8-14, *B*). These defects were not drilled to bone and were only a debridement of the leveling of the edges adjacent to the avulsed articular cartilage.

If the defect produced is superficial and less than full-thickness articular cartilage, it can be quite symptomatic with continued exfoliation of the articular incongruous edges. An arthroscopy plus intra-articular shaving (debridement of these articular lesions that are not through the full thickness of the cartilage) have prompted healing as early as 2 months, as seen by repeat arthroscopic examination (Fig. 8-15).

It should be noted that in severe degenerative arthritis in older people, articular lesions debrided down to bone have not been seen to resurface as they have in younger patients and young adults. Also, multiple drilling has been carried out in patients with osteochondritis dissecans, and healing of these articular defects has been seen and demonstrated both by arthroscopy and x-ray examination, at 6 to 12 weeks (Fig. 11-3, *D*).

Fissures in the articular cartilage have been observed with second-look arthroscopy. Some have stayed the same, others have healed, and others have fragmented and degenerated in as little time as 4 months.

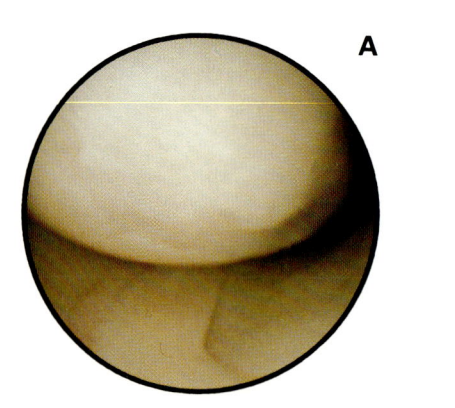

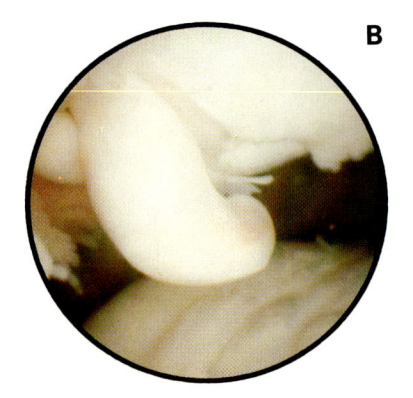

FIG. 8-15

A Arthroscopic view taken 2 months following acute injury and partial articular cartilage avulsion *not* down to bone. Intra-articular shave was performed, healing was complete, and patient had no inflammatory signs 2 months following injury.
B Arthroscopic view of chondronecrosis diffuse in 16-year-old boy, including patella and all articular surfaces. Notice large chunk of necrotic material hanging down from patella and degenerative change beyond femoral condylar surfaces.

REFERENCES

1. Krause, W., Pope, M. N., Johnson, R., Weinstein, A., and Wilder, D.: Mechanical changes in the knee, postmeniscectomy, J. Bone Joint Surg. (Br.) **57**(4):570, 1957.
2. Noble, J., and Hamblen, D. L.: The pathology of the degenerative meniscus lesion, J. Bone Joint Surg. (Br.) **57**(2):180, 1975.
3. Scapinelli, R.: Studies on the vascularity of the human knee joint, Acta Anat. **70**:305, 1968.
4. Tirgari, M.: The surgical significance of the blood supply of the canine stifle joint, J. Small Anim. Pract. **19**:451, 1978.

Chapter 9

Meniscal disease

Normal meniscus
Torn meniscus
Degeneration of the meniscus
Peripheral detachment
Discoid meniscus
Retained meniscus
Bucket-handle tear
Hypermobile meniscus
Postoperative evaluations

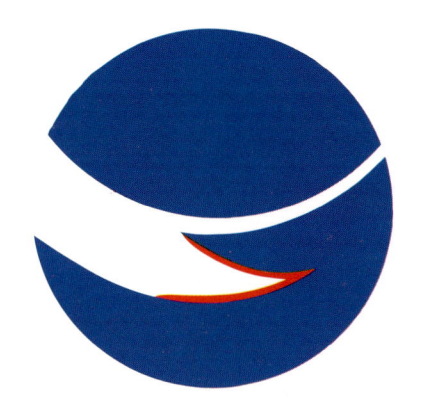

NORMAL MENISCUS

The meniscus is in service of the articular cartilage, and, unless it is violating the articular cartilage, meniscectomy should be avoided. In some patients, peripherally detached menisci or cystic degeneration within the menisci produces symptoms such that meniscectomy is clinically indicated. Arthroscopy with local anesthetic has provided an easy and safe method of examining patients with knee problems thought to be meniscal abnormalities. Observation of meniscal degenerations and their concomitant natural history has prevented a number of unnecessary meniscectomies.

The posteromedial and posterolateral approaches have revealed a surprisingly high number of meniscal abnormalities not visible on anterior inspections of the joint. Coexisting loose bodies in other compartments of the joint do not go unrecognized. Many can be managed arthroscopically by vacuuming the joint and thus avoiding a second arthrotomy. In some situations where there was certainty that an abnormality was located in a particular compartment of the joint, arthroscopy showed either that it was the opposite compartment which was involved or that there was a concomitant opposite compartment injury. The surgical plan was changed accordingly. Arthroscopy has saved patients unnecessary arthrotomy in areas where there was no meniscal abnormality. On the other hand, arthroscopy has revealed unsuspected lesions and has dictated an appropriate arthrotomy.

TORN MENISCUS

Arthroscopically there are four circumstantial signs of a torn meniscus (Fig. 9-1).

A normal meniscus has a sharp inner border, whereas an inner border that appears rounded off suggests a tear within the meniscus. A markedly rounded off meniscus is usually indicative of a bucket-handle tear.

The vertical and horizontal dimensions of the meniscus increase in size with degeneration. A large girth suggests a tear within the meniscus. Degeneration occurs first within the meniscal substance (Fig. 9-2, A). Breaking through of the clefts to the "skin" of the meniscus permits visualization of the tear.

Another circumstantial sign of a torn meniscus is a pileup of synovium around the synovial-meniscal reflection (Figs. 9-1 and 9-4, C). Normally transition is flat. If the meniscus is mobile and is catching and pulling off of its attachment, an exhaustive search for a meniscal tear should be made.

If the articular surface of the femur is roughened adjacent to the tibial spine, a tear of the posterior horn of the meniscus should be suspected (Fig. 9-1). This area will be localized and not diffuse. The condylar area is viewed with the knee in flexion. When the knee is extended, the area impinges on the posterior horn. When the tear is not visible anteriorly, it often can be identified by posterior puncture.

When any of these four signs exist, complete anterior and posterior inspections plus probing must be carried out to discover the torn meniscus.

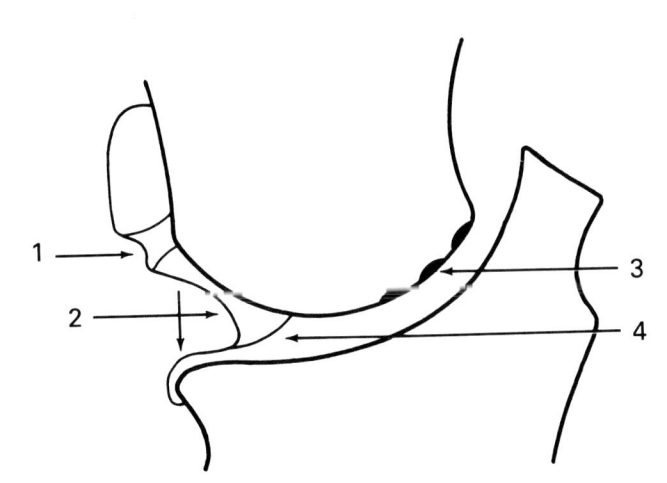

FIG. 9-1. Four circumstantial signs of torn meniscus. When any one is present arthroscopically, thorough search must be made for meniscal abnormality. *1,* Pileup of synovium at meniscal-synovial reflection probably exists secondary to abnormal motion of meniscal attachment below. *2,* Increased anteroposterior or horizontal diameter of meniscus probably reflects interstitial separation of collagen bundles of meniscus. *3,* Localized area of degenerative arthritis adjacent to tibial spine suggests posterior horn tear of meniscus in that compartment. Separate posteromedial or posterolateral inspection is obligatory to rule out lesion not visualized anteriorly. *4,* Rounded off inner border of meniscus suggests either parrot-beak tear or old tear of mensicus.

Diagnostic arthroscopy of the knee

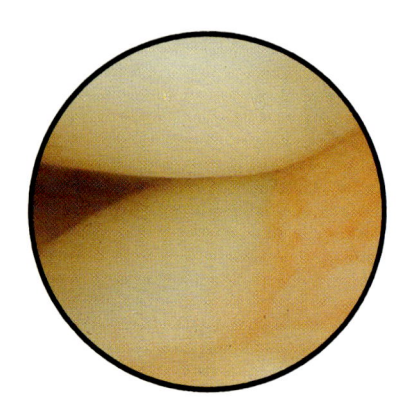

FIG. 9-2

A Pileup of synovium at meniscal-synovial junction suggests tear somewhere in meniscus.

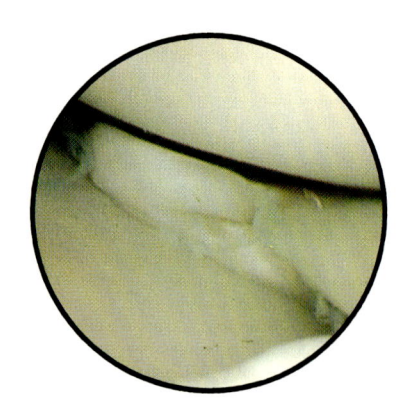

B Rounded inner border of meniscus or thickening in vertical or horizontal dimension is sign of disruption of meniscus.

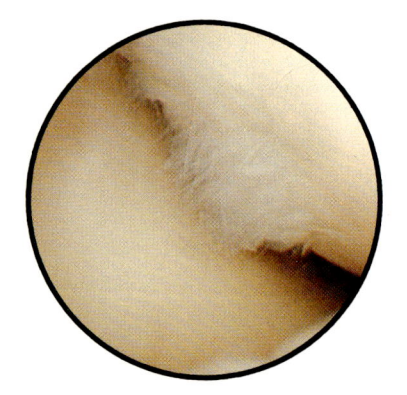

C Injured articular cartilage on femoral condyle adjacent to tibial spine alerts arthroscopist to posterior horn tear not seen from anterior view.

Meniscal disease

DEGENERATION OF THE MENISCUS

The stages of degeneration observed arthroscopically in the meniscus are outlined in Chapter 8. Fringe tears can mimic meniscal tears clinically (Fig. 8-2). These lesions, when identified arthroscopically, do not require surgical intervention; the synovial fluid cleanses them, and they are absorbed by the synovium, rendering the patient asymptomatic. It should be noted that this is an early sign of degeneration and that in later years a torn meniscus may develop, with separation of the collagen bundles.

Some patients have had clinical signs and symptoms of a torn meniscus but normal arthroscopic findings. Within 4 to 6 months, because of persistent symptoms, repeat arthroscopy carried out with local anesthetic showed a complete tear in an area easily visualized in the previous arthroscopic examination. It is my opinion that these patients had interstitial separations of the collagen bundles, with deformation of the meniscus causing the symptoms. Because the lesion had not broken through the surface of the meniscus, it was not visualized arthroscopically. It would not have been seen on an arthrogram either because there was no separation of the meniscus for the dye to move into.

We have observed patients with meniscal symptoms and deformation of the meniscus but no complete tears (Fig. 9-3). This is especially noticed in the posteromedial and posterolateral horns of the menisci. Meniscectomy is unnecessary if the symptoms are tolerable. In those patients who choose meniscectomy for symptomatic reasons, I have seen marked histologic degeneration in the area of the deformation. Undoubtedly the meniscus had undergone previous injury without complete separation. It should be restated that every effort should be made to discourage meniscectomy unless the articular surface is being damaged.

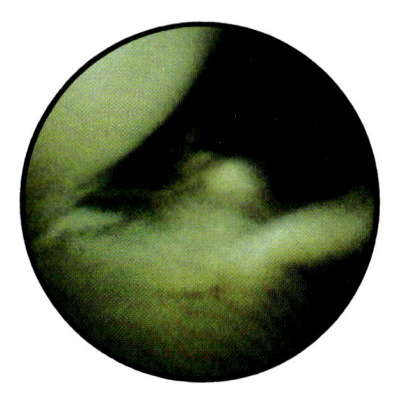

FIG. 9-3. Photograph taken with Needlescope. Posterior medial compartment via transcutaneous puncture shows deformation of posterior horn of meniscus with some "rose-petaling" effect of disruption of meniscal tissue on its surface. Femoral condyle is to left.

PERIPHERAL DETACHMENT

An acute peripheral detachment is easily identified (Fig. 9-4, A). It is important to inspect the area of the meniscal-synovial reflection in acute injuries. In hyperextension injury the separation can be off the anterior horn. In some rotational injuries, especially with a torn anterior cruciate ligament, the area at the tibial collateral ligament will have a separation approximately ½ to 1 inch in length, which can only be visualized with penetration of the endoscope into this area while valgus stress is applied.

In some patients no meniscal injury was visible anteriorly and the diagnosis was substantiated by posterior inspection. The separation was not seen initially with posterior puncture but only with slow retraction of the endoscope and angulation toward the tibial collateral ligament (Fig. 9-4, B). This again emphasizes the importance of posterior inspections. The same has been so for the posterolateral corner near the attachment of the popliteus tendon, because it goes through its synovial sheath posteriorly and laterally to the lateral meniscus. Peripheral detachments are not necessarily accompanied by degeneration of the meniscus.

The meniscal tissue may show hemorrhage deep to its surface. This represents a tear into the substance. Removal must be performed according to individual need. Many of these lesions may heal if they have a peripheral attachment (Fig. 9-4, D and E).

DeHaven[1] has reported some well-documented early results of meniscoresis. I have attempted to allow small peripheral detachments in adolescents to heal themselves. They will seal down in a couple of months, but they may remain painful and attenuated. If patients are very active, they are prone to complete tears within the next several months[2] (Fig. 9-4, C).

The ability to inspect these peripheral lesions arthroscopically encouraged me to treat patients in their early teens conservatively. My clinical impression that peripheral detachments would seal down and become asymptomatic has not been borne out, and existing clefts with synovial proliferation along the medial meniscus have been easily identified. Therefore, when there is peripheral detachment of the meniscus, especially with ligamentous injury, meniscoresis at the time of the injury reduces overall morbidity.

Meniscal disease

FIG. 9-4

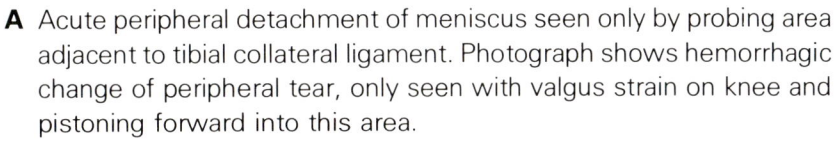

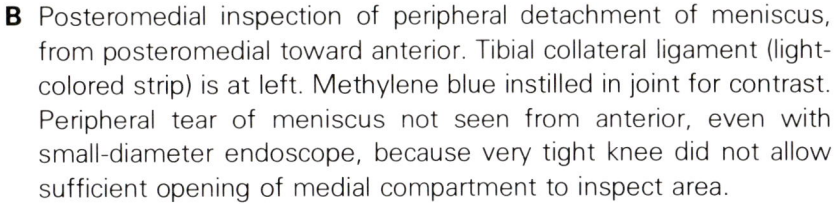

A Acute peripheral detachment of meniscus seen only by probing area adjacent to tibial collateral ligament. Photograph shows hemorrhagic change of peripheral tear, only seen with valgus strain on knee and pistoning forward into this area.

B Posteromedial inspection of peripheral detachment of meniscus, from posteromedial toward anterior. Tibial collateral ligament (light-colored strip) is at left. Methylene blue instilled in joint for contrast. Peripheral tear of meniscus not seen from anterior, even with small-diameter endoscope, because very tight knee did not allow sufficient opening of medial compartment to inspect area.

C Old peripheral detachments or tear of menisci evident by sulcus at synovial-meniscal reflection or buildup of synovium in area. Lesion correlates well with patient's symptoms of pain and instability.

D Gross anatomic specimen shows hemorrhage within posterior horn that was visualized arthroscopically.

E Open meniscectomy had been performed, and inspection into tear through meniscus from its posterior attachment was observed.

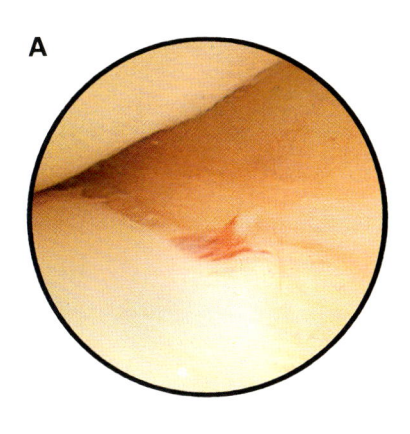

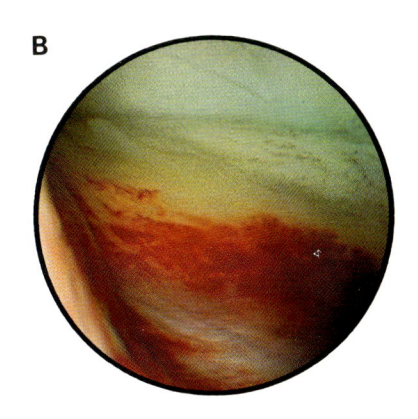

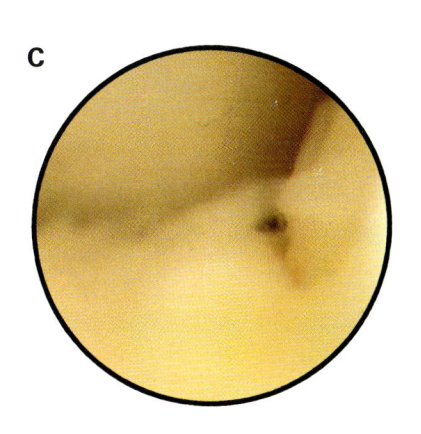

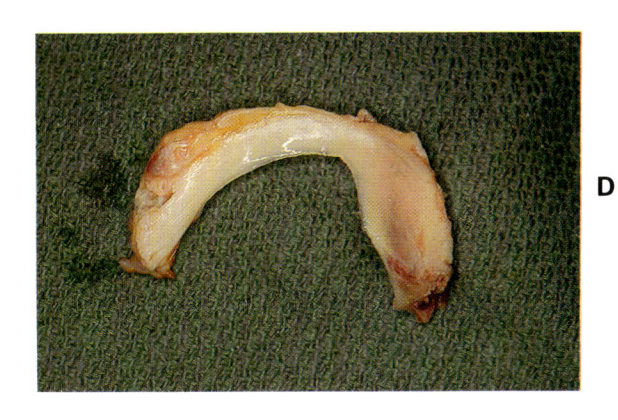

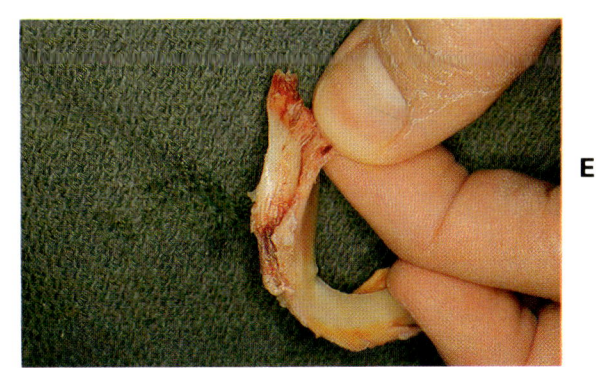

Diagnostic arthroscopy of the knee

DISCOID MENISCUS

The discoid meniscus is usually lateral. If its superior surface is not disrupted, the diagnosis may be overlooked because one interprets the superior meniscus surface as the tibial plateau. Difficulty in entering the narrow lateral joint space should increase suspicion of a discoid meniscus. The same would hold true for the rarer medial occurrence. The variations of discoid meniscus are from a thickening and a rounded inner edge to a total filling of the compartment. A central tear cannot be visualized from the superior surface view (Fig. 9-5). Arthroscopic resection can reshape the meniscus without total removal.

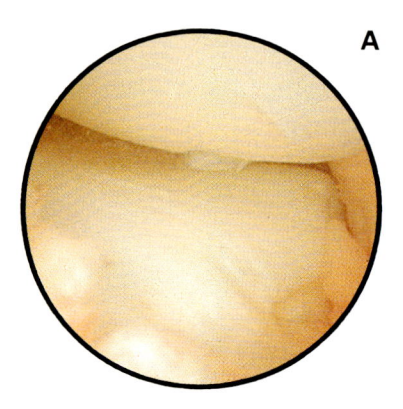

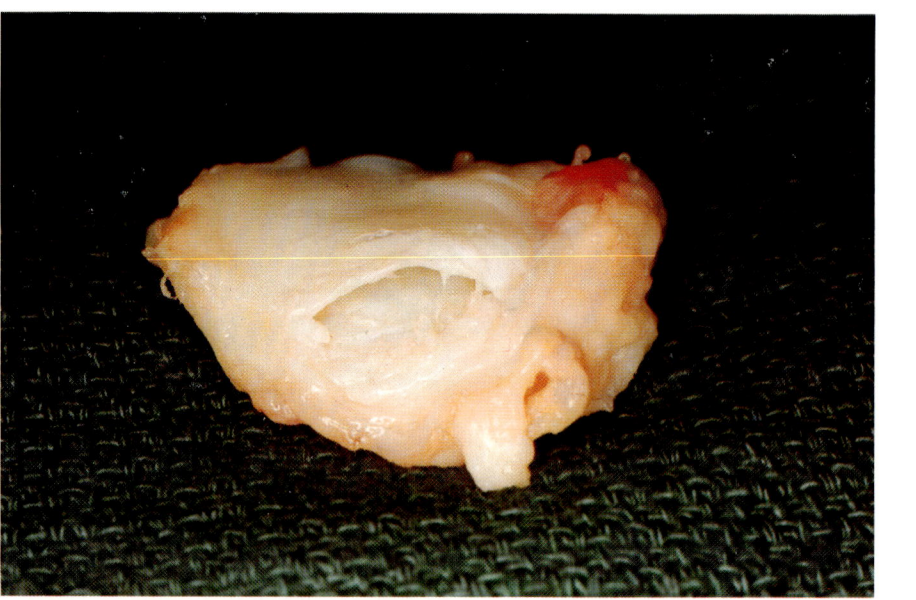

FIG. 9-5. A, Discoid meniscus usually fills entire compartment, most often laterally. Frequently symptomatic. Although tear may not be seen arthroscopically, horizontal cleft tears commonly produce symptoms. **B,** Discoid meniscus with degeneration and horizontal cleft tear within. Lesion would not have been identified arthroscopically because it had not broken through skin of meniscus, nor would it be identified by arthrogram; yet it was symptomatic, producing complaints of instability.

Meniscal disease

RETAINED MENISCUS

Patients have been referred for arthroscopic evaluation because symptoms persisted after short anterovertical arthrotomy for resection of the meniscus. A typical syndrome includes a partial tear of the anterior cruciate ligament, a short anterovertical arthrotomy, and a retained posterior meniscus. Histologic sections show that this is not a regenerated meniscus but actually an incompletely excised posterior horn. The medial compartment is most commonly affected. When these retained menisci are long standing in the presence of mild instability, degenerative changes are virtually always present, frequently manifested by the presence of loose bodies. Many of these patients had a tear of the posterolateral meniscus that was not identified at the time of arthrotomy but could have been seen, had a comprehensive arthroscopy been carried out prior to surgery.

For the first 10 years of my practice I subscribed to meniscectomy carried out at the level of vascularity, that is, complete meniscectomy of all degenerative meniscal tissue. I was trained to resect the meniscus, leaving a narrow supporting rim near the collateral ligament, and to make every effort to remove any posterior existing or potential irregular meniscus. This is not a total meniscectomy into capsular tissues (Fig. 9-6). I experienced 10 years of satisfactory clinical results.

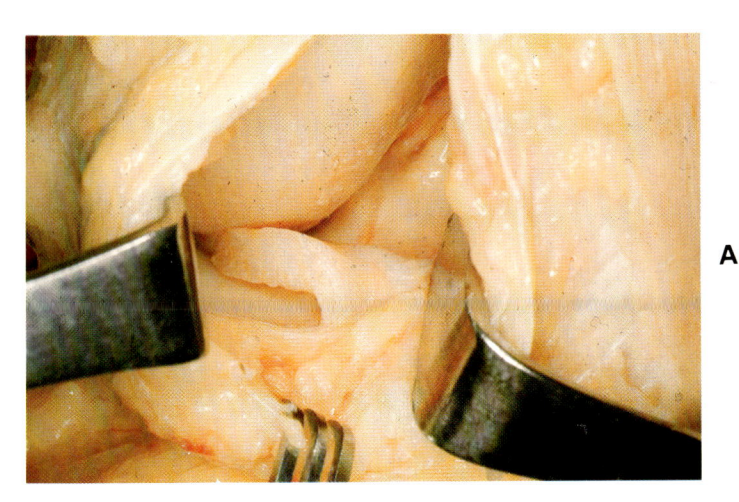

FIG. 9-6

A Level of resection on amputation specimen. Capsule is not violated. Small rim of meniscus remains in area of tibial collateral ligament for support.
B Arthroscopic view taken 10 years after subtotal meniscectomy.
C Reshaped meniscus in same patient 10 years after subtotal meniscectomy.

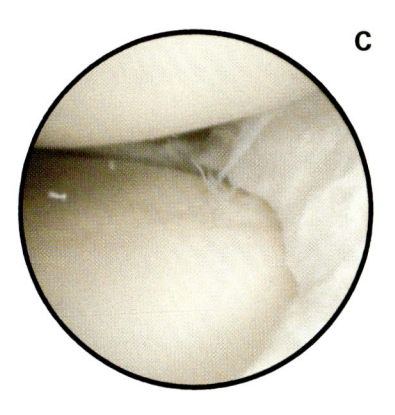

Diagnostic arthroscopy of the knee

Meniscectomy done at the level of vascularity allows regeneration of fibrous tissue. Meniscectomy done in the absence of vascularity allows only the irregular inner border of the regenerative meniscus to persist. This principle is partially true. The vascularity does come into the meniscus farther than I thought. This has been demonstrated in vivo, after subtotal arthroscopic meniscectomy. (See Chapter 8.)

Resection of a retained posterior meniscus will alleviate the symptoms if degenerative changes or loose bodies do not exist. When a retained meniscus is accompanied by rotary instability or loss of the cruciate ligament and medial supporting structures, resection of the posterior horn with a reconstructive procedure is indicated to reduce the progressive morbidity.

How is a retained posterior horn symptomatic? First, if there are degenerative or cystic changes in the existing rim, they can produce symptoms. Second, the posterior rim may be abnormally mobile, especially in the presence of ligamentous instability. Arthroscopic selective meniscectomy, that is, excision of all the abnormal and abnormally mobile meniscal tissue, removes the symptoms, and second-look arthroscopy shows a reshaped posterior meniscus rim (Fig. 9-7).

The posterior meniscal separations are perpendicular to the articular surfaces of the tibia and therefore are not visible anteriorly. It should be noted that in the presence of a torn anterior cruciate ligament or a ligamentous injury related to the medial compartment the possibility of an occult posteromedial or posterolateral meniscal tear increases. Therefore, whenever a completely or incompletely torn cruciate ligament is identified, potential posterolateral and posteromedial meniscal separations should be suspected; posterior puncture techniques are encouraged. The retained posterior tear can thus be avoided.

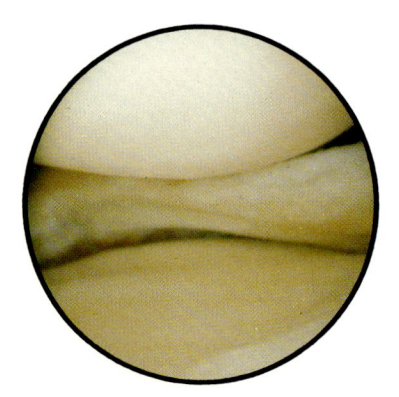

FIG. 9-7. Postoperative view of subtotal arthroscopic medial meniscectomy after 7 months in asymptomatic patient.

Meniscal disease

BUCKET-HANDLE TEAR

One of the difficult lesions for the uninitiated arthroscopist to identify is the bucket-handle tear (Fig. 9-8). Clinically, diagnosis is simple. Arthroscopically, because the mass of the meniscus is in the intercondylar notch, it interferes frequently with the penetration of the endoscope and blocks the view. After a few bucket-handle tears in the notch are seen, their diagnosis becomes easier. Some patients with a complete bucket-handle tear that is all the way in the notch will not have the usual lack of range of motion, making clinical diagnosis difficult.

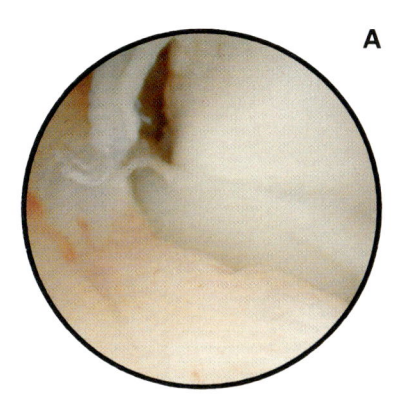

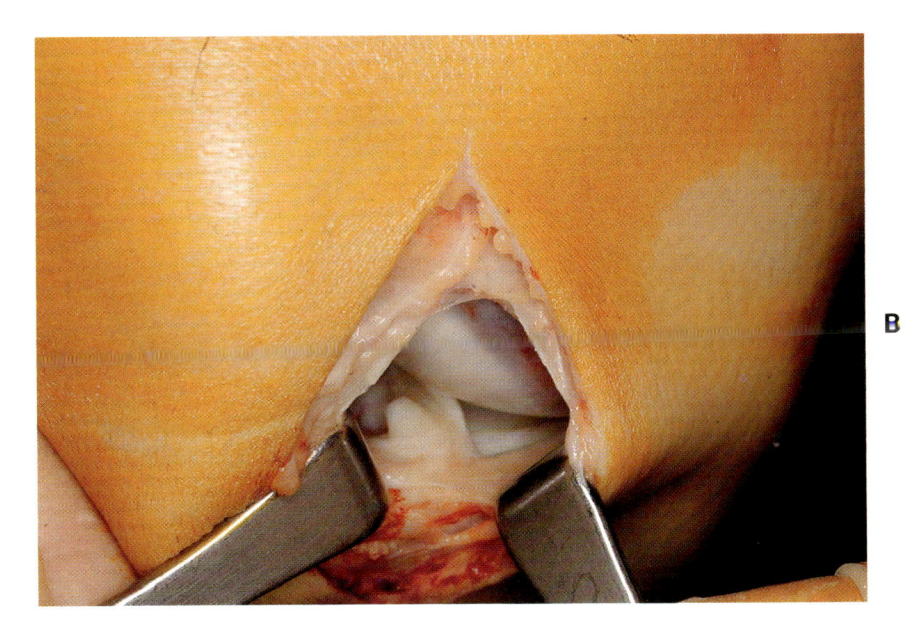

FIG. 9-8

A Arthroscopic view of a bucket-handle tear in intercondylar notch. Sometimes mass of displacement notch interferes with arthroscopic technique and should increase one's suspicion of possibility of tear, especially if there is only a small rim after passing by overlooked bucket-handle tear.
B Bucket-handle tear seen at time of arthrotomy.

HYPERMOBILE MENISCUS

Many patients have had meniscectomies for so-called hypermobile menisci. Arthroscopy has provided an opportunity to evaluate this condition and discern that there is no underlying tear within the meniscus. I have seen menisci that were clinically hypermobile and have confirmed the diagnosis at arthroscopy with manipulation of the knee. Attenuation of the coronary ligaments can allow the meniscus to become increasingly mobile and symptomatic. This can occur in patients who have normally hypermobile joints; the increased natural laxity of the joint allows increased mobility of the menisci. Unless the meniscus is injuring the articular surface, I advise against meniscectomy. The abnormality should be explained to the patient, and he should be assured that he does not have a meniscal tear or articular cartilage damage. Most patients will accept the diagnosis and modify their activities accordingly, thus avoiding meniscectomy.

POSTOPERATIVE EVALUATIONS

Postoperative arthroscopic evaluations are most commonly asked for in those patients who have had open meniscectomy through a short anterovertical approach. These patients often have an abnormal posterior horn of the meniscus, most often with concomitant degenerative condylar changes or loose bodies.

I have observed patients after a complete arthroscopic examination and medial meniscectomy, who, during the 8 to 10 weeks after surgery, have incurred a relatively minor knee injury with meniscal symptoms in the opposite compartment. I was hesitant to believe there was anything more than a tear of fibrous tissue; however, in several patients a second tear of the opposite meniscus has been observed this early in the postoperative course. Therefore any patient who has undergone a meniscectomy, but who has any meniscal symptoms postoperatively or slow rehabilitation, is a candidate for arthroscopy with local anesthetic to evaluate the intra-articular status.

These evaluations have shown that synovitis following arthrotomy is usually subsequent to degenerative arthritis with fine debris in the joint. (See Chapter 8.) Unexplained synovitis following arthrotomy is a clear indication for arthroscopy, at which time the existence of any other articular abnormality can be identified. Most often there are loose bodies in the joint, which can be vacuumed out during arthroscopy, preventing morbidity and prolonged rehabilitation.

The theory that synovitis is secondary to lack of patient initiative in progressive quadriceps exercises has been dismissed. In fact, arthroscopic inspection after arthrotomy shows that patients who are rehabilitated with vigorous and almost abusive progressive quadriceps exercise universally develop degeneration of the patellofemoral articulation with loose bodies. This most often occurs if activity is initiated within 6 weeks after surgery. During this time the articular surfaces are most succulent and more prone to injury due to the compressive and shearing forces of heavy progressive quadriceps exercises. For this reason, I have restrained patients in the healing phases from that type of activity and have initiated isometric quadriceps exercises until there is maturation of the fibrous tissue and no inflammatory signs about the joint. Then increased activity is certainly safe.

In a number of patients who erroneously were instructed or believed that the joint would heal faster with exercise, condylar injury or loose bodies have resulted. Thus I instruct patients to let the wound heal first; then work for range of motion and isometric strength; and then, following maturation and healing, work for increased power.

REFERENCES
1. DeHaven, K.: Personal communication, 1979.
2. Shneider, D. A., and Johnson, L. L.: Peripheral detachment of the meniscus: arthroscopic evaluation and clinical correlation, Orthop. Rev., Sept. 1977.

Chapter 10

Patellar disease

Chondromalacia
Dislocation
Subluxation
Osteochondritis dissecans
Acute fracture
Old fractures
Ruptured tendon
Contusion of the knee
Postoperative evaluation
    Patella baja
    Metallic prosthesis
    Subtotal patellectomy
    Patellectomy
Bipartite patella
Peripatellar synovitis

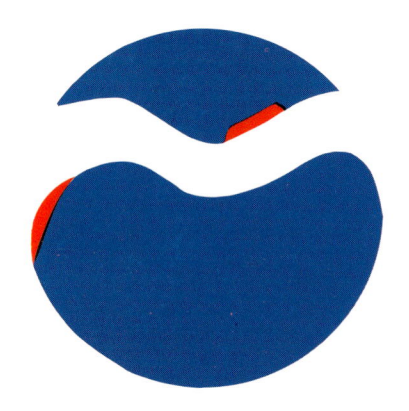

Arthroscopy has confirmed the clinical diagnosis in a high percentage of patients with patellar conditions, as opposed to meniscal lesions, which have a rather low incidence of exact correlation. Patellar conditions are relatively straightforward. However, some conditions clinically interpreted as torn menisci or torn ligaments have been arthroscopically established as patellar abnormalities.

The patella can be viewed in most patients through an anterolateral puncture. Very gentle retraction of the endoscope is necessary to bring the patella into tangential view. If there is any compromise in the inspection from below due to obesity, scar tissue, or osteophytes on the patella, a suprapatellar examination is indicated. (See Fig. 3-31.) If the patella is at all suspect as the primary site of abnormality, a suprapatellar examination is routine. If a dislocation of the patella is suspected, inspection from above is from the lateral side. Routinely, the patella is inspected from the medial side because it is technically easier. With the patient's thigh in external rotation, the patellofemoral articulation can be viewed from above. It is possible to see the undersurface of the patella, the suprapatellar pouch, and the fat pad.

With the patient under local anesthesia, dynamics of the knee joint can be observed while the patient contracts the quadriceps mechanism or by flexion and extension. An artifact is produced by distension of the capsule from saline in the joint. Therefore interpretations of patellar gliding are not completely valid. Inspection from an inferolateral portal normally makes the patella appear to overhang the lateral femoral condyle; this is not to be interpreted as a sign of malalignment of the patella. It should be noted that during quadriceps compression the tongue of the fat pad moves proximally under the patella. It is

Patellar disease

unusual for this to be symptomatic when palpated with the endoscope under local anesthesia or during quadriceps compression. Resection of the fat pad fronds under local anesthesia during patellar shaving demonstrated that this area was anesthetized. This is not so for the synovium in the suprapatellar pouch, which is quite sensitive.

Endoscopic palpation of the patellar surface can be carried out with local anesthesia. It produces no pain, even in chondromalacia. The sensation of crepitus is more often correlated to palpation of the femoral surface opposite the patella.

CHONDROMALACIA

Many patients are thought clinically to have chondromalacia of the patella (Fig. 10-1) because their pain is in the area of the patella or because with flexion and extension they have crepitus in the kneecap. They may complain of pain while walking up and down stairs or after prolonged sitting. The physical examination may produce pain in the patellar area, with quadriceps tightening against resistance applied to the patella.

Chondromalacia of the patella is a common diagnosis arthroscopically, but not every patient who has these symptoms has chondromalacia (e.g., many young girls who have no pathologic abnormality and an absolutely smooth, firm patella).

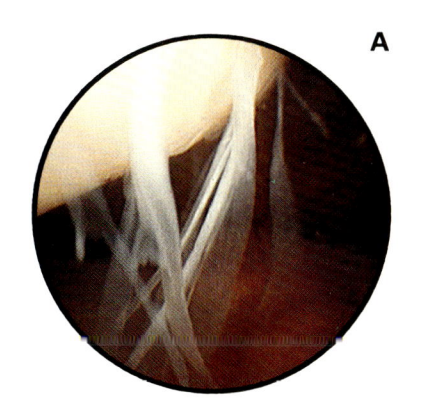

FIG. 10-1
A Chondromalacia of patella, bacon-strip type. Filmy articular strips can come off patella, especially at superior pole. These frequently are free in joint. Compare with Fig. 10-2.
B Chondromalacia of patella with saw-tooth type appearance of shaggy loose articular cartilage.
C Severe chondromalacia of patella with crabmeat-like material hanging down.
D Peripatellar synovitis with considerable vascularity in villous formation.

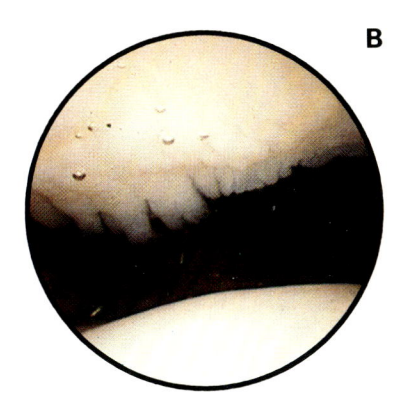

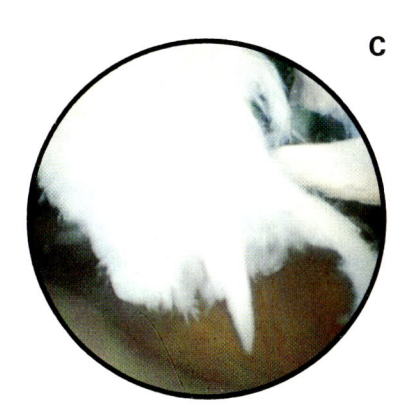

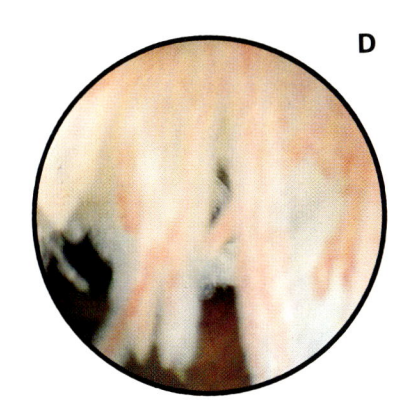

Diagnostic arthroscopy of the knee

In those patients who have some symptoms of chondromalacia as well as pain referred to the medial joint line, the differential diagnosis can be challenging. Arthroscopic examination with local anesthetic establishes the diagnosis. Most frequently, patients with this symptom complex and medially referred pain have chondromalacia patellae. Only a few have a torn meniscus, and some have loose bodies throughout the joint (Figs. 10-2 and 10-3). These can be vacuumed out, reducing the symptoms.

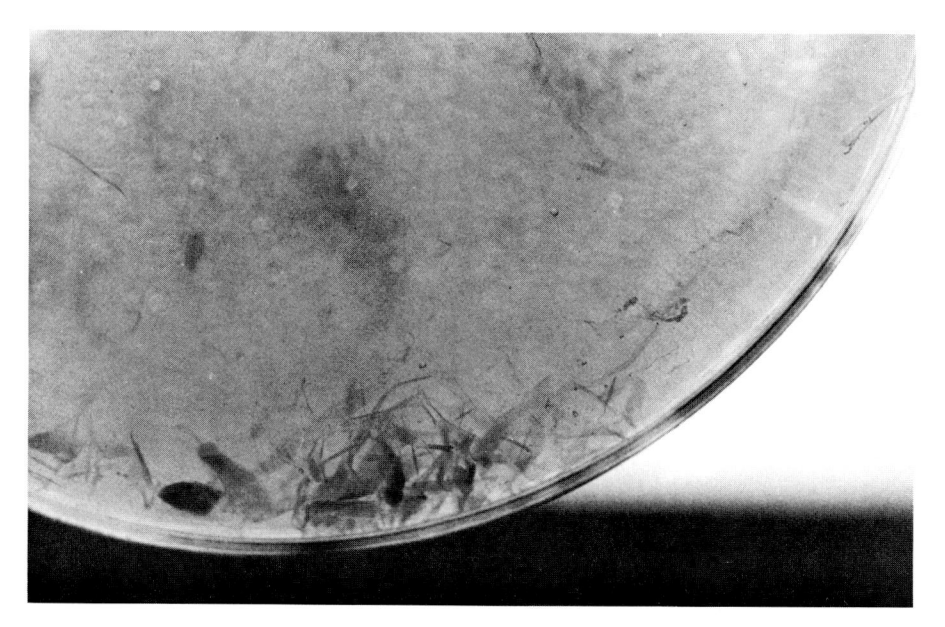

FIG. 10-2. Loose articular fragments off patella, such as seen in Fig. 10-1, A.

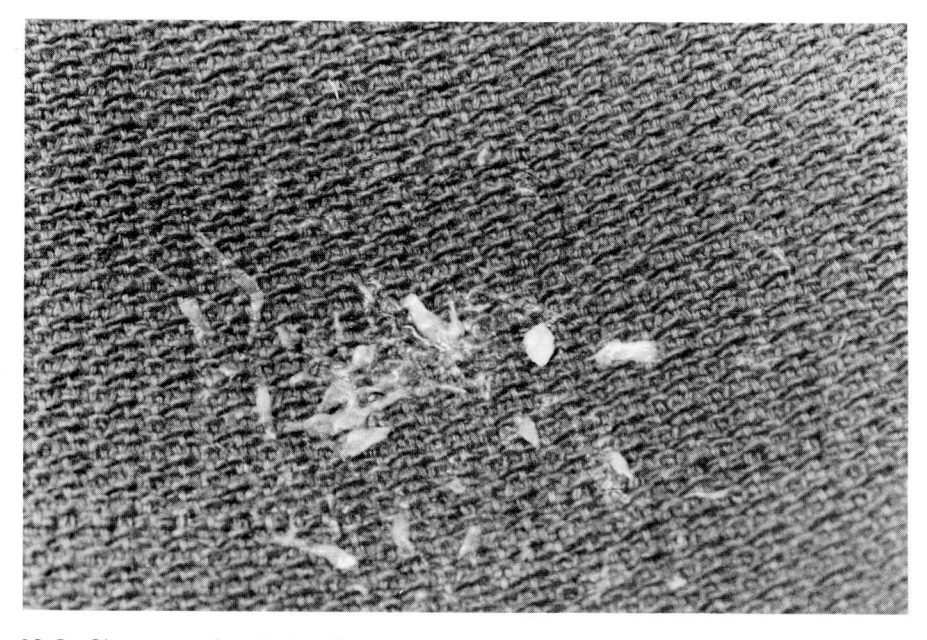

FIG. 10-3. Close-up of articular fragments strained onto towel for closer observation. Material must be absorbed by joint, producing discomfort.

Patellar disease

Confirmation of the diagnosis by arthroscopic direct visualization increases the physician's confidence in a conservative treatment program and engenders acceptance on the part of the patient or the patient's parents.

DISLOCATION

Dislocation of the patella is to be suspected in virtually any injury of the knee (Fig. 10-4). In a series of patients, ligamentous and torn menisci were suspected prearthroscopically, but the defects of dislocation of the patella were observed at the time of inspection of the joint. Arthroscopy has increased my suspicion that patellar conditions mimic meniscal or ligamentous abnormalities.

A defect in the lateral femoral condyle may be identified arthroscopically (Fig. 10-4, B). A piece of bone may be knocked out of this area in acute dislocations of the patella. The loose body invariably is in the lateral sulcus and is engulfed by the synovium in a couple of weeks. Occasionally there can be a patellar injury with acute dislocation of the patella (Fig. 10-4, C). Lateral joint tenderness may mimic a torn lateral meniscus.

Arthroscopy with local anesthetic is of special value in confirming a diagnosis of acute dislocation of the patella and dictating the appropriate treatment. The presence or absence of loose bodies can be established. Many articular injuries do not involve enough bone to show up well on roentgenograms, and even when a large loose body is involved, the x-ray examination may be compromised because of the patient's discomfort. Acute dislocation of the patella with a chunk of articular cartilage in the joint increases morbidity and prolongs rehabilitation. In some patients under local anesthesia, I have elected to remove the loose body arthroscopically with a Jaws modified pituitary rongeur. In others, the extent of the soft tissue tear was so evident that I recommended surgical repair.

At surgery for chronic dislocations of the patella, the articular defect can be seen over the lateral femoral condyle, with depression and abrasion of the surface. There may also be loose bodies in the posterior compartment; thus posterolateral inspection is important to their detection and removal. In addition, concomitant torn anterior cruciate ligaments and torn menisci may be seen in recurrent dislocation of the patella.

The lesion in the lateral femoral condyle is in a surprisingly low position (Fig. 10-4, A). The knee must be in approximately 90° flexion for the depression or articular fracture to occur with patellar dislocation. Therefore, during physical examination of the patient it is important that the test for hypermobile patella or dislocation of the patella be done with the knee at 90° flexion rather than complete extension. Some patients who in no way have clinical dislocations of the patella have very mobile patellae in complete extension, because the quadriceps expansion is taut in flexion. Other patients have no suggestion of mobility in the extended position or even a particularly high-riding patella; yet when the knee is brought down to 90° flexion and force is applied to move the patella laterally, they will grimace, confirming the presence of acute dislocation.

Diagnostic arthroscopy of the knee

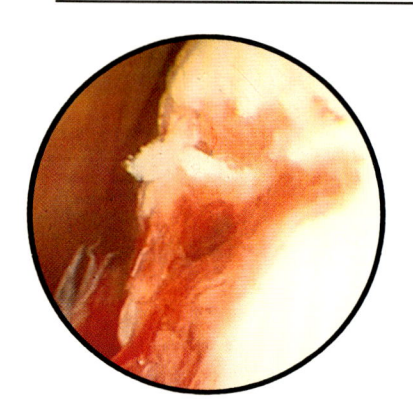

FIG. 10-4. Acute dislocation of patella.

A Hemorrhagic defect of articular fracture as seen in tangential view of lateral femoral condyle. This is usually one finger breadth superior and lateral to lateral meniscal-synovial reflection.

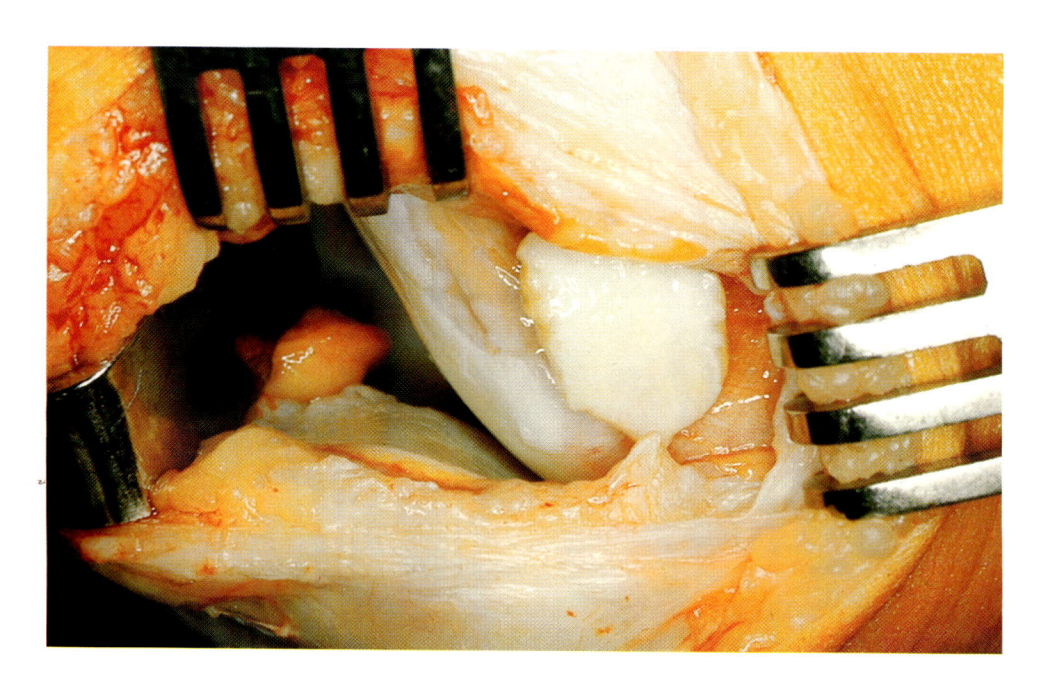

B Defect of lateral femoral condyle at time of surgery. Articular fragment engulfed in synovium laterally on lateral femoral condyle. Notice that knee is in 90° flexion for patella to shift out in this area.

C Arthroscopic view of same patellar defect.

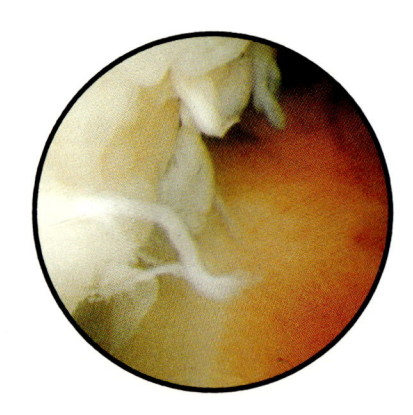

Patellar disease

SUBLUXATION

Subluxation of the patella is a common and frequently unsuspected abnormality. Review of my series shows that in a number of patients articular defects and depression of the lateral femoral condyle suggested a diagnosis of patellar subluxation long before it was clinically suspected. In addition, potential subluxation of the patella may be suspected in girls with knee symptoms, especially patellar, but no clinical evidence of a defect in the lateral femoral condyle. In a number of such patients in whom arthroscopic findings were normal, subluxation was confirmed within a year. Patients should be advised to watch for the manifestation.

OSTEOCHONDRITIS DISSECANS

Osteochondritis dissecans is a rare lesion of the patella that can be seen and managed arthroscopically. X-ray examination shows the defect best from the skyline view (Fig. 10-5, A). The arthroscopic view from the suprapatellar puncture shows the separate piece (Fig. 10-5, B).

My experience has been to simply remove that piece. Recently I have not noted any necessity to drill or curette down to bleeding bone as formerly had been anticipated. The defect heals over nicely with reactive fibrous tissue.

ACUTE FRACTURE

Arthroscopy can assist in diagnosis of an acute fracture of the patella (Fig. 10-6, A). It may not be possible to establish by x-ray examination the amount of

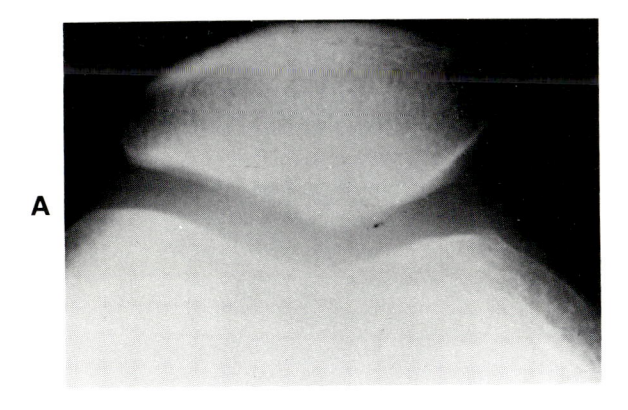

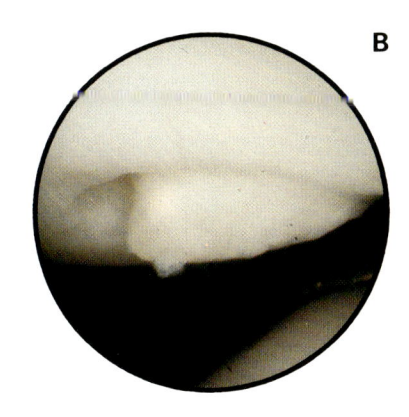

FIG. 10-5

A X-ray skyline view of patella with osteochondritis dissecans. Notice the defect at apex of patella.
B Arthroscopic view of suprapatellar pouch showing loose osteochondritic piece of patella in same patient.

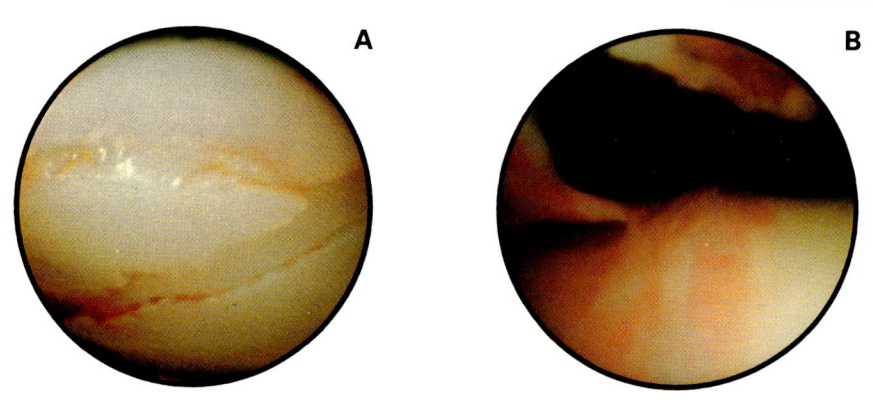

FIG. 10-6

A Arthroscopic view of minimally displaced intra-articular fracture of patella not requiring open reduction.

B Simple undisplaced fracture of patella with considerable morbidity related to fibrous adhesions coursing from patella to adjacent joint structures. X-ray examination of joint showed minimal changes; articular changes were considerable. Arthroscopic transcutaneous resection improved patient's mobility.

separation or displacement of the patellar surfaces. Arthroscopy with local anesthetic can establish the amount of disruption of tissue. Frequently there is an alteration of the articular surface not seen on the roentgenogram, and there may be loose articular pieces in the joint that can only be identified and removed arthroscopically.

Not every fractured patella need be examined arthroscopically, but there are those selected cases where it can help plan treatment.

The morbidity following a fracture of the patella may be aggravated by intra-articular fibrous adhesions (Fig. 10-6, *B*).

OLD FRACTURES

Some patients with old fractures of the patella have benefited from arthroscopic examination. It has been possible to establish complete union of the articular surfaces or an existing chondromalacia of the patella at the fracture line. It is not uncommon to have symptomatic fragmentation of articular surfaces at the area where even a moderately displaced patellar fracture existed.

Some patients have been arthroscopically evaluated for medicolegal purposes.

RUPTURED TENDON

Some patients have dysfunction of the knee secondary to either a new or old ruptured quadriceps or patellar tendon. It is especially important in reconstructive surgery to assess the entire intra-articular status of the joint. If no abnormality is detected by arthroscopy, arthrotomy is not indicated, and repair of the tendon can proceed, with surgery limited to the lesion itself. The fibrosis from extended surgery is avoided, and the rehabilitation time is shortened.

CONTUSION OF THE KNEE

I have seen patients who had direct blows to the area of the knee develop hemarthroses or suspected articular fracture of the patella. A direct blow to the synovium against the end of the femur can produce a hematoma and effusion, which can mimic a ligamentous injury. There is decreased range of motion. The diagnosis is easily established arthroscopically, and the appropriate conservative rehabilitation measures can be instituted.

It is possible that a direct blow to the patella will not fracture the osseous substance but only the articular surface. Diffuse stellate bursting fractures of the articular surface, with considerable morbidity, have been seen in athletes who have fallen on hard surfaces. There was no evidence of articular fracture. Debridement of the articular material shortened rehabilitation.

Other patients have had degenerative articular lesions but no fracture, the result of a severe direct blow to the patella. Many of these conditions are diagnosed only by arthroscopy, and these patients are excellent candidates for intra-articular shaving of the patella (Fig. 10-1, C).

POSTOPERATIVE EVALUATON
Patella baja

Postoperative evaluations have been carried out in patients with patella baja who have had aggressive Hauser reconstruction of the knee with considerable pain (Fig. 10-7). One of the causes of pain following an aggressive Hauser procedure may be compression of the fat pad between the patella and the tibia; subtotal resection may give relief of symptoms. In one patient with mild chondromalacia of the patella a recess of the plug of bone resulted in remission of symptoms, and patellectomy was not indicated. Another patient had only minimal chondromalacia of the distal pole of the patella and a rather large fat pad. An arthrotomy was carried out. The screw was removed from the tibia; the fat pad, which was massive and compressed in the intercondylar notch, was excised; and the roughened distal pole of the patella was shaved. This rendered the patient asymptomatic.

Metallic prosthesis

Complications have been seen in patients with metallic patellar prostheses. One patient had marked chondromalacia of the intercondylar notch, with pain on palpation in that area; removal of the prosthesis was recommended. A second patient had a painful knee without chondromalacia on the intercondylar notch; further conservative treatment was suggested.

Subtotal patellectomy

Evaluation of a variety of subtotal patellectomies has shown that the remaining articular surface was markedly fragmented and degenerated, that there was tilting of the patella in the junction between the patella and the patellar surfaces, or that the surfaces were irregular and symptomatic. Definitive treatment can only be based on arthroscopic evaluation and pathologic findings.

Diagnostic arthroscopy of the knee

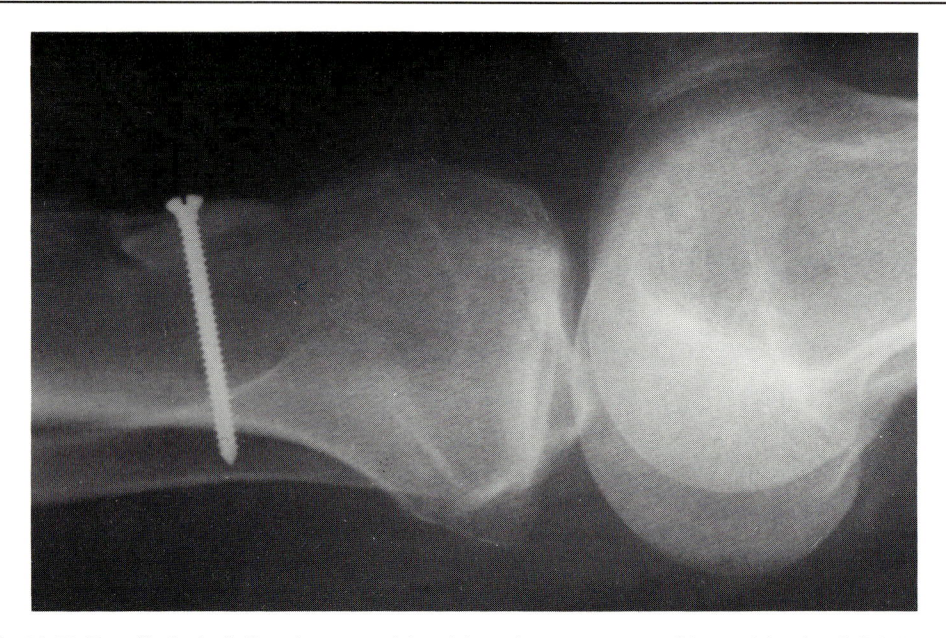

FIG. 10-7. Patella baja following considerable advancement of bony block of tibial tubercle. When this knee was brought into flexion, patella virtually abutted the tibial condylar surface.

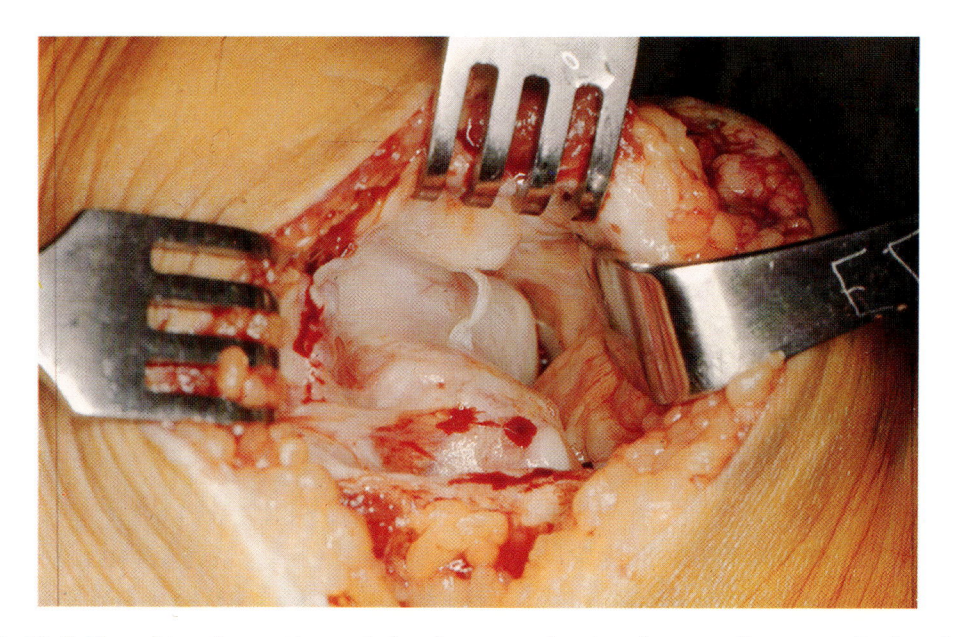

FIG. 10-8. Tag of tendinous tissue following tenorrhaphy after patellectomy. Patient had traumatic patellar fracture and subsequently developed catching and popping in joint. Arthroscopy demonstrated the lesion eroding intercondylar notch of the femur, which was removed by arthrotomy. This type of lesion could be removed by transcutaneous arthroscopy.

Patellectomy

Some patients who have had patellectomies have complained of pain or catching in the area of the arthrotomy or the site of the anastomosis of the quadriceps and patellar tendon. In one patient a rather large piece of tissue was hanging from the anastomosis, causing it to catch in the joint during extension and flexion (Fig. 10-8). Excision of the large mass of tissue rendered the patient asymptomatic. The diagnosis could not be established other than by arthroscopy.

BIPARTITE PATELLA

Most patients with bipartite patella and symptoms have no chondromalacia or articular separation in the area of the defect. Sometimes a differential diagnosis between the fracture and bipartite patella can only be confirmed arthroscopically.

In two patients with x-ray evidence of bipartite patella, severe pain over years was managed conservatively without benefit. Arthroscopic examination showed marked chondromalacia at the junction of the nonunion site. A subsequent arthrotomy and excision of the extra ossicle, which in fact was a nonunion site all the way through the articular surface, gave remission of symptoms.

PERIPATELLAR SYNOVITIS

In peripatellar synovitis long villae of synovium, very much like fringe, surround the patella. These synovial tags are not rheumatoid but degenerative in morphologic character. They can catch between the patella and the femoral surfaces, and often the tips hemorrhage and swell. Universal remission of symptoms has been achieved with conservative treatment, including isometric exercise and salicylates. Peripatellar synovitis is one anatomic explanation for knee discomfort in young girls (Fig. 10-1, *D*). If the tissue is massive and accompanies patellofemoral degeneration, arthroscopic resection is performed.

Chapter 11

Condylar disease

Fractures
Degenerative changes
Loose bodies
Degenerative synovitis
Osteochondritis dissecans
Osteochondral defects
Preoperative evaluations
Postoperative evaluations

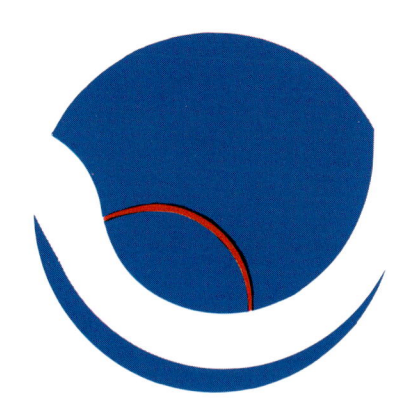

Arthroscopy provides a method of observation of the articular cartilage not available by any other method. By the time a roentgenogram shows juxta-articular hypertrophic bony changes, articular cartilage disease is usually far advanced. Still, the x-ray examination does not reveal whether there is regenerated articular surface, complete loss of articular surface, or raw ebonated bone. The presence or absence of most loose bodies cannot be identified except by arthroscopy.

FRACTURES

The existence of an intra-articular fracture of the knee joint with ligamentous injury can be determined by arthroscopy. Inspection of the joint can establish the amount of displacement and the presence or absence of concomitant intra-articular ligamentous or meniscal tears. For example, if a patient has a medial plateau fracture with displacement sufficient to warrant reduction by open surgery, there may be an accompanying lateral compartment tear or cruciate ligament tear. The amount of surgical dissection necessary to reduce the fracture can be limited by knowledge obtained arthroscopically. The meniscus need not be unnecessarily removed to reduce an

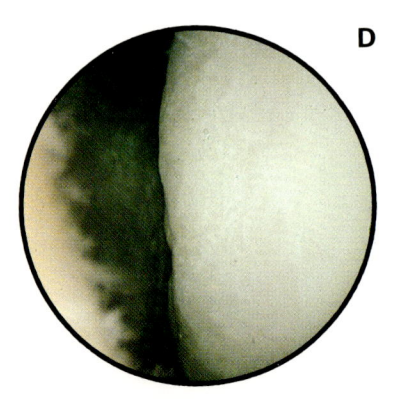

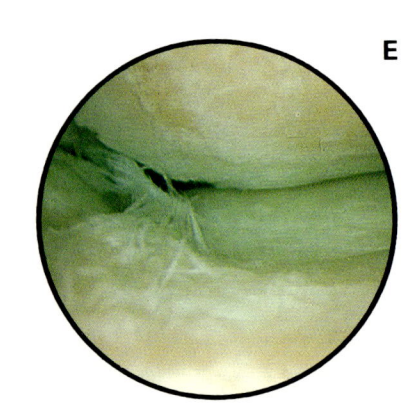

Condylar disease

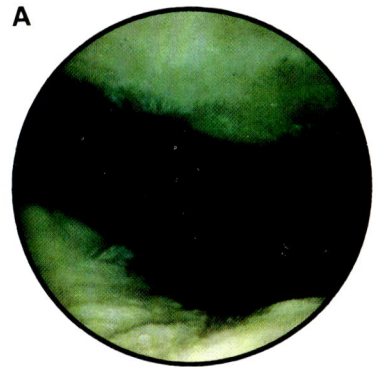

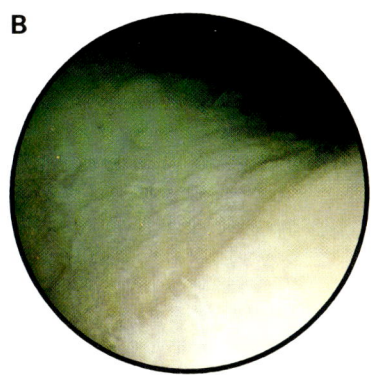

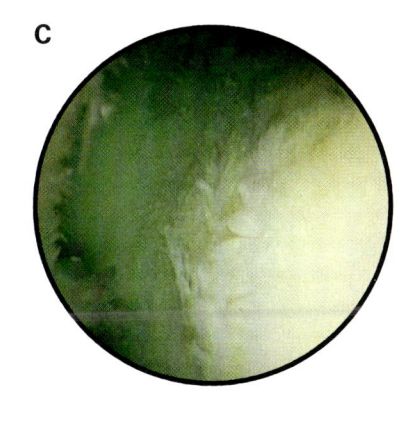

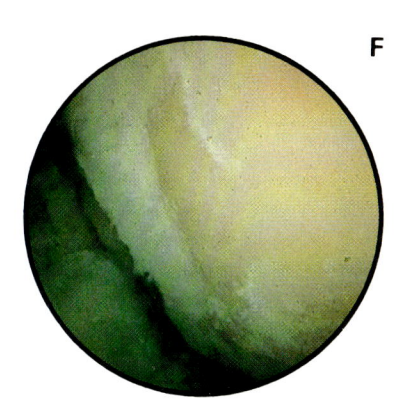

FIG. 11-1

A Motion is involved in arthroscopy. Starting superiorly, view under patella; view intercondylar notch from medial. Juxta-articular surfaces are markedly degenerated.

B With slight retraction of endoscope, view now encompasses only intercondylar notch, with loss of articular surface. Methylene blue is in joint. Patella is not seen.

C Farther down intercondylar notch, fat pad comes into view at left.

D Endoscope moved up to tangential surface of femoral condyle. Synovial wall is at left. Articular surface of condyle at periphery has good regenerated cartilage.

E Inspection along lateral compartment shows complete degeneration of articular surfaces and degenerated torn meniscus.

F Absence of bone on medial femoral condyle, which appears yellow.

G Intercondylar notch shows degenerated synovial tissue over anterior cruciate ligament. No loose bodies.

H Entire medial compartment with degenerative meniscus and loss of articular surface on both femur and tibia.

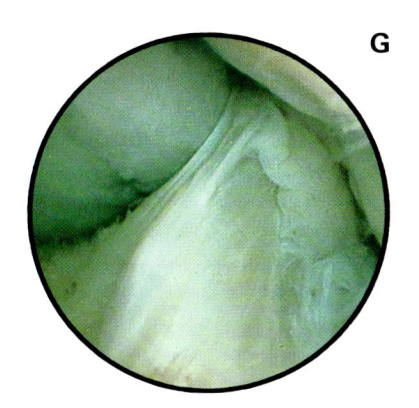

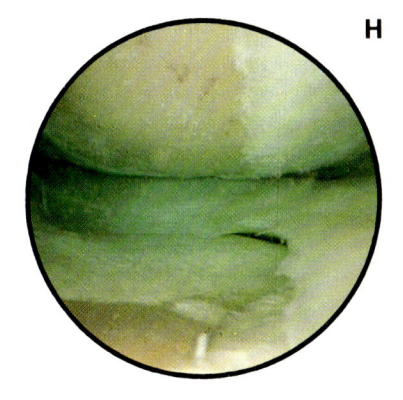

Diagnostic arthroscopy of the knee

FIG. 11-2. Hypertrophic spurring on medial femoral condyle adjacent to patella in progressive degenerative arthritis.

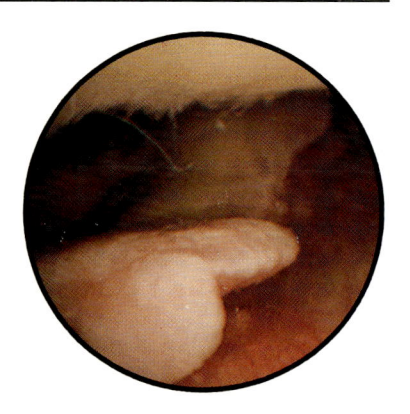

intra-articular fracture. In a fracture where radiologic findings secondary to magnification are overread, arthroscopy can demonstrate that the separation is minimal. Surgery is avoided, and casting is all that is required.

DEGENERATIVE CHANGES

Degeneration of the articular cartilage can vary from early bacon-strip fragmentation, as seen in the patella, to convolutions. (See Fig. 10-1.) Further degeneration will show exposed yellow bone (Fig. 11-1). The synovium in degenerative arthritis can be acutely inflamed (see Chapter 9), or there can be a very fine filamentous degenerative change, especially in the posterolateral compartment.

The main value of diagnostic arthroscopy in degenerative arthritic disease is in establishing the exact status of the disease or in evaluating it from an investigative standpoint (Fig. 11-2). Arthroscopic surgical methods have provided new approaches to these conditions. (See Chapter 18.)

LOOSE BODIES

Loose bodies are more common than is clinically expected. The easy access to visualization of the joint by arthroscopy with the patient under local anesthesia, preceding arthrotomy with general anesthesia, has shown a surprisingly high incidence of loose bodies. These often mimic other conditions, such as a torn meniscus. Many loose bodies can be managed arthroscopically, either by removing them with various sized cannulas and vacuuming (see Chapter 8) or by removing larger loose bodies with the Jaws modified pituitary rongeur (Fig. 11-3, *A*).

The natural course of loose bodies is for them to be absorbed in the synovium. In a patient with a large number of loose bodies the synovium will actually engulf the articular material. A synovectomy may be indicated.

DEGENERATIVE SYNOVITIS

Acute nonrheumatoid synovitis with considerable inflammation occurs with an acute degenerative process with multiple fine loose bodies in the joint. Arthroscopy and removal of these loose bodies reverses the process and renders the patient asymptomatic. Sometimes an arthroscopic synovectomy is performed.

Condylar disease

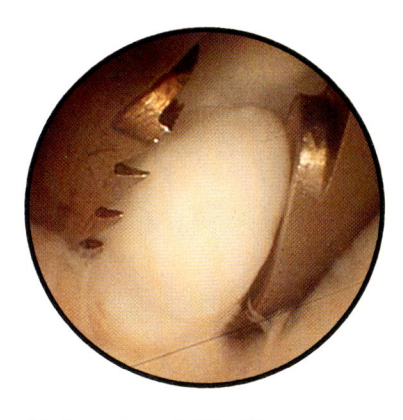

FIG. 11-3

A Loose body in posteromedial compartment being removed by Jaws modified pituitary rongeur.

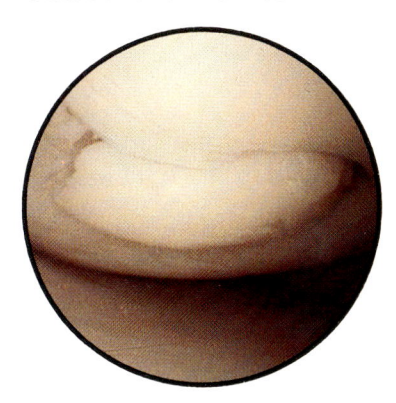

Osteochondritis dissecans.

B Area of osteochondritis dissecans separated from articular surface.

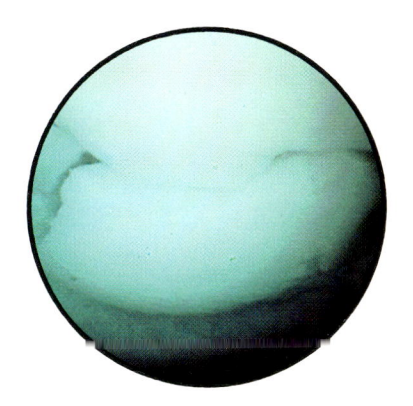

C Methylene blue can help to clearly delineate articular separation, especially in situations less subtle than this.

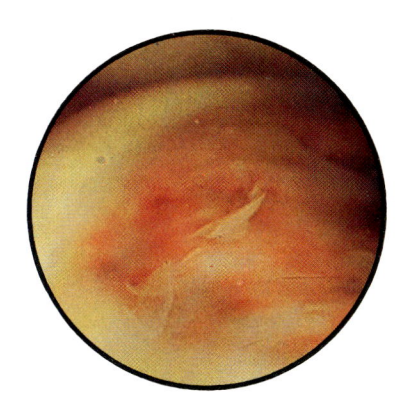

D Large defect created surgically down to raw bleeding bone, 6 weeks prior to this intra-articular photography.

183

OSTEOCHONDRITIS DISSECANS

The management or investigation of osteochondritis dissecans is facilitated by arthroscopy (Fig. 11-3, B and C). In new patients with osteochondritis dissecans the usual procedure is to inspect the area of the defect with the patient under local anesthesia. Staining with methylene blue indicates whether the articular surface is intact. It is also possible to palpate the area and establish whether there is loosening or pain, which can affect management. If the defect is intact and painless, conservative treatment and immobilization will usually result in healing in 6 months. If the defect is small and loose, surgical removal is indicated, with sharp excision of the bed down to bleeding juxta-articular bone. Arthroscopic surgical techniques permit removal or debridement, reduction, and fixation with or without drilling. (See Chapter 18.)

If a defect has not healed after a number of months, repeat arthroscopy with local anesthetic can be carried out.

OSTEOCHONDRAL DEFECTS

Defects of the articular surface of the knee can occur from trauma or surgery. In acute dislocations of the patella, loss of the articular surface of the lateral femoral condyle is common. (See Fig. 10-4, C.) Some patients lose large portions of the articular surface of the patella as well.

In patients with articular cartilage injuries from bucket-handle tears of the meniscus, or osteochondritis dissecans, a sharp surgical excision perpendicular to the articular surface is indicated for removal of the soft loose fragmented articular surface. Small lesions will heal within 6 weeks. Larger lesions (1 inch) may take 12 to 14 weeks before the vascularity of the bed of the lesions dissolves and becomes fibrocartilaginous. Restriction of weight-bearing activities until these defects have healed reduces morbidity. Healing, as seen arthroscopically, correlates well with the absence of inflammatory symptoms. (See Fig. 11-3, D.)

PREOPERATIVE EVALUATIONS

Arthroscopy is potentially beneficial in evaluating tibial osteotomy or total-joint resurfacing because it can verify the presence or absence of articular cartilage. Raw bone in a compartment, not yet manifested by roentgenographic changes, or a torn meniscus is probably a contraindication to shifting weight to the unaffected compartment. In the future, arthroscopy should provide a method of more refined selection of patients for tibial osteotomy. Evaluation of articular cartilage injury can show symptomatic hypertrophic osteophytes without marked change in the articular surface or meniscus. Patients with such injuries may be candidates for Magnusson "house cleaning" at the time of surgery.

Intra-articular shaving under arthroscopic control has shown promise in salvaging degenerative knee joints and prevented, at least temporarily, total-knee replacements.

Arthroscopic evaluation of a patient who is a candidate for so-called total-knee replacement can establish the presence or absence of articular surfaces.

The necessity for unicompartmental or bicompartmental resurfacing may be reevaluated. Potentially, the existence of patellar disease could influence the decision to resurface a patella.

POSTOPERATIVE EVALUATIONS

Violation of the articular cartilage is the most serious injury that the knee joint can undergo. Arthroscopic evaluation in patients who underwent surgery for an injury to meniscal or ligamentous tissue, but whose morbidity increased over the subsequent weeks and months, often shows articular cartilage injury. Simple meniscal injury without evidence of articular cartilage injury at the time of surgery has been seen. Within 6 to 8 weeks, effusion and discomfort developed. Arthroscopic examination showed articular cartilage dissection off the femoral condyle. It is presumed that there was a shearing injury to the articular cartilage at the time of the meniscal injury, but that it was not evident at the time of arthrotomy because the articular cartilage was not vascular and the patient had a low metabolic rate. This injury was identified only by arthroscopy at a later date, and loose bodies were removed from the joint.

Good results have been achieved without arthrotomy by transcutaneous methods. (See Chapter 8.)

Chapter 12

Extrasynovial lesions

Torn ligaments
    Anterior cruciate
    Tibial collateral
    Posterior cruciate
    Lateral complex injury
Chronic instability
Cysts
Ankylosis
Osgood-Schlatter disease
Preoperative evaluations

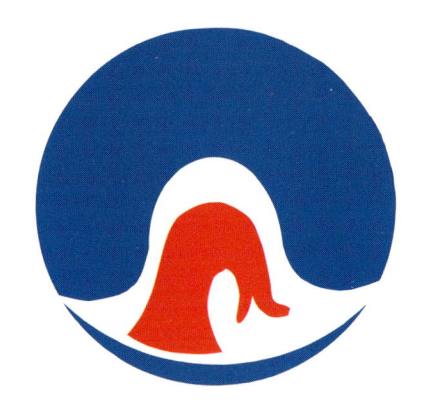

TORN LIGAMENTS
Anterior cruciate

A torn anterior cruciate ligament is a rather common injury (Fig. 12-1). It was present in 15% of 962 knees reviewed. It was a less common finding in the total patient population examined diagnostically under local anesthesia but was seen in 30% of 162 consecutive knees of patients examined under general anesthesia over a 1-year period. Series IV had a 13% incidence.

The clinical diagnosis of a torn anterior cruciate ligament can be difficult because of the existence of pain and hemarthrosis and resultant muscular guarding on the part of the patient. Unless there is an accompanying stretch of the lateral or medial supporting structures or gross instability of all structures, the presence of cruciate ligament injury can be masked.

The arthrogram is virtually inept as an aid in diagnosing torn anterior cruciate ligaments. A completely torn ligament not violating the synovial sheath does not allow dye filling. The roentgenogram provides poor circumstantial evidence.

Arthroscopy offers the only accurate method of assessing the status of the anterior cruciate ligament. It is possible to visualize the covering and the presence or absence of hemorrhage and to pull the tibia forward on the femur to observe the effect on the anterior cruciate ligament. Often the area of separation of attenuated old tears or acute tears can be seen by performing a drawer test during arthroscopy.

The so-called isolated anterior cruciate ligament tear has been the subject of debate by clinicians over the years. Prior to arthroscopy the joint could not be assessed to the extent that is possible now by anterior and posterior visualization. Such injury is considered isolated if there is no other abnormality that necessitates either arthroscopic treatment or arthrotomy. Ten percent of patients in Series IV could be considered to have so-called isolated anterior cruciate ligament injury.

Extrasynovial lesions

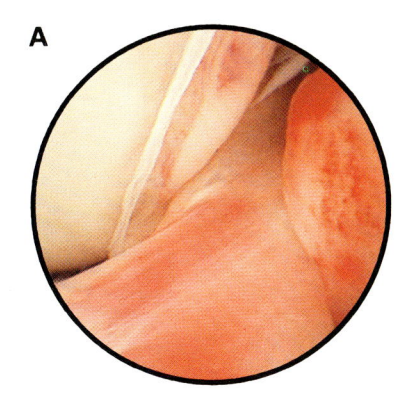

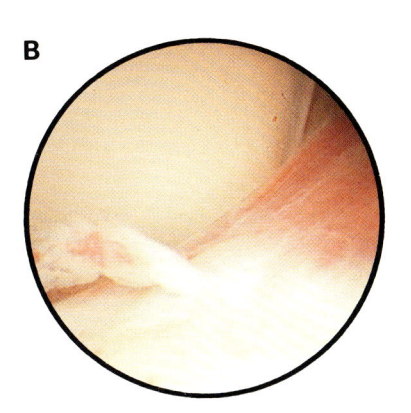

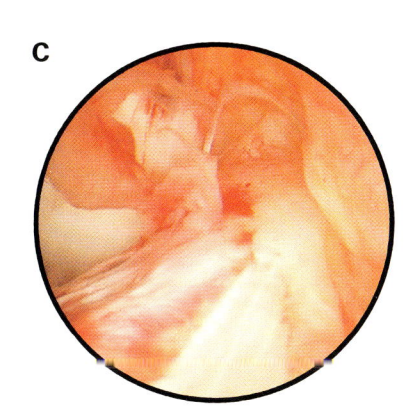

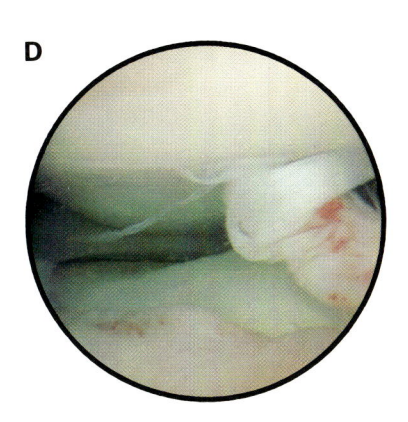

FIG. 12-1

A Torn anterior cruciate ligament does not show any gross separation. Hemorrhage appears to be subsynovial and interstitial. However, complete disruption of anterior cruciate ligament not evident from this view. Separate posterolateral puncture showed vast majority of cruciate ligament, which necessitated excision to remove symptoms.

B Common anterior cruciate ligament abnormality is extrusion of portion of ligament through slit in synovium. This eventually absorbs and rounds off. Small one is asymptomatic.

C Complete disruption of anterior cruciate ligament, with fragment completely off pole.

D Anterior cruciate ligament caught in anterolateral compartment. This may clinically mimic torn lateral meniscus.

E Complete disruption of anterior cruciate ligament. Old complete disruption will show hemorrhage around it for up to 12 weeks following injury, but ligamentous tissue itself is avascular and contracted.

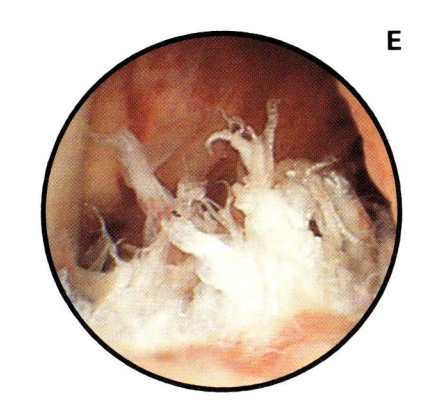

It is exceedingly rare in isolated cruciate ligament injury not to observe at least some hemorrhage in the wall of the posteromedial or posterolateral joint through posterior puncture; it is difficult to visualize this by anterior arthrotomy or anterior arthroscopy. The hemorrhage is frequently extrasynovial and involves the capsular tissues. (See Fig. 12-5, D.) Often hemorrhage disseminates to the posterior horn of the meniscus or the synovial attachment, yet there is no visible separation of the meniscus. Arthroscopic findings support the concept that when an injury is of such magnitude that it results in hemorrhagic change or tissue separation of the anterior cruciate ligament, there invariably is hemorrhage and tissue disruption in the capsular structures of the joint.

Eighteen of 113 patients examined in Series III who had anterior cruciate ligament injuries, either new or old, had degenerative changes of the joint or loose bodies from existing degeneration. Clinical instability was universally accompanied by the presence of a torn or attenuated anterior cruciate ligament; however, it should be noted that gross instability is not solely dependent on the presence or absence of the anterior cruciate ligament, but on the capsular supportive structures (e.g., the tibial collateral ligament on the medial side).

A torn anterior cruciate ligament accompanied or mimicked another condition in 25 of the 34 patients in our first series. At the time of examination the ligaments were torn in such a way that they could not be repaired, or the evaluation came at a time when absorption of the ligament did not render it repairable. It is important that a torn anterior cruciate ligament was not clinically recognized in many situations where it was seen arthroscopically. This supports the concept of early diagnosis in any suspected ligamentous injury, which is now possible by arthroscopy. Clinical instability may exist with partial cruciate injury (Fig. 12-2).

An accompanying meniscal injury is very common. In a second series of patients, seen from September, 1975, to September, 1976, meniscal injury accompanied anterior cruciate ligament tears in 49% of those examined under local or general anesthesia. This association should prompt awareness that when the preoperative diagnosis shows a torn meniscus, preparation should be made for necessary ligament repair or compensatory capsular reconstruction.

Of all patients in the two series, about half had extrasynovial and ligamentous injury and half had meniscal, patellar, or condylar disease.

In Series III, when the anterior cruciate ligament was torn, the patient had a 50% chance of degenerative arthritis. Thirty-nine percent of the patients had a torn meniscus, and an additional 34% had had a previous meniscectomy.

Shneider[3] reviewed a selected group of our arthroscopy patients. He picked 295 patients with a torn anterior cruciate ligament observed at arthroscopy by the anterior portal. A complete tear of the anterior cruciate ligament was found in 169 patients, and the remaining 126 had partial or stretching injuries. The average age in the series was 25 and men predominated.

If the single anterior inspection did not show an abnormality of the respective meniscus, then a separate transcutaneous approach was made to ei-

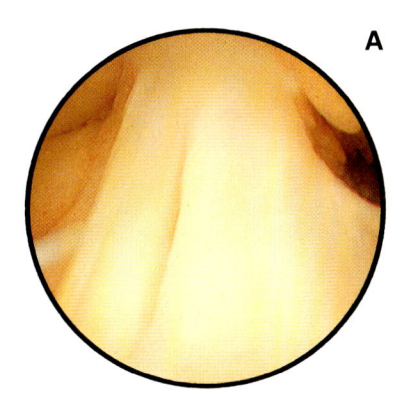

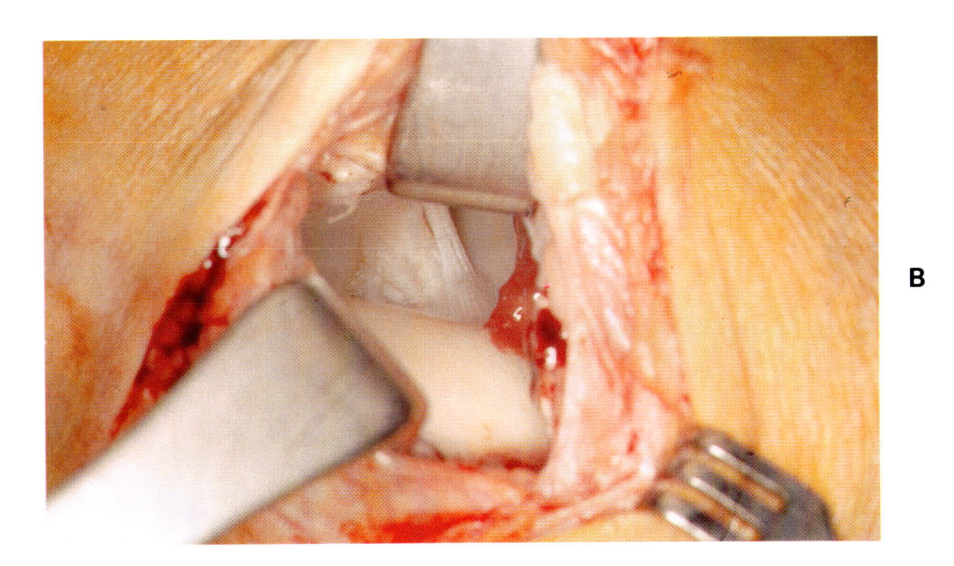

FIG. 12-2

A Longitudinal separations of cruciate ligament fibers, with loss of synovial covering and cabling of individual bundles, is sign of old partial tear. Although ligament is intact, instability demonstrates lack of ligament integrity.
B Gross anatomic specimen of same lesion.

ther the posteromedial or posterolateral compartment. The Needlescope was used in most patients.

He found an isolated tear of the anterior cruciate ligament in 16% of the patients, that is, there was no meniscal, or other ligamentous, or capsular injury observed either clinically or by arthroscopy, including the separate posterior punctures.

The medial meniscus was torn in 70% of these patients. The posterior puncture was necessary to make the diagnosis in 36% of patients in this group. The anterior cruciate ligament tear and medial meniscus tear without the lateral meniscal injury occurred in 57 patients (19%).

The lateral meniscus was torn in 70% of these patients; the separate posterior inspection was necessary to make the diagnosis in 32% of this group.

Diagnostic arthroscopy of the knee

The incidence of anterior cruciate tear and lateral meniscal tear without a medial meniscal injury was 19%.

Both menisci were torn in 51% of patients with a torn anterior cruciate ligament.

The importance of the separate posterior punctures is emphasized when 36% of the medial meniscal injuries were only seen from posterior and 32% of the time when the lateral meniscus was torn.

The concomitant existence of cruciate ligament injury and degenerative arthritis, either suspected preoperatively or observed in patients with instability, points out the importance of the integrity of the anterior cruciate ligament. Many loose bodies that accompany this type of degenerative change can be observed only by posterior puncture. Articular loose bodies can be removed with the arthroscope, thus reducing morbidity without opening the compartment. In a few situations we have been able to arthroscopically remove large pieces of anterior cruciate ligament in either the posteromedial or posterolateral compartments, thus eliminating the need for arthrotomy.

The management of specific anterior cruciate ligament abnormalities depends on the discretion and experience of the surgeon. Arthroscopy provides a definitive evaluation on which surgical judgment can be based.

Tibial collateral

Arthroscopy provides an excellent means of evaluating a patient with tibial collateral ligament injury (Fig. 12-3). Tenderness and pain over the tibial collateral area, increased by valgus stress, in the absence of palpable defect or marked instability probably indicate an underlying torn meniscus. In the presence of hemorrhage this diagnosis cannot be well established by arthrography but can be confirmed arthroscopically. Rapid rehabilitation therapy can be instituted if there is no instability or intra-articular lesion. Arthroscopy dictates appropriate early surgical intervention if there is internal derangement.

If the patient has a torn tibial collateral ligament and a palpable defect in that area, arthroscopic examination can discern any intra-articular abnormality

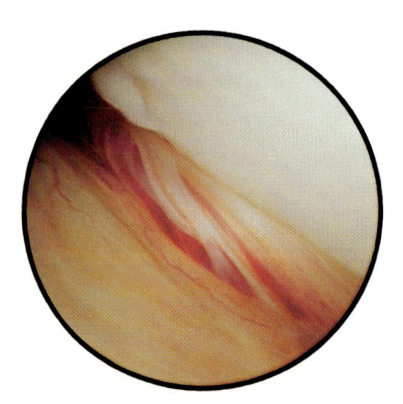

FIG. 12-3. Torn tibial collateral ligament tissue drawn inside joint adjacent to medial femoral condyle.

Extrasynovial lesions

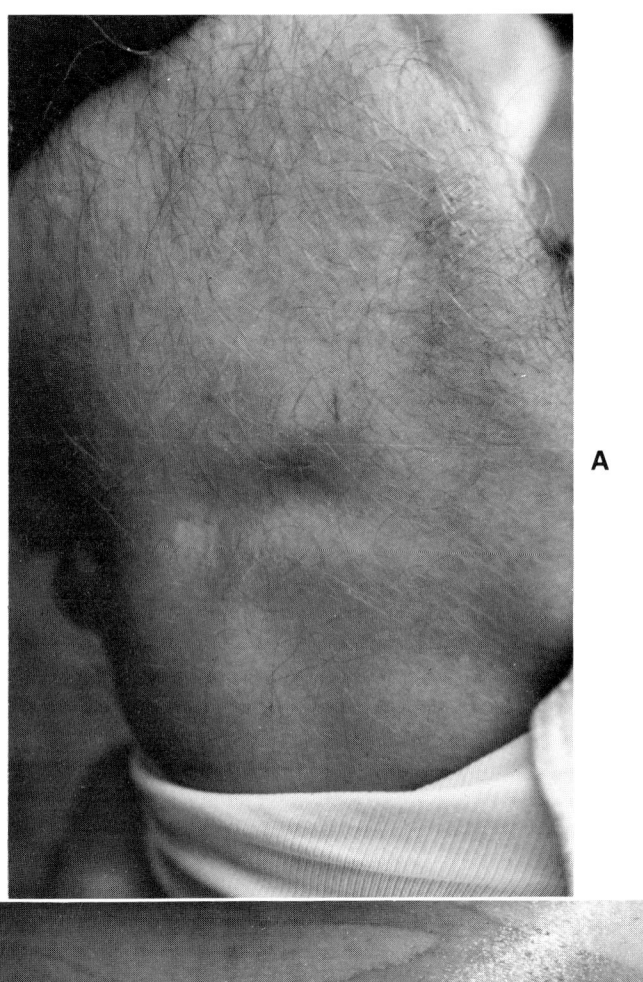

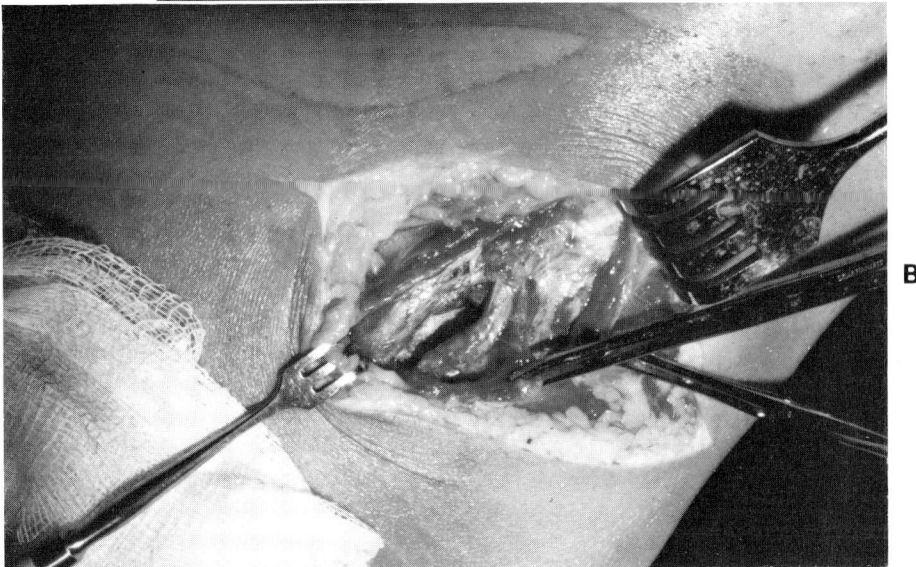

FIG. 12-4. **A,** Torn tibial collateral ligament with sucking in of medial joint tissues during valgus stress immediately after acute injury. **B,** Limited surgical exposure is possible when arthroscopy has ruled out other lesions.

that is amenable to surgery. If the lesion is well localized to the tibial collateral ligament off the femur and there is some instability, surgical exploration can be localized to that area and the repair carried out, resulting in rapid rehabilitation. An extensive arthrotomy is not necessary for joint exploration; it can be accomplished by arthroscopy (Fig. 12-4).

Posterior cruciate

Isolated tears of the posterior cruciate ligament can be visualized by posteromedial puncture. It is not uncommon to see hemorrhage in that ligament without posterior instability. Isolated complete disruption of the posterior cruciate ligament can be confirmed at arthroscopy. I have seen two patients with complete absence of posterior cruciate ligament after injury and absorption.

Anteriorly, the view of the posterior cruciate ligament is partially obscured by the anterior cruciate ligament. However, in the total absence of the anterior cruciate ligament the posterior cruciate ligament is well defined and easily visualized anteriorly.

In the presence of both anterior and posterior cruciate ligament injury without complete detachment, marked subsynovial hemorrhage makes arthroscopic determination somewhat difficult from anterior puncture in the intercondylar notch. Therefore posteromedial inspection is essential in evaluating the status of the acutely injured posterior cruciate ligament in the absence of gross instability (Fig. 12-5, A to C).

Lateral complex injury

The popliteus tendon can be visualized anterolaterally where it attaches to the femur. Avulsion of the tendon in that area has been identified. The normal course of the tendon is down through a sheath posterior and lateral to the meniscus. With anteromedial puncture a small-diameter endoscope can be passed obliquely across the lateral compartment, and the popliteus tendon can be seen under and posterior to the meniscus. (See Fig. 7-2.)

Posterolateral inspection shows the popliteus tendon as it courses obliquely behind the meniscus. This area can house small loose bodies. In many instances the arthroscope can be introduced in this posterolateral sheath, and loose bodies can be vacuumed from the compartment. Disruption of the popliteus tendon along its course in the sheath has been visualized.

Arthroscopy has not been of particular value in diagnosing ruptures of the fibular collateral ligament and iliotibial band. They can be identified only by the presence of retrosynovial hemorrhage.

CHRONIC INSTABILITY

The evaluation of a patient with chronic instability of the joint can be enhanced by arthroscopy. The examination can clearly determine the extent of intra-articular abnormality and degenerative changes within the joint. Worn articular surfaces adversely affect the prognosis. The presence of retained menisci can be determined, and surgical management can be planned. The presence of anterior cruciate ligament fronds caught in the joint can be identified

Extrasynovial lesions

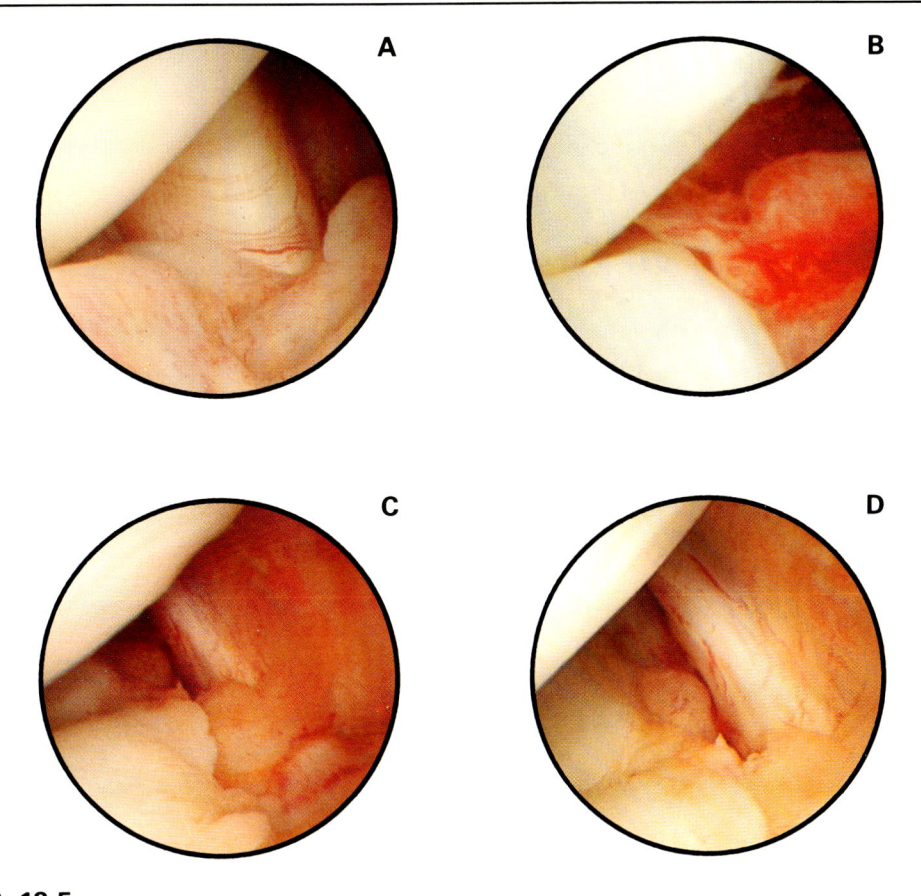

FIG. 12-5

A Posteromedial view of normal posterior cruciate ligament. Notice close position of meniscus to femoral condyle.

B Posteromedial view of capsular hemorrhage but without tear of posterior cruciate ligament. This type of capsular injury often accompanies what otherwise would have been considered an isolated anterior cruciate injury.

C Partial torn posterior cruciate ligament in resting position. Notice meniscus sagging off femoral condyle.

D Same patient as in **C** but with posterior drawer sign being performed. Notice posterior displacement of tibia on femur and narrowing of femoral attachment of this ligament.

and is amenable to arthrotomy at the time of reconstruation. (See Fig. 12-1, D.) Loose bodies can be removed through the arthroscopic cannulas.

There are some situations in which arthroscopic intra-articular inspection provides definitive information on which to further advise the patient of his problem, its surgical correction, and prognosis. When the arthroscopic inspection demonstrates no intra-articular abnormality that requires surgical intervention, the reconstructive procedure can proceed without the joint being entered.

The existence of abnormal posterior medial meniscal horns with partial cruciate ligament tear and degenerative arthritis is the most common problem associated with instability. Patients requiring reconstructive surgery can be accurately advised preoperatively of the surgical design. Often these patients have some apprehension because of multiple previous surgical procedures. Arthroscopy also can establish the presence or absence of torn menisci or abnormalities in the opposite compartment. If an existing lesion were unnoticed, prognosis would be hampered. Selective or subtotal arthroscopic meniscectomy can be performed, thus avoiding the arthrotomy. An extracapsular reconstructive procedure may be performed without the added morbidity of the exploratory arthrotomy. (See Chapter 9.)

Chronic lateral instability of the anterolateral rotary type with lateral pivotal shifts is minimized in the absence of the lateral meniscus. The mechanism of the lateral pivotal shift is accentuated in the presence of a meniscus.

When a major problem is on the lateral side, arthroscopy establishes not only the status of that compartment but also the necessity for surgery on the medial compartment of the knee.

CYSTS

Baker cysts are often associated with rheumatoid synovitis or chronic degenerative arthritis with loose bodies. Occasionally they are seen with a retained posterior horn with degenerative erosion of the posterior tibial condyle. The opening to the Baker cyst may be visualized arthroscopically from the posteromedial compartment, and the inside of the cyst can be inspected. In some patients there is unidirectional flow of fluid from the joint to the Baker cyst, as demonstrated by the placing of methylene blue in the joint. This dye flows into the cyst but does not flow back to the posteromedial compartment. Debris of an articular nature has been seen within Baker cysts. In cases where the cyst is secondary to another pathologic condition, correction of the condition will not eliminate the cyst. Resection of the cyst and removal of the articular debris are necessary for remission of symptoms.

Meniscal cysts are reported most commonly on the lateral side,[1] but I have seen several on the medial side. To save a patient unnecessary meniscectomy whenever possible, arthroscopy has been carried out. If there is no visible abnormality of the meniscus, the cystic mass is resected down to the meniscus. If the meniscus is not markedly degenerated at the entry site of the cyst, meniscectomy is not performed. However, a degenerative meniscus or considerable disruption of meniscal tissue with extension of the cyst to the meniscus warrants a meniscectomy. Currently I am following the progress of three patients who had resection of meniscal cysts without meniscectomy. One patient developed subsequent degenerative torn meniscus within 6 months; the other two patients have had no symptoms for 3 years.

The arthroscopic means of selective meniscectomy has permitted resection of the degenerative meniscal tissue. On two occasions the intra-articular shaver resection decompressed and allowed entry into the cyst for careful debridement. The cysts have not recurred in 1 year's time.

Juxta-articular ganglion cysts can occur adjacent to the knee and mimic meniscal cysts. If arthroscopy demonstrates no intra-articular abnormality, the cyst is resected. Because these cysts do not track down to the menisci and go to the synovial paratendinous tissue, no arthrotomy or meniscectomy is necessary.

ANKYLOSIS

A few patients have developed ankylosis of the knee despite exhaustive physical therapy after previous multiple surgical procedures.

With the patients under general anesthesia, arthroscopy was performed to assess the interior of the joint and establish that there was no internal derangement causing the lack of motion. In the past, if no abnormality was found, the joint was manipulated and physical therapy was initiated, to the considerable benefit of the patient. It should be noted that arthroscopy provided confidence to both the physician and the patient that there was no offending intra-articular lesion and that surgical exploration and adhesiotomy were not necessary. Rehabilitation was relatively short.

When adhesions span the joint space, the arthroscopic resection has relieved pain and resulted in increased range of motion. This prevented the morbidity associated with manipulation or arthrotomy.

OSGOOD-SCHLATTER DISEASE

A few patients with Osgood-Schlatter disease have had some referred knee complaints and an extra ossicle in the area of the tibial tubercle. With the patients under general anesthesia, arthroscopy was carried out to establish that no intra-articular abnormality existed. The extra ossicle of the tibial tubercle was excised, and rehabilitation therapy was instituted with absolute confidence that no underlying intra-articular abnormality went unnoticed.

PREOPERATIVE EVALUATIONS

Patients with acute gross disruption of ligamentous structures, whose knees are essentially disarticulated, do not require arthroscopic examination to assess the joint. Instillation of saline in the joint does not maintain distension because of the capsular disruption.

There are patients with suspected or established ligamentous injuries in whom the presence or extent of the lesion is not easily established clinically. Such patients may have discomfort enough that they tighten the quadriceps muscle, making evaluation by x-ray examination and arthrogram difficult.

If hemarthrosis is present, arthrogram interpretation can be compromised. Hemarthrosis is not a contraindication to arthroscopy.[2] The method that I have outlined of vacuuming the joint and instilling a 50-ml bolus of saline allows these joints to be inspected. It may be necessary to completely remove the blood and reinstill saline seven to ten times to cleanse the joint. Furthermore, it might be necessary during viewing to instill saline under pressure from the syringe through the K-52 catheter and along the cannula to clear the area immediately in front of the viewing lens. It would be an unusual situation in which persistence did not result in an adequate and comprehensive evaluation, even continuous irrigation.

REFERENCES

1. Becton, J. L., and Young, H. H.: Cysts of the semilunar cartilage of the knee, Arch. Surg. **90:**708, 1965.
2. DeHaven, K. E.: Acute injury to the knee. In American Academy of Orthopaedic Surgeons: Symposium on arthroscopy and arthrography of the knee, St. Louis, 1978, The C. V. Mosby Co.
3. Shneider, D. A., and Johnson, L. L.: Arthroscopic findings associated with the torn anterior cruciate ligament, Paper presented at the Annual Meeting of the American Orthopedic Sports Medicine Society, Innsbrook, Fla., July, 1979.

Chapter 13

Synovial disease

Synovial plica
Rheumatoid arthritis
Degenerative arthritis
Pigmented villonodular synovitis
Osteochondromatosis
Gout
Pseudogout
Reiter syndrome
Hemangioma
Psoriatic arthritis
Hemorrhagic synovium
Alkaptonuria
Foreign bodies
Pedunculated nodular synovitis
Infection
Postoperative evaluations

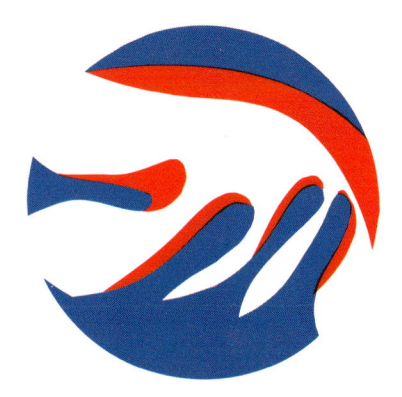

Arthroscopy provides easy access for direct visualization of the morphologic characteristics of the synovium. The suprapatellar pouch has the most abundant synovial surfaces for visualization. It may be possible with continued experience to characterize the various rheumatologic conditions by their arthroscopic synovial morphology.

A number of patients have undergone diagnostic evaluations by arthroscopy for synovial disease in which the cause was not clear and the extent of the disease was not established. It has been possible to biopsy the synovium, either with direct vision or blindly when the condition is diffuse (Fig. 13-1). Synovial

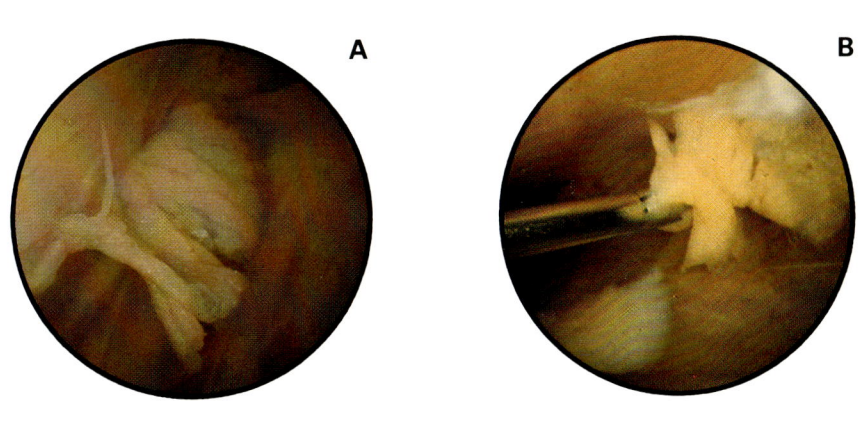

FIG. 13-1

A Pedunculated lesion of synovium visualized in suprapatellar pouch.
B Biopsy performed under local anesthesia and direct visualization.

Diagnostic arthroscopy of the knee

fluid evacuated from the joint is useful for cell-block examination, which may show sheets of synovial tissue or articular debris, and tissue diagnosis. (See Fig. 8-2.)

SYNOVIAL PLICA

Folds in the synovium are common in the knee joint. The two most common folds are the suprapatellar (Fig. 13-2) and the medial shelf (Fig. 13-3). I have seen a lateral shelf on three occasions. These were a mirror image of the more common medial plica but not asymptomatic. There is a normal, yet rarely mentioned, fold in the lateral sulcus above the popliteus sheath (Fig. 13-4).

Fibrous adhesions occur in many areas following arthrotomy and should not be confused with a normally existing synovial fold (Fig. 13-5). Also, I have

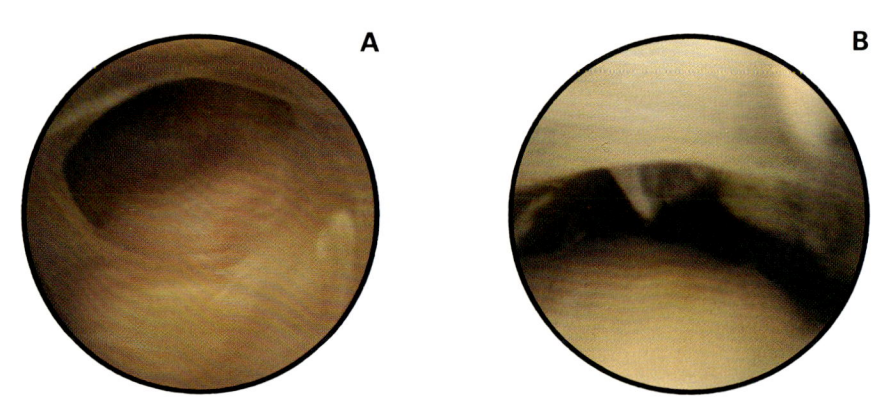

FIG. 13-2

A Suprapatellar pouch showing large suprapatellar plica seen above patella.
B Progression with arthroscope brings medial wall with suprapatellar plica into closer view.

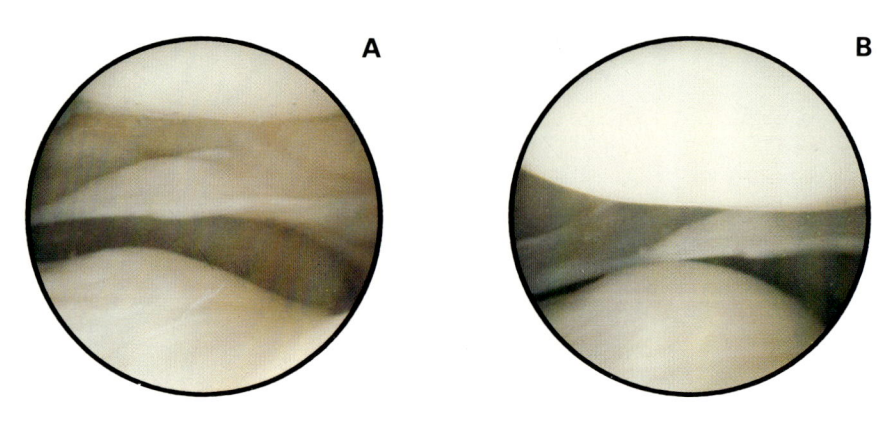

FIG. 13-3

A Patella above and femoral condyle below. Medial shelf is between.
B With decompression, plica comes down on femoral condyle.

Synovial disease

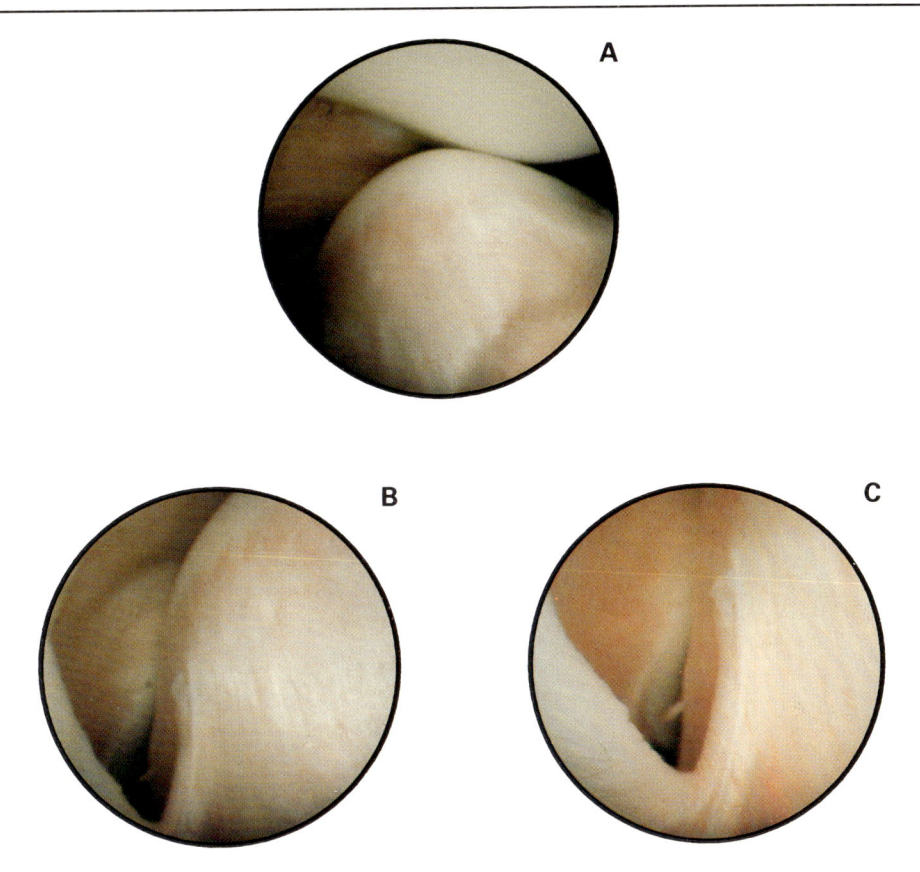

FIG. 13-4

A Lateral patellofemoral articulation.
B Arthroscope moves into lateral sulcus and synovial fold in that area comes into view.
C Normal synovial fold in the lateral sulcus immediately above popliteus fossa.

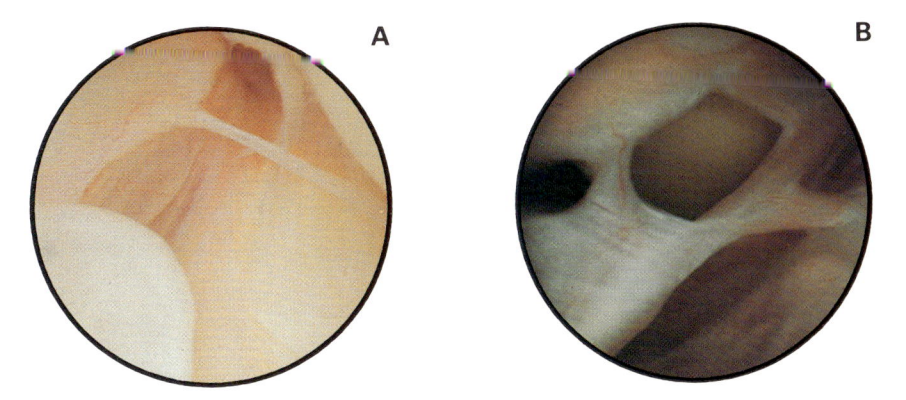

FIG. 13-5

A Fibrous scar tissue often follows surgical procedures on joint and should not be mistaken for normal synovial folds.
B Fibrotic adhesions can be considerable. These may respond to arthroscopic resection.

Diagnostic arthroscopy of the knee

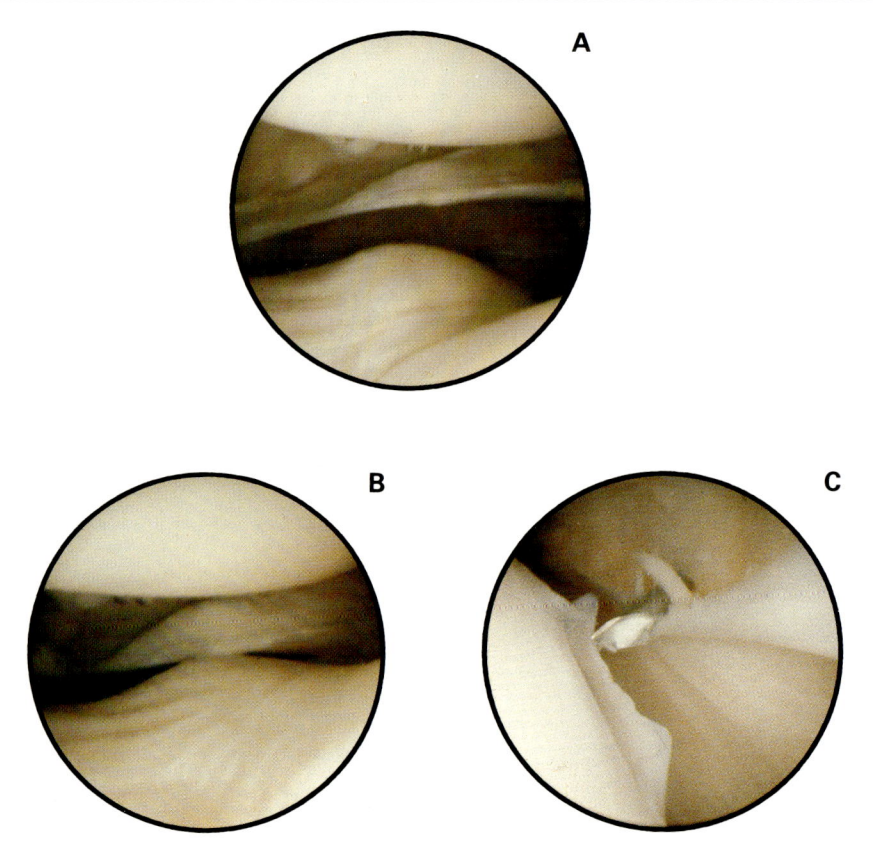

FIG. 13-6

A Medial shelf, or plica, is at right and patella is above.
B With flexion, medial shelf moves across or impinges on medial femoral condyle to the right.
C With extension, lesion can be seen on femoral surface. Look for possible erosion opposite on patella or thickness of plica.

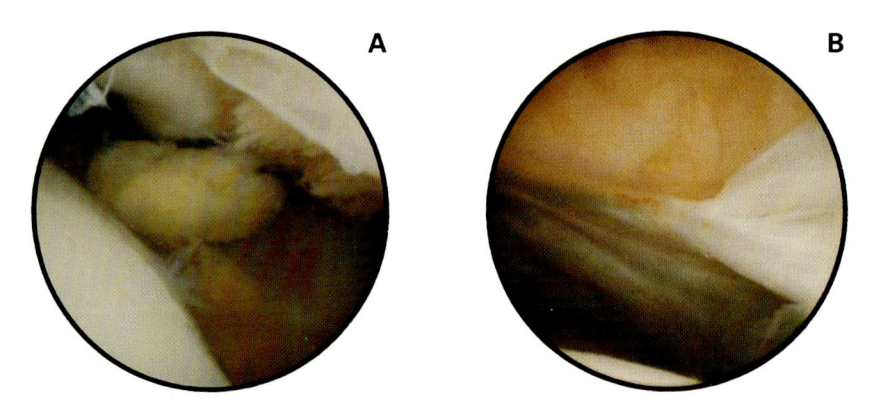

FIG. 13-7

A Nodular synovitis following traumatic rupture of medial shelf plica.
B Regenerated medial shelf seen 11 months after arthroscopic resection of asymptomatic plica.

seen one plica that was circular and looked like the brim of a hat with synovium pouching out the center. This was located on the anterior femur just above the patellar joint.[3]

A normal anatomic structure may become clinically symptomatic, that is, a hypermobile meniscus or a snapping iliotibial band over the greater trochanter. So it is with the suprapatellar and medial shelf plicae. Pathologic status is best determined by arthroscopy under local anesthesia. It is possible to visualize the position, shape, thickness, and any possible erosion of either the adjacent femur or patella. Gradual decompression (Fig. 13-3, B) and a passive range of motion assist in determining whether this lesion is to be incriminated (Fig. 13-6). The sine qua non is the ability to correlate, under local anesthesia, whether the patient recognizes tugging or popping of this structure as the exact duplication of his symptoms.

Arthroscopic section or resection is simple and technically pleasing, especially as one starts intra-articular surgery. In fact, it is difficult to resist removing them, especially the medial shelf. If one adheres to the aforementioned criteria, very few will be identified as the cause of clinical symptoms. In over 1,000 arthroscopies under local anesthesia the medial shelf in only four patients was determined to be actually symptom producing.

I have observed one spontaneous rupture of the medial shelf with a resulting localized traumatic nodular synovitis (Fig. 13-7, A). I also have seen three regrown medial shelves after resection. These patients were under general anesthesia for possible arthroscopic meniscectomy. No meniscal lesion was found. Therefore the medial shelf was resected too, but not through the medial synovial wall. The patient did not improve, and a repeat arthroscopic examination showed a normal knee except for the regrown medial shelf (Fig. 13-7, B). The area of scar was not symptomatic and was not resected. Enthusiasm for plica resection should be tempered by the possibility of fibrous regeneration.

RHEUMATOID ARTHRITIS

Rheumatoid arthritis is a varied condition (Fig. 13-8). We have examined patients with negative results on serum tests and relatively low sedimentation rates but whose histories suggested rheumatoid arthritis. Arthroscopy has been of benefit in establishing the diagnosis. With an established diagnosis, arthroscopy serves to follow the progress of medical treatment or to establish the extent of the articular damage. Watanabe[3] reported the clinical benefits of arthroscopy and lavage of rheumatoid joints.

Rheumatoid arthritis is characterized by long, fingerlike, projective villi with rounded ends, with a single blood vessel tracking up each villus (Fig. 13-9, A and B). The surface area of these villi is considerable. The tips of the villi frequently have fibrinoid exudate (Fig. 13-9, C), which can be selectively stained with methylene blue. The wall has an extremely prominent vascular pattern of linear blood vessels, which accounts for the erythema accompanying this condition. There is considerable cloudiness in the joint when first entered, and cleansing of synovial fluid is essential for good visualization. Often a tuft of

Diagnostic arthroscopy of the knee

RHEUMATOID ARTHRITIS

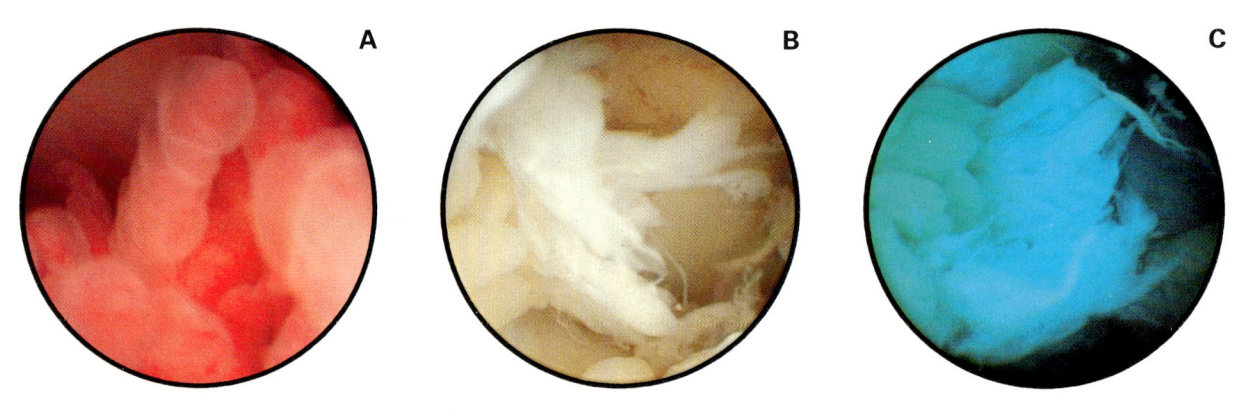

FIG. 13-8

A Rheumatoid arthritis with a marked inflammatory component.
B Rheumatoid arthritis with villous fibrinoid exudate.
C Methylene blue injected into joint defines villi.

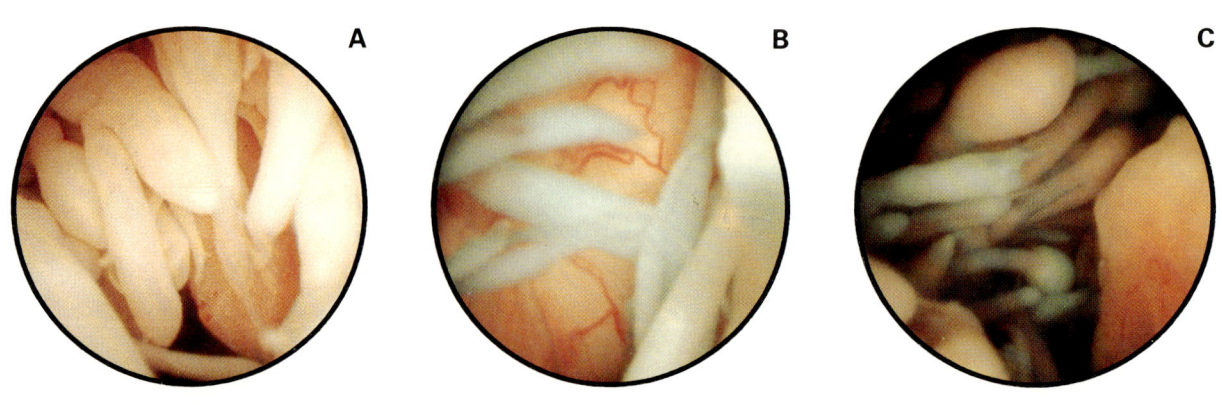

FIG. 13-9

A Rheumatoid arthritis with marked fibrinoid dumbbell protrusions from villi.
B Same knee with marked vascularity in wall of joint.
C Rheumatoid arthritis with methylene blue staining of fibrinoid exudate.

Synovial disease

synovium is caught in the joint, usually between the patella and the femur, and becomes hemorrhagic.

Arthroscopy has been used to inspect joints of patients who have had synovectomies. It is not unusual, in spite of excellent medical management, to see regrowth of synovium of a similar type as early as 6 months following knee joint synovectomy, but the villi are smaller and more fibrotic. Synovectomy by arthroscopic surgical technique is an excellent method of treatment. I have performed this on shoulders and knees. There is immediate rehabilitation. (See Chapter 20.) Second-look arthroscopy has shown no regrowth, for as long as 19 months in one case.

DEGENERATIVE ARTHRITIS

In degenerative arthritis the villi are rather fine and fimbriated. They are multiple, diffuse, shorter, and less round than those in rheumatoid arthritis (Fig. 13-10, A). This type of change is most common when there are loose bodies free in the joint. In some patients loose bodies have been engulfed so extensively throughout the synovium that a synovectomy was required to ablate the offending foreign body from the articular surfaces. (See Figs. 8-2 and 13-10, B.) Early arthroscopic removal of loose bodies precludes this progressive synovitis.

Another form of degenerative arthritis is an acute inflammatory nonrheumatoid arthritis. The patient may have a degenerative meniscus and perhaps mild tibia vara with degenerative compartment changes. Acutely inflamed joints appear the same as infected joints (Fig. 13-11). The presence of loose bodies can be established arthroscopically. They can be vacuumed from the joint, reversing the process.

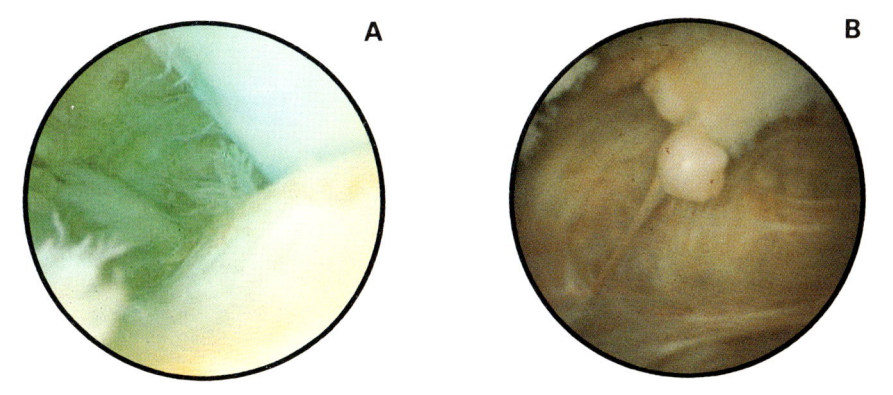

FIG. 13-10. A, Posterolateral compartment with marked proliferative villous synovitis seen in chronic degenerative changes, usually in presence of loose bodies. **B,** Engulfing of articular cartilage within synovium in degenerative synovitis.

Diagnostic arthroscopy of the knee

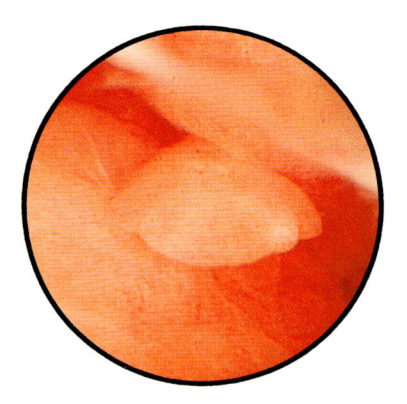

FIG. 13-11. Acute inflammation of joint, whether septic or due to degenerative changes, has extremely vascular synovium but without many villi.

PIGMENTED VILLONODULAR SYNOVITIS

Pigmented villonodular synovitis (Fig. 13-12, *A* and *B*) has been observed with surprising frequency. It was suspected in one patient, but in others degenerative arthritis was diagnosed. Arthroscopic findings are classic and descriptive. Although there are no articular changes in the early stages, longstanding pigmented villonodular synovitis is accompanied by loss of articular tissue (Fig. 13-12, *B* and *C*). With arthroscopy, invasion of the articular cartilage can be determined. The patient can be advised of the possibility of recurrence and the existence of degenerative changes that will affect the prognosis.

This condition is traditionally treated by total synovectomy (Fig. 13-12, *D* to *F*). Arthroscopic synovectomy has been beneficial, especially in recurrences following open synovectomy.

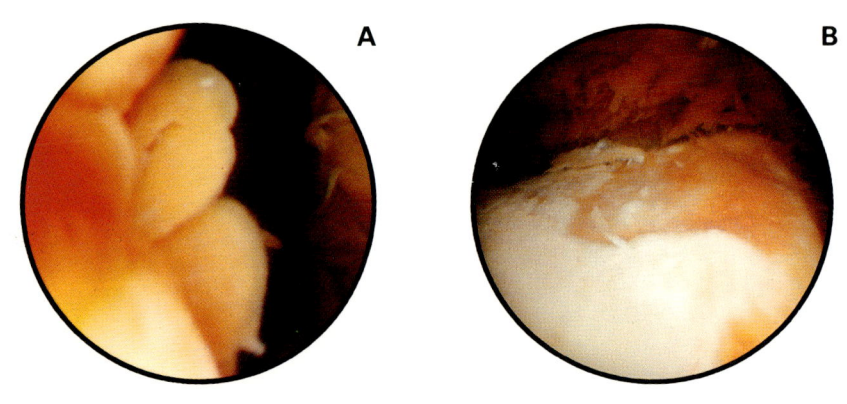

FIG. 13-12

A Arthroscopic view of pigmented villonodular synovitis.
B Arthroscopic view of erosion of articular cartilage and pigmented villonodular synovitis.

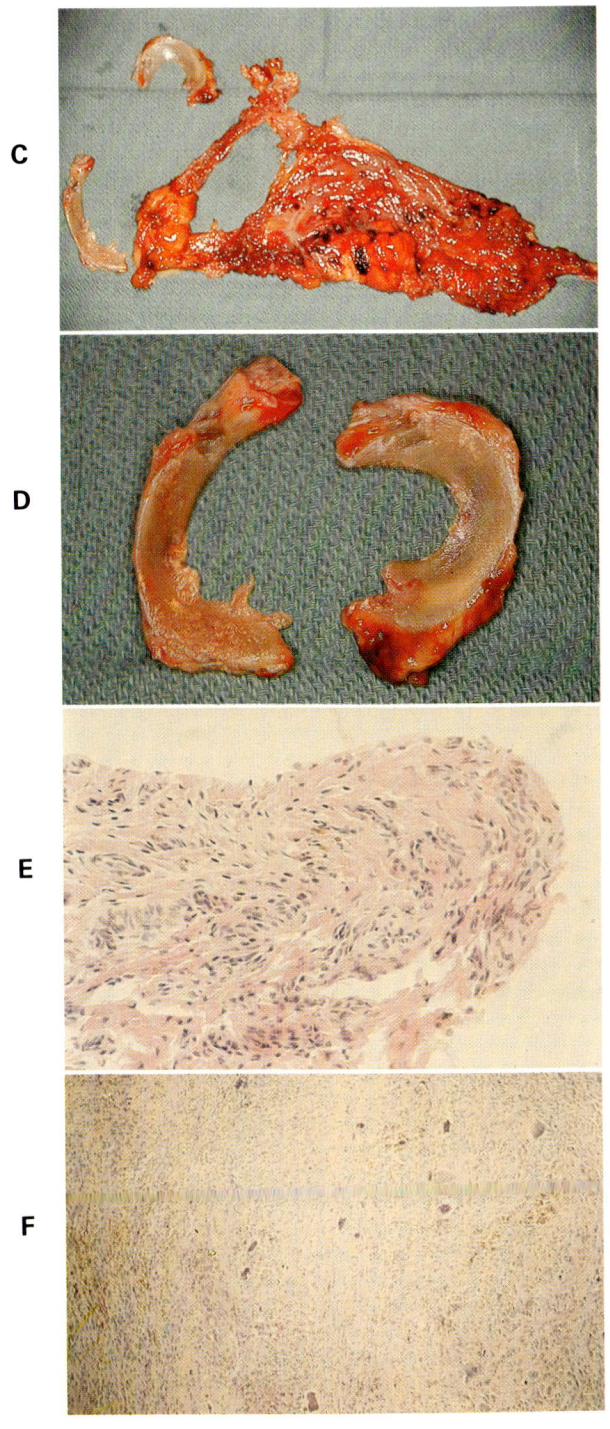

FIG. 13-12, cont'd

C Gross anatomic specimen at time of synovectomy showing marked synovial changes with erosion of articular cartilage to bone.
D Menisci removed by conventional open total synovectomy.
E Gross anatomic specimen of synovium removed in pigmented villonodular synovitis.
F Photomicrograph of synovial tissue showing fibrous proliferation and hemosiderin pigmentation.

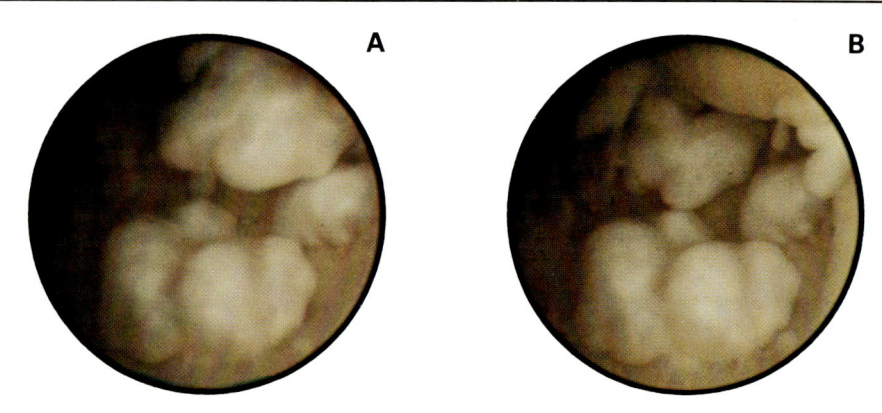

FIG. 13-13

A Synovial osteochondromatosis showing budding of articular metaplasia to cartilaginous tissue.

B Osteochondromatosis with budding synovial bodies as well as loose bodies.

OSTEOCHONDROMATOSIS

Osteochondromatosis has been observed in four patients (Fig. 13-13). In one, the nidus of the metaplasia was easily identified in the suprapatellar pouch and around the fat pad. It was especially important that there were multiple loose bodies in the posterolateral compartment. Because the thigh usually rests in external rotation, gravity carries the loose bodies to the posterolateral compartment. Also, the posterolateral and posteromedial compartments had areas of metaplasia. It was recommended to the referring surgeon that synovectomy be carried out, but also that the posteromedial and posterolateral compartments be opened to excise the areas of metaplasia to prevent recurrence.

Two patients had virtually hundreds of small osteochondromatous loose bodies. No metaplasia was observed in the synovium of the other compartments. For that reason, the joints were not opened, but all loose bodies were vacuumed from the joints with large cannulas. Histologic section identified these as osteochondromatoses. Because no metaplasia was identified in the synovium and because of the absence of articular disease, no arthrotomy was carried out. Both patients have remained asymptomatic for over a year.

A very satisfactory result was achieved by arthroscopic synovectomy after recurrence following open synovectomy. (See Chapter 20.)

It is interesting to note that these multiple loose bodies differ from those of diffuse degenerative arthritis. In osteochondromatosis, loose bodies are not absorbed by the synovium. The synovial metaplastic areas have a budding appearance and shed the loose bodies rather than engulf them.

GOUT

Acute gouty arthritis can exist in the absence of an elevated uric acid level or family history of the disease. There may be acute nonarticular arthritis of a knee joint. Arthroscopic findings are classic,[2] including marked inflammation and considerable villi proliferations. Tophaceous gouty deposits within the villi appear very much like crystals and are highlighted by the light on the arthro-

Synovial disease

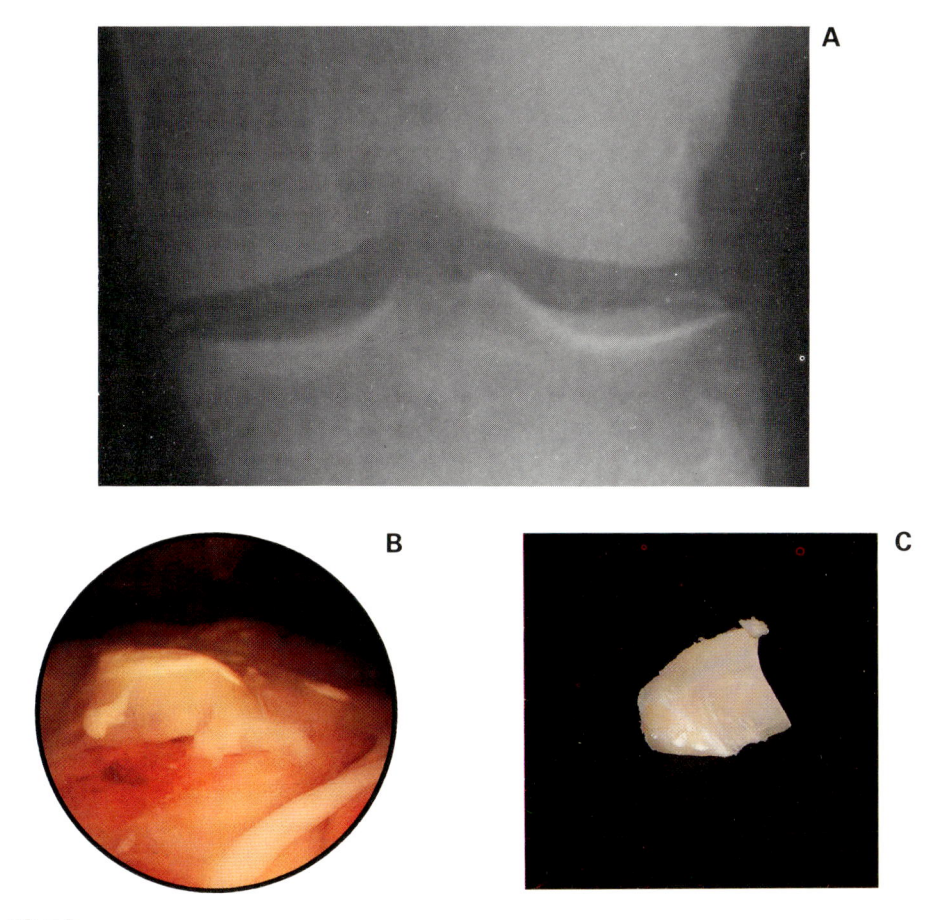

FIG. 13-14

A X-ray film of patient with pseudogout showing calcification of articular and meniscal tissues.
B Pseudogout shows calcium pyrophosphate crystals and plaques throughout synovial tissue. Vacuuming of joint and irrigation provide visual and pathologic diagnosis. Biopsy can be done with direct visualization to establish histologic diagnosis by polarized light on crystals.
C Cross section of meniscus in pseudogout.

scope; the eye is attracted to these deposits, and diagnosis is easily made. Confirmation can be made by direct-vision biopsy and histologic inspection or polarized-light arthroscopic identification.

PSEUDOGOUT

Pseudogout has been observed arthroscopically in four patients (Fig. 13-14, *B*). The calcium pyophosphate crystals are deposited in plaques, as opposed to the more isolated crystals seen in acute gout. The synovium is quite inflamed adjacent to the plaques. X-ray examination may show mineral deposition in the articular or meniscal tissue (Fig. 13-14, *A* and *C*). Direct biopsy provides material for polarized-light diagnosis. Biopsy can also be performed. Lavage of the joint at the time of arthroscopy is more than adequate treatment for a rather dramatic response.

Diagnostic arthroscopy of the knee

REITER SYNDROME

Reiter syndrome has been observed in one patient with acutely inflamed joint in which the mucosa appeared very much like that seen in streptococcal infections. There were no articular changes in the joint and no villi. The joint had virtually hundreds of pieces of fibrinoid exudate, which were selectively stained with methylene blue for identification and confirmed by histologic section. Vacuuming out these fibrinoid exudates resolved the synovitis sooner than would have been expected from the natural history of the condition (Fig. 13-15).

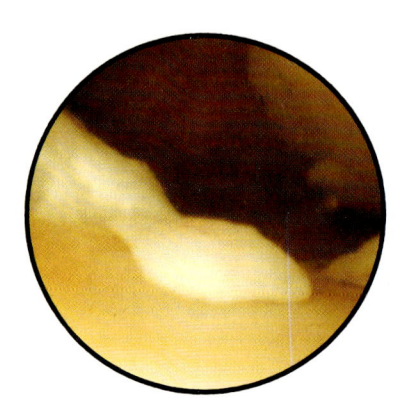

FIG. 13-15. Arthroscopic view of Reiter syndrome with loose fibrinoid bodies in joint.

HEMANGIOMA

Hemangioma was seen in a 19-year-old boy who had had multiple undiagnosed hemorrhages in his knee over time. Arthroscopic examination showed a synovial lining very much like that seen in pigmented villonodular synovitis. Suprapatellar pouch inspection showed a large mass of hemangiomatous tissue with considerable fibrous bands. There was not much reactive synovitis except for the pigmented villi. Resection of the hemangioma rendered the patient asymptomatic (Fig. 13-16).

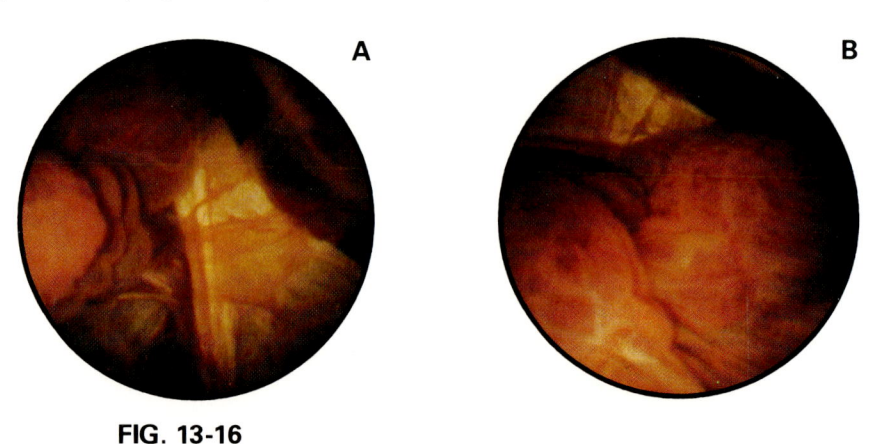

FIG. 13-16
A Synovial hemangioma in suprapatellar pouch.
B Close-up view of vascular abnormality of synovium.

Synovial disease

PSORIATIC ARTHRITIS

Psoriatic arthritis (Fig. 13-17) has a unique morphologic pattern. There is a marked arboretum of villi, which appear very lacy. Considerable vascular budding is seen within the wall of the synovium as well as in the arboretum of the tissue. Debris in the joint is fibrinoid but very shaggy, appearing like seaweed. It selectively stains with methylene blue. In contrast, in rheumatoid arthritis the fibrinoid exudate is on the tips of the villi, giving a dumbbell appearance. In Reiter syndrome these loose bodies are rather round and flat.

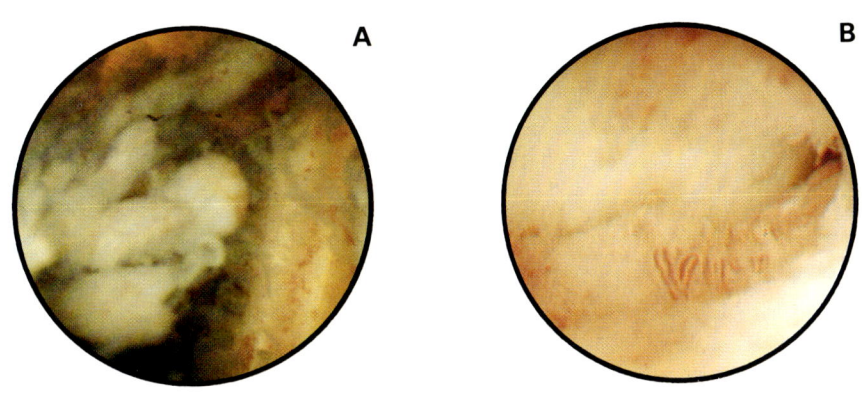

FIG. 13-17

A Psoriatic arthritis with lacelike synovial proliferation.
B Vascularity with rabbit-ear appearance of synovium in psoriatic arthritis.

HEMORRHAGIC SYNOVIUM

In any arthroscopic examination, attention should be paid to synovial hemorrhage (Fig. 13-18), especially in the area of the fat pad. This is usually indicative of a torn anterior cruciate ligament or an acute dislocation of the patella. On occasion, hemorrhagic synovium has been seen with contusion or parapatellar synovitis (Fig. 13-18, B). In the latter condition a shaggy fringe-type material about the patella catches within the patellofemoral junction, resulting in hemorrhage. Hemorrhage of pedunculated synovium has been seen in rheumatoid arthritis. Acute hemorrhage has a different characteristic and is easily identified morphologically.

ALKAPTONURIA

Alkaptonuria may produce a degenerative joint disease manifested by synovitis and even loose bodies (Fig. 13-19). These patients have a deficiency of homogentisic acid oxidase in the liver and kidneys. There are ochre deposits in the collagen tissue, hence the name *ochronosis*. Arthroscopically there is deposition in the meniscus (Fig. 13-19, A) and a coallike deposition that erodes the articular cartilage (Fig. 13-19, B and C). The clinical diagnosis is easily made in older patients by inspection of the earlobe (Fig. 13-19, E).

Diagnostic arthroscopy of the knee

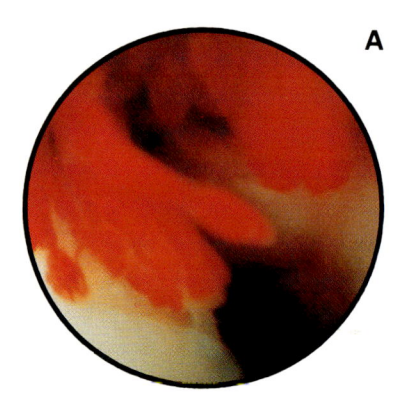

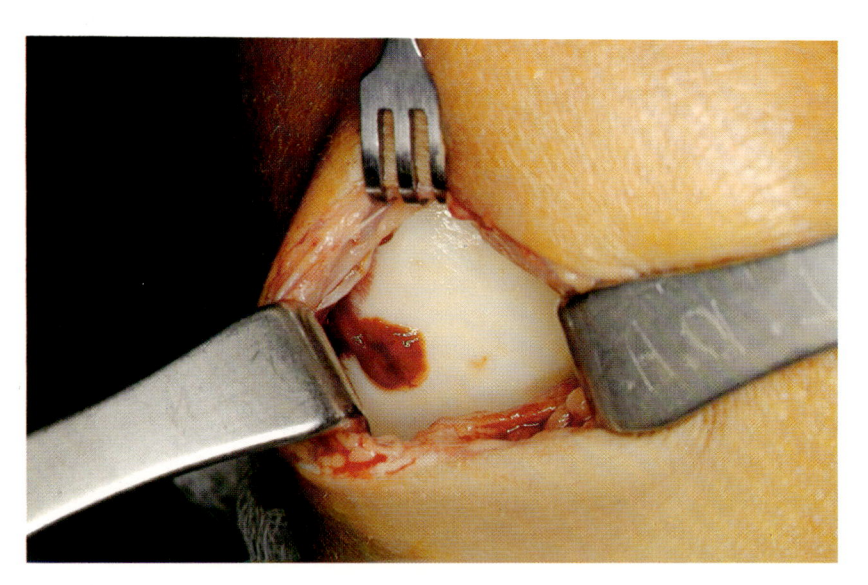

FIG. 13-18

A Subsynovial hemorrhage will disseminate into villi. If in fat pad, it usually indicates tear of anterior cruciate ligament. Acute dislocation of patella will show subsynovial hemorrhage as well.
B Traumatic pedunculated hemorrhagic synovium that mimicked torn medial meniscus. This was found prior to use of arthroscopy in my practice. At this time it could have been diagnosed and managed arthroscopically.

Synovial disease

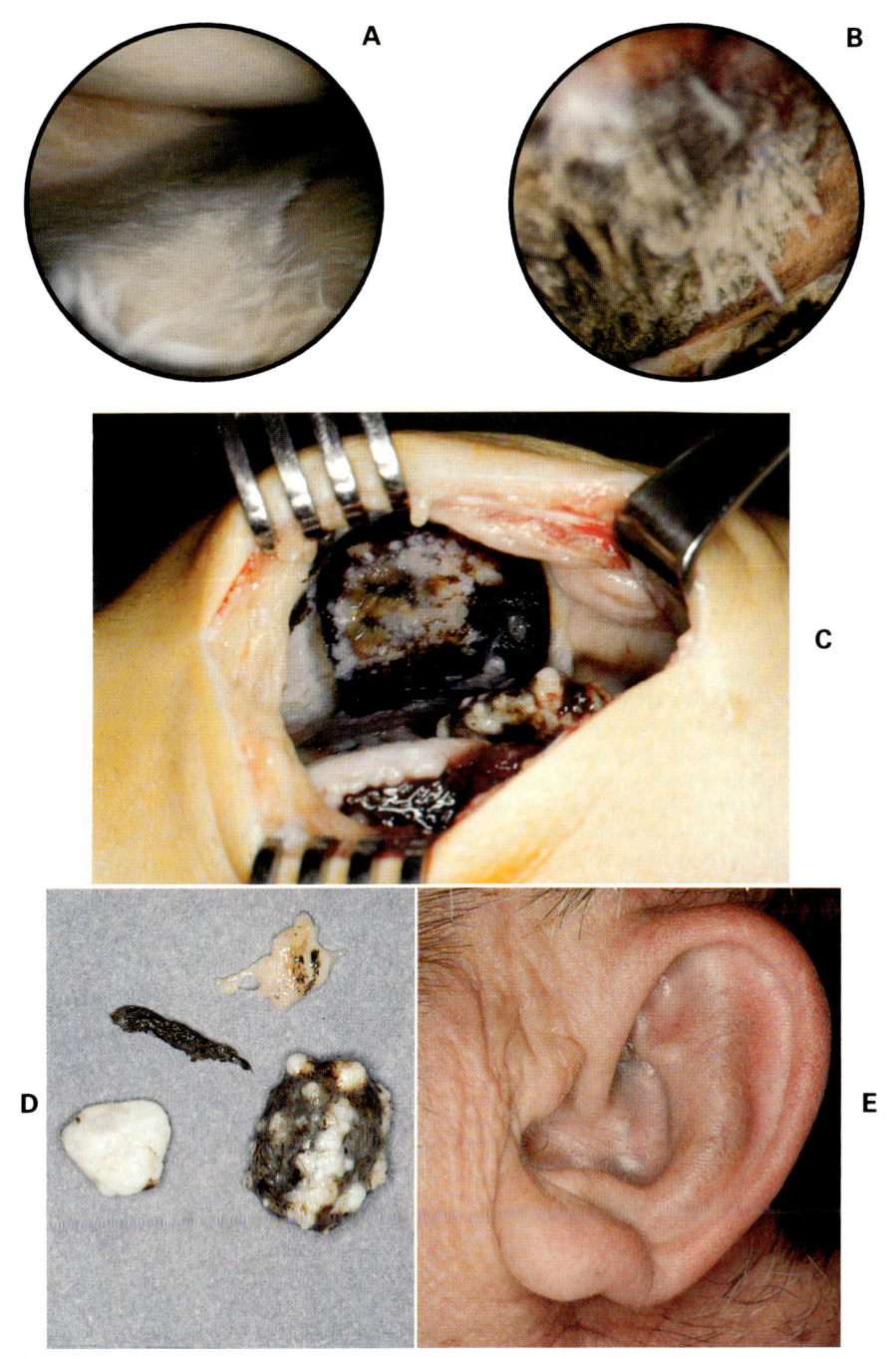

FIG. 13-19

A Ochronosis deposition in medial meniscus.
B Charcoal or chalklike destruction of articular cartilage of knee joint in patient without alkaptonuria.
C Same patient at arthrotomy showing changes in synovium and loose body in articular cartilage.
D Gross anatomic specimen of loose bodies and synovial and necrotic material removed from joint.
E Alkaptonuria is clinically identified by the bluish black pigment deposition in hyaline cartilage of ear.

FOREIGN BODIES

Persistent synovitis has been seen in some patients after penetration of the knee by an object (e.g., pieces of wood or nonradiopaque matter). With arthroscopy, injury or abrasion can be visualized in the joint and foreign bodies engulfed in the synovium can be identified. Local synovectomy is the treatment of choice.

PEDUNCULATED NODULAR SYNOVITIS

Several patients have had palpable loose bodies in the knee. Arthroscopy showed pedunculated nodular synovitis, which was resected arthroscopically. There has been no recurrence in these patients.

INFECTION

Some patients have had acute knee infection in which the synovium appeared identical to that seen in streptococcal mucosal infection. Cultures showed positive findings, and in one patient the infection was indeed due to *Streptococcus* organisms. I have not seen acute gonococcal arthritis arthroscopically.

Arthroscopy aspiration for analysis and culture, along with copious irrigation, can prevent the need for drainage by arthrotomy in some patients.

POSTOPERATIVE EVALUATIONS

Inspection of the joint in patients who have had total-knee replacement has not been particularly fruitful. We have documented photographically the regrowth of synovium in a patient who had had a geometric total-knee prosthesis for 18 months. She had catching and popping between the condylar surfaces, which was easily identifiable arthroscopically with active and passive motion. Injection of cortisone into the joint has rendered the patient asymptomatic for 2 years.

Some patients with Waldius total-knee prostheses have been seen because they had pain. Due to the very tight fibrotic sac, examination is difficult, and it has not been possible to tell whether there was cement loosening; therefore arthroscopy was not of much benefit.

I have been particularly hesitant in recommending that arthroscopy be performed routinely in patients with total-knee prostheses because of the risk of infection. One patient with a suspected low-grade infection had loosening of a Waldius prosthesis. During arthroscopy hemarthrosis developed, resulting in acute exacerbation of the subclinical infection. Arthrotomy and drainage were necessary. The prosthesis was subsequently removed.

REFERENCES

1. McKusick, V. A.: Heritable disorders of connective tissue, ed. 4, St. Louis, 1972, The C. V. Mosby Co.
2. O'Connor, R. L.: The role of arthroscopy in the management of crystal synovitis, J. Bone Joint Surg. **56**:206, 1974.
3. Watanabe, M., and Takeda, I. H.: Atlas of arthroscopy, ed. 3, Berlin, 1979, Springer-Verlag.

PART TWO

ARTHROSCOPIC SURGERY OF THE KNEE

Chapter 14

Surgical instrumentation

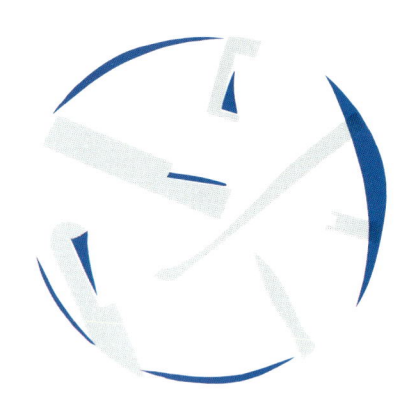

Development of powered instrumentation
 History
 Intra-articular Shaver System
 Further improvements
 Summary
Surgical equipment and instruments
 Visual equipment
 Positioning equipment
 Surgical Assistant
 Saline inflow
 Outflow
 Draping
 Other equipment
 Needle
 Surgical hand tools
 Hand cutting instruments
 Operating arthroscopes
 Intra-articular Shaver System
 Golden Retriever

DEVELOPMENT OF POWERED INSTRUMENTATION
History

Arthroscopy is a surgical procedure. Further manipulation or removal of intra-articular structures appropriately falls under the heading of arthroscopic surgery. The simple procedures of removing loose bodies or sectioning synovial folds by transcutaneous methods have been performed over the years by arthroscopists. Watanabe[10,11] performed the first resection of meniscal tissue by arthroscopic control in 1962. Jackson and Dandy[6] had advocated a partial meniscectomy by arthroscopic means or open arthrotomy if not technically possible by the former method. O'Conner[8] developed instrumentation and an arthroscopic technique for the resection of meniscal tissue. He also advocated the partial meniscectomy. Metcalf[7] has performed more than 600 arthroscopic partial meniscectomies in the past few years with uniformly good results.

Oretorp and Gillquist,[9] in Sweden, have developed instrumentation and techniques for arthroscopic surgery, especially the total meniscectomy. Carson[2] has reported the total resection of the posterior half of the meniscus.

All these methods involved a transcutaneous procedure performed under direct arthroscopic visualization coupled with manual tools for biting and cutting tissue.[5,9,11] These procedures are demanding technically. Initially, considerable time is required to accomplish the removal of even a portion of the meniscus. The multiple passes may result in "scuffing" of the articular surfaces, even with a smooth instrument.

Arthroscopic surgery of the knee

A few follow-up examinations, after a partial meniscectomy, have been reported.[6,8]

Development of powered instrumentation was mandatory to make arthroscopic surgery a viable, useful technique in the hands of orthopedic surgeons. Powered instrumentation was designed to meet the following criteria:

1. An operative time comparable to that of conventional methods
2. Attention to:
    a. Aseptic technique
    b. Adequate exposure
    c. Tissue cutting under tension
    d. Gentleness with tissue
3. An operative environment allowing a comfortable position for the surgeon, plus freedom of both hands for operative manipulation
4. Last, but not least, less morbidity than and results comparable to, if not better than, conventional methods.

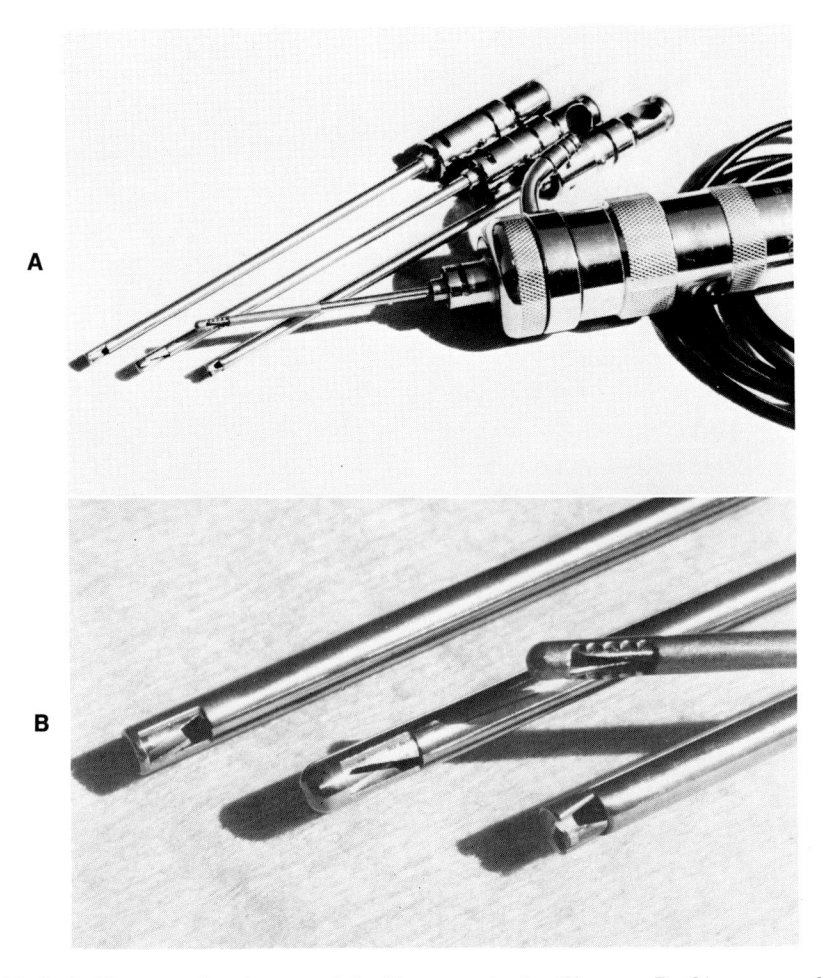

FIG. 14-1. A, First production model of Intra-articular Shaver. **B,** Close-up of cannulas.

Surgical instrumentation

In 1975, discussions were held with biomedical engineers to choose a pathologic model for developing a system of intra-articular power instrumentation. Because of the nature of meniscal tissue and the small potential space of the compartment, a staged approach was planned toward the development of meniscectomy instrumentation. The main requirement was adequate space for manipulation of both an arthroscope and the power instrumentation.

Severe chondromalacia of the patella seemed to provide the ideal model for this type of development. First, the patella is in the largest potential space in the knee joint, the suprapatellar pouch. Most orthopedists are familiar with this area from their experience with aspiration within the knee joint. Also, chondromalacia heretofore was not treated successfully by arthrotomy and knife blade shaving.[1,12] There was considerable down side safety in attempting arthroscopic surgery. An open operation could always be performed. Also, it seemed unlikely that the results of treatment would be worse after arthroscopic surgery.

Thus an attempt was made to develop an instrument that would both cut and remove tissue from the articular surfaces of the patella. This instrument ultimately became known as the Intra-articular Shaver System (Fig. 14-1).

Intra-articular Shaver System

The first model was a hand-operated, battery-powered, unidirectional, rotating-cutting suction device (Fig. 14-2). At that stage of development the procedure took so long that the operator developed considerable hand fatigue, as well as other problems incurred with this new technique. The system was then modified with a foot-pedal control with reverse and forward cutting modes. This had a definite advantage over the single mode of rotation because some tissues tend to fold one way or another and can be cut better from the opposite direction by reversing the rotation.

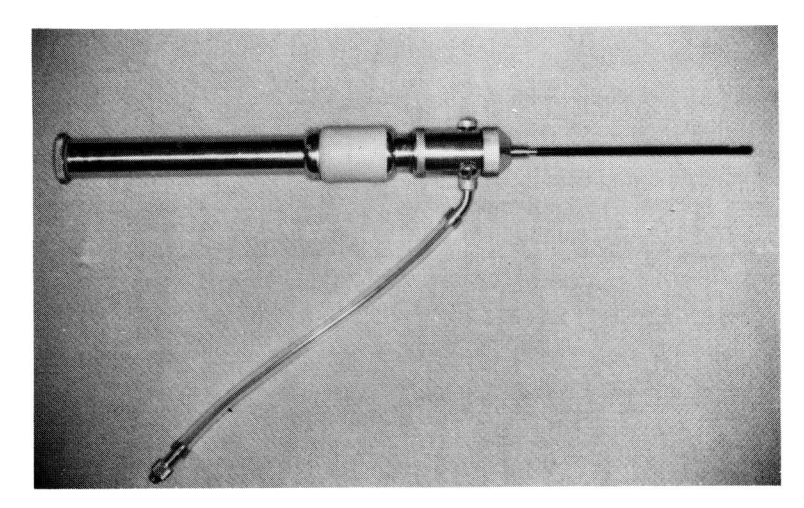

FIG. 14-2. Prototype of Intra-articular Shaver was hand-activated model.

Visualization was essential. Initially these procedures were controlled by direct visualization. This required flexion of the physician's back and loss of use of the hand that held the arthroscope. A video monitor system was introduced and solved this problem. Video has continued to be an integral dimension of this arthroscopic surgical technique.

Adequate joint distension is important to arthroscopic visualization; it took on a greater role with arthroscopic surgery. The inflow of saline was originally regulated with a heart-lung machine. This permitted calibration of pressures and flow. The patient's fluid intake and output were measured preoperatively and postoperatively because of the considerable infusion of saline. Because the potential problem of saline absorption had no clinical effect on the cardiovascular or other systems, intake and output measurements were abandoned. Next, the cost of regulating inflow with an expensive heart-lung pump could be eliminated. Consultation with urologic surgeons revealed that the same flows could be achieved with 6 liters of saline elevated 1 m above the patient. The flow and pressures were carefully calibrated to the openings and tubes of the Intra-articular Shaver System. The room suction in my operating room measured at 15 inches of mercury.

The last dimension to be considered technically was the RPM of the motor. My initial impression was that a higher RPM would be better. By trial and error I learned that approximately 150 RPM in air or 100 RPM in saline was perfect for the calibrated system to create tension in tissue for excision. Also, a slower RPM was important so that the window could stay open long enough to draw the material into the opening for excision.

At this stage the instrument was safe and useful and would cut articular debris off the patella, although it was more efficient at cutting peripatellar synovium. The inability to cut deeply on the articular tissue was discouraging, and measures were considered to make the instrument more aggressive. While this was being attempted the patients were experiencing remarkable relief from crepitus as well as the elimination of pain and effusion. Therefore second-look arthroscopies were in order (Fig. 14-3, C). They demonstrated healing of the patellar articular surfaces to an extent not as yet thought possible with "inadequate" shaving or debridement. The patella was not drilled to bleeding bone as was previously thought necessary to achieve healing.[4]

Thirteen of the initial 72 patients reviewed have submitted to second-look arthroscopy and showed coalescence of the articular cartilage. Subsequent histologic sections have shown a flow of fibrocartilage from the articular cartilage. (See Chapter 8.) It fills in the spaces and coalesces the defects. No further attempt was made to make the original Intra-articular Shaver head more aggressive for articular cartilage.

Experience with the Intra-articular Shaver was encouraging clinically, in my chondromalacia patella model. The first stage provided the hydrodynamics, the basic equipment, and the technical abilities and coordinated team approach. As a bonus, a simple, safe, effective method of treating severe chondromalacia became a reality.

Surgical instrumentation

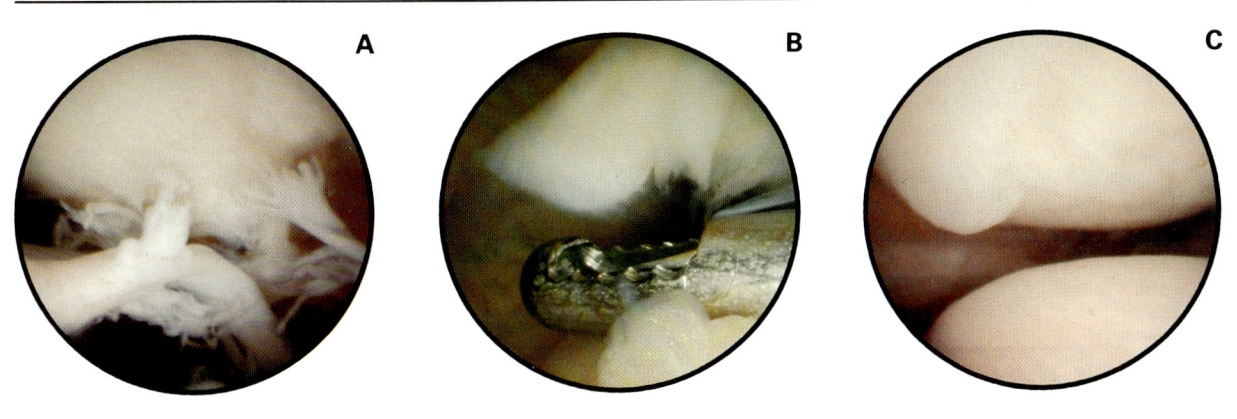

FIG. 14-3

A Arthroscopic views of severe chondromalacia patellae.
B Intra-articular Shaver cutting debris from patella.
C Two years after intra-articular shave of patella.

Further improvements

The original Intra-articular Shaver would debride only the most degenerative meniscal flap tear. Improved cutting was finally possible in January, 1978, with the design of the keyhole shape and the subsequent development of the cutter. This design permitted cutting at the end, corner, and side. The first arthroscopic meniscectomy with this instrument was performed May 17, 1978. Initially, cutting was slow because of metal deformation and fatigue. That was solved with improved metals. By September, 1978, arthroscopic total meniscectomy by powered instrumentation was possible but required approximately 50 minutes of surgical time. Subtotal arthroscopic meniscectomies were accomplished in less time.

Still, two major problems existed. The 4-pound television camera was too heavy for the assistant to hold for extended periods. Second, visualization was often compromised by lack of joint space opening. Two major additions to our armamentarium facilitated operative arthroscopy, especially in the medial and lateral compartments. First was the addition of the articulated viewing arm connecting the endoscope to a suspended television camera (Fig. 14-4). It greatly reduced the fatigue of the first assistant. This device was developed by Professor Wittmoser of West Germany and Professor Hopkins of England. It is modified by the Karl Storz Company. They are available in 5, 3, and 2 articulations, with the cost increasing for more articulations. The greater the number of articulations, the less illumination transmitted. This occurs because illumination is lost at every glass interface.

Second was the development of a mechanical means of securing the thigh—the Surgical Assistant (Fig. 14-5). This instrument secured the distal femur but permitted a few millimeters more opening of the joint space. The view of posterior horns was excellent, and space for the entrance of instruments was created. This also eliminated fatigue on the part of the second assistant and the relief person and eliminated the often moving target.

Arthroscopic surgery of the knee

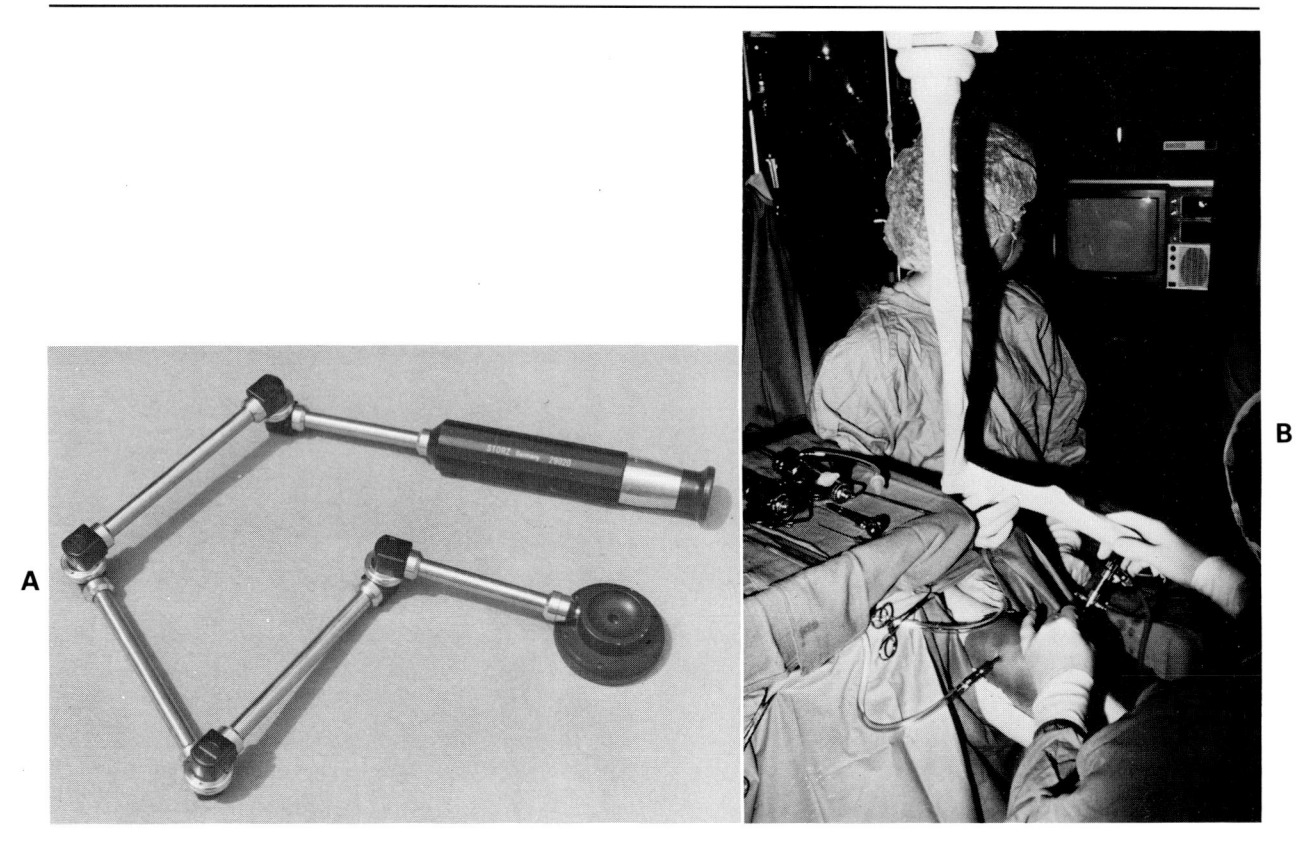

FIG. 14-4. A, Articulated viewing device suspended between camera and television. **B,** Covered with sterile stockinette.

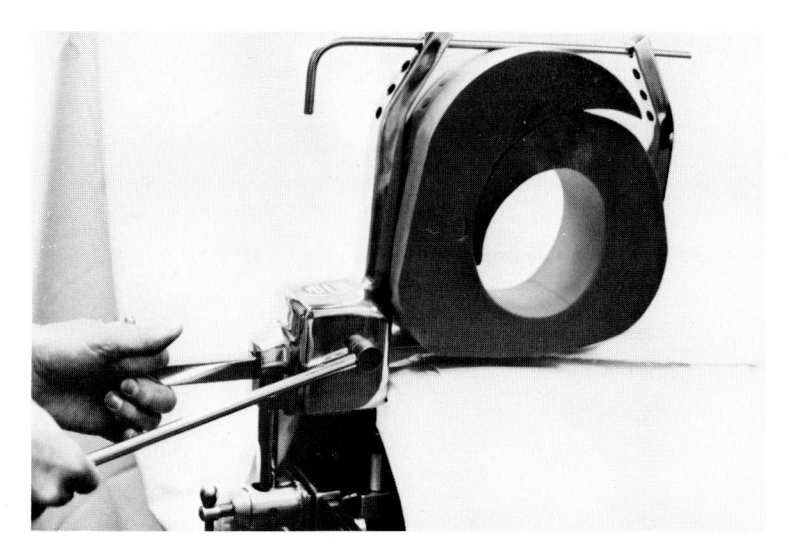

FIG. 14-5. Surgical Assistant is 17-pound metallic frame with foam insert that attaches to operating room table and provides excellent stability of proximal thigh. It is secured by pumping handle of mechanism and then locking.

Surgical instrumentation

The criteria were met to promote arthroscopic surgery. By the fall of 1978, arthroscopic surgery was performed in all compartments, including the intra-articular shave of the patella, sectioning of synovial lining, removal of loose bodies, and meniscectomy without the enormous technical effort necessary by manual instrumentation. The Intra-articular Shaver System was a reality.

Summary

As exciting as all this seemed to be, arthroscopic surgery is no more advanced than the automotive industry was at the time of the Model T Ford. There were many horses and buggies that could outrun the Model T. So it is with knee joint surgery. Many orthopedists do not consider using so much time and effort when a conventional arthrotomy can accomplish the same results.

Like the automotive industry, arthroscopic surgery will change in time. There are many surgeons who feel they can perform an open operation or arthrotomy much faster than by arthroscopic means. Some arthroscopic surgeons say the manual biting of the tissues is faster for them. It is my conviction that the former methods will pass away.

SURGICAL EQUIPMENT AND INSTRUMENTS

A surgeon's instrumentation must be excellent and will require a significant investment. Fortunately, I have been able to purchase this equipment over a period of time. The cost has been nearly $30,000 including breakage and replacement. It will not be less for any other arthroscopist.

It is possible to compromise for this type of surgery and eliminate the purchase of some major item or link in the system. I recommend, however, that the serious arthroscopist or arthroscopic surgeon purchase the best equipment and have no weak link. Do not be delayed by waiting for a better model next year. We hope for better tools but do not wait for them.

The following material describes the many different tools and instruments being used in arthroscopic surgery. The system has been developed by purchasing existing surgical instruments, modifying others, and creating new ones. There is no one company or source that provides the entire package.

This material is not a "consumer report." No effort has been made to evaluate every instrument on the market. This list merely reflects those which appeared the best at the time this system was developing and have proved satisfactory in my hands.

Visual equipment
Arthroscopes

Types of arthroscopes are discussed in Chapter 2. I have been using the 4-mm, 30° inclined Storz scope with a 5-mm sheath for my surgical work. The Needlescope is used for diagnostic work and auxiliary posterior punctures that are occasionally necessary to accompany the surgical procedures. The larger diameter Storz model provides an excellent actual field of view, apparent field of view, brightness, and clarity. The larger scope that carries more light down its channel with the fiberoptic cable and more back through its larger lenses is

221

Arthroscopic surgery of the knee

necessary because of the loss of light that occurs within the articulated viewing device. The 30° inclined view facilitates operative work. A powerful light source, as mentioned in Chapter 2, is essential.

Articulated viewing device

The articulated viewing device (Fig. 14-4) is a linkage of glass prisms that allows angulation and rotation by the nature of the mechanical connections. It provides a link between the ocular of the arthroscope and the suspended television camera. It is expensive but has excellent optical clarity. Thus it is not necessary for an assistant to hold a heavy video camera and its cord connection to the monitor system. (See Chapter 15.) It is not sterilized, even in ethylene oxide, because of potential deterioration. It is covered with a sterile stockinette.

My initial experience was with the five-articulated projection onto television for teaching and research purposes. Since then I have acquired a three-articulated viewing device. It transmits 30% more illumination and has a significantly reduced cost, but it is too short to be suspended and must be covered with a sterile stockinette and placed on the Mayo stand.

Television

The television plays a very important role in arthroscopic surgery (Fig. 14-6). It allows a comfortable position for the surgeon and frees both hands for manipulation. The art of operating while viewing a video screen has not been difficult to learn. The added benefits of encouragement and interest for the operating room personnel have been immeasurable.

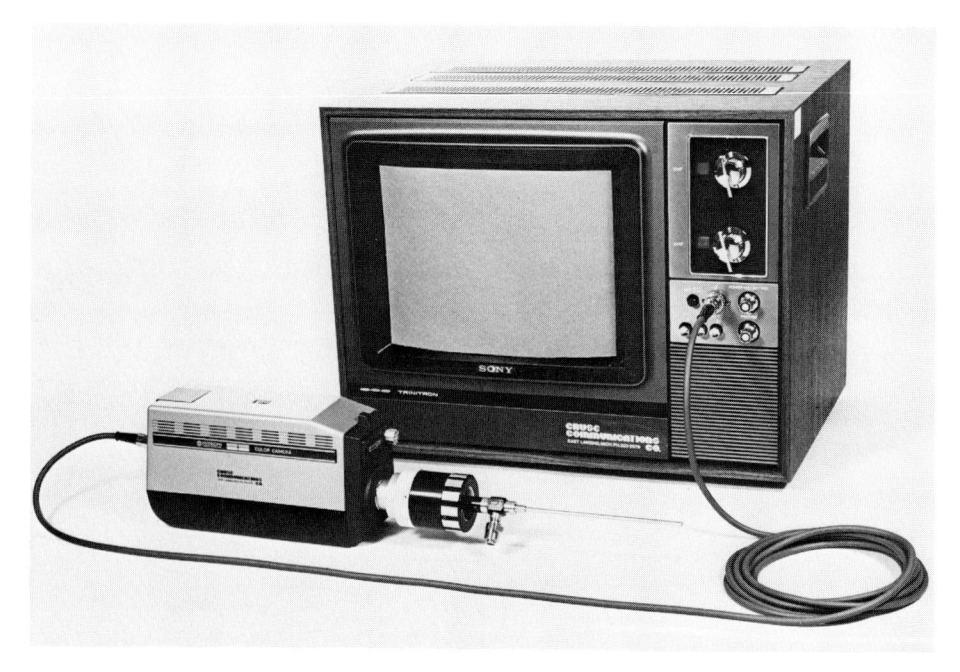

FIG. 14-6. Video monitoring is important part of arthroscopic surgery. This system has been especially modified for arthroscopist's needs. (Courtesy Cruse Communications, East Lansing, Mich.)

Surgical instrumentation

Camera

I have been using a Hitachi 9025 camera that is approximately 6 years old. There are many new developments in video. An effective, relatively inexpensive way to accomplish video viewing is with a video camera customized with a direct connection to a television monitor (Fig. 14-6). Simultaneous recording is excellent for teaching and research and can be accomplished with a professional ¾-inch, or the more economical ½-inch, cassette system (Fig. 14-7). The recording quality of both systems is equal. At most professional meetings a ¾-inch player is used. Surgeons with ½-inch material would have to convert to ¾ inch for some presentations. Until there are miniaturized video cameras producing adequate light and in color, it seems necessary to continue using the intra-articular viewing device and the suspended camera system. High-cost medical units have not produced any better image.

Positioning equipment

A standard operating room table with the ability to break down at the foot is recommended. The Clark attachment on the operating table (Fig. 14-8) holds the Surgical Assistant fixation bar.

Surgical Assistant

The Surgical Assistant* is a 15-pound surgical steel frame with a specially designed closed-cell foam insert and a crossbar (Fig. 14-9). It eliminates the inconsistency that occurs when the thigh is held or secured by a human assistant. It also provides an excellent fulcrum for opening into varus or valgus position and internal and external rotation under the exacting control of the surgeon. To date, there have been no means to provide this proximal fixation

---

*Instrument Makar, Inc., 4536 S. Hagadorn, East Lansing, Mich. 48823.

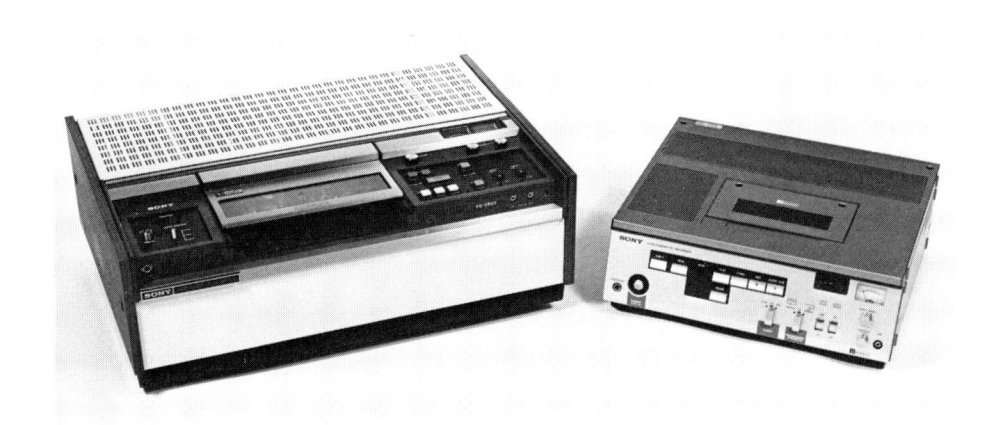

FIG. 14-7. Television recorders can be either professional ¾-inch or ½-inch Betamax type for home use.

Arthroscopic surgery of the knee

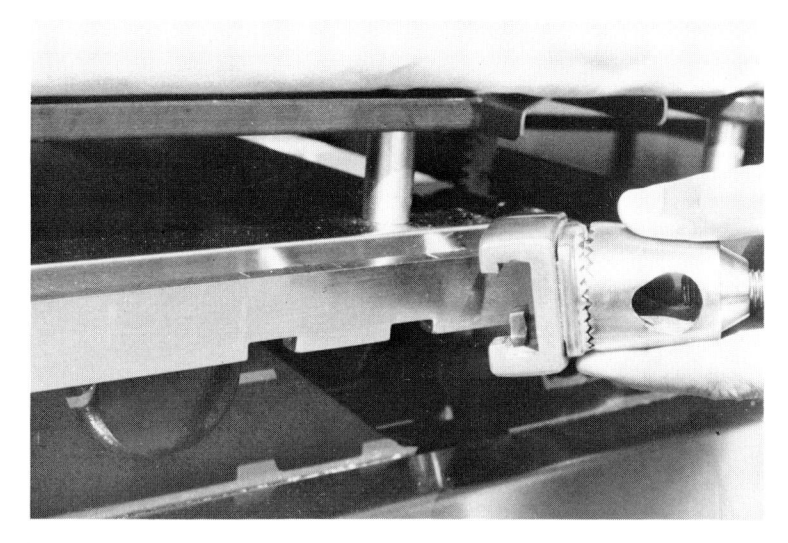

FIG. 14-8. Clark attachment is generally used for stirrups suspension but also to accommodate Surgical Assistant for arthroscopic surgery.

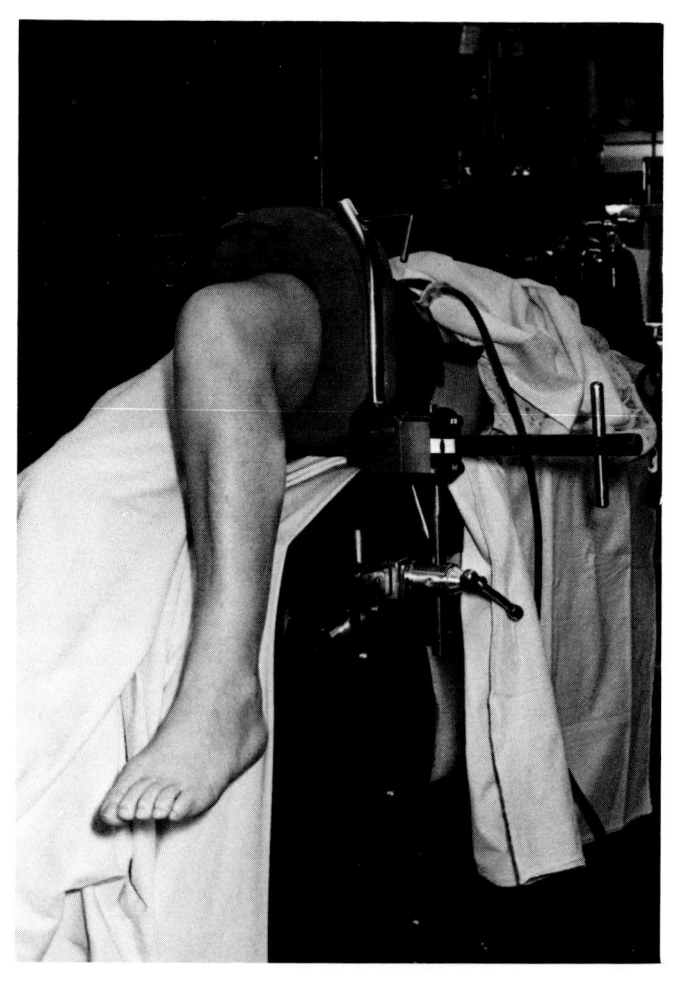

FIG. 14-9. Surgical Assistant is tightened around leg approximately 4 to 6 inches above superior aspect of patella. Normal circular circumference of thigh has changed to quadrilateral configuration for better fixation of distal thigh.

Surgical instrumentation

that allows the maximum opening on all compartments of the knee. Just as in other kinds of surgery, one should not be cutting or resecting in an area that is outside his field of vision. A mechanical assistant allows a 1- or 2-mm greater opening, a mechanical advantage for direct visualization into the compartments of the knee heretofore not able to be viewed by other means.

The closed-cell foam inserts are washable and have excellent cleanability. Their durability has been proved in more than 1500 cases. They are not steam autoclavable and would enlarge and deform if that was attempted. There is some compression of the foam, but not enough deformation to interfere with its function.

The special feature of the locking device cam is the ratchet mechanism by which one can tighten the device more than would be possible by mechanical means or pressure. The T-bar is pulled as the cam level performs the tightening.

Some surgeons who use the Surgical Assistant have encountered compromised space between the upper portion of the patella and the attachment of the Surgical Assistant below the tourniquet, especially in short, overweight women. These surgeons favor this system because they do not use video; thus the head must be put down next to the knee joint, from which position it can bump into or contaminate the Surgical Assistant. They have solved the problem in one of two ways. The first is to put the Surgical Assistant high on the thigh and the tourniquet below, which eliminates the mass of the Surgical Assistant down near the patella or knee joint. The other method is to attach the tourniquet in its normal position, apply the Surgical Assistant around the tourniquet, and then inflate the tourniquet. Neither method has caused any neurovascular complications to date, according to the reports I have received.

I have not found it necessary to use those methods on any patient yet because the regular use of the arthroscope attached to the articulated viewing device does not occupy that type of space and does not cause any difficulty in either viewing or performing a lateral release or patellar surgical procedure from this comprehensive setup.

Saline Inflow

The inflow is created by 6 liters of saline suspended on an IV pole. I also use a special circular sandbag to secure the base of the IV pole; when the bags are full and elevated to a considerable height, this system could topple over (Fig. 14-10). The 4.2-mm cannula system of the Intra-articular Shaver is also necessary for the inflow conduit.

Outflow

The outflow tubing attached to the shaver should be as short as possible yet provide some freedom of motion for the surgeon. Long, coiled outflow tubes between a wall vacuum and a collecting bottle are a disadvantage and can reduce the force.

A large collecting bottle that holds many gallons is beneficial in the initial, long surgical procedures (Fig. 14-11). A collection bag is taped to the inflow

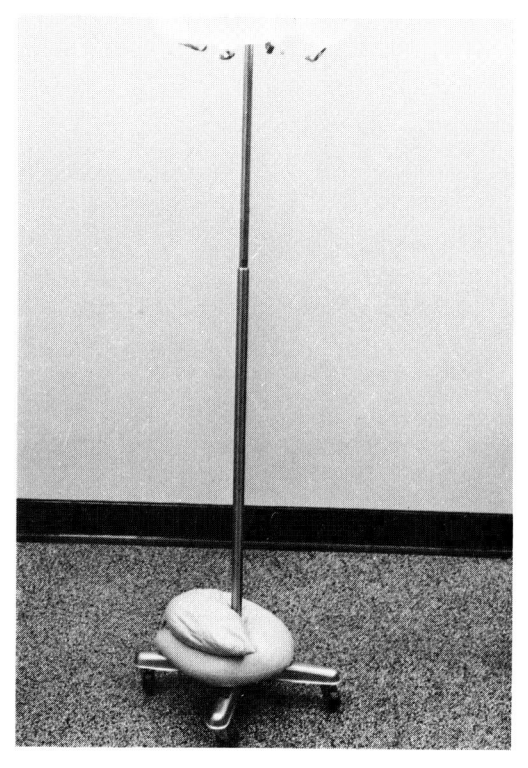

FIG. 14-10. Circular sandbag around base of most IV poles will prevent accidental tipping, since weight is elevated high above floor.

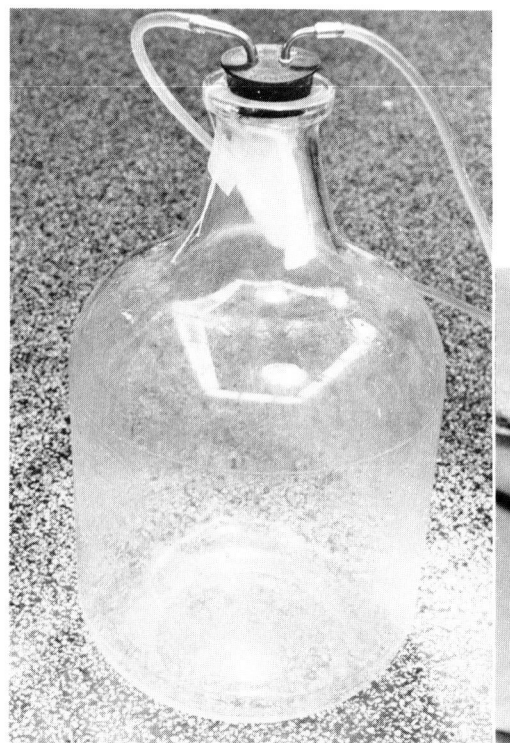

FIG. 14-11. A, Large suction bottle accommodates even longest procedure and abundant saline usage. Collection bag is placed in top of suction bottle; thus decanting of all fluid is not necessary at end of procedure. **B,** Suction tube showing pieces of debrided articular material being removed from joint.

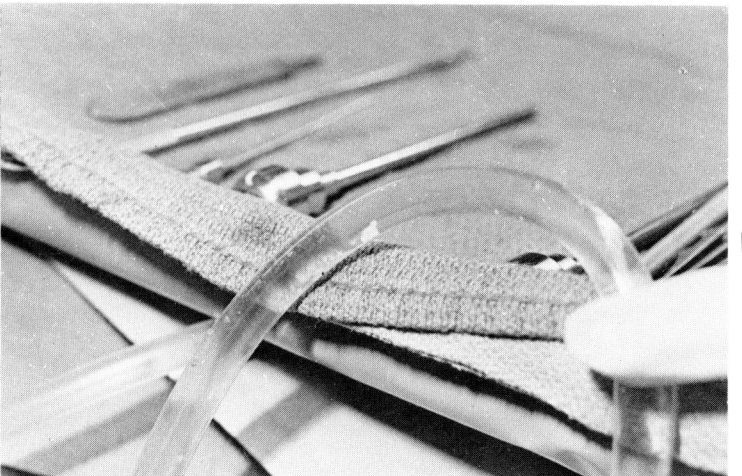

Surgical instrumentation

and collects the resected material. Thus it is not necessary to decant large amounts of saline to collect the specimen.

Draping

The commercially available drape with the plasticized stockinette, as well as plastic drapes with adhesive seals and water-impervious paper drapes with absorption qualities, are used. Water-impervious gowns are used for the physician's comfort, as are a plastic drape and a paper shoe cover in case of the inevitable spillage of saline.

Other equipment

One or two Mayo stands, depending on the procedure, a back table for instruments, and a stool for the surgeon are required. (See Chapter 15.) A separate table or stand is necessary for the power unit as well as one for the light source.

Needle

A No. 18 spinal needle is essential for locating the transcutaneous portal of entry.

Surgical hand tools
Probe

The probe is perhaps the most basic hand instrument for arthroscopy and especially arthroscopic surgery. The Dandy probe, used in other disciplines, has been adopted by arthroscopic surgeons. The Oretorp probe has excellent design for handling (Fig. 14-12). It has calibration marks near the end of the probe for intra-articular measurements. Both are of good size and

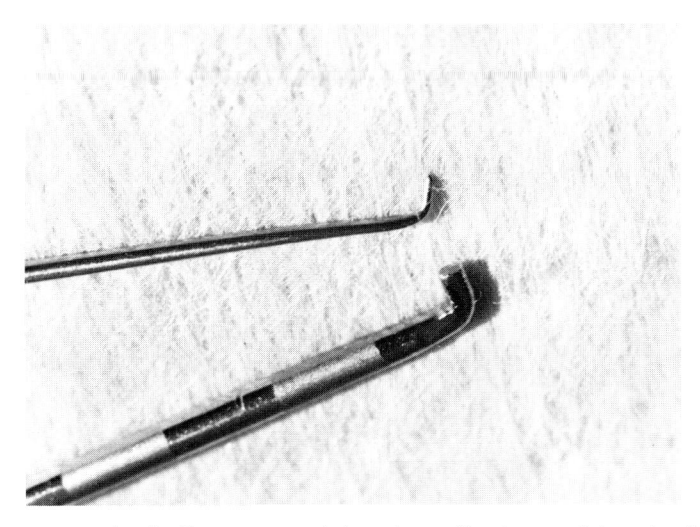

FIG. 14-12. Larger probe is Oretorp model and smaller is special probe for arthroscopic surgery.

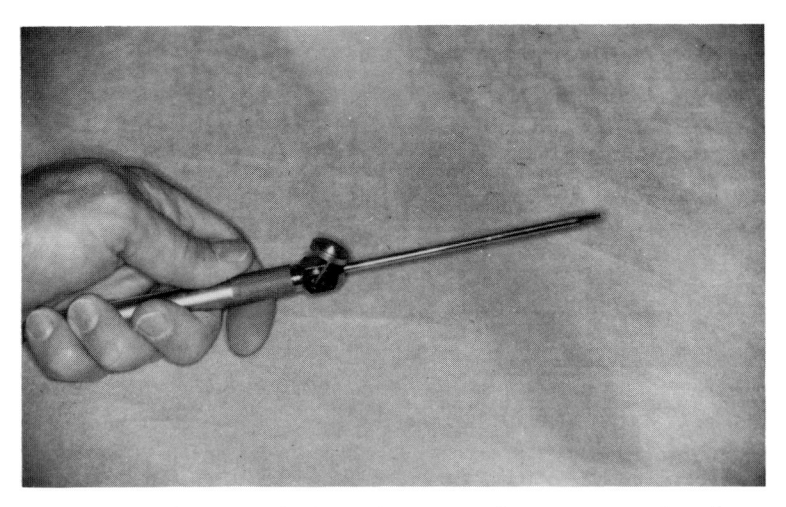

FIG. 14-13. Oretorp knife blade is based on excellent concept but has rather large handle that limits moving into posterior compartment.

excellent design for this type of work. Sometimes the smaller one is preferred because of access into tight spaces. Both are smooth enough so that they do not abrade the joint. With them the surgeon can elevate the meniscus or draw the posterior horn of the meniscus forward to inspect for clefts that otherwise might not be seen.

An arthroscopic hand instrument set is available. There are two probe designs that fit the Intra-articular Shaver System. One is large, similar to the Dandy or Oretorp; the other is small, which I find more valuable in the small recesses and for palpation, as well as for hooking small loose bodies or small indentations of the menisci (Fig. 14-12).

Knives

There are a number of different knife blades and handles available. The most basic is the modified handle made by the Beaver Company, which attaches readily to their blades (Fig. 14-14). The Beaver No. 67 is a conventional knife blade most useful for cutting soft tissue. It is preferred for lateral release. The No. 64 Beaver blade is rounded on the end yet has sharpness all the way around the end. It is excellent for incising the meniscus but is ineffective for lateral release. The Beaver blades have a potential for breaking.

The handle and disposable knife blade can enter the cannula system. The cannula may be retracted completely off the knife blade or lead the handle through the tissue with the blade in the knife for ease of manipulation. Of course, it can also be left in place and just retracted a bit. The advantage of completely removing the cannula from the knife blade is that it removes any possibility of leakage of saline.

Unfortunately, disposable blades are of necessity attached to a stock handle with a rather large diameter. This can limit access to the joint. Often during viewing of the tip of the blade the handle abuts the articular surface. They are the sharpest disposable blades at an economical price available at this time.

Oretorp has introduced a rather ingenious retractable blade system (Fig.

Surgical instrumentation

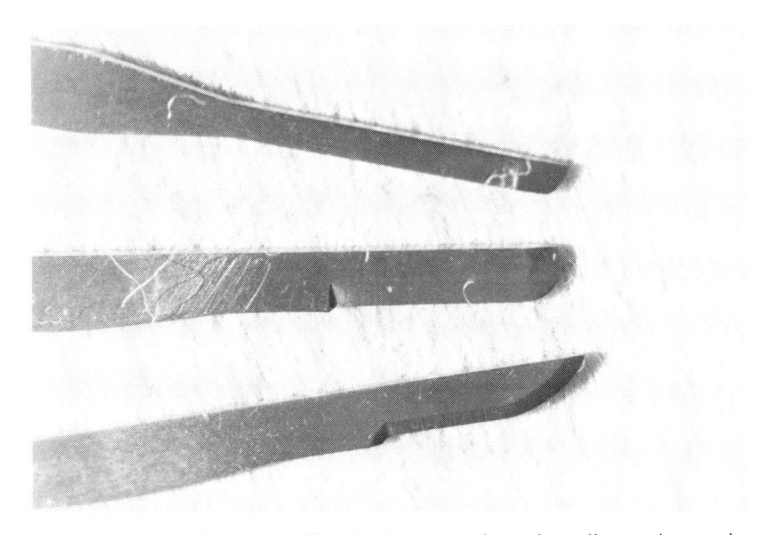

FIG. 14-14. Disposable miniature knife blades attach to handle and are sharp. They are brittle and can break.

14-13). The retractability is its best feature. The disadvantage is the high cost of the blades ($25). After one steam autoclaving they lose their maximum sharpness. There are three shapes, which is an advantage, but the cost at this time has limited their practicality. Also, the size of the shaft that holds the knife blade is similar to that of the Beaver handle; this limits its access to all areas (Fig. 14-14). The more recently produced blades are thicker to reduce breakage potential (Fig. 14-15).

A variety of other miniature knife blades has been developed for transcutaneous surgery (Figs. 14-15 and 14-16). The specific shapes of these blades fit specific arthroscopic surgical needs. They have replaced the Beaver handle or Oretorp retractable system because of their smaller size and graduated handle. Their small size facilitates access to the posterior compartments and intercondylar posterior horn area not reachable by any of the blades just mentioned. Also, their transcutaneous route leaves only minimal punctures, similar to the needle laceration for arthrocentesis, and the puncture wounds do not result in leakage of saline. They have microhurled handles for excellent gripping, and they can be passed through a cannula or used percutaneously. They are disposable but reusable with gas sterilization. However, steam sterilization can greatly reduce their effectiveness. Cidex soaking is acceptable. They are malleable, less brittle, and magnetic.

The No. 711 IM blade is for plica resectioning. The No. 747 is like a miniature traditional meniscotome. It is used to release the posterior horn of the bucket-handle tear. The 764 and 767 blades have replaced the similar shaped Beaver blades in our system because their shape allows them to glide under the condyle and reduces breakability.

IM blades are used to release or develop meniscal tissue for resection. There are some positions in which the Intra-articular Shaver cannot be positioned to resect the meniscal tissue, and the knife blade can develop those edges.

Arthroscopic surgery of the knee

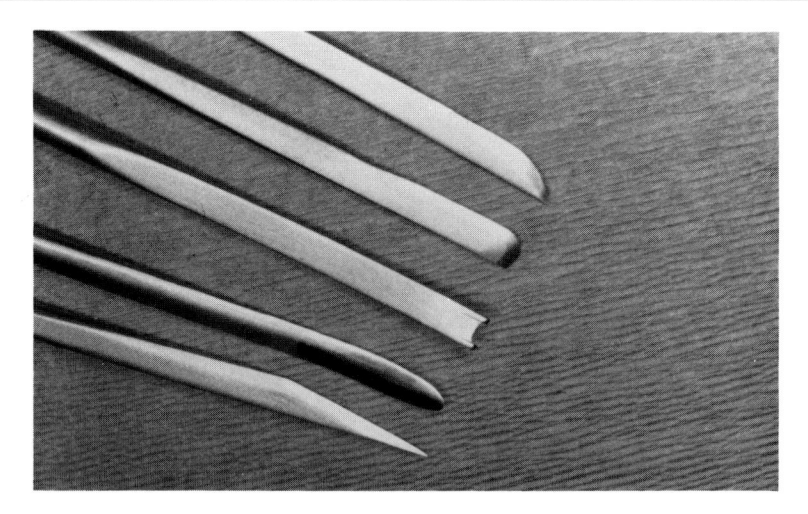

FIG. 14-15. IM microblades are available in five sizes. From top to bottom they are: No. 711, for sectioning synovial plicas; No. 761, which has two sharp edges and is slightly curved; it is excellent for balancing anterior horn of meniscus, for resection of posterior horn tears, and reshaping of posterior meniscus; No. 747, miniature Smiley type, traditionally used for meniscal surgery, especially for longitudinal tears and posterior detachment of bucket-handle tears; No. 764, designed to resect anterior horns of menisci with bucket-handle tears and sectioning base of flap tears and some posterior horn meniscal tears; No. 767, used in arthroscopic lateral release under direct visualization.

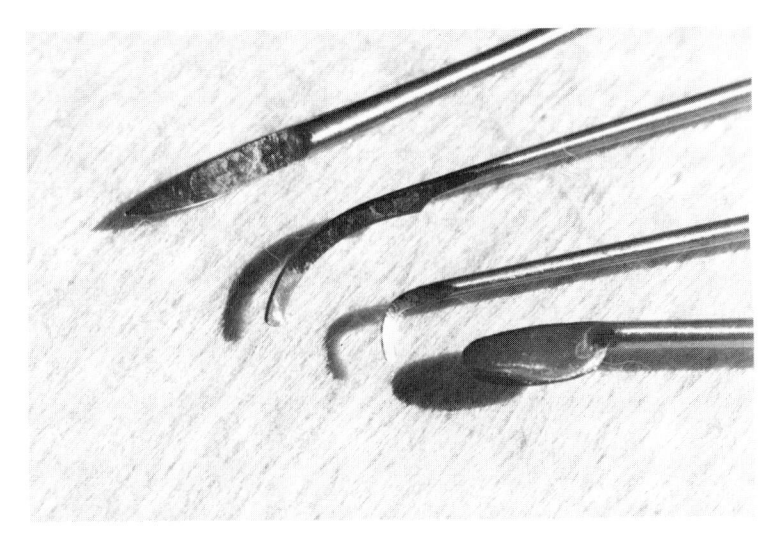

FIG. 14-16. Multiple small knife blades in various shapes are available for specific tasks in intra-articular surgery.

Surgical instrumentation

An oblique-angled end-cutting meniscotome (IM blade No. 761) is used to release the most extreme posterior horn of the meniscus.

Graspers

Among the instruments used for grasping, the Jaws Jr. and the standard Jaws are good choices in the treatment of loose bodies. (See Fig. 2-10.) The smaller one passes through the cannula system; the larger one is for larger loose pieces but will not pass through the cannula system.

The Schlessinger Grasper, a multitooth clamp made by the George Tieman Company, has excellent teeth (Fig. 14-17). It is sturdier than any other grasper I have used. It is best for grasping meniscal tissue and some tenacious loose bodies. It also has the capacity to bite through some areas of tenacious meniscal tissue. Another type is a sliding grasper for holding a released anterior portion of a bucket-handle tear (Fig. 14-18). Thus it is not necessary to hold onto a clamp. It is self securing and allows the meniscus to be brought up under tension; yet it eliminates having to squeeze some instrument or hold grasping forceps with a towel clip.

There is a miniature grasper with teeth for reaching in to grasp small fragments of meniscus, especially in the posterior horn (Fig. 14-19). It is of considerable value when using transcutaneous knife blades to resect or trim in the area of the posterior horn or extreme posterior attachment of the meniscus.

The grasping forceps that accompany the Oretorp system have a space between the graspers, which makes them ineffective in holding onto the meniscus. Also, the graspers that accompany other systems do not have the strength or power of the Schlessinger model.

Miniature harpoon

A fishhook or miniature harpoon can assist in grasping small pieces in tight areas of the knee for cutting and removal.

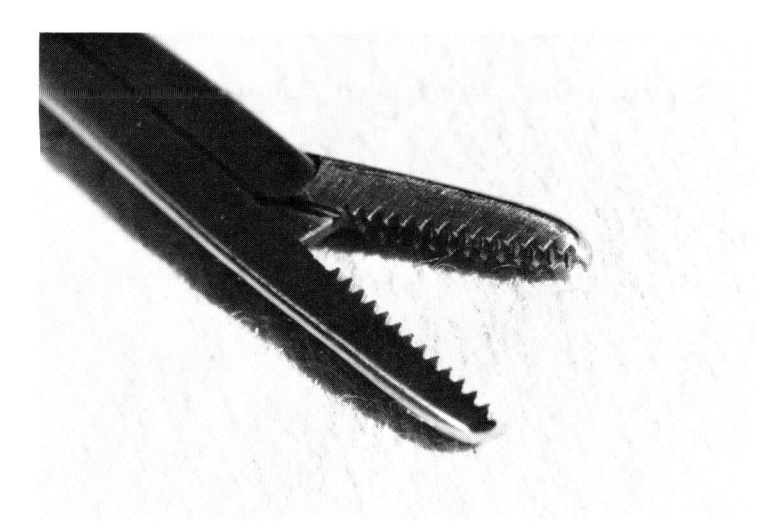

FIG. 14-17. Schlessinger Grasper is excellent and durable for meniscal work and loose bodies. (Courtesy George Tieman Co.)

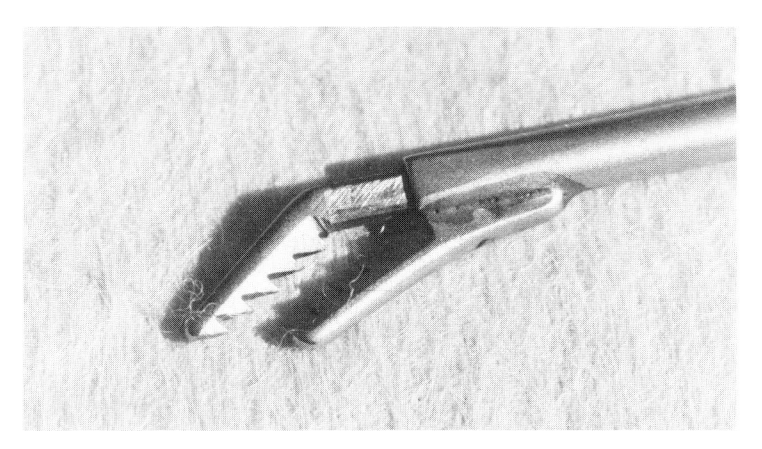

FIG. 14-18. Secured grasper is used to attach to anterior horn and eliminates need for continued grasping with hand or attachment of towel clip to keep manual clamp closed.

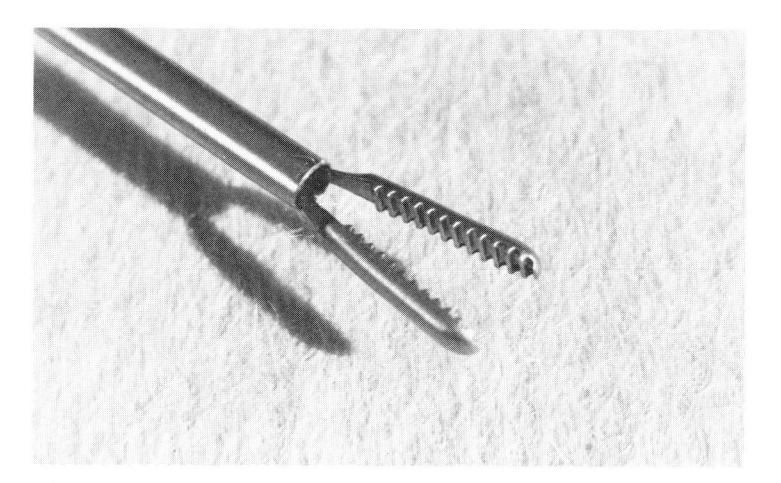

FIG. 14-19. Miniature grasper facilitates removal of meniscal and loose bodies from closed spaces, especially posterior compartment.

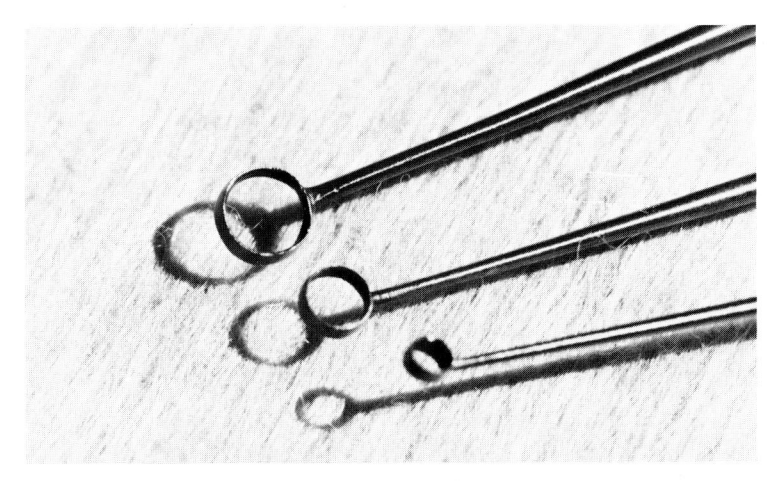

FIG. 14-20. Curettes come in various sizes and can be used on articular cartilage to shape edges or debride loose material too tenacious for other means.

Curettes

Curettes of various sizes are available from many companies (Fig. 14-20). Miniature curettes are helpful in some areas of osteochondritis in articular injury. They will not cut meniscus, but they will allow one to curette the articular surfaces.

Curettes that go through the interchangeable cannula system can provide a sense of palpation not possible with the Intra-articular Shaver. They are used as a preliminary means of identifying the extent of the lesion of the femoral condyle or patellar surface and to elevate tenacious areas not accessible to the Intra-articular Shaver. They also can be an advantage in removing cartilaginous surfaces of a bed of osteochondritis dissecans. Their use can be followed with the Intra-articular Shaver System to suck and debride.

Hand cutting instruments
Basket forceps

The basket forceps have been a standard part of arthroscopic surgery for the subtotal meniscectomy, plica, and resecting portions of articular cartilage. I rarely use them. The 3- or 5-mm basket forceps can grasp thin meniscal articular tissue and nibble away and remove that tissue or prominence effectively. The disadvantage is that a 5-mm size, which is bigger and stronger, cannot fit into the posterior compartment. The 3-mm size, which may have limited access, takes a smaller bite, is not as strong, and is more vulnerable to breaking. The cost of these instruments is considerable, and unless a physician is sponsored by a manufacturer, the replacement cost is prohibitive for instruments so fragile.

The other disadvantage of basket forceps is that the bite produces a piece of material that floats free in the joint, diminishing viewing possibilities like a snowstorm. Caspari[3] has shown that many pieces remain in the joint in spite of lavage. This diminished view could result in scuffing of the articular cartilage or inaccurate resection of meniscus.

The Oretorp basket forceps (Fig. 14-21), although somewhat large (5 and 3 mm), have a 10-year guarantee against breakage. They seem to be the most economical purchase for an instrument used only occasionally.

The basket forceps have been superseded, in my experience, by the Intra-articular Cutter for flap tears and rims of menisci. The Intra-articular Cutter removes each piece from the joint via the suction system; thus viewing is not obstructed, as it is with the basket forceps. I find basket forceps useful on the most extreme posterior horn when end cutting is necessary. The bits must be small and multiple and carefully removed.

Scissors

Currently there is a variety of scissors in both 5- and 3-mm sizes. The 5-mm models are too large for any meaningful cutting that could not otherwise be done by knife blade. On occasion there is some advantage in using the 3-mm scissors in the posterior horn. However, they are fragile and work on a pin system. Unfortunately, most scissors are nonmagnetic steel, and if a por-

Arthroscopic surgery of the knee

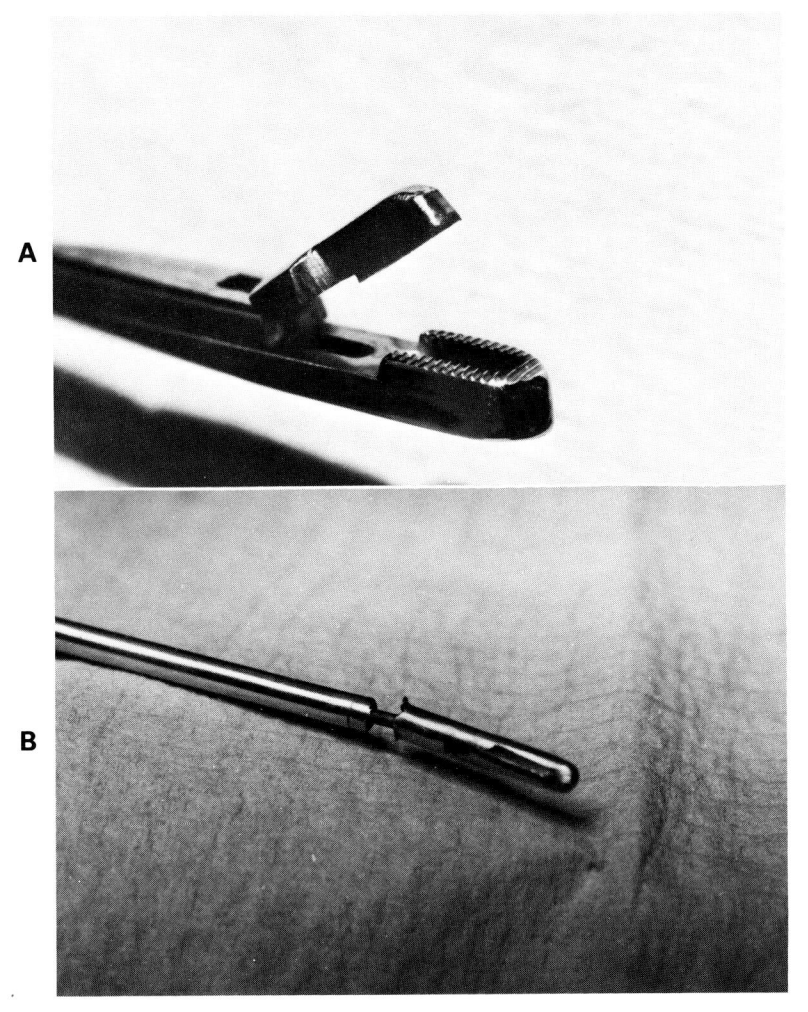

FIG. 14-21. A, Oretorp basket forceps are durable and guaranteed for 10 years. **B,** Some forceps might be too fragile to grasp tenacious material, which results in breakage.

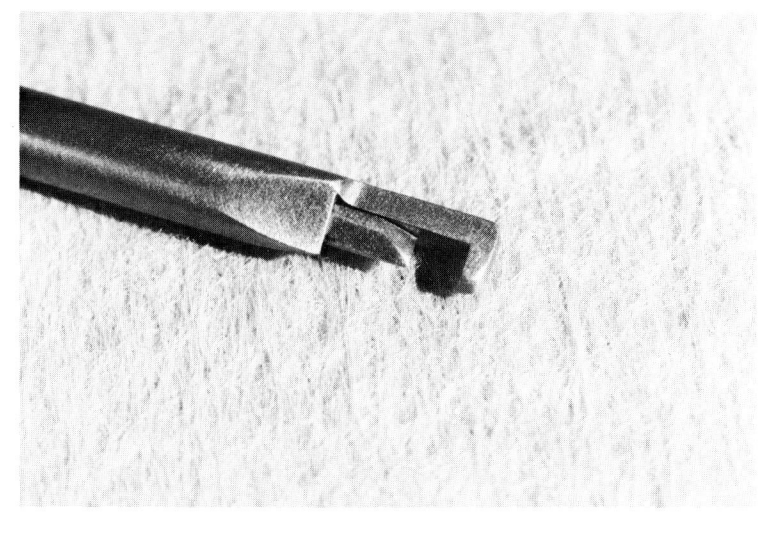

FIG. 14-22. Guillotine forceps are more durable than scissors for cutting meniscal tissue.

Surgical instrumentation

tion breaks off, it is difficult to retrieve it. Any large bite or attempt to resect a considerable portion of a normal meniscus just results in fracture of the scissors. That is not only expensive, but also renders the instrument useless for the procedure.

Guillotine forceps can replace the scissors in many instances. They are less prone to fracture, are rarely dull, and will cut heavy tissue (Fig. 14-22). Still, I prefer the IM blades for most of these maneuvers.

Operating arthroscopes

O'Connor introduced the "operating arthroscope." It is a modification and shortening of the laparoscopes used in gynecology. The advantage of this system is that it allows for visualization of the instrumentation directly in front of the endoscope; therefore one does not have to develop any skills of triangulation to find the instrument at any point in space. It probably has its greatest usefulness in grasping a loose body in either the suprapatellar pouch or the anterior chambers. Also, it can section a plica, an anterior horn, or the bucket-handle portion of a torn meniscus.

The disadvantages, in my judgment, outweigh the advantages. The endoscope is large and requires a considerable opening of the knee. Although the instrument is placed immediately in front of the arthroscope, it does not have any mobility beyond that which the arthroscope permits, or just a forward and backward action. One of its serious disadvantages is the position required for the arthroscopist. The operator must bend over, assuming an uncomfortable body position. Also, the instruments have to be placed superior and posterior to the operator's head, resulting in marked external rotation, extension, and elevation of the shoulder during manipulation. Besides being uncomfortable, it is a rather poor position for eye-hand coordination. The potential for contamination is great. This instrument has limited usefulness in arthroscopic surgery.

Intra-articular Shaver System

The Intra-articular Shaver System consists of a battery-powered, electric motor-driven, rotating cutting, suction device. The cutting tip consists of two tubes, one inside the other. The outer tube is fixed and has a window at the end; the inner tube has an oblique sculptured open end and rotates off the motor drive. (See Fig. 14-1.)

The Intra-articular Shaver System has its own set of cannulas. They have a 4.2-mm inside diameter and accommodate the arthroscopic hand instrument sets as well as the original Intra-articular Shaver, Cutter, and the various interchangeable cutting heads. Also, the cannula system allows interchangeability of portals without removal of the cannulas (Fig. 14-23).

A "little shaver" was designed with a 3-mm outside diameter and the similar cannula system for other joints, such as the shoulder, elbow, and ankle (Fig. 14-24). This is considered in more detail in Chapter 21.

An advance in the Intra-articular Shaver System is the interchangeability of the heads. The same basic motor is used. A drain case is attached, and each head design is now replaceable in the same basic motor drive and housing (Fig.

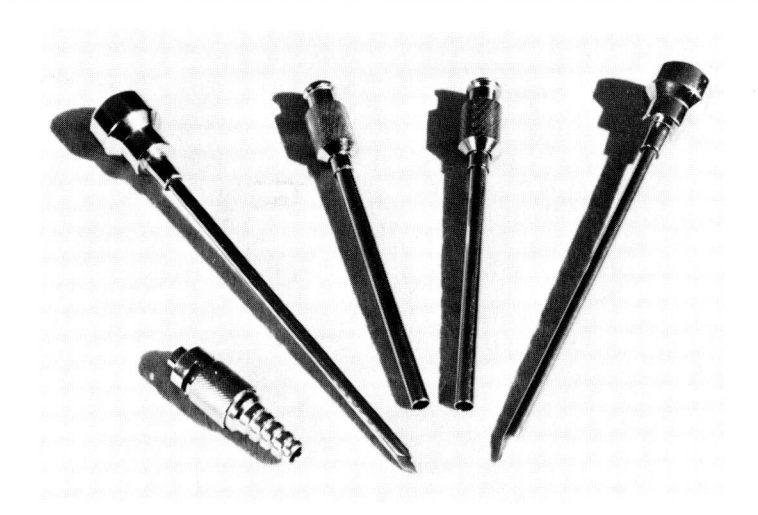

FIG. 14-23. Multiple cannula system of Intra-articular Shaver affords passage of loose bodies by suction or vacuuming. Also, multiple instruments can be inserted without repeat passages through tissue, which could create edema from microtrauma.

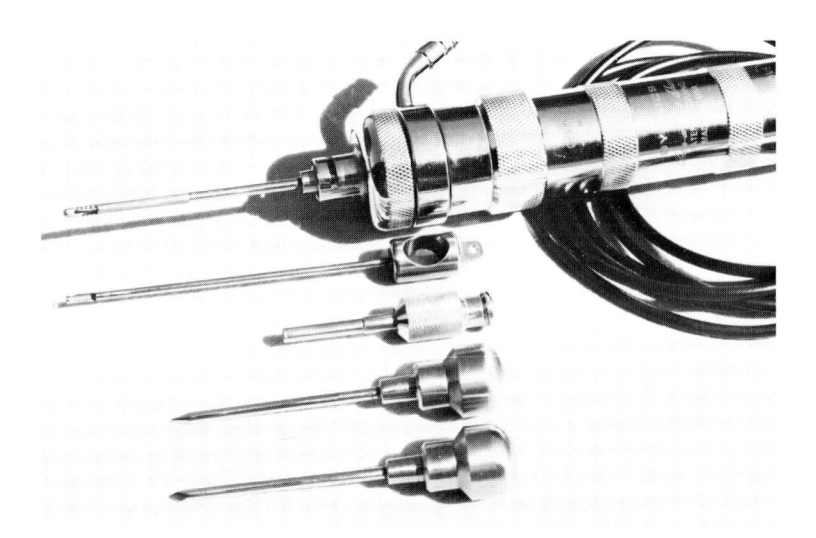

FIG. 14-24. Little Shaver, 3 mm in diameter, is valuable in shoulder and ankle joints for intra-articular shaving.

14-25, *A* to *C*). The meniscus cutter is used for cutting more tenacious intra-articular material.

The technical problem arises in placing meniscal tissue within the opening or mouth of the meniscus cutter, given the space limitations of arthroscopic surgery. Cutting is ineffective in areas that are difficult to get an angle on to free meniscal material into the cutter. Therefore a knife blade is used in conjunction with the meniscus cutter to develop the edges that would readily be brought in by suction and resection of posterior horn flap tears and plica. It is accomplished through the system.

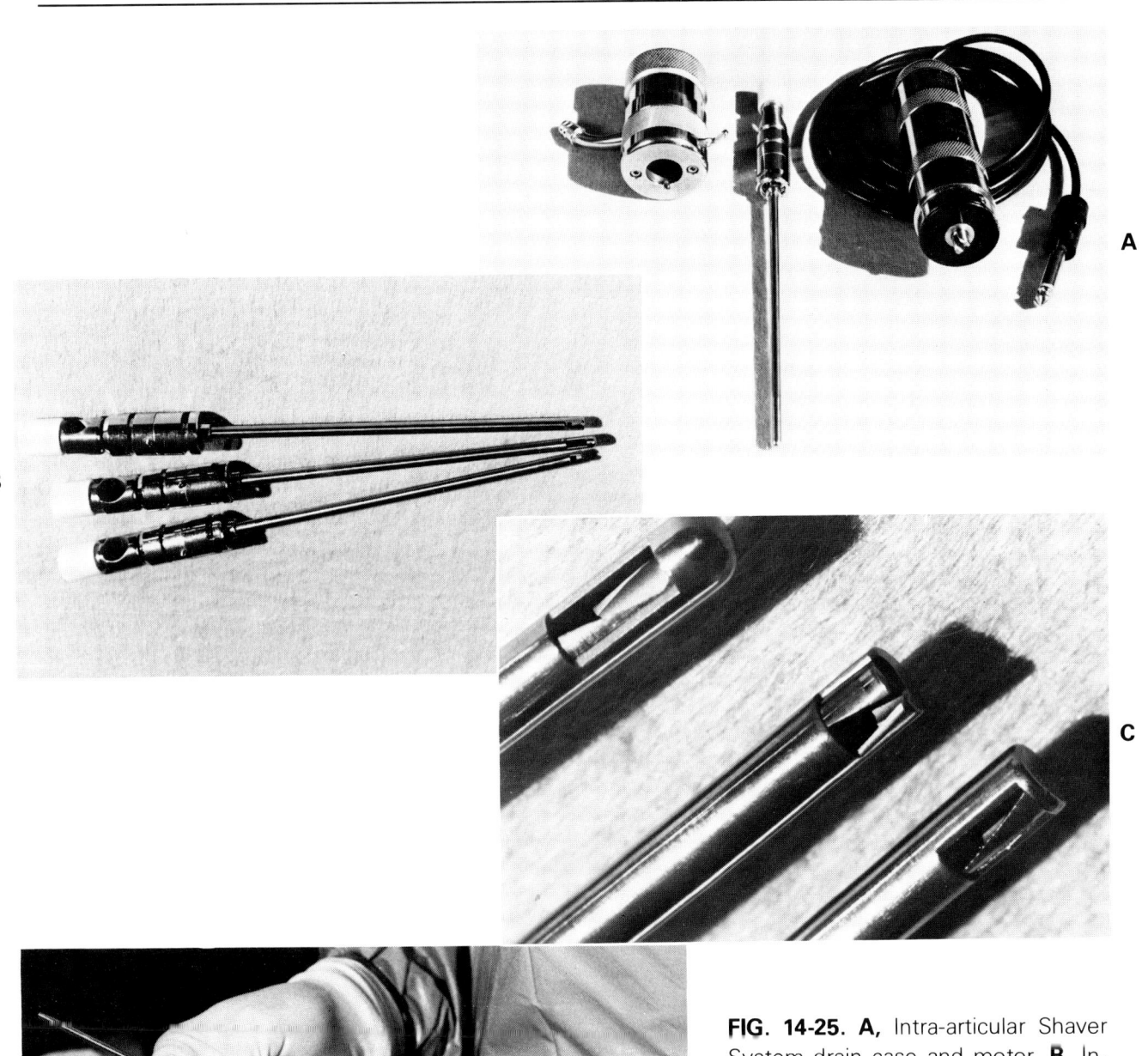

Surgical instrumentation

FIG. 14-25. A, Intra-articular Shaver System drain case and motor. **B,** Interchangeable blades. **C,** Close-up of Intra-articular Shaver superior, Intra-articular Cutter in middle, and Intra-articular Trimmer below. **D,** Intra-articular Shaver System has quick release from the crank case to accommodate interchangeable heads. Instruments are manufactured by Dyonics, Inc., Woburn, Mass.

Arthroscopic surgery of the knee

The third replaceable type of blade is the Trimmer. It is adapted for the intercondylar areas and cleans up the small debris after arthroscopic meniscectomy. It may be used in the small joints and has a high-efficiency, long-lasting, sharp cutting edge (Fig. 14-25, A to C).

The most recent addition to the Intra-articular Shaver System is a drill attachment (Fig. 14-26). This provides a means of placing multiple drill holes in a condylar defect or articular bed. In addition, it is possible to gain fixation with Kirschner-type wires.*

A rechargeable battery accompanies the shaver. There is one attachment

---

*Guhl wire, Richards Manufacturing, Memphis, Tenn.

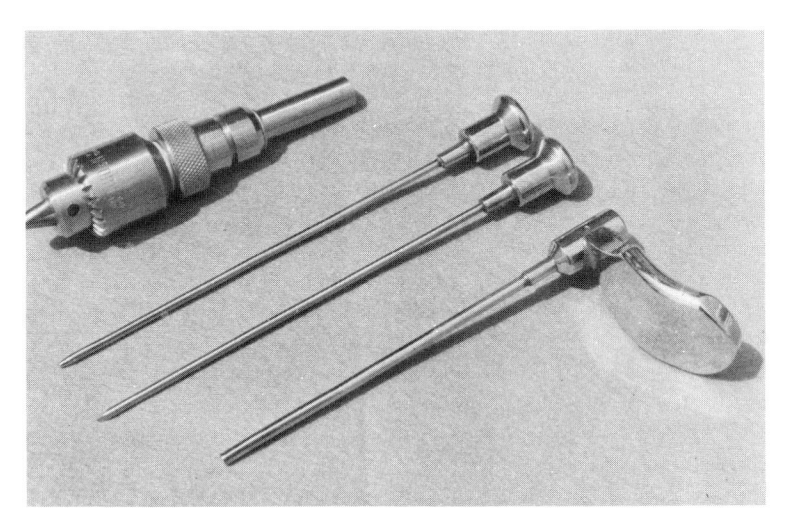

FIG. 14-26. Drill chuck has quick release and is useful in cases of osteochondritis dissecans.

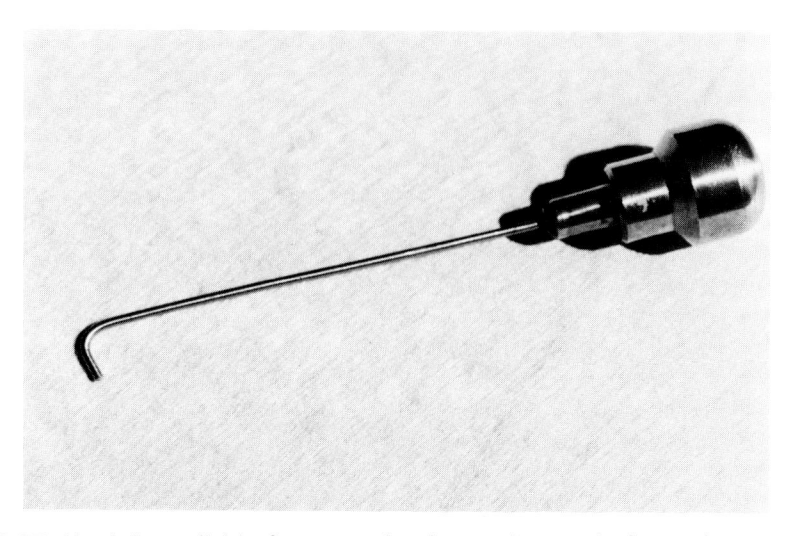

FIG. 14-27. Hook is available for removing internal cannula from shaver system.

Surgical instrumentation

for the sterile plastic insulated wire to the motor drive. A second plug is unsterile and attaches to the foot pedal on the floor. The foot pedal allows both forward and reverse activity of the rotation of the Intra-articular Shaver.

Another part of the system is a small hook for removal of the inner cannula that sometimes, with a perfect fit, can be difficult to reach or remove (Fig. 14-27).

This system has been carefully calibrated in RPM, the size of the openings of the window, the inner cannula, and the saline flow. The original calibrations were calculated on an infusion heart-lung machine. This is elaborated on in Chapter 16. The Intra-articular Shaver System has been designed to accommodate not only the power instrumentation but also various hand tools (Figs. 14-16; 14-18 to 14-20).

At this date the Intra-articular Shaver System has an established place in arthroscopic surgery. With the advancement of the technology and the improvement of the quality of the metals, there is virtually unlimited expression in various types of cutter heads for various types of tasks in the field of arthroscopic surgery. Many additional designs are currently under development.

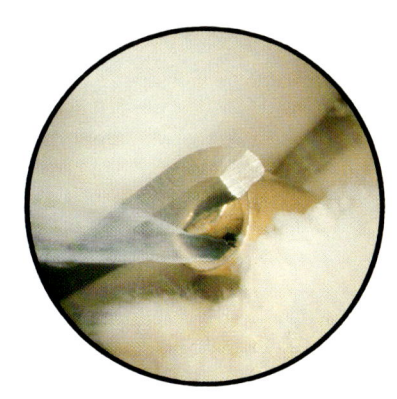

FIG. 14-28. Golden Retriever is magnetized sucker for retrieval of magnetic, metallic loose fragments.

Golden Retriever

It is important that all the instrumentation used in the joints have some magnetic quality. A magnetized suction instrument can bring any small pieces from accidental fracture into view for easy retrievability. The Golden Retriever is a sucker with a powerful small magnet within. It uses two forces to assist in retrieving small metallic foreign bodies from the joint (Fig. 14-28).

REFERENCES
1. Bentley, G.: The surgical treatment of chondromalacia patellae, J. Bone Joint Surg. **60B**:74, 1978.
2. Carson, R. W.: Arthroscopic meniscectomy, Orthop. Clin. North Am. **10**(3):619, 1979.
3. Caspari, R.: Personal communication, 1980.
4. Ficat, R. P., and Hungerford, D. S.: Disorders of the patello femoral joint, Baltimore, 1977, The Williams and Wilkins Co.

5. Ikeuchi, H.: Surgery under arthroscopic control (discoid meniscus) "R", Rev. Int. Rheum. **33**:57, 1976.
6. Jackson, R. W., and Dandy, D. J.: Arthroscopy of the knee, New York, 1976, Grune & Stratton, Inc.
7. Metcalf, R.: Personal communication, 1980.
8. O'Connor, R.: Arthroscopy, Philadelphia, 1977, J. B. Lippincott Co.
9. Oretorp, N., and Gillquist, J.: Transcutaneous meniscectomy under arthroscopic control, Int. Orthop. **3**(1):19, 1979.
10. Watanabe, M., Arthroscopy, the present state, Orthop. Clin. North Am. **10**(3):505, 1979.
11. Watanable, M., Takeda, I. H., and Ikeuchi, H.: Atlas of arthroscopy, ed. 2, Berlin, 1969, Springer-Verlag.
12. Wiles, P., Andrews, P. S., and Devas, M. B.: Chondromalacia patellae, J. Bone Joint Surg. **38**3:95, 1956.

Chapter 15

Basic principles of arthroscopic surgery

How to learn
Triangulation
Concepts of joint irrigation, inflows, and outflows
Expectations
Patient selection and preparation
Surgical technique
    Technical concepts
Team approach
Baisc setup for patellar shaving
    Patient positioning and preparation
    Circulating nurse
    Control of the extremity
    Outflow system during operation
Lateral release technique
Comprehensive arthroscopic surgical technique
    Patient positioning and preparation
    Placement of the inflow cannula
    Positions for arthroscopic surgery
    Placement of the arthroscope
    Preoperative arthroscopic diagnostic examination
    Probing
    Puncture sites for surgical instrumentation
    Patella and patellofemoral shaving
Summary

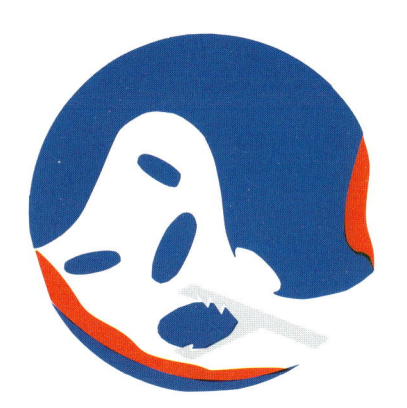

HOW TO LEARN

Arthroscopy and arthroscopic surgical techniques are valuable clinical tools for patient care. Diagnostic accuracy is high, the surgical methods produce minimal morbidity, and a strong pathophysiologic basis has been established. There have been excellent results.

Arthroscopy itself is technically difficult to master. An inherent skill of eye-hand coordination is essential. This specific skill is certainly unrelated to intelligence and even normal surgical skills. It is similar to an inherited ability of musical pitch or tonal memory. Practice can improve one's skills no matter what the starting point.

How does one best go about embarking on this new surgical adventure? It would be wise to attend one of a variety of arthroscopic seminars given by individuals or by the American Academy of Orthopaedic Surgeons and the International Arthroscopy Association. Second, direct observation of someone familiar with and skilled in arthroscopy and arthroscopic surgery plays a role in the comprehension of this type of surgery.

At the present time, arthroscopic surgery is a continuing education experience for orthopedists in clinical practice. It is difficult, at best, to instruct residents or even those at the fellowship level. A certain fundamental knowledge and experience that goes with clinical practice is necessary to appreciate the value of these techniques and their results.

The best current means of learning arthroscopic surgery is to begin with the simple procedures and advance to the more complex. The following chapters present the chronologic and technical progression that I have followed. This step-by-step outline develops the how and why of different methods.

After having attended instructional courses, read the available materials, and reviewed television teaching tapes, an orthopedic surgeon is still not ready to perform a procedure. I recommend procuring above-the-knee amputation specimens and having them frozen until there is time available to set up the instrumentation and irrigation systems. Practice is not dependent on the time restriction found in actual surgical situations.

After viewing teaching material with the operating room staff, the surgeon should perform a dry run with the staff in the operating room so that all staff members understand their responsibilities.

The last preparation is to allow plenty of time for the first cases; both the surgeon and the patient should be prepared that conventional treatment by "opening" the joint may be required. Initially it took me and my staff 90 minutes just to set up the operating room. The procedures took at least that long. Now we are able to complete even the more complex arthroscopic surgical procedures in less than an hour, including room turnover time. The effort and concentration demanded are such that we do not like to perform over six procedures per day. The energy needed to maintain a high level of proficiency can be exhausted after 6 to 8 hours of this kind of surgery.

Surgeons should schedule their procedures so that adequate time is available—an estimated 2 hours; thus the anesthesiologist and/or other surgeons who are to use that particular operating room subsequently will not be kept waiting.

TRIANGULATION

The skill of triangulation is an integral part of the arthroscopist's abilities. It is difficult to find a second instrument in the joint. Triangulation is picking a point, 1, the lesion; viewing from point 2; and using an instrument from point 3. After basic arthroscopic skills are mastered, biopsy of synovium and loose body removal techniques should be learned. Then advancement to other intra-articular arthroscopic procedures may commence. The intra-articular shaving of the patella for severe chondromalacia is recommended as a next logical step. The space is large and accommodates both the arthroscope and other instruments that can be brought into view. Sectioning, or resectioning a plica when indicated, could be a next step; then, meniscectomy, chondroplasty, and synovectomy. Last, the fixation in osteochondritis dissecans and a combination of arthroscopic surgical procedures with extrasynovial repairs in instability can be considered.

Basic principles of arthroscopic surgery

Concepts of joint irrigation, inflows, and outflows

The traditional arthroscopist used a small inflow needle in the suprapatellar pouch to distend the joint. The Verres needle was used either for inflow or, in some cases, outflow. In the latter situation the arthroscopist attached a saline inflow to the arthroscope within the joint. It drained out of the small Verres needle.

These techniques seem unnecessary. The alternative method is described in Chapter 3. The simpler system of entering the joint with the arthroscope and distending the joint eliminates the need for the inflow and outflow tubes.

When surgical arthroscopic procedures were developed, the traditional method had some carryover. Some surgeons performed arthroscopic surgery with inflow and outflow needles in the suprapatellar pouch, inflow and outflow attachments to the arthroscope, and suction outflow from the Intra-articular Shaver System. These elaborate techniques were unnecessary and, in fact, inefficient.

With the Intra-articular Shaver System a large amount of saline flowed through a 4-mm cannula from the plastic tubing attached to 6 liters of saline elevated 1 m above the patient. The Intra-articular Shaver's cannula and/or the Shaver itself in operation under suction served as the outflow. A secondary decompression needle for outflow from the suprapatellar pouch was not only unnecessary but also decompressed the joint, resulting in lack of distension for visualization as well as lack of flow to draw the tissue under tension into the Intra-articular Shaver for resection.

In diagnostic surgery a suspended inflow and outflow setup is not necessary, and saline can be managed by inflow and outflow through the arthroscopic cannula. In addition, when there is inflow through the cannula at the time of viewing, a turbulence of the tissues is produced in front of the arthroscope. This is somewhat distracting for visualization, especially during arthroscopic surgical work.

The surgical saline system has been simplified to the 4-mm inflow cannula from anterior, lateral, and inferior to the patella for the basic intra-articular shaving technique; or, in the more comprehensive setup, the inflow comes through the Intra-articular Shaver cannulas (4 mm) to the medial aspect of the suprapatellar pouch. *No other inflows or outflows are necessary.*

There is some value during diagnostic observation of the joint to use decompression. Suction is attached to the arthroscopic spigots. The inflow is cut off. The mobility of the meniscus in both the distended and the decompressed state may be evaluated (Fig. 15-34).

EXPECTATIONS

Discouragement is likely if one's expectations exceed what is possible. The surgeon may find that he does not want to spend the time and energy necessary in adding this demanding, new dimension to his speciality. At that point he might choose not to be involved; but if he does go ahead, he can expect to have many discouraging moments in learning this new technique. Given the desire to do so, all the best available equipment, and adequate training in these techniques, the surgeon can learn these new methods. After 6 or 12 months of continued case experience, there are noticeable and satisfying improvements in one's technical ability. Part of this is due to the familiarity with the procedure; some is due to the continued introduction to new equipment; but, for the most part, the surgeon is gaining confidence and competence, which certainly reward him for his efforts.

Another factor to consider when learning arthroscopic surgery is the resistance and even resentment on the part of certain colleagues. This attitude frequently results from prejudice, lack of familiarity with the procedure, and lack of knowledge of any of its potential benefits. There may also be some hesitation on the part of the operating room personnel to change their routines. This can usually be overcome by the arthroscopist's enthusiasm. The anesthesia department is conditioned to the time involved in learning arthroscopy. With adequate preparation and care not to underschedule cases, they will be more amenable to participation, and surgeons who anticipate following the arthroscopy will not be delayed. The administrative staff of the hospital, who are concerned with running a business, will probably be cooperative if they understand, from the start, the significant initial expense and how it can be weighed against the attractive revenue-producing increase in outpatient surgical flow. The cost to the hospital can be somewhat circumvented if the arthroscopist purchases his own equipment. These instruments are vulnerable to wear and breakage, so personal ownership ensures optimal care.

PATIENT SELECTION AND PREPARATION

The best approach in patient selection is a candid discussion with the patient, with the surgeon sharing knowledge, opinions, and level of experience with this type of surgery. The patient is informed that this type of surgery is available, that it is in a developmental stage (but beyond the experimental stage), that it is a viable clinical tool, and that the early results are very encouraging. No effort is made at salesmanship, and the patient is given a patient information sheet on arthroscopic surgery. Patients are encouraged to weigh the information with which they have been presented against the alternative conventional methods. Also, I advise them of individuals who have more experience than myself, so that they can avail themselves of their consultation and treatment. This approach has met with a favorable reception. As one gains abilities and confidence, it is still important to follow this approach, although enthusiasm may make that difficult.

Arthroscopic surgery is not a substitute for physician-patient relationships or clinical examination. Also, it is not an all-encompassing form of treatment.

Basic principles of arthroscopic surgery

It is a new and exciting tool for the care of patients with knee problems.

Color-coded instruction sheets allow physicians to recall case generalities in the absence of a complete record.

As mentioned, I have given patients, in addition to personal contact and instruction, an arthroscopic surgery patient instruction sheet (Fig. 15-1), which has been of considerable value in making a statement about arthroscopic surgery and answering any potential questions. Note the indication that, although every reasonable attempt is made to perform the surgery arthroscopically, I have reserved the right to perform the technique by conventional meth-

---

ARTHROSCOPIC SURGERY
PATIENT INFORMATION SHEET

BACKGROUND:
Technologic advances in recent years have permitted surgical procedures to be performed inside joints without opening by traditional methods.

The advent of a small diameter viewing device called an arthroscope has given doctors the capacity to inspect the interior of human joints by direct vision. Hence, their diagnostic capacity and accuracy has been greatly advanced in recent years. Photographic recording on slides, movies, and television have become routine through these miniature lens systems.

Just as miniaturization has come into electronics, i.e. small calculators, radios, TV's, the same is so in surgery. In fact, it comprises a subspecialty known as microsurgery.

Arthroscopic surgery has become a reality. It combines the ability to view inside the joint with a small telescope (arthroscope), even to recording simultaneously on television with manipulation of microsurgical instruments.

PRESENT STATE OF THE ART:
In the past two years, in cooperation with industry, medicine has been given even more efficient, effective, safe, motorized instrumentation.

The first such instrument is called an Intra-Articular ShaverR. It provides the capacity to shave or smooth roughening areas within the joint.

The second such instrument has been designed to remove torn cartilages without opening the joint.

Your anticipated surgery will include utilization of one or all of the above new advances, depending upon your specific joint problem.

ANESTHESIA:
Your arthroscopic procedure may be performed under general or perhaps local anesthesia. This choice of anesthesia depends upon your general physical condition, the complexity of your problem, and the judgment of your surgeon and/or anesthesiologist.

Often it is in your best interest to have the diagnostic portion of the procedure performed under local anesthesia with an anesthesiologist standing by to administer medication. This affords you, the patient, the safety of local anesthesia and early discharge from the hospital, yet provides the flexibility of administering a general anesthetic as necessary to complete the surgical procedure safely and with maximum patient comfort. A general anesthetic may be administered depending on the findings and indicated surgical procedure. A general anesthetic ususally allows a same day discharge from the hospital.

A hospital admission may be advised in certain instances for out of town patients, or when a medical condition dictates. The stay will usually be a day or so.

INSTRUCTIONS:
Enclosed are directions to the Ingham Medical Center, and general instructions concerning your preparation.

Following surgery, you will be given a prescription for pain medicine (codiene compound), unless you are allergic. There will be a dressing upon your joint that may be removed the next day. Small paper tapes may cover the small points of entry into your joint. You may place a bandaid upon your skin as necessary. You may use your limb within the tolerance of your comfort. You may shower or bathe 48 hours following surgery. Your joint may feel bruised or full of fluid, but this should decrease in a few days. Any question of unusual pain, swelling, or fever should of course be reported to us immediately.

The complexity of any individuals surgery will vary with the severity of the condition. The simple diagnostic procedure has the least patient discomfort. The internal releasing of tight tissue for dislocating knee caps may be uncomfortable and result in swelling and bruising. The latter surgery may also require a knee splint.

With any surgery or penetration of the body there is some discomfort, be it drawing a sample of blood from the arm. It is no different with arthroscopic surgery. In spite of the discomfort you may experience, you may be assured that it is less than by open surgery.

Every reasonable attempt will be made to perform the surgery arthroscopically but when indicated open surgery by conventional methods may be performed.

If there are any questions please phone, write or ask us personally.

Thank you,

Lanny L. Johnson, M.D.

FIG. 15-1. Arthroscopic surgery patient information sheet. (Color code: white; see above.)

ods. Selection of a case depends on the surgeon's ability to perform such techniques. I recommend starting with the simple procedures first.

The patient's general condition certainly has to be considered. The principal problem that has interrupted the scheduling of patients, in my practice, is hypokalemia. It is not unusual for surgical candidates to be taking antihypertensive medication without potassium supplements. Thus I routinely check the serum potassium level at the time the patient is examined, at 1 week, and at 1 day before any scheduled surgery.

The selection of anesthesia depends on the surgeon's skills, the cooperation of the patient, and the nature of the lesion. Often, in just a diagnostic situation, as outlined in earlier chapters, I perform an outpatient local diagnostic arthroscopy with a Needlescope to sort out patients who do not have definite, positive physical findings to match their complaints. For a patient who has a suggestion of an intra-articular abnormality, such as a plica, I use stand-by anesthesia and perform the examination under local anesthetic to have a clinical correlation with the intra-articular abnormalities. If the case is simple to manage, surgery is performed under local anesthesia. If it is then observed to be complex, the patient is already prepared, and the anesthesiologist, who is standing by, administers the general anesthesia.

It has not been necessary to use preoperative medication except in patients for whom I anticipate having to use a general or spinal anesthetic. There is no contraindication to the use of narcotics or tranquilizers to ensure patient comfort. For patients in whom a complex lesion requiring intra-articular surgery has been determined, a general anesthetic is administered.

The greater part of my arthroscopic surgery is performed on an outpatient basis in a general hospital. Experience has shown that the first case of the day should be a patient who has been admitted to the hospital. I generally select one for whom a hospital admission may have been indicated anyway for general medical reasons. Thus I avoid tardiness in starting the daily schedule.

SURGICAL TECHNIQUES

The basic skills of arthroscopy must be mastered prior to embarking on arthroscopic surgery. The technique of basic arthroscopic examination is outlined in Chapter 3. These skills are transferred into the techniques of arthroscopic surgery.

TECHNICAL CONCEPTS

Asepsis, hemostasis, and gentleness are time-honored principles of surgery. It is not different in arthroscopic surgery. In addition, good exposure and visualization are essential. These principles are fulfilled somewhat differently during arthroscopy and arthroscopic surgery. Distension of the joint is an important common denominator, without which any visualization would be compromised, regardless of the technique used. The best, most powerful light source with high quality new cables and light bulbs is necessary. Stability of the thigh and maximal opening of the joint spaces, either medial or lateral, are best achieved with the use of the Surgical Assistant.

Basic principles of arthroscopic surgery

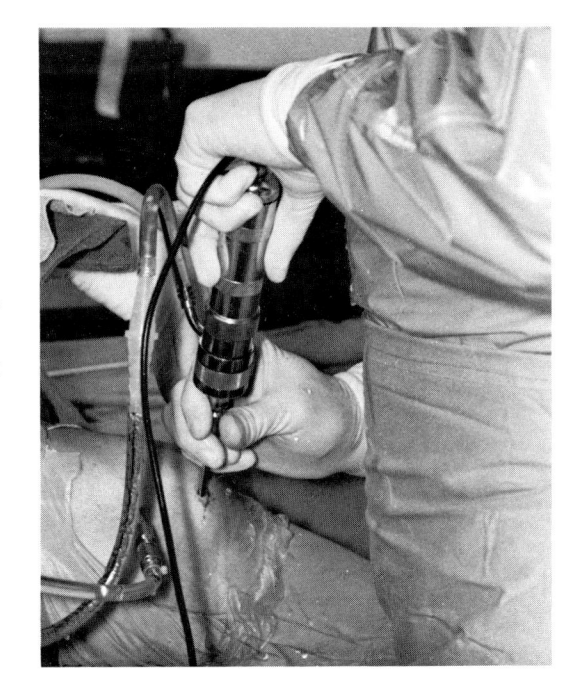

FIG. 15-2. Commitment to use both hands during arthroscopic surgery is essential. Nondominant hand should assist dominant hand during early training and/or fatigue.

A comfortable position for the surgeon, with both hands free in front and the upper extremities in a resting position, is achieved during arthroscopic surgery with the use of the arthroscope attached to the television camera with an articulated viewing device. Bimanual dexterity is essential for smooth and successful technical achievement. One need not be ambidextrous. At first it may be uncomfortable to perform some primary manipulations with a nondominant hand. But it is necessary to learn to use a nondominant hand in a primary way. For example, if one is doing a right knee lateral meniscectomy, the arthroscope is viewing from the medial side, and the instrumentation is coming in from a lateral portal, it is necessary to use the left hand for the primary resection. The arthroscope is held in the right hand, since it would be clumsy to try to work with the right hand. Initially, the nondominant hand should hold the cutting instrument and the dominant hand should come over and support it (Fig. 15-2). With time, one can learn to use the nondominant hand with facility. On occasion, with fatigue or late in the day, the control may diminish some, and support for fine manipulative movements may be necessary with the dominant hand again.

The surgical setup can be divided into three methods: (1) the basic setup is used for intra-articular shaving of the patella; (2) arthroscopic lateral release is possible with either organizational setup; and (3) the comprehensive surgical setup permits all types of arthroscopic surgery, as well as many conventional knee joint procedures. Although the original setup is somewhat antiquated compared with the later ones, it is an excellent way to train the operating room staff and the arthroscopist in these techniques with considerable patient safety. The comprehensive surgical setup and technique are for the more complex cases and an experienced team and surgeon.

Arthroscopic surgery of the knee

Team approach

Every variable and condition should be organized and planned to maximize the surgeon's efficiency at the time of the procedure. A team approach to this type of work is mandatory. It behooves the surgeon to develop some interest and enthusiasm for this type of procedure. If he does not have it, then the others in the operating room will not. Recent surveys at various arthroscopic seminars have shown that 90% of orthopedic surgeons have a different, untrained assistant for their procedures. Every effort should be made to have a trained and preferably the same assistant for every procedure. This may mean the hiring of a new employee by the surgeon or the hospital. Hospitals frequently have renal and heart teams, but orthopedists have always been expected to "go it alone." It is time for the arthroscopic surgeon to change this.

The team approach is essential to a smooth arthroscopic surgical procedure. Each person's responsibilities should be discharged without overlapping of assignments but with mutual support and cooperation.

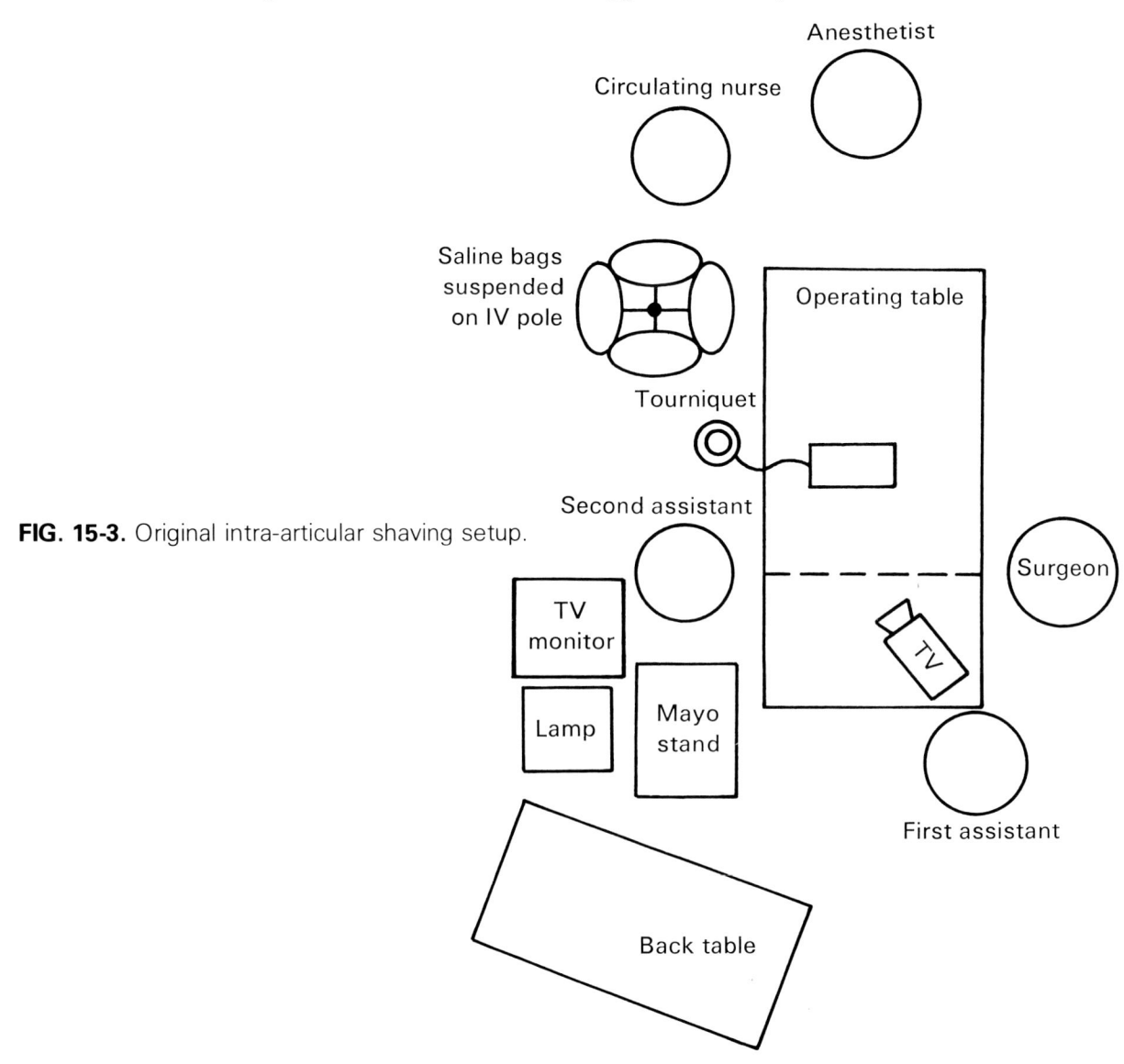

FIG. 15-3. Original intra-articular shaving setup.

BASIC SETUP FOR PATELLAR SHAVING
Patient positioning and preparation

The patient is placed in the supine position on the operating room table (Fig. 15-3). The anesthetic may either be general or infiltrated local (1% lidocaine). A diagnostic arthroscopy should then be performed (Fig. 15-4).

The tourniquet is placed high on the thigh. An Esmarch bandage is placed on the lower extremity. The wrap is removed, and a skin preparation is performed. A sterile drape is placed to expose that same area around the knee. After an opening is made in the stockinette, a folded sheet is placed under the ankle to elevate that extremity above the opposite extremity; this gives better access to the medial aspect of the joint (Fig. 15-5).

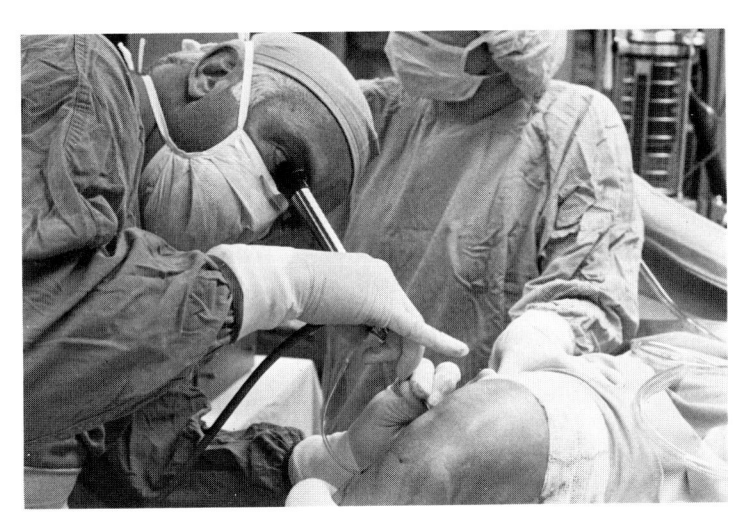

FIG. 15-4. Diagnostic arthroscopy should precede any articular surgery.

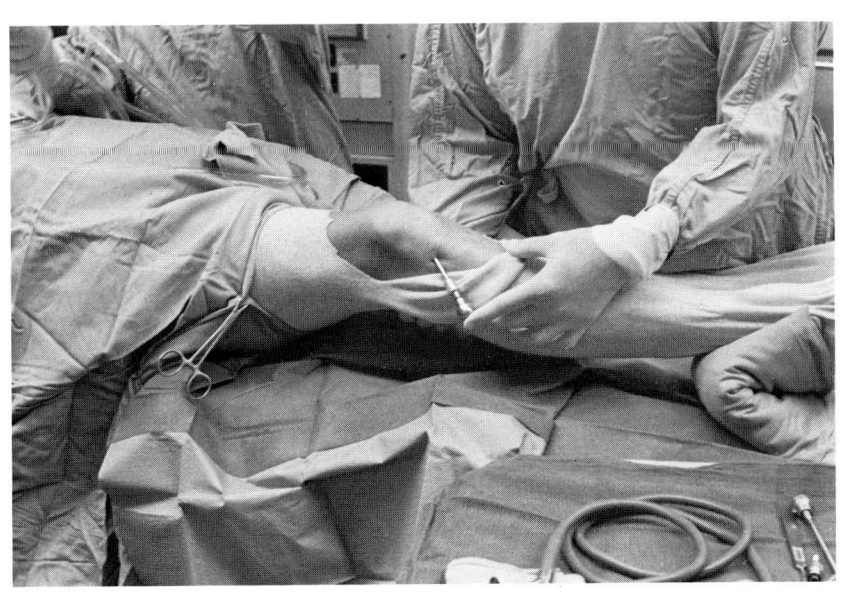

FIG. 15-5. Folded sheet is placed under heel of extremity to be operated on for elevation above opposite knee, making approach easier.

Circulating nurse

The foremost responsibilities of the circulating nurse are control of the television recording and saline infusion. Monitoring the patient under local anesthesia and assisting the anesthesiologist as instructed when a general anesthetic is delivered are also important.

RESPONSIBILITIES

During setup
1. Turn on lights.
2. Set up skin preparation materials.
3. Set up saline infusion.
4. Check suction outflow and collection system.
5. Prepare and position television monitor recorder.
6. Confirm patient's name tag and review medical record.
7. Position patient on operating table.
8. Assist anesthesiologist and patient monitoring.
9. Deliver autoclaved equipment to back table.
10. Secure tourniquet and inflate on command.
11. Hold patient extremity for skin preparation.
12. Secure light cable to source.
13. Bring in shaver power source, turn on switch, secure cable, and place foot pedal.
14. Assist with sterile draping of television camera and cable.

During procedure
1. Assist anesthesiologist; monitor patient if under local anesthesia.
2. Maintain adequate saline inflow.
3. Control video recording.

After procedure
1. Deflate tourniquet.
2. Assist anesthesiologist.
3. Help patient to recovery room.
4. Label specimens and complete records.
5. Assist with room changeover.

Second assistant

The main responsibilities of the second assistant are setup, instrument organization, and control of inflow and outflow.

RESPONSIBILITIES

During setup
1. Set up back table.
2. Set up Mayo stand.
3. Assist in draping patient.

During procedure
1. Organize instrument table.
2. Control inflow and outflow.

Basic principles of arthroscopic surgery: basic setup for patellar shaving

After procedure
1. Clean equipment for autoclaving.
2. Assist in room.

First assistant

The main duties of the first assistant are care of the arthroscope and holding the attached television camera.

RESPONSIBILITIES

Before arthroscopy
1. Assist in setup of back table.
2. Remove arthroscope from Cidex and cleanse.
3. Assist with skin preparation and draping.

During procedure
1. Assist with instrument positioning.
2. Hold television camera.

After procedure
1. Cleanse arthroscope and place in Cidex.
2. Assist with room change.

At end of day
1. Clean and secure all equipment in containers and cabinets.

Control of the extremity

The extremity is controlled during surgery by varus and valgus positioning and a combination of flexion, extension, and external and internal rotation. There are some operating room tables that do not lower as much as others, and some larger patients make control of the extremity difficult. In those cases, where the table will not be lowered as much as necessary, the surgeon would have to push with his thigh while on tiptoe. This can be corrected easily by a small amount of a reverse Trendelenburg positioning on the operating room table, which effectively lowers the Surgical Assistant and facilitates control of the extremity with both feet on the floor.

The lateral inferior portal is used for the inflow tract. First the sharp trocar in the cannula brings the instrument through the capsule; then a blunt trocar in the joint penetrates up under the patella; and then the cannula is moved into the lateral sulcus (Fig. 15-6, A). The blunt trocar is removed and an adapter for the attachment of the inflow cannula is attached (Fig. 15-6, B).

Six liters of saline (two 3-liter bags) are suspended 1 m above the patient and attached by a sterile Y tube. The tubing is attached to the inflow cannula adapter (Fig. 15-7, A). The joint is then distended. The inflow plastic tubing is then secured to the stockinette with a towel clip (Fig. 15-7, B). This keeps the inflow cannula in the lateral sulcus.

When the joint is distended, it is possible to bring an arthroscope in from the anterior medial side and inferior to the patella (Fig. 15-8). This site is medial to the normal anteromedial portal because the knee will be in extension. The desired direction of entry is parallel, and below the patella view across to

Arthroscopic surgery of the knee

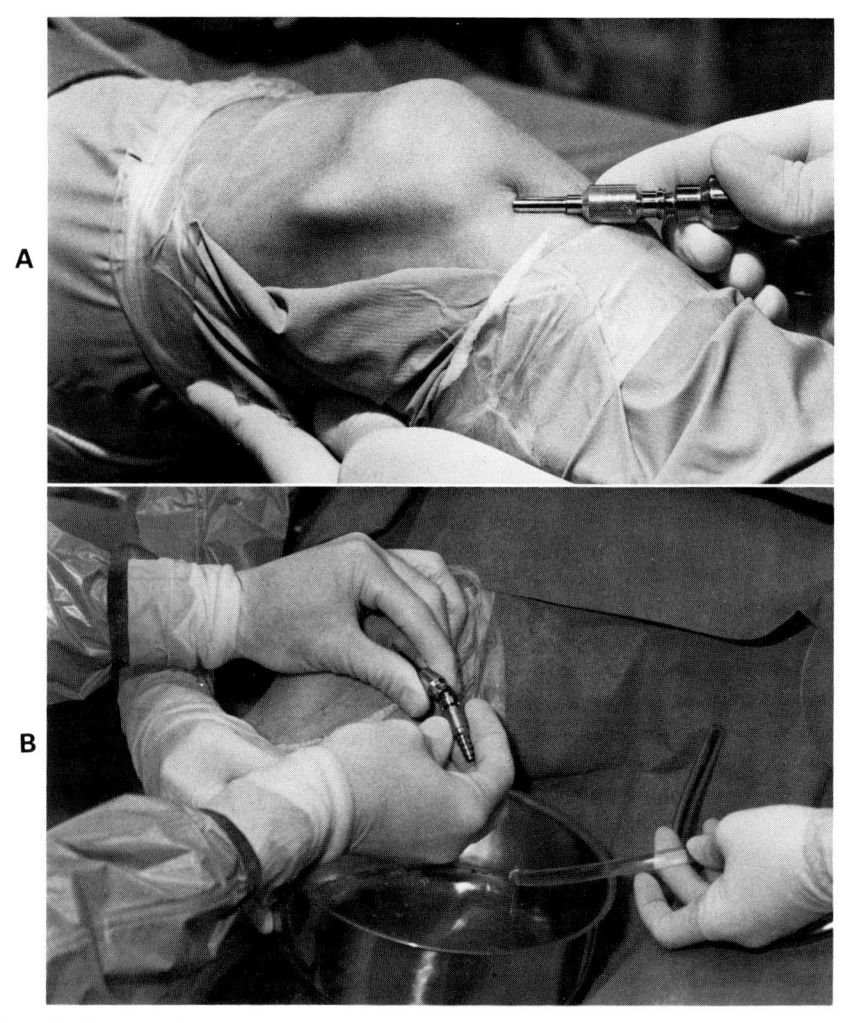

FIG. 15-6. A, Cannula is placed in the lateral sulcus, removing it from area under patella where surgery is anticipated. **B,** Adapter is attached to cannula.

the lateral side. The arthroscope is inserted in a standard fashion. Direct inspection confirms the entry and position before the attachment of the television camera.

The television is covered with a sterile stockinette. A plastic drape is placed around the camera itself to protect it from saline soaking. Scissors open the end of the stockinette so the adapter can attach to the television camera. The now unsterile scissors are discarded and the television camera is attached to the arthroscope (Fig. 15-9). The extreme tip of the stockinette covering the television cable is secured with tape. The interior of the joint is then inspected, and the suprapatellar pouch structures are brought into view (Fig. 15-10).

A No. 18 spinal needle enters from the superior and medial aspects, parallel to the patellar surface. This trial entry ensures that the Intra-articular Shaver will be in excellent position for patellar shaving. It may take several placements to make exact contact parallel with the patella. Attention is turned to outside the joint. The skin is lanced with a No. 11 blade at the point of needle

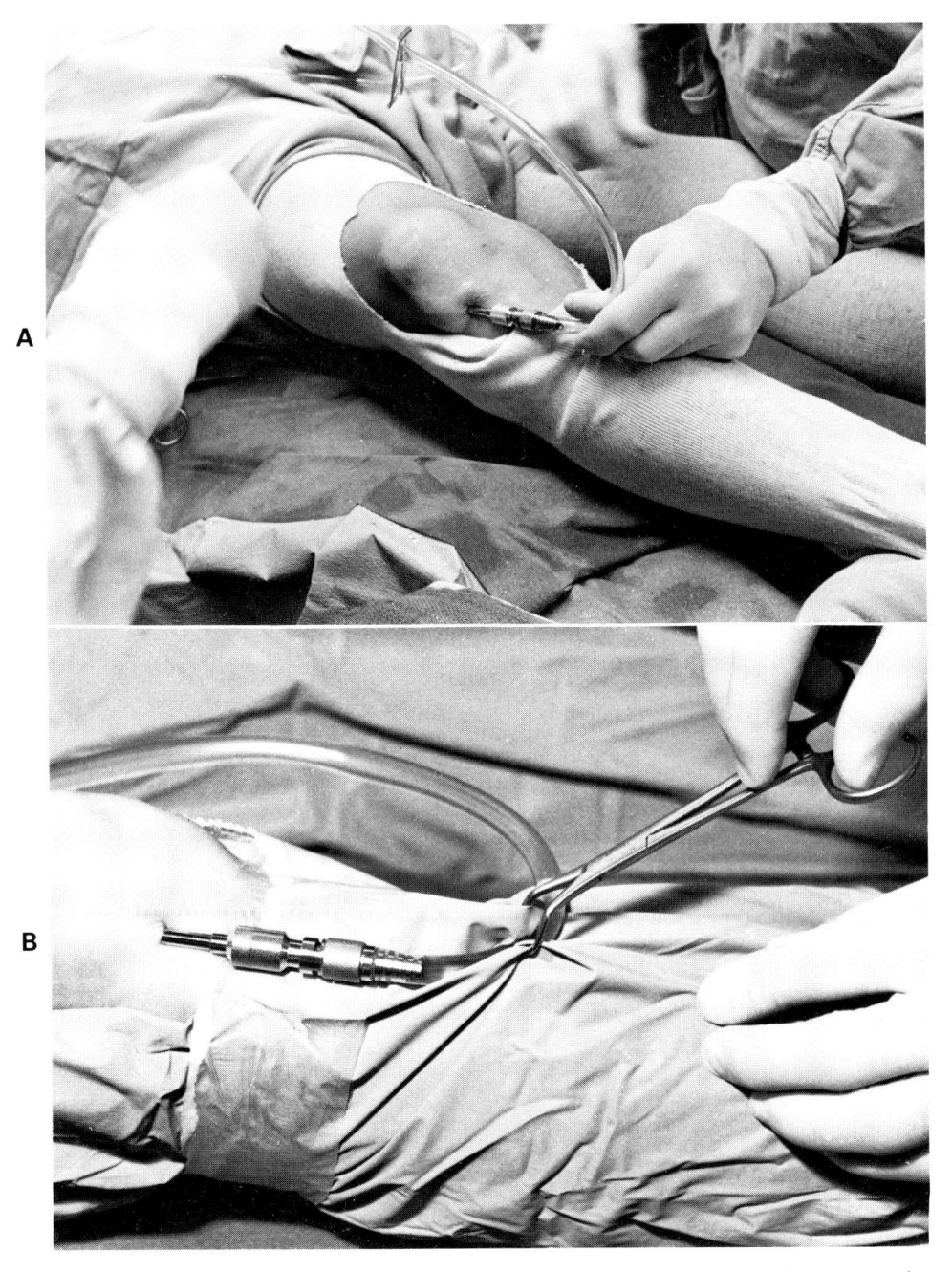

Basic principles of arthroscopic surgery: basic setup for patellar shaving

FIG. 15-7. A, Tubing is attached to inflow. **B,** Towel clip secures inflow cannula and tubing so that inflow cannula will not pop out of lateral sulcus.

Arthroscopic surgery of the knee

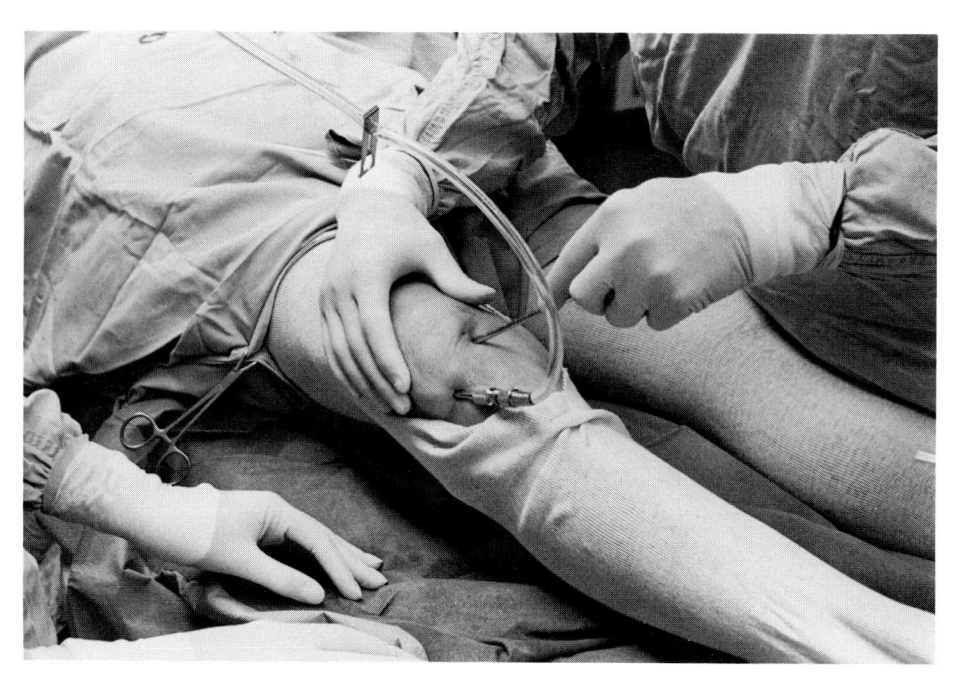

FIG. 15-8. Arthroscope is placed after distension has been achieved. Position is somewhat lateral to normal diagnostic arthroscopic puncture site.

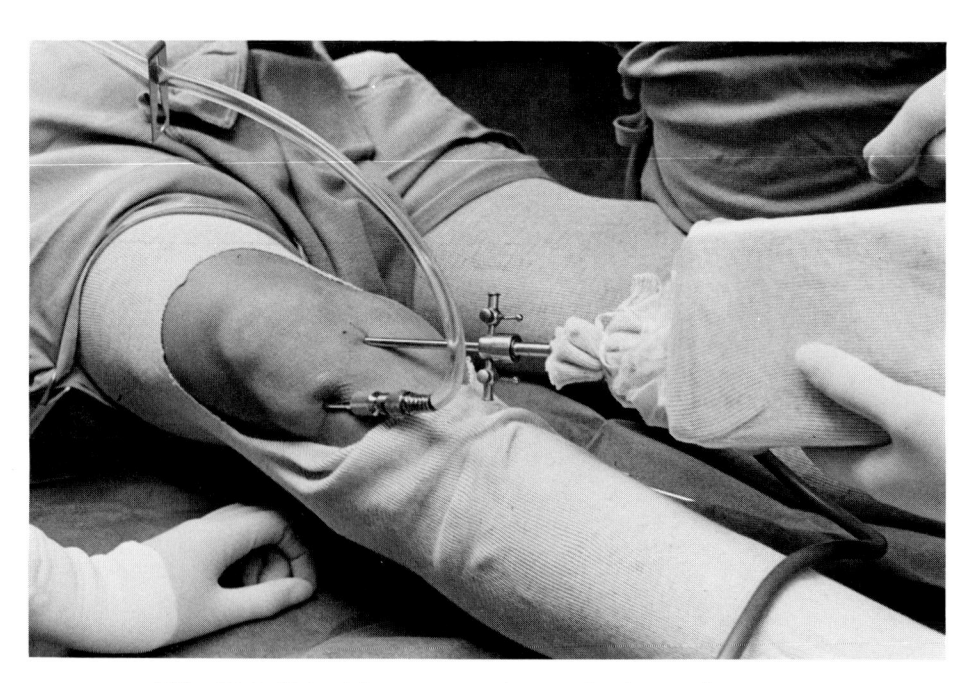

FIG. 15-9. Television camera is attached to arthroscope.

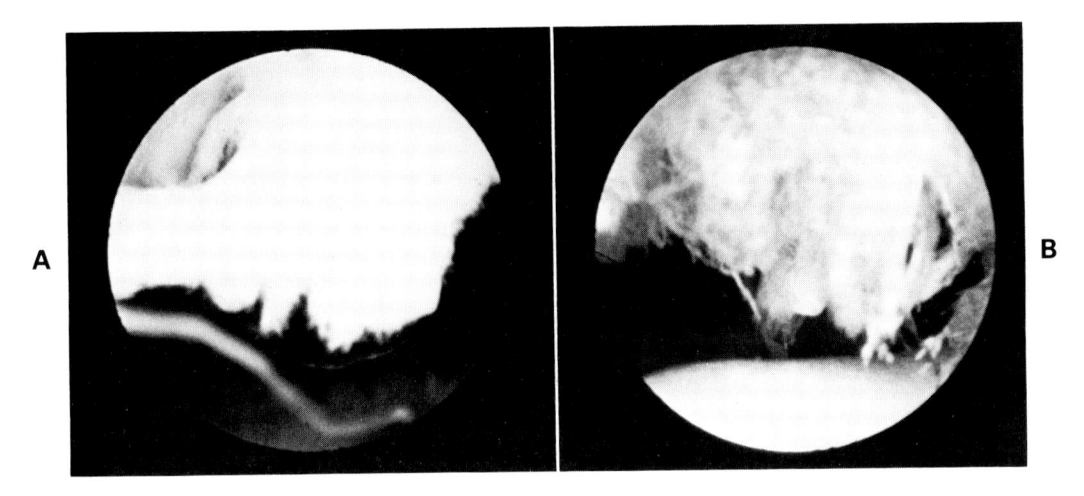

Basic principles of arthroscopic surgery: basic setup for patellar shaving

FIG. 15-10. A, Suprapatellar pouch shows marked degenerative change of patella. **B,** Peripatellar synovitis is evident in this arthroscopic view.

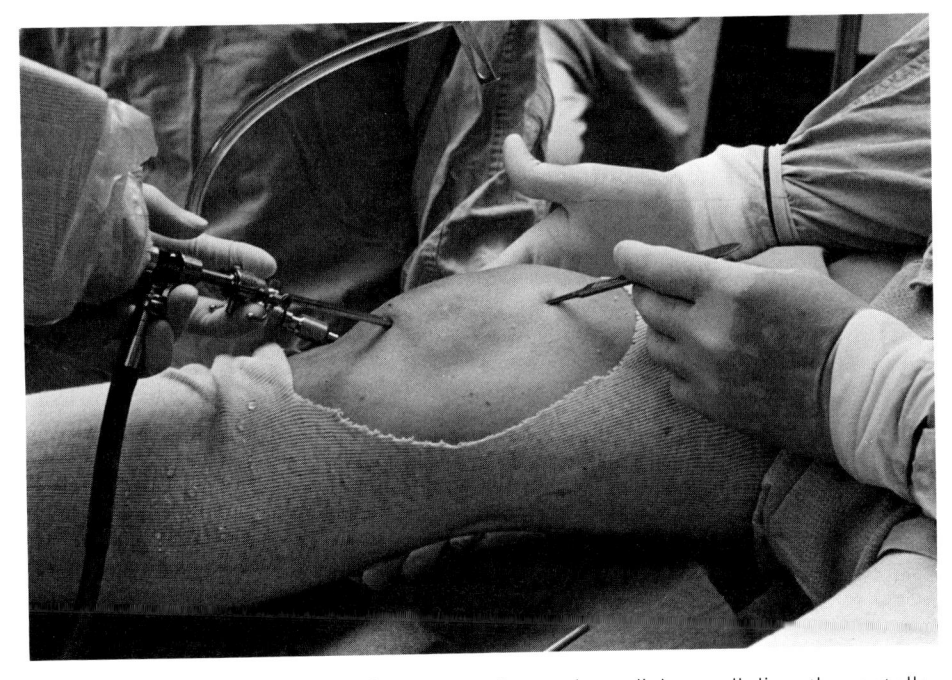

FIG. 15-11. Trocar is placed from superior and medial, paralleling the patella.

insertion (Fig. 15-11). A sharp, and then a blunt, trocar enters the joint in the same plane as the needle. The trocar is removed and replaced with the Intra-articular Shaver instrument shaft. The cannula is then rotated to lock in place on the Intra-articular Shaver.

Outflow system during operation

The outflow system is attached by normal operating room suction tubing to the spigot of the Intra-articular Shaver. The electric cord is attached to the power source. After the power source is turned on, the instrument is activated by the forward and reverse foot pedal. This can be covered with a plastic bag for protection from saline spillage and corrosion.

Arthroscopic surgery of the knee

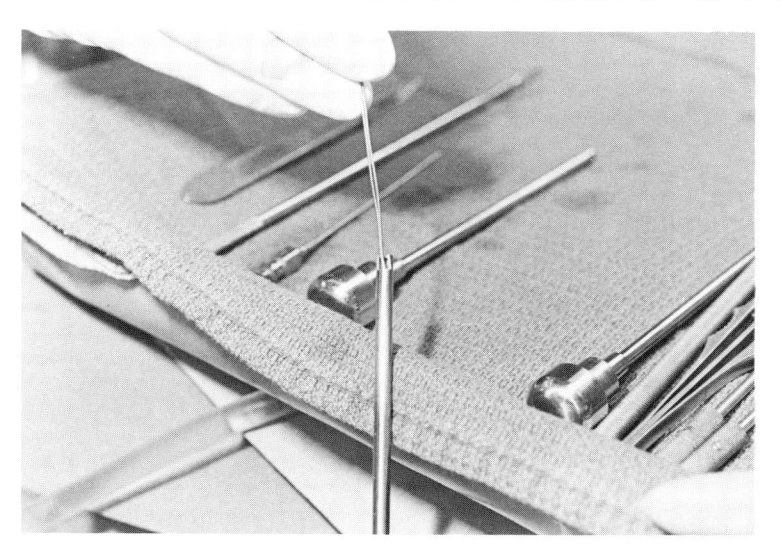

FIG. 15-12. Intra-articular Cutter cannula is unplugged by passage of folded wire through it. Effective intra-articular shaving can now be accomplished.

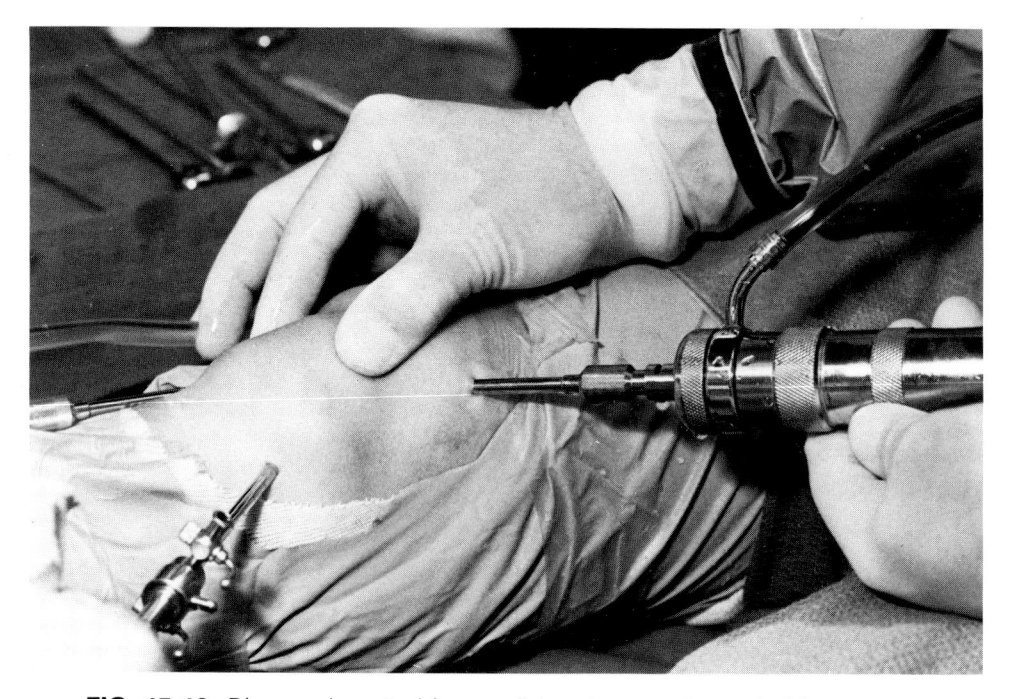

FIG. 15-13. Bimanual control is possible when assistant holds camera.

Because there is a rotating motion and alternating opening and closing of the window of the shaver, there is a chugging effect of the material down through the suction system. This material eventually ends up in the small "tobacco bag," which is taped to the inflow area on the large vacuum bottle. The tubes should be short and the pressure maintained at approximately 381 mm Hg.

In some instances the material can block the Intra-articular Shaver System. This occurs if a large piece is caught or if it is a hard bony material. This

Basic principles of arthroscopic surgery: basic setup for patellar shaving

stops the flow and effective action of the Intra-articular Shaver System or Cutter. When this occurs, the material in the instrument should be removed, and a No. 18 wire that is folded on itself is passed down through the orifice of the cutter to clear the channel (Fig. 15-12).

After the preceding instructions have been carried out, the intra-articular shaving can commence. A bimanual control of the patella facilitates this by not only tipping the patella but also by some compression of the patella to enable shaving down into the patellar surface (Fig. 15-13).

In some cases there is reactive parapatellar synovitis. Resection of that tissue is important therapeutically. It also may be necessary, in some patients,

---

POST OPERATIVE PATIENT INFORMATION
INTRAARTICULAR SHAVING CHONDROPLASTY

Your operation was performed by arthroscopic methods. The interior of your joint was visualized with a small telescope. The diagnosis was established and the appropriate surgery was performed with special micro-instruments.

DRESSING: A soft dressing has been applied to your knee. This compression dressing should be comfortable and absorb any leakage of fluid and/or blood. Although the dressing may become moist or blood stained, this is not usually a cause for alarm. We have not experienced any hemorrhage or excessive bleeding in our patients.
   The dressing may be removed safely at anytime. Routinely, the dressing is removed the day after surgery, and the appropriate number of bandaids are applied. The bandaids may be utilized over the next several days.

PAIN: Upon discharge you should secure a prescription for pain medication. Usually this will be Tylenol with **codiene.** Please inform us of any known drug allergy. **Codiene** may produce nausea and/or a fine skin rash. In that case, the medication should be discontinued and our office contacted for an alternate medication. The application of an ice pack to the knee will decrease swelling and discomfort in the first 48 hours. Please do not use aspirin, as it may increase bleeding in the first few days.

WOUNDS: The small points of entry may be sore and develop bruising over the next several days. This bruising will eventually disappear and does not require any special care.

BATHING: The sensation of "splashing" of fluid in the joint is not a cause for concern. It represents residual fluids from surgery, and they will absorb. It will be safe to shower 48 hours following surgery. Bathing or soaking should be delayed for several days. Cleansing of the skin adjacent to the small wounds with soap and water may be performed with the first dressing change.

ACTIVITY: Crutches may be necessary for comfort in the first week following surgery. You may step upon your surgical leg when comfortable. Active motion and tightening of quadricep muscles (the muscles on front of the thigh) should start the day of surgery. A twice a day activity (10-15 min.) for motion and muscle contraction should continue through three weeks.
   Swimming and bicycling are permissable as tolerated. Jogging, running, or stop and go sports should be deferred for 6 or 8 weeks. Heavy weight lifting should be delayed for 4 months.

RESULTS: Preliminary reports as well as our experience have shown arthroscopic surgery produces results equal to, if not better than surgery performed by open, conventional methods. The benefits are in less discomfort, risk, and scarring for the patient.
   We frequently remind patients that although the external incisions are small, they still have had an operative procedure inside their joint. Experience has shown that internal healing takes several weeks. In fact, complete healing to mature tissue may take three months. At that time most patients have a decrease in pain and swelling.

PRECAUTIONS: If you develop any fever (101 F° or above), unexpected pain, redness, or swelling in your legs, please contact our office for consultation or examination. TELEPHONE (517) 351-7450.

Thank you,

Lanny L. Johnson, M.D.

FIG. 15-14. Postoperative intra-articular shaving instructions. (Color code: green; see p. 245.)

to remove the fronds of the fat pad that comes up under the patellar surface. This provides clear viewing of the patella. If a suprapatellar plica or medial shelf appears to be diseased, then the Intra-articular Shaver can be used to remove these structures as well. (See Chapter 20.)

It should be noted again that the Intra-articular Shaver will cut only diseased articular material and will not debride normal cartilage. After the intra-articular shaving has been determined to be as complete as possible from that portal, the television recorder is placed on pause. The inflow tubing is released from the anterolateral inferior portal and interchanged with the Intra-articular Shaver portal. The Intra-articular Shaver is then moved into the cannula that was for the inflow. The areas of articular cartilage not available for resection are now removed from the new angle. Further debridement is carried out. This allows a more complete removal of all the articular debris. (Other articular surfaces are discussed later.)

At the conclusion of the procedure no sutures are necessary. A simple compression dressing of gauze and sterile cotton wrap (Webril) is applied. The postoperative instructions are given on a prepared color-coded (green) sheet (Fig. 15-14), and the patient is discharged.

LATERAL RELEASE TECHNIQUE

The setup for the lateral release technique is identical whether using the original patellar shaving setup or the comprehensive surgical organization.

The inflow cannula is in the lateral portal, inferior to the patella. The portal for the knife entrance is superior and medial to the patella. This was the portal

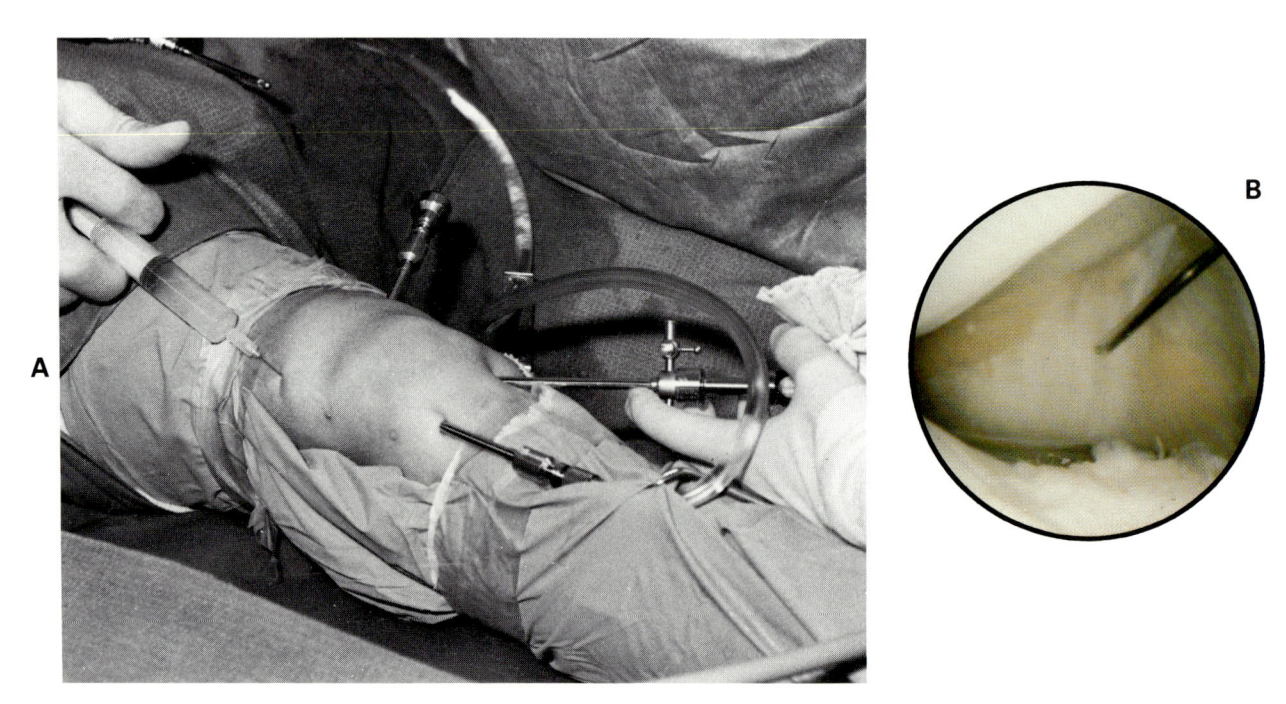

FIG. 15-15. A, Bupivacaine (Marcaine) is injected along capsule and into synovial tissue on anticipated site of lateral release. **B,** Arthroscopic view identifies position of needle. It is then retracted, and tissue is infiltrated with 0.25% plain Marcaine.

Basic principles of arthroscopic surgery: lateral release technique

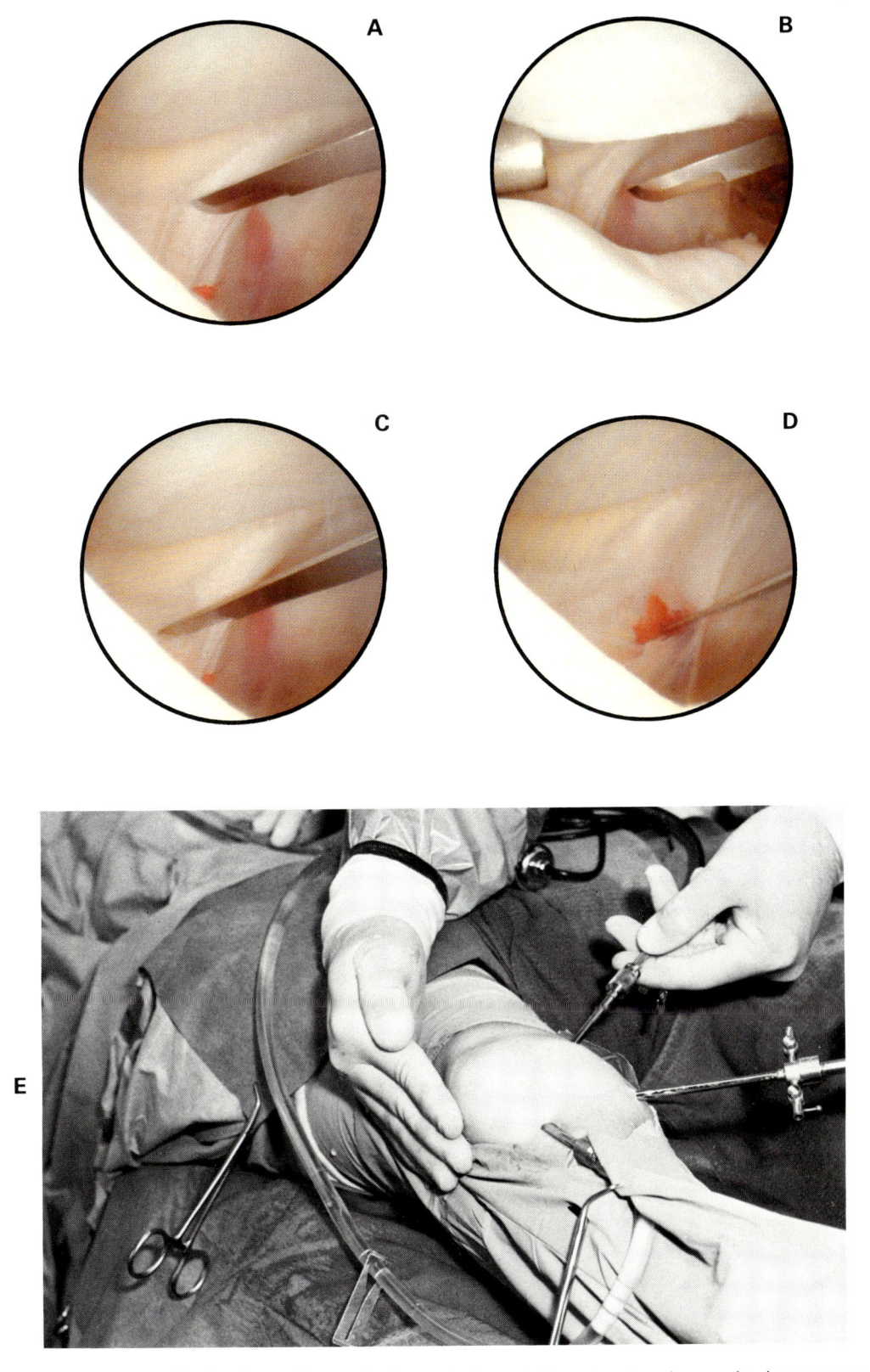

FIG. 15-16. A to **D**, Cutting of lateral release is from inflow tract and superior into vastus lateralis muscle; it releases superior lateral corner of quadriceps attachment to patella. **E**, Outside palpating hand assists in determining depth of lateral release.

Arthroscopic surgery of the knee

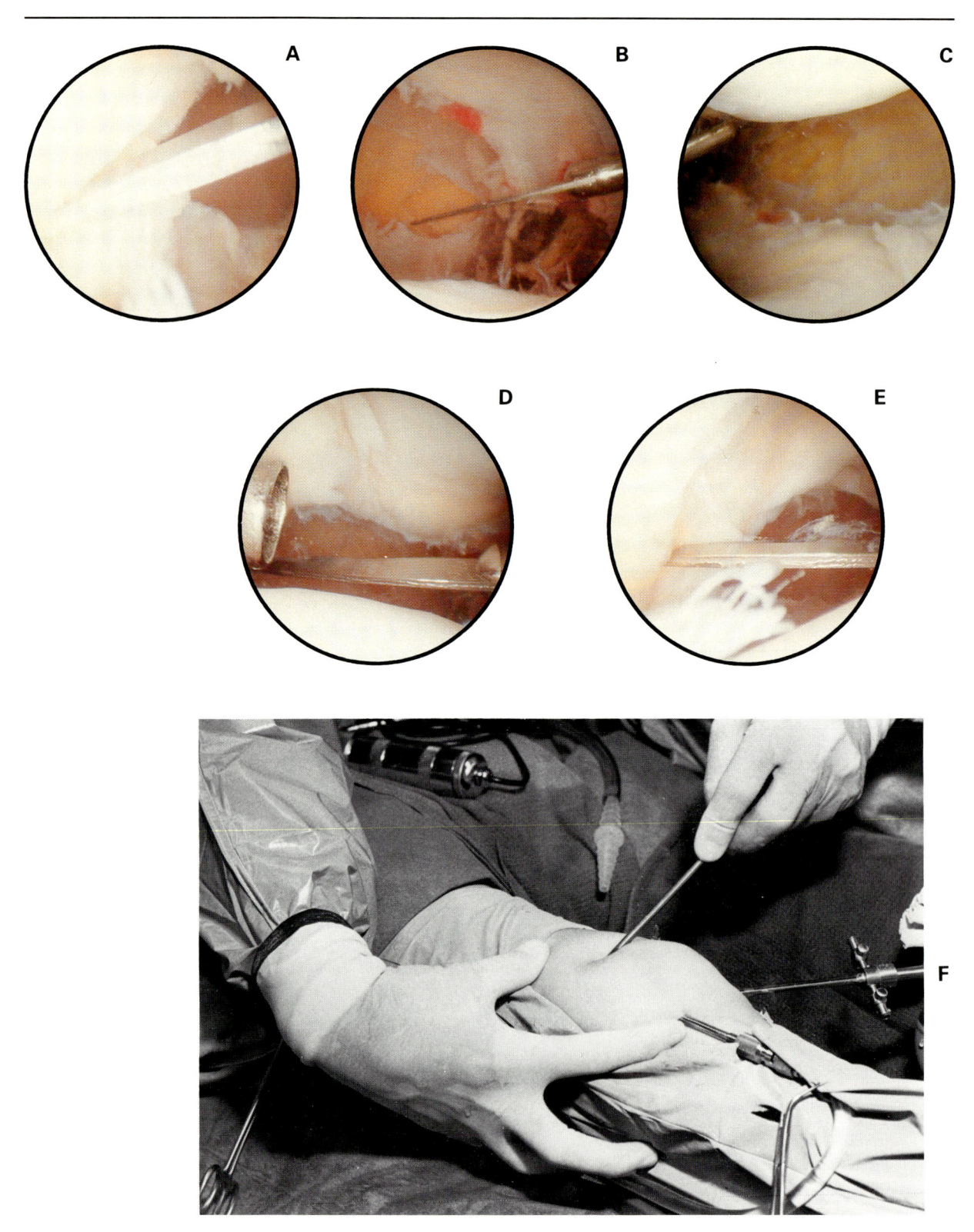

FIG. 15-17

A to **E,** Arthroscopic views of progression of lateral release, both proximal and distal. **F,** Outside hand can palpate extent of lateral release by using cannula and visualization from inside to determine adequacy and extent of this lateral release.

of the shaver in the original setup and the site of the inflow cannula in the universal setup. The inflow portals and operative portals may have to be rearranged, depending on the starting organization.

Marcaine, 0.25%, is injected in the lateral capsular tissues (Fig. 15-15). This maneuver is facilitated by placing the needle into the lateral joint for exact location by video viewing. The anticipated area of the capsular incision is determined for anesthetic infiltration. The needle tip is withdrawn from inside the joint and angled to infiltrate the capsule. No intra-articular anesthesia has been necessary, even when the operation is performed under local anesthesia. Lidocaine, 1%, may be added for faster anesthesia when local anesthesia is chosen.

First, the cannula may have to be located with blunt trocar insertion and viewing from a video screen. The knife is inserted through the cannula. After the anesthesia has infiltrated in the exact area of the lateral release, the incision is begun on the easily identifiable lateral bands (Fig. 15-16). The depth of the incision is regulated by direct arthroscopic vision but also by palpation with the opposite hand from outside the knee (Fig. 15-16).

The extent of the release is from the inflow cannula below and into the vastus lateralis muscle superiorly and a portion of the quadriceps tendon (Fig. 15-17). The perspective can be distorted if only the arthroscopic view is used. Therefore placement of the knife, or better, the cannula, at the superior extremity of the incision outlines the exact extent when palpated with the outside control handle. This outside control handle assists with the depth of the inside incision to the synovium and capsule. Also, it relieves the necessity of cutting across the quadriceps tendon with the altered perspective of the inclined arthroscopic view.

To review, this incision goes through the synovium and capsule, but does not violate the yellow subcutaneous tissue. The extent is from the inflow cannula inferior into the vastus lateralis muscle and tendon to release the lateral corner attachment to the patella.

The instruments may then be removed. The patella should be easily and gently manipulated to a position of medial displacement. This verifies the effectiveness of the release. No sutures or paper skin tapes are needed. In fact, with swelling, a skin tape may produce a skin blister. The puncture wounds heal readily. The compression dressing with a lateral pad is applied. The tourniquet is released until a flush appears in the foot, which is then reelevated. The tourniquet apparatus accompanies the patient to the recovery room, and the foot remains elevated 20 minutes. The tourniquet is released. This technique allows blood to fill the small vessels and then clot without continued intravascular pressure, and it seems to limit the bleeding. The anesthesiologist can control the discomfort from the tourniquet during the recovery period with a narcotic.

Large ice bags (double thickness to prevent leakage) are applied in the recovery room and go home with the patient (Fig. 15-18). A splint is applied prior to discharge (Fig. 15-19). The patient or relative is given color-coded (yellow) postoperative instructions (Fig. 15-20).

Arthroscopic surgery of the knee

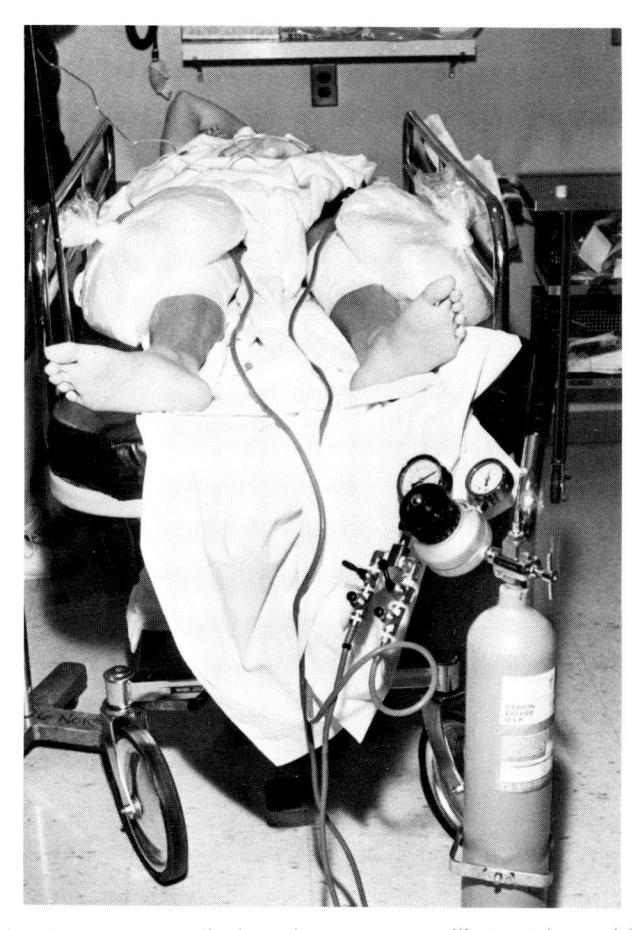

FIG. 15-18. Ice bags are applied to decrease swelling and provide anesthesia.

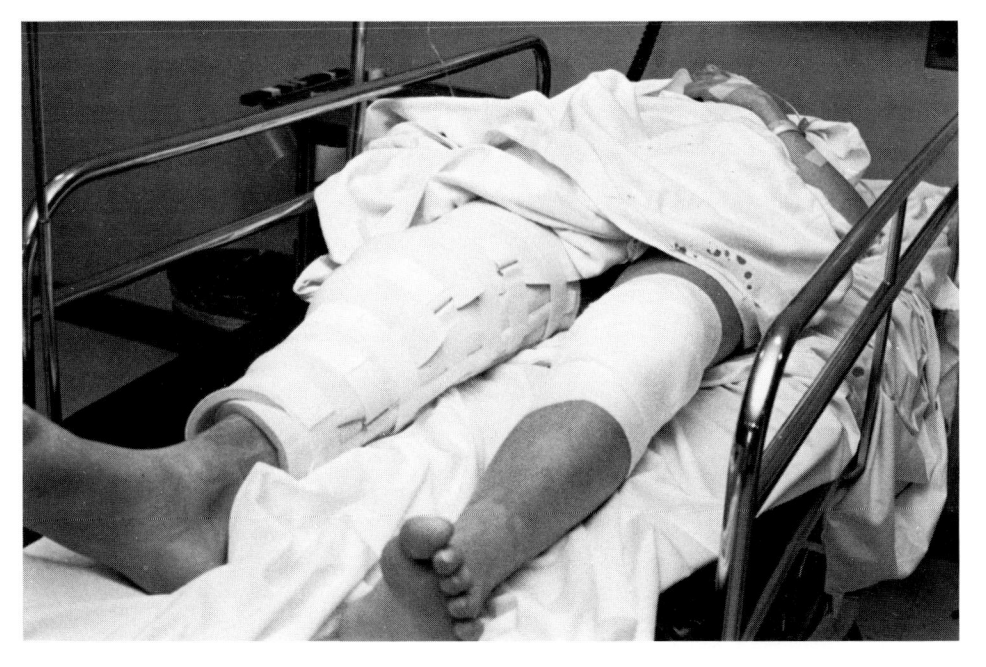

FIG. 15-19. Patient is discharged with commercially available disposable soft splint.

Basic principles of arthroscopic surgery: comprehensive setup

---

POST OPERATIVE PATIENT INFORMATION
LATERAL RELEASE

Your operation was performed by arthroscopic methods. The interior of your joint was visualized with a small telescope. The diagnosis was established and the appropriate surgery was performed with special micro-instruments.

DRESSING: A soft dressing has been applied to your knee. This compression dressing should be comfortable and absorb any leakage of fluid and/or blood. Although the dressing may become moist or blood stained, this is not usually a cause for alarm. We have not experienced any hemorrhage or excessive bleeding in our patients.

A splint has been applied to your knee for your comfort. You may adjust it to accomplish this need. The splint will be worn most of the time the first week. The next two weeks it will be used for sleep and going out of the house. After three weeks it should not be necessary.

PAIN: Upon discharge you should secure a prescription for pain medication. Usually this will be Tylenol with **codiene.** Please inform us of any known drug allergy. **Codiene** may produce nausea and/or a fine skin rash. In that case, the medication should be discontinued and our office contacted for an alternate medication. The application of an ice pac to the knee will decrease swelling and discomfort in the first 48 hours. Please do not use aspirin, as it may increase bleeding in the first few days.

The bruising may be rather large on the back and outer side of the thigh, knee, and into the calf and leg. Also, there may be a large bulge to the outer side of the knee cap. Experience has shown that this resolves within a few weeks.

WOUNDS: The small points of entry may be sore and develop bruising over the next several days. This bruising will eventually disappear and does not require any special care.

BATHING: The sensation of "splashing" of fluid in the joint is not a cause for concern. It represents residual fluids from surgery, and they will absorb. It will be safe to shower 48 hours following surgery. Bathing or soaking should be delayed for several days. Cleansing of the skin adjacent to the small wounds with soap and water may be performed with the first dressing change.

ACTIVITY: The splint will be used for three weeks. You may walk on the leg with/or without crutches. Muscle tightening exercises will "milk" swelling out of the extremity and assist healing. Bending of the knee should commence at one week. It will go slow at first.

Swimming and bicycling may be possible after three to six weeks. Expect three months to return to more vigorous sports.

RESULTS: Preliminary reports as well as our experience have shown arthroscopic surgery produces results equal to, if not better than surgery performed by open, conventional methods. The benefits are in less discomfort, risk, and scarring for the patient.

We frequently remind patients that although the external incisions are small, they still have had an operative procedure inside their joint. In your case, a releasing incision of about three inches. Experience has shown that internal healing takes several weeks. In fact, complete healing to mature tissue may take three months.

PRECAUTIONS: If you develop any fever (101 F⁰ or above), unexpected pain, redness, or swelling in your legs, please contact our office for consultation or examination. TELEPHONE (517) 351-7450.

Thank you,

Lanny L. Johnson, M.D.

FIG. 15-20. Postoperative lateral release instructions. (Color code: yellow; see p. 245.)

COMPREHENSIVE ARTHROSCOPIC SURGICAL TECHNIQUE

The original position for intra-articular shaving procedures presented some difficulty with surgery in other compartments. As a result, a system was developed to provide ease in every type of arthroscopic procedure. As with the technique for a comprehensive examination or the technique for intra-articular shaving of the patella, the comprehensive arthroscopic surgical procedure has specific positions for the equipment, instrumentation, and functions for persons of the team (Fig. 15-21).

Arthroscopic surgery of the knee

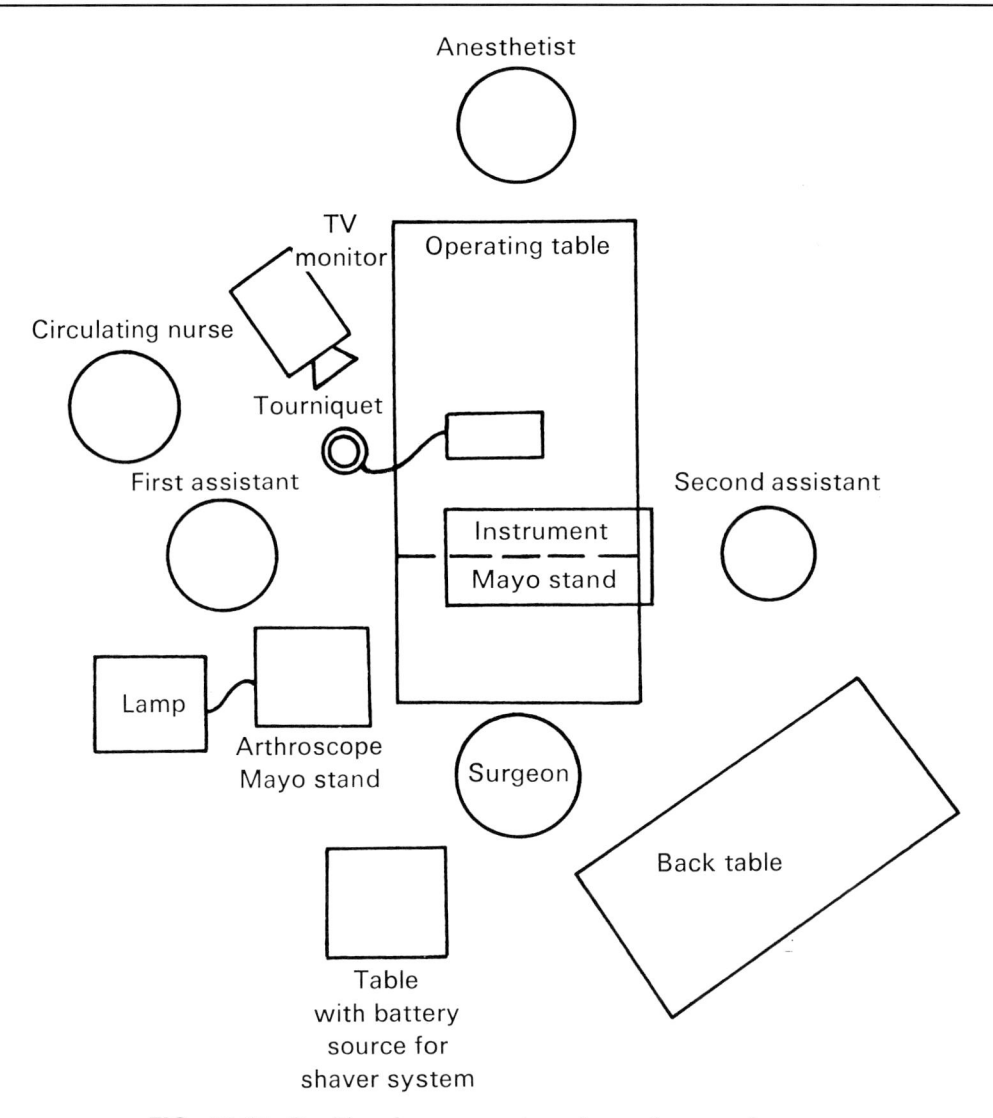

FIG. 15-21. Position for comprehensive arthroscopic surgery.

Patient positioning and preparation

The patient is placed in the supine position on a regular operating room table. The operating room table is moved so that the television camera on the light frame is just above the lateral side of the operative knee. A general anesthetic is preferred. It has been possible to perform simple meniscal resections under local anesthesia. After satisfactory anesthesia has been achieved, a tourniquet is placed high on the thigh and an elastic wrap is placed on the lower extremity. The tourniquet is elevated to 500 mm Hg, and the elastic wrap is removed.

The Clark attachment secures the Surgical Assistant to the operating room table (Fig. 15-22, *A*). The foam insert is placed around the thigh, and both are set into the stainless steel bracket of the Surgical Assistant. It is placed so as to conform to the thigh at approximately 4 to 6 inches above the superior aspect of the patella. The superior bar is placed across at the appropriate level to eliminate superior dislodgement from the Surgical Assistant during valgus or varus

Basic principles of arthroscopic surgery: comprehensive setup

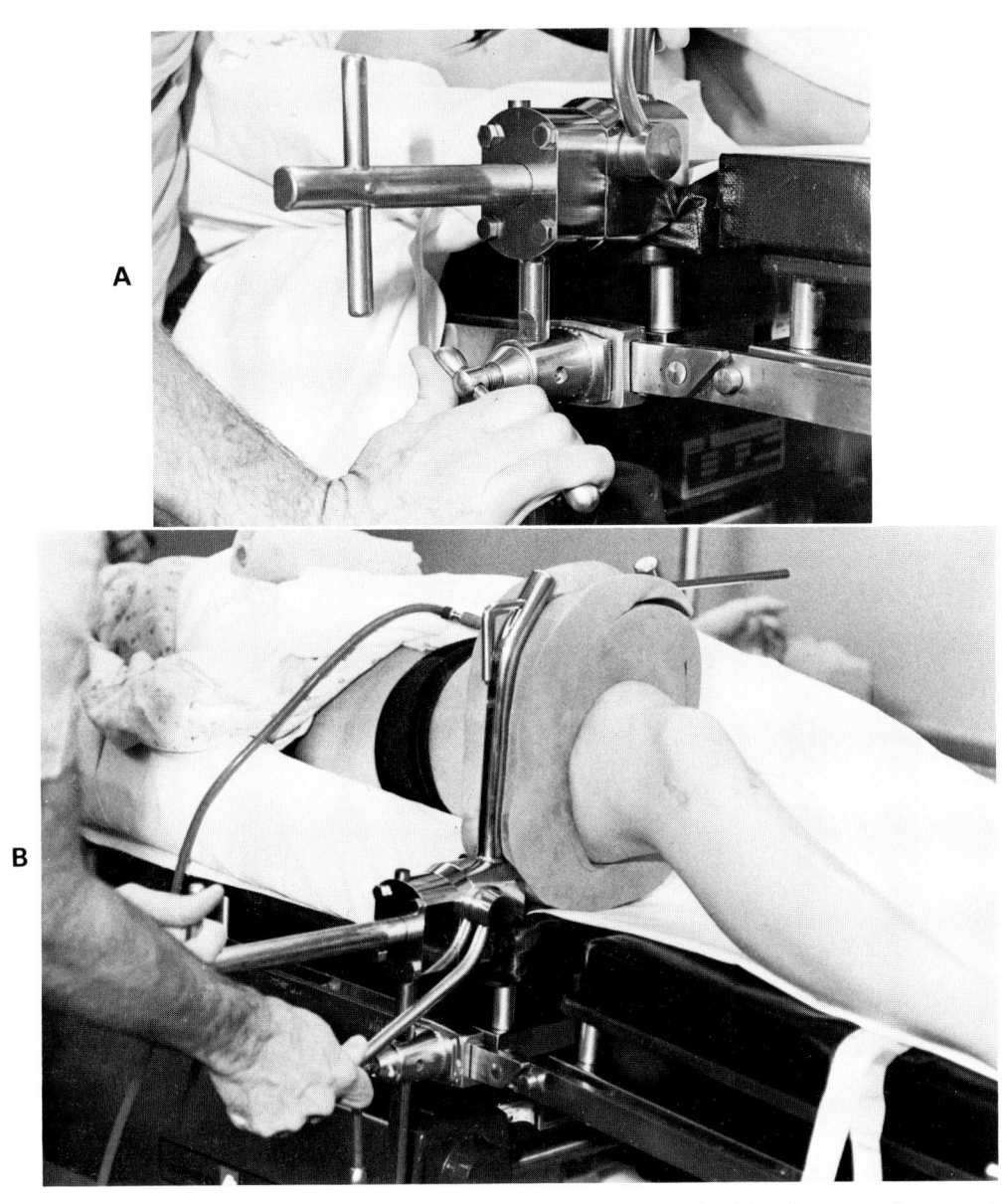

FIG. 15-22. A, Clark stirrup accessory, which attaches Surgical Assistant to the standard operating table. **B,** Surgical Assistant is secured to patient manually and with pumping of cam action lever.

stress. Compression is then achieved by pulling with one hand on the arm of the Surgical Assistant; the last few tightenings of the Surgical Assistant are accomplished by pumping the cam locking mechanism (Fig. 15-22, *B*). It is secured by depressing the handle of the locking mechanism.

A quadrilateral containment is achieved with this mechanical surgical device. This contour prevents rotation of the thigh with varus or valgus stress. The foam insert prevents slippage on the skin and the subsequent rotation. Open surgical procedures are easily performed without changing this position. High tibial osteotomy is especially facilitated by the Surgical Assistant.

Arthroscopic surgery of the knee

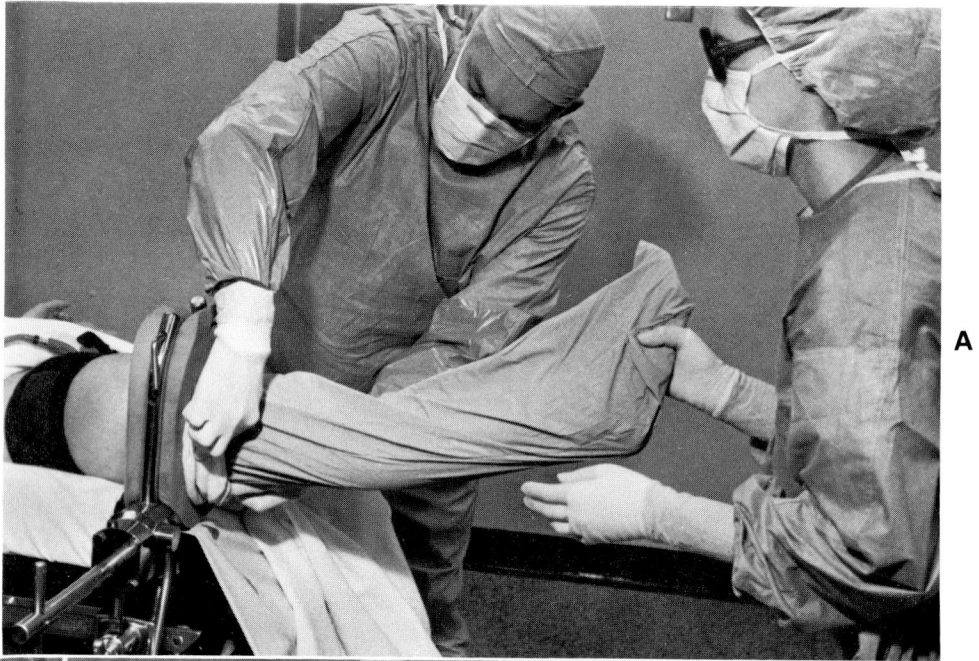

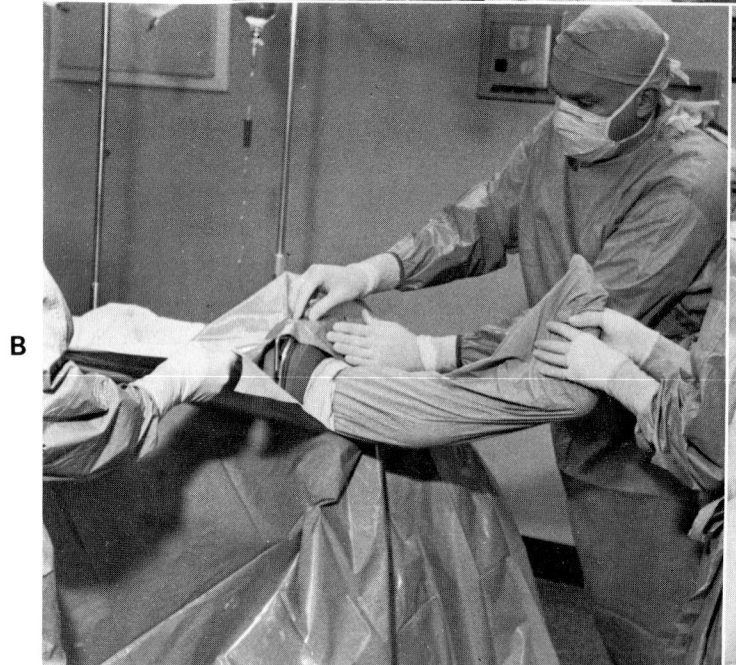

FIG. 15-23. A, Leg is draped up to Surgical Assistant. **B,** Plastic draping with adhesives seals off unsterile areas. **C,** Final draping is accomplished with absorbent disposable paper drape.

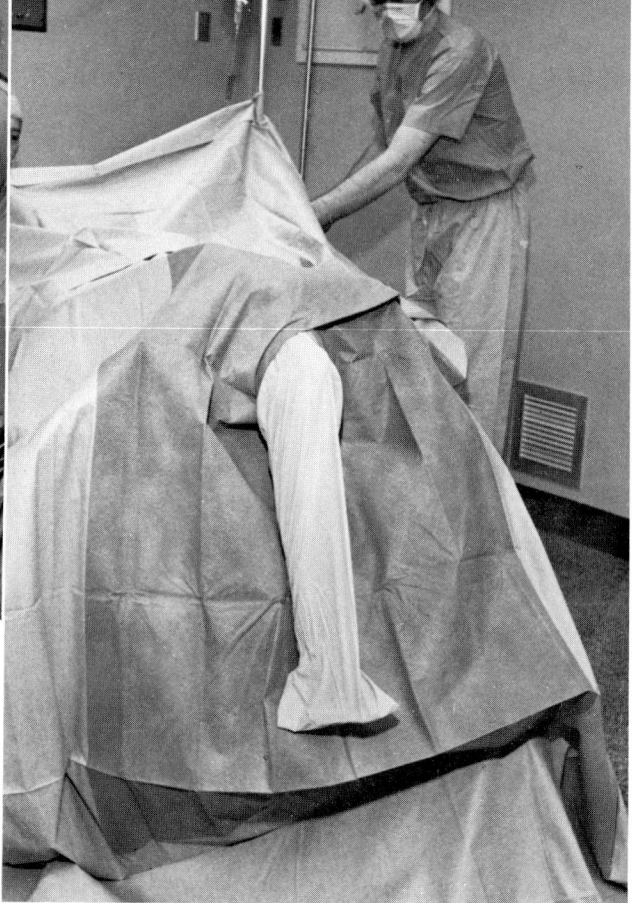

Basic principles of arthroscopic surgery: comprehensive setup

It should be noted that the measured pressure within the Surgical Assistant has been between 250 and 300 mm Hg. There is a potential tourniquet effect. It should not be left in place any longer than a normal pneumatic tourniquet. If a surgical procedure lasts longer than 1½ hours, I recommend that the tourniquet be released along with this instrument. It does not have to be completely removed. After sufficient time (15 to 20 minutes) the tourniquet could be reelevated, and the Surgical Assistant could be retightened. Redraping is not necessary for either of these maneuvers.

There have been no cases of neurovascular compression. We have had two instances of partial tear of the tibial collateral ligament in a man 74 and a woman 76 years of age. This occurred while pushing against the leg during debridement of a degenerative medial compartment. There was some minimal tenderness over the tibial collateral ligament and no clinical instability. No exploration was necessary at the time of surgery or later.

A skin preparation is applied to the knee and proximal leg. The sterile elasticized stockinette is brought over the lower extremity and tightly up against the foam insert of the mechanical Surgical Assistant (Fig. 15-23, A). A plastic drape, with adhesive, is placed tightly around the proximal portion of the thigh and over the Surgical Assistant foam insert to form a very clear and tight plastic seal about that area (Fig. 15-23, B). This is followed by the paper drape (with absorbent facing) up around the leg and overlapping itself superior to the thigh and over the patient's body. The final drape is placed superiorly as a shield for the patient's head and the anesthesiologist (Fig. 15-23, C).

The first assistant brings in the first Mayo stand with the arthroscopic equipment alongside the knee to be operated on (Fig. 15-24). The second assistant brings in the second Mayo stand with the instrumentation opposite the knee to be operated on. It is placed in a position above the patient's thigh and torso (Fig. 15-25).

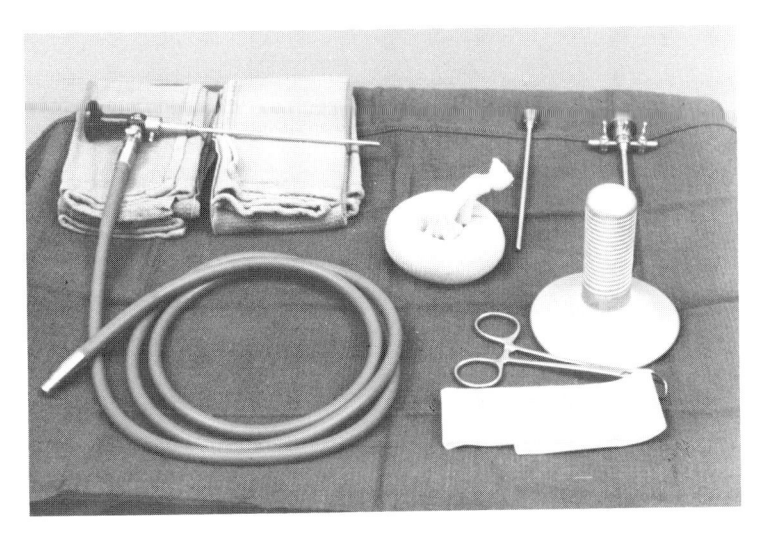

FIG. 15-24. Arthroscopic Mayo stand contains arthroscope, sterile light handle, small strip of drape to attach stockinette to arthroscope, articulated viewing device, and arthroscope and light cable.

Arthroscopic surgery of the knee

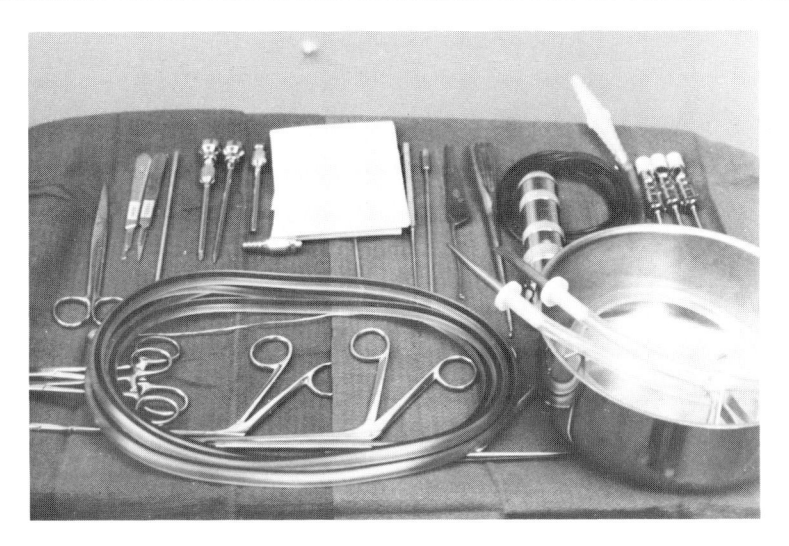

FIG. 15-25. Surgical Mayo stand includes Intra-articular Shaver System with its accessory hand instrumentation.

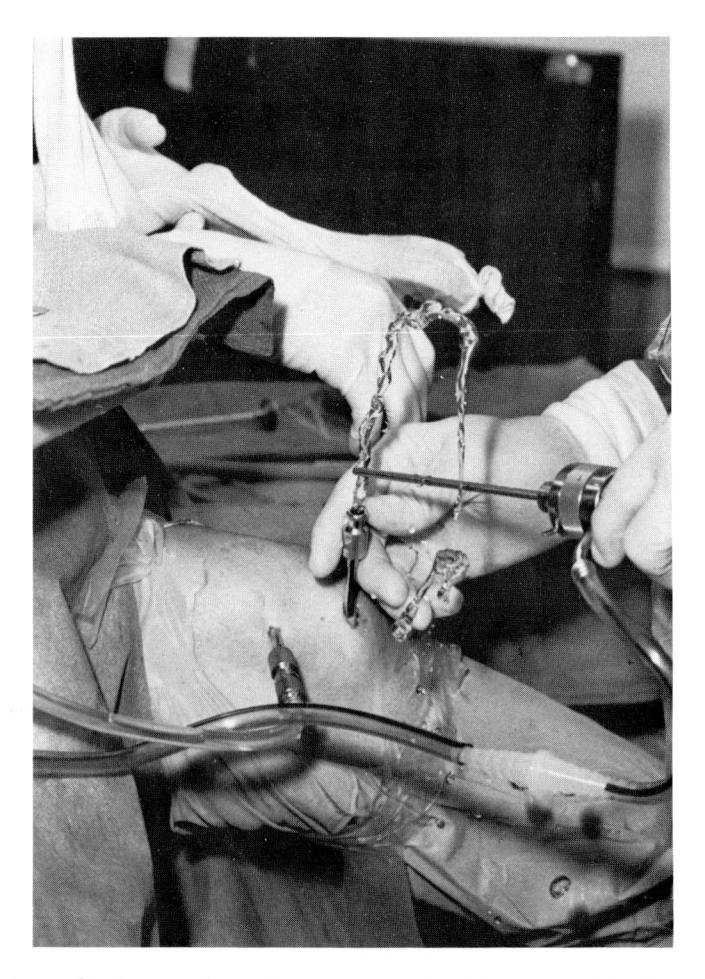

FIG. 15-26. Tubes of inflow and suction come under Mayo stand to the operative site.

Basic principles of arthroscopic surgery: comprehensive setup

The operating table is placed so that the extremity to be operated on is exactly under the light and suspended television camera. The operating table should be lowered as much as possible without potential contamination of the sterile, draped foot of the patient. It is elevated to a height that allows the surgeon maximal control of the extremity.

The surgeon is protected from dampness by a plastic apron. A sterile sheet is placed around the waist down to the ankles. This catches any saline spills and prevents running of saline down the plastic into the shoes or onto the floor. It also prevents the leg from slipping against the loose-fitting gown. The stool may be covered as well. The surgeon assumes a position in front of the patient's extremity. The foot of the patient rests on the surgeon's lap or just down in the sterile area between the patient and the surgeon.

The second assistant hands the Y tubing to the circulating nurse. This is attached to the two 3-liter bags of saline hanging from the IV pole. The base of the IV stand is secured with a doughnut-shaped sandbag. The air bubbles are removed from the system; the suction is then handed off superiorly to the circulating nurse. Both these tubes come under the second Mayo stand, which secures them and prevents dislodgement (Fig. 15-26). They are also removed from the operative field and will not interfere with any movement of the surgeon or the assistants.

The first assistant unravels the 2-inch sterile stockinette and covers the articulating device. This is then attached to the television camera, which is suspended from the operating room light for control of the video system and the articulated viewing device. The light cable is handed to the circulating nurse, who attaches it to the light source.

The surgeon opens the area of the stockinette over the knee. There are two strips of 3-inch-wide plastic adhesive on the second Mayo stand. One is used to secure the lower end of the opening and is wrapped around circumferentially so that saline will not run down inside the rubberized stockinette. The second strip is used to secure the paper drape above the superior aspect of the knee.

Placement of the inflow cannula

The inflow cannula is placed medial and slightly superior to the patella (Fig. 15-27, *A*). The skin is lanced with a No. 11 blade. A sharp trocar and the cannula pierce the skin, subcutaneous tissue, and fascia. The sharp trocar is exchanged for a blunt trocar, and the joint is entered. The entry is made so that the cannula comes down under the patella and over to the lateral-inferior side. When entry is confirmed, the cannula is retracted and allowed to rest perpendicular to the long axis of the knee in the suprapatellar pouch superior to the patella. The adapter for the inflow tubing is attached (Fig. 15-27, *B*). A sterile basin is brought in under the cannula at the medial aspect of the knee. The tubing of the inflow passes under the second surgical Mayo stand and is attached to the inflow cannula and its adapter (Fig. 15-27, *C*). The joint is distended.

The inflow from a Verres needle or one of the small spigots on the arthroscope is inadequate for distension and subsequent Intra-articular Shaver Sys-

Arthroscopic surgery of the knee

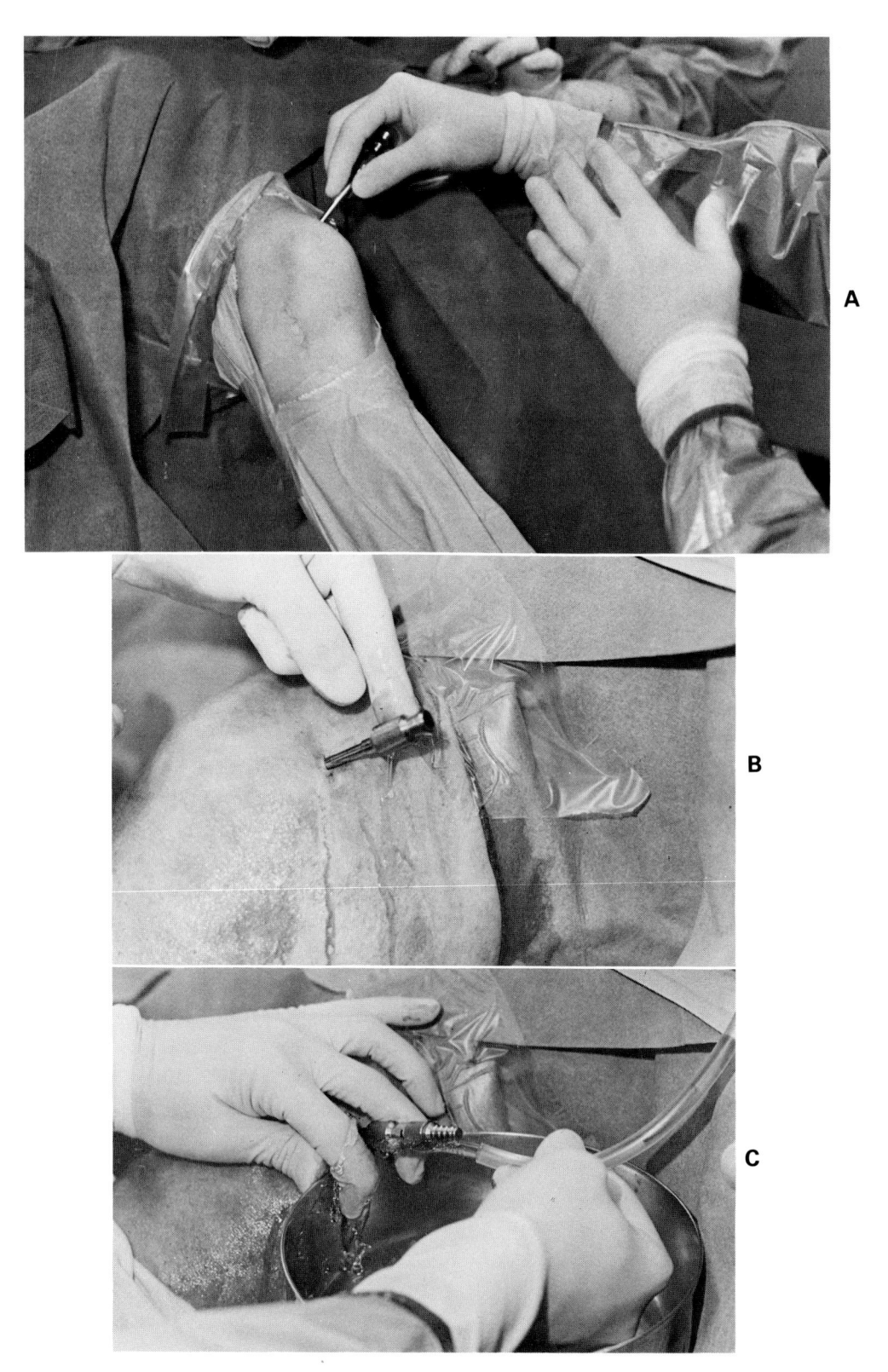

FIG. 15-27. A, Inflow cannula is placed superior and medial to patella. **B,** Inflow tubing adapter is attached. **C,** Inflow tubing comes down under table to anterior medial superior part near patella.

Basic principles of arthroscopic surgery: comprehensive setup

tem operation. The traditional inflow via the endoscope should be abandoned, since it causes turbulence in front of the scope and wiggling of synovial tissues, which distracts from the viewing.

Positions for arthroscopic surgery

Each compartment can be operated on by a change in body position and the interchangeability of the arthroscope and the instrument portals. The suprapatellar pouch is operated on with the knee in extension and the arthroscope either coming from the lateral side or reversed and coming in medially with the instrumentation from the opposite portal.

The medial compartment is inspected with a valgus strain placed on the knee with the lateral thigh or body. Sometimes, to achieve the exact flexion or extension position, this necessitates rising onto the toes of the extremity applying the pressure. Reverse Trendelenburg position of the table helps.

From a sitting position the surgeon can view the anterior chambers and the intercondylar notch and withdraw the endoscope and the instrumentation. Maximal distension must be available for anterior chamber surgery.

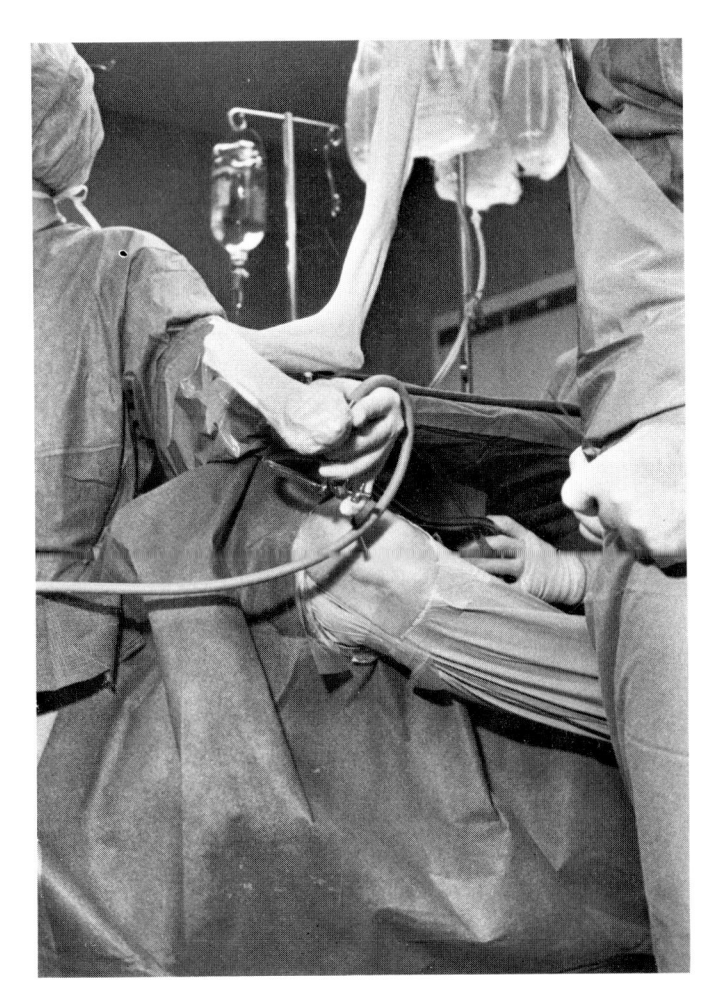

FIG. 15-28. First assistant holds arthroscope so surgeon can manipulate leg and/or surgical instruments.

Arthroscopic surgery of the knee

An interchangeability is possible by moving the arthroscope medially and bringing the cannula system into the lateral portal. The Intra-articular Shaver is then placed into the lateral portal. The surgeon stands on the lateral side of the extremity and applies a varus force to the knee.

The instruments may be held with one hand and the arthroscope with the other, giving the surgeon ultimate control of both instruments. This is possible because of the Surgical Assistant and the control the surgeon has of the knee and extremity. In some situations the surgery is facilitated by the first assistant holding and securing the arthroscope (Fig. 15-28). This reduces the fatigue of the surgeon and also frees his second hand. The second hand may be used to control the Intra-articular Shaver or other instruments. When it is necessary to use the nondominant hand and one does not have the control or the endurance, the dominant hand may have to assist. This also can be helpful in small manipulations.

When the assistant is holding the arthroscope and attaches the articulated viewing device, it frees the second hand of the surgeon to apply valgus strain or internal or external rotation to the extremity.

The foot opposite the direction in which the force is being applied to the patient's leg remains on the floor. The extremity closest to the leg is used to control the foot pedal. Forward and reverse controls are possible.

Placement of the arthroscope

The usual placement of the arthroscope in this comprehensive surgical setup is anterolateral (Fig. 15-29), which is facilitated by the placement of the

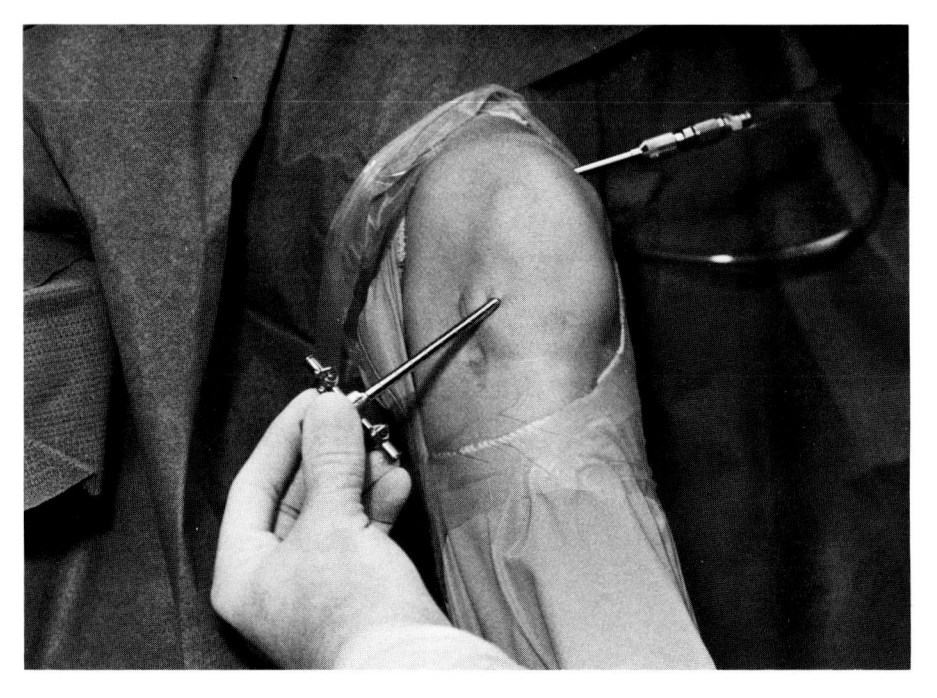

FIG. 15-29. Arthroscope is placed anterior and lateral and inserted toward intercondylar notch.

Basic principles of arthroscopic surgery: comprehensive setup

first Mayo stand. In addition, the light source is lateral to the operative knee. If it is known or suspected that the patient has a torn lateral meniscus, then the initial entry of the arthroscope is from the anteromedial portal. None of the other positions of tables or equipment is modified; only the arthroscopic entry site is changed.

The skin is again lanced with a No. 11 blade. (See Fig. 7-8, A.) A sharp, and then a blunt, trocar enters the joint. This puncture should be lateral to the tip of the patella. Aim to the medial side of the joint. A placement into the intercondylar notch is best. A move up under the patella obliquely to about 30° will carry the synovium back onto the shank of the arthroscopic cannula if necessary. If the placement is too midline, it goes through the fat pad. The fat pad can easily retract over the end of the arthroscope and obscure viewing. If it is too low, the tough meniscus tissue interferes with mobility. Neither is desirable. The outflow of saline from the cannula confirms entry (Fig. 15-30). If at this time there is blood or cloudy fluid in the joint, it is easily vacuumed out by bringing the suction tube to the end of the arthroscopic cannula and cleansing all compartments.

The arthroscope is placed in the joint by the surgeon. It is secured by the first assistant. The first assistant then passes the suspended stockinette-covered articulating viewing device and a pair of scissors to the surgeon.

The surgeon opens a ½- to ¾-inch hole in the stockinette with the scissors. The unsterile scissors are then passed out of the operative field. The stockinette is stretched slightly and placed over the ocular attachment of the arthroscope,

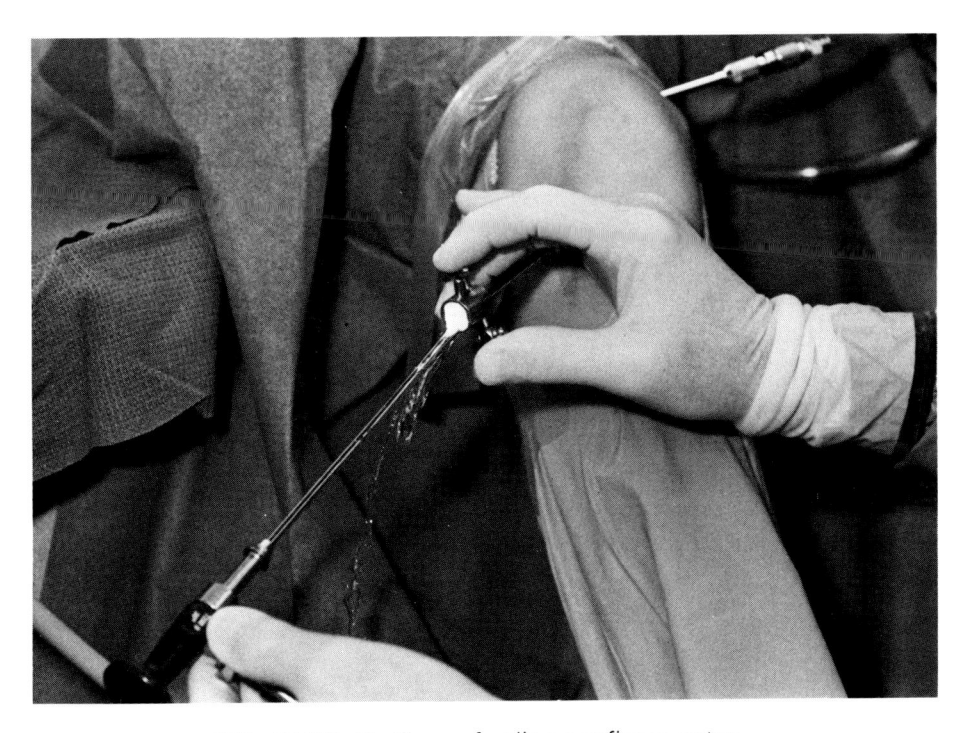

FIG. 15-30. Outflow of saline confirms entry.

Arthroscopic surgery of the knee

and the articulating viewing device is secured to the arthroscope. A 1½-inch-wide strip of adhesive plastic is then wrapped in a figure eight around the stockinette attachment to the arthroscope (Fig. 15-31). This prevents any slippage of stockinette so that the surgeon can handle this area with facility and not have any resultant contamination.

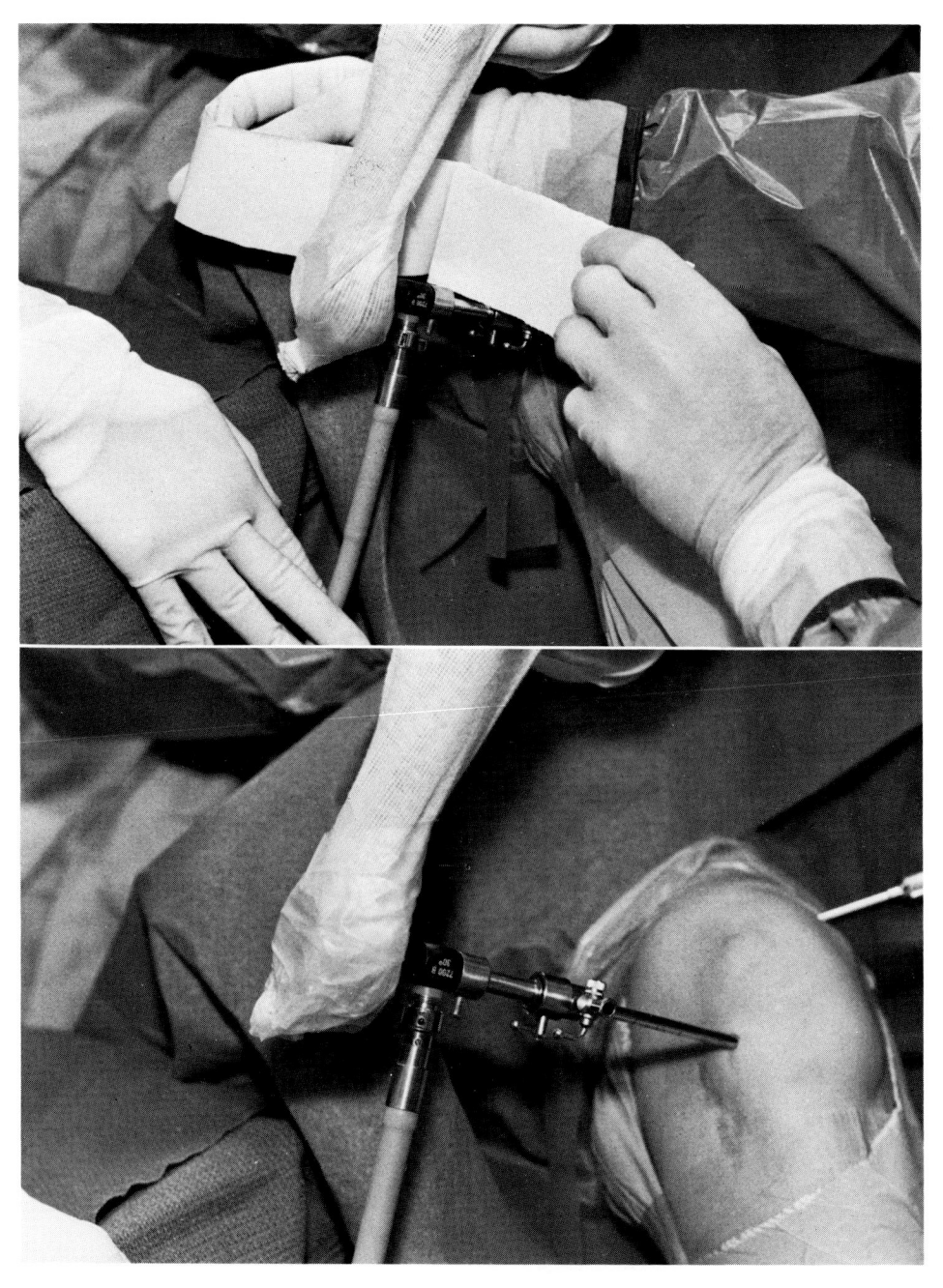

FIG. 15-31. Arthroscope attached to articulated viewing device; 1½-inch strip of sterile plastic adhesive secures stockinette and articulated viewing device to arthroscope with figure eight maneuver.

Basic principles of arthroscopic surgery: comprehensive setup

Preoperative arthroscopic diagnostic examination

In most cases a previous arthroscopic examination has not been accomplished. Therefore a comprehensive examination is performed and recorded on videocassette immediately prior to any arthroscopic surgery. The environment created for the arthroscopic surgery by the Surgical Assistant and the inflow of saline, which are preparatory to the surgical dimension of the procedure, facilitate the preliminary diagnostic arthroscopy. Therefore the initial part of every arthroscopic surgery procedure is documentation of the arthroscopic findings. This then allows the surgeon to plan and design the surgical portion of the operation, which will immediately follow the diagnostic arthroscopy.

Anatomic areas

Suprapatellar pouch. The arthroscope is manipulated into the suprapatellar pouch. Either the patella or the inflow cannula is a good landmark for orientation. It may be necessary to rotate the articulating viewing device at the attachment to the television camera to square the video picture. A recording is made of the arthroscopic findings. (See Chapter 7.) Next the patella is inspected. Retraction with slight angulation aids identification of the intercondylar notch. Rotation of the inclined view helps demonstrate this area. It is possible, by advancement and rotation of the arthroscope, to visualize both the medial and lateral sulci adjacent to the suprapatellar pouch. In the lateral sulcus there are often loose bodies. It is also possible to see the popliteus tendon and sheath from the lateral vantage point (Fig. 15-32).

The patellar surface can be palpated by using the opposite hand on the inflow cannula when viewing the patella (Fig. 15-33). Palpation with the side of the cannula gives a sense of the softness of the articular surface. If there is a break in that articular surface of the patella, the depth can be evaluated by palpating with the cannula.

A move is then made to the medial compartment following the tangent of the medial femoral condyle. The knee is quite distended at this time, so this is generally easily accomplished. This is the appropriate time to inspect for a medial synovial shelf or any erosions or osteophytes on the femoral condyle.

Medial compartment. The surgeon stands and places valgus force on the patient's leg with his hip or thigh. It is then possible to see the articular surface of the femur, and with flexion and extension the entire surface is visualized. The meniscus is identified, as are the condylar surfaces. It should be noted that the knee is in the distended position, and the meniscus is displaced peripherally from its normal resting location. Suction applied to the arthroscope, with the inflow clamped off, brings the meniscus back into position. A combination of flexion and extension, varus and valgus stress, and internal and external rotation is produced to visualize the entire compartment.

Intercondylar notch. The seated surgeon then visualizes the intercondylar notch. The arthroscope best visualizes the anterior cruciate ligament if it is moved to the lateral side of the membranous ligament. The posterior cruciate ligament's femoral attachment may be seen from this vantage point. A drawer sign can be performed to study the dynamics of the cruciate ligaments.

Arthroscopic surgery of the knee

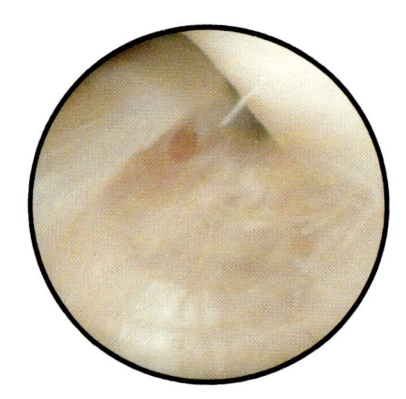

FIG. 15-32. Arthroscopic view of popliteus sheath from inferior and lateral.

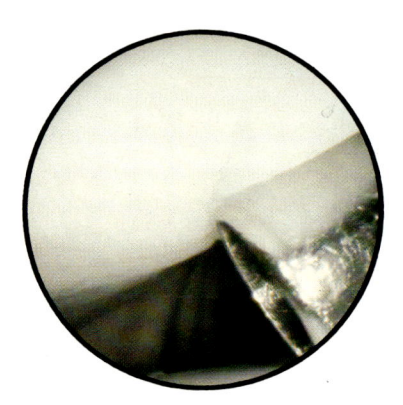

FIG. 15-33. Arthroscopic view of patella. Surgeon palpates surface with inflow cannula that is superior and medial.

Lateral compartment. The arthroscopist stands and changes body position to the lateral side of the extremity. A varus force is applied with pressure against the leg. Both hands are still free for manipulation. The lateral compartment visualization is accomplished by flexion and internal rotation of the leg as well. This can be as much as 90°, depending on the patient. This somewhat duplicates the cross-legged position or the "figure 4" position used in open surgery. Visualization of the tibial plateau is possible with the cross-legged position.

Posterolateral compartment. Gentle manipulation of the endoscope, in most patients, allows entrance into the posterior lateral compartment over the extreme posterior horn. A rotational move laterally shows the popliteus sheath from the superior aspect of the meniscus. Visualization of the popliteus under the meniscus is readily accessible. The meniscus is traced to the most extreme anterior horn with retraction of the arthroscope and rotation of the 30° inclined view to anterior.

The inflow is then clamped off, and suction is applied to the arthroscopic spigots to move the meniscus into its more normal, nondistended position. The lateral meniscus has great mobility. With the inflow cut off and suction applied, the meniscus will virtually collapse and obliterate the entire lateral compartment (Fig. 15-34). The suction is turned off and the inflow opened. Redisten-

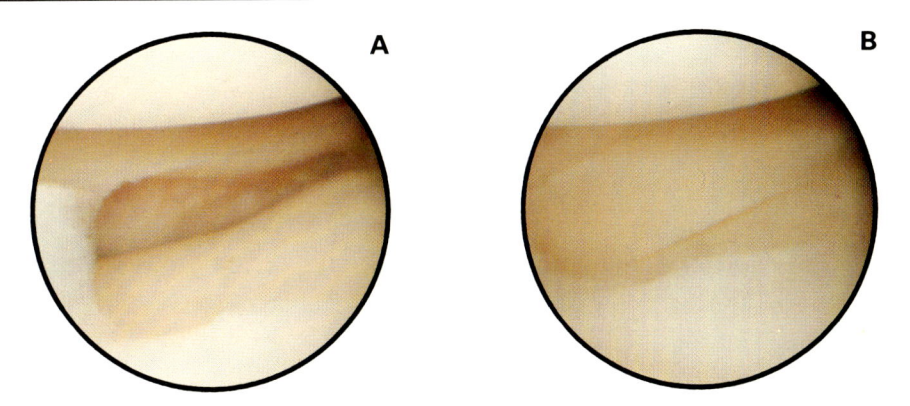

Basic principles of arthroscopic surgery: comprehensive setup

FIG. 15-34

A There is considerable mobility to lateral meniscus, seen here in maximal distension.
B With inflow clamped off and suction applied to arthroscope spigot, lateral meniscus collapses inward from posterior and anterior, hinging immediately anterior to popliteus tendon.

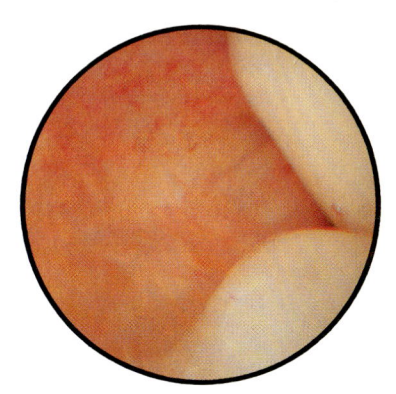

FIG. 15-35. Posterior medial horn of meniscus can be seen by modified Gillquist approach from anterior and lateral without changing to 70° inclined scope.

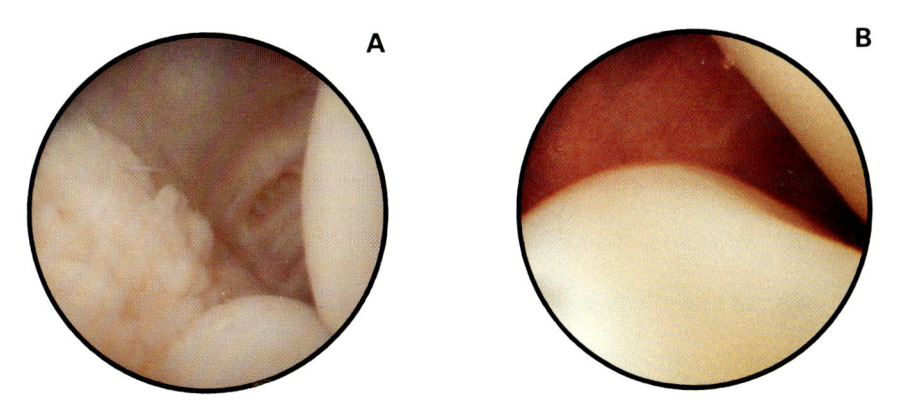

FIG. 15-36

A Interchange of 30° to 70° inclined scope shows medial wall of joint and meniscus.
B With internal rotation of the tibia on femur, meniscus drops off femoral condyle to better view its superior surface for any tears.

sion is accomplished. Sometimes acute flexion and varus strain, especially in a fat or scarred knee, will bring the capsular tissues down and around the femoral condyle to such an extent that the flow of saline is obliterated. The varus strain and flexion have to be relaxed momentarily to redistend the lateral compartment.

Posteromedial compartment. The arthroscope then courses back and views the medial compartment adjacent to the tibial spine, and, with manipulation of both the extremity and the arthroscope, entry can be made into the posteromedial compartment. With a 30° inclined arthroscope, rotation of that instrument provides a view across the posterior horn (Fig. 15-35). In some instances it is necessary to exchange the arthroscope for the blunt trocar to make the entry adjacent to the tibial spine into the posteromedial compartment. Occasionally the 30° incline view may not provide adequate visualization of the entire compartment, and an interchange with the 70° oblique scope, as recommended by Gillquist, is necessary (Fig. 15-36).

Probing

At this juncture, if there is no intra-articular abnormality demonstrated or only a suspicious area, then probing is indicated. The Oretorp probe is an ideal size to elevate the meniscus and probe under and over it (Fig. 15-37). One may be sure there is no subtle cleft by forceful palpation with the rounded edge of the probe on the superior aspect of the meniscus. Also, the probe may be moved back into the posterior compartment to grasp the posterior horn of the meniscus to bring it forward. The posterior horn of the medial meniscus should not displace forward; it is firmly attached in the normal knee.

The anterior cruciate ligament may be probed to identify any looseness that was not evidenced by the drawer sign. It is possible to evaluate the exact position of the tear and determine amenability to any surgical repair.

In the lateral compartment, probing easily elevates the lateral meniscus. It is possible to place the probe in the popliteus sheath, which should not be mistaken for a tear. (See Fig. 15-32.) The lateral meniscus has more mobility than the medial. Using the centimeter markings on the Oretorp probe gives one a standard by which to measure mobility.

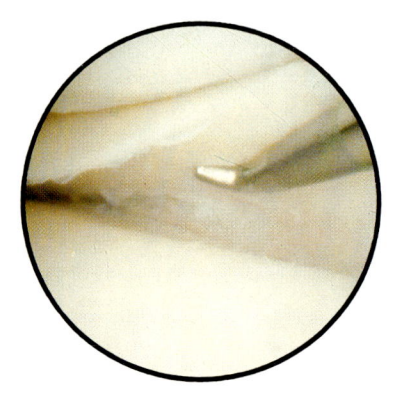

FIG. 15-37. Probing meniscus is standard procedure to assist visualization and evaluate mobility.

Basic principles of arthroscopic surgery: comprehensive setup

If, at that juncture, the patient shows no indication of a need for either arthroscopic or open surgical procedure, the anesthesiologist is so instructed, the equipment is removed, and sterile dressings are applied.

Separate posteromedial or posterolateral approaches are indicated when the area has not been visualized from the anterior approach. (See Chapter 3.) This is performed with the Needlescope to reduce joint puncture leakage.

Puncture sites for surgical instrumentation
Medial compartment

If a torn medial meniscus was easily seen by arthroscopic viewing and the remainder of the arthroscopic examination has been normal, the medial compartment is viewed from the lateral approach. The surgeon stands to the medial aspect of the leg, and valgus strain is applied. No conscious effort is made to predetermine the external site of puncture into the medial compartment. This site is determined by the internal view. It is very difficult to pick the external skin puncture site and have it be correct, given the variety of shapes and sizes of knees. The surgeon visualizes the medial wall of the joint arthroscopically and palpates the medial aspect of the patient's knee to identify a place immediately superior to the meniscus, as seen from the arthroscopic view.

Attention is then turned to where the finger was palpating, and a 3-inch, No. 18 spinal needle is placed into the joint at this juncture (Fig. 15-38). Care is taken to place the needle between the neurovascular bundles, as seen by transillumination (Fig. 15-39). This technique avoids nicking a branch of the cutaneous nerve. The site is slightly medial through the capsule and angulates posteriorly as it enters through the synovium. This method requires palpation and inspection from the inside, and then needle placement is performed from the outside.

With the spinal needle, one should be able to manipulate between the medial compartment in such a way that the entire meniscal lesion can be palpated. A "dry run" maneuver with the needle ensures access at the time of resection. Also, the needle should be in a position so that flexion or extension of the knee gives access for the correction of any articular abnormality. Replacement of the needle or direction is performed until a perfect position is achieved. Manipulation of the needle will establish access to all the anticipated surgical sites, yet the skin or capsule is not violated.

When a medial femoral condylar shave is indicated, the needle placement will be higher and more medial than for a posterior meniscal tear.

The cannula is taken in hand, and the needle is removed. The surgeon watches and conceptualizes the spatial relationships in which the needle was placed. A No. 11 blade lances the skin, and the cannula and sharp trocar pierce the capsule. This is exchanged for a blunt trocar to enter the joint (Fig. 15-40). This will be the exact same course that the needle followed and will be in perfect position for the operative manipulations. The cannula and blunt obturator are seen on the television monitor.

After the cannula has been placed, access to that compartment has been established. The variety of surgical instruments may be passed through those

Arthroscopic surgery of the knee

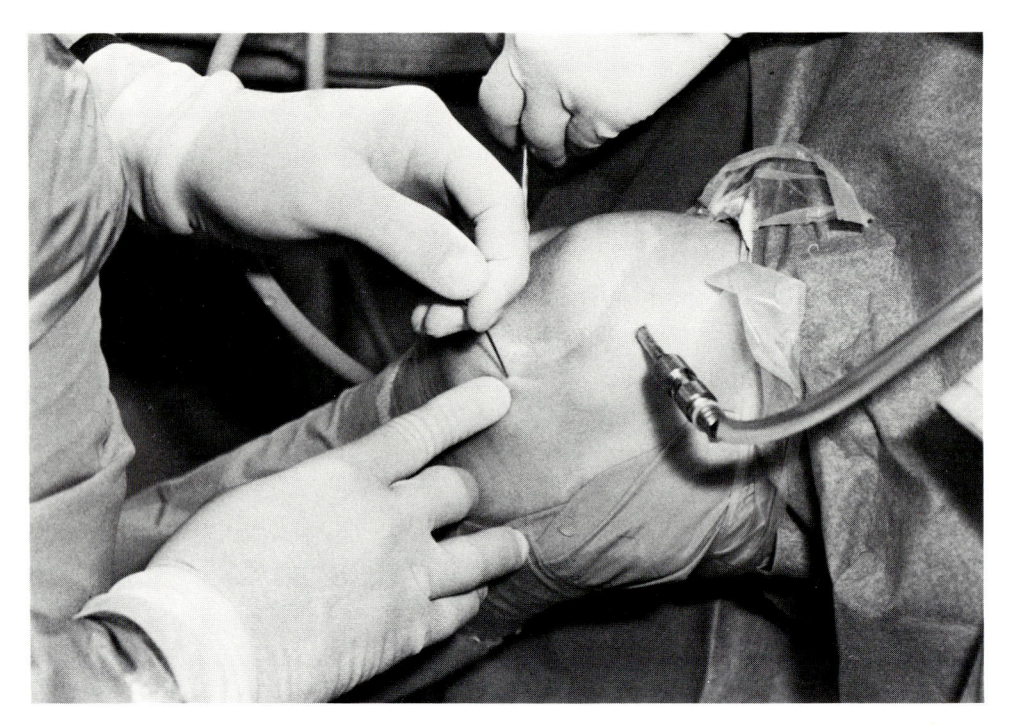

FIG. 15-38. Palpation of medial wall from outside helps in selecting site for placement of No. 18 spinal needle.

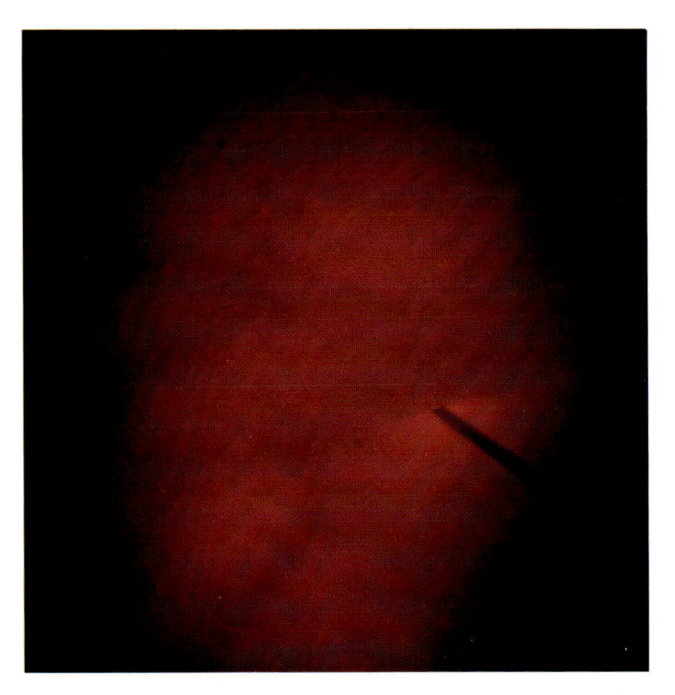

FIG. 15-39. Transillumination of neurovascular bundles aids selection of site for needle and cannula placement, where they will not nick suprapatellar branch of saphenous nerve.

Basic principles of arthroscopic surgery: comprehensive setup

channels without violating, stretching, or again manipulating the capsule beyond the opening the 4-mm cannula has provided.

It is possible to place knife blades, probes, specially designed forceps, and cutting devices, as well as the variety of instruments that accompany the Intra-articular Shaver, through this portal (Fig. 15-41). The portal may also be used for interchangeability with the arthroscope or the saline inflow system. In

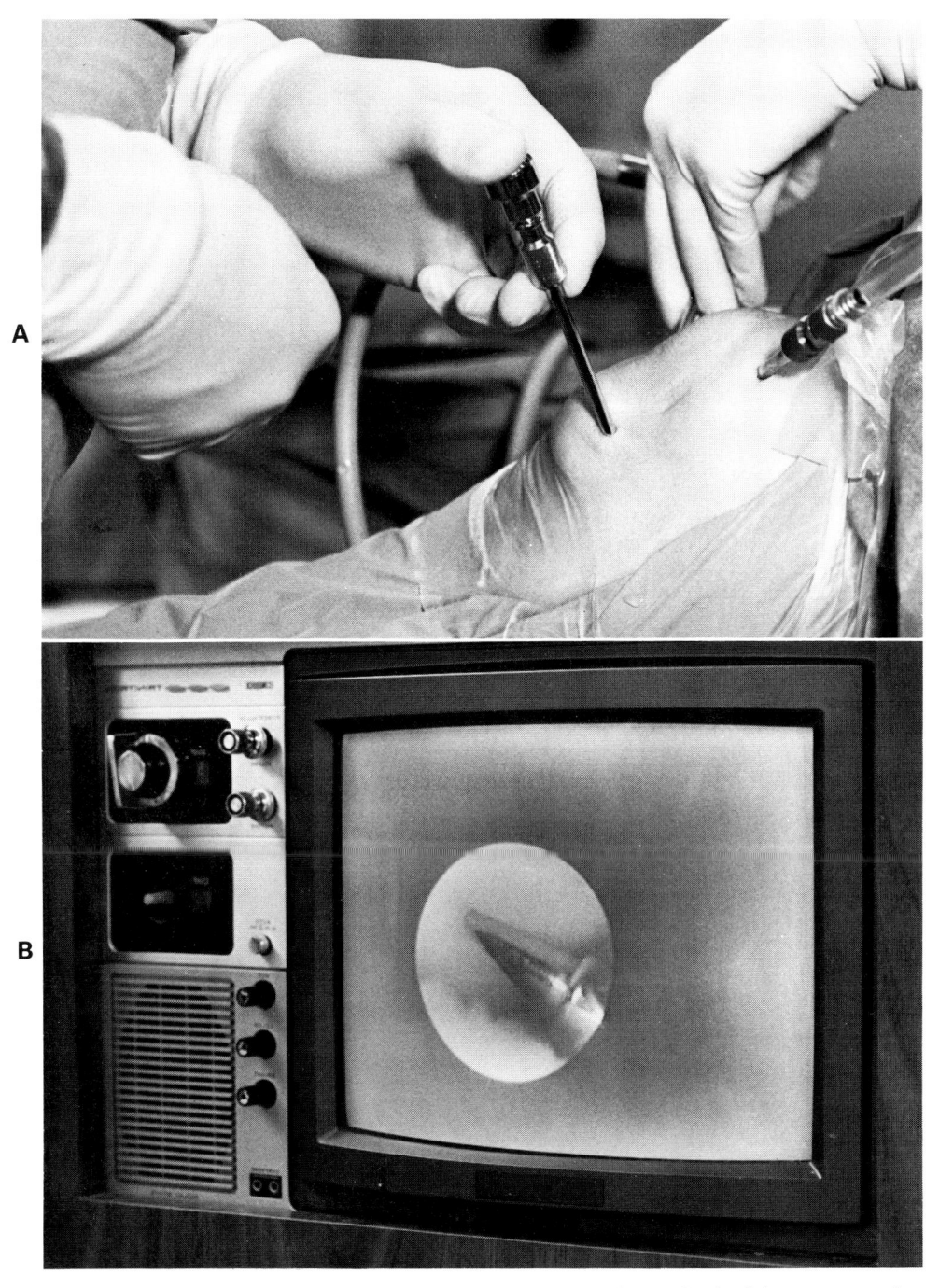

FIG. 15-40. A, Blunt cannula is placed from outside. **B,** View of television screen shows blunt cannula in medial compartment.

Arthroscopic surgery of the knee

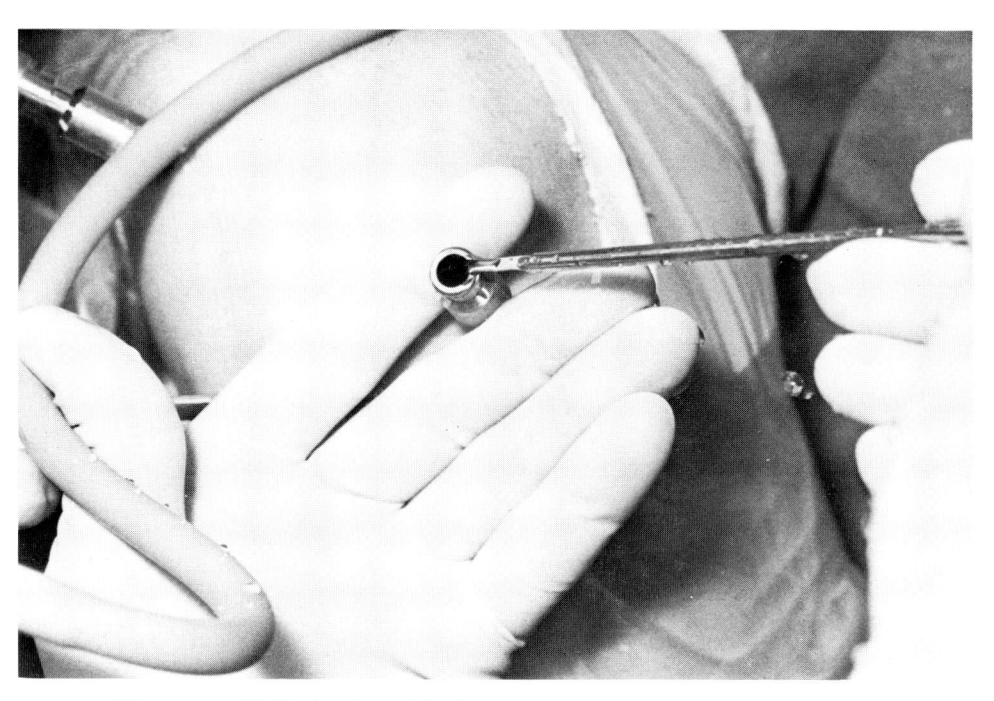

FIG. 15-41. Knife is placed in Intra-articular Shaver cannula system.

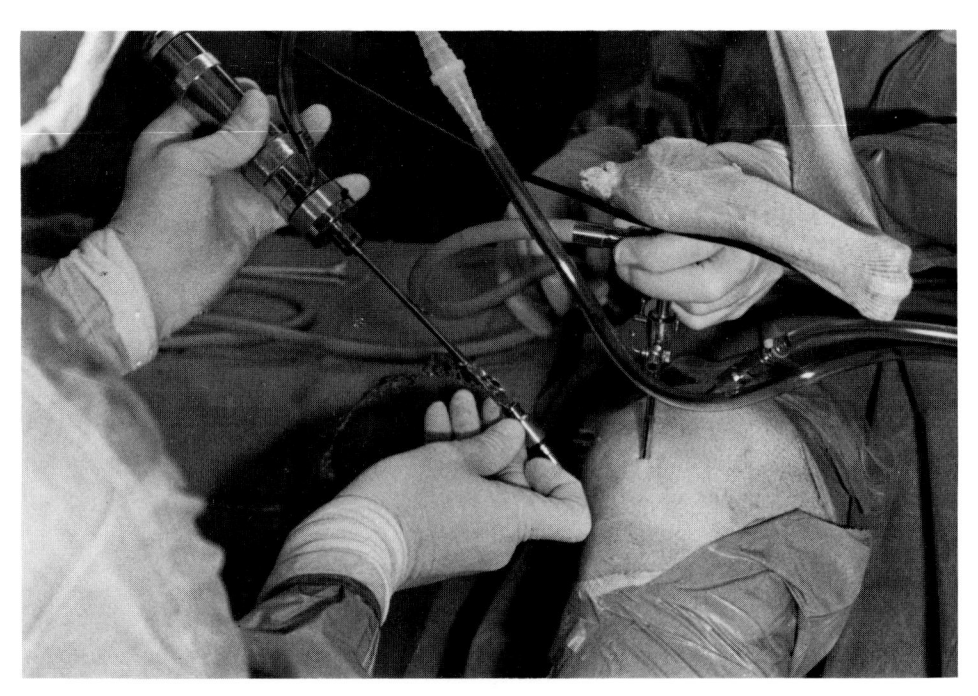

FIG. 15-42. Surgery within lateral compartment is facilitated by surgeon standing to lateral side of thigh and applying varus force. Arthroscope is brought in from medial and instrumentation cannula from lateral.

Basic principles of arthroscopic surgery: comprehensive setup

addition, if the portal is not being used, a blunt probe can be placed into the cannula to secure that position while the procedure is carried on in another compartment of the knee.

The same basic techniques and principles apply to whichever compartment is being approached surgically.

Lateral compartment

The lateral compartment is exposed by a varus strain on the knee and by flexion. The arthroscope is changed to the medial position, and the instrumentation comes in from the lateral side (Fig. 15-42). Because of the anatomy of the knee, it is possible, with flexion and rotation, to easily expose and operate on all the lateral meniscus, including its posterior rim, when the leg is held in the Surgical Assistant under general anesthesia. This type of opening has not been possible without the Surgical Assistant. Varying degrees of internal and external rotation, flexion and extension, and varus strain are possible in combination to create the necessary arthroscopic view and surgical approach.

Patella and patellofemoral shaving

The original method of patellar shaving was greatly facilitated by the straight leg position. It is possible to create the same space by bringing the leg up into extension and leaving the inflow cannula superior. With redirection of the arthroscope and the cannula system to the superior portion of the joint and by using the technique of triangulation, the patella can be visualized from the lateral side and shaved from the medial. Also, it is possible to debride the intercondylar notch opposite the patella when it is involved (Fig. 15-43).

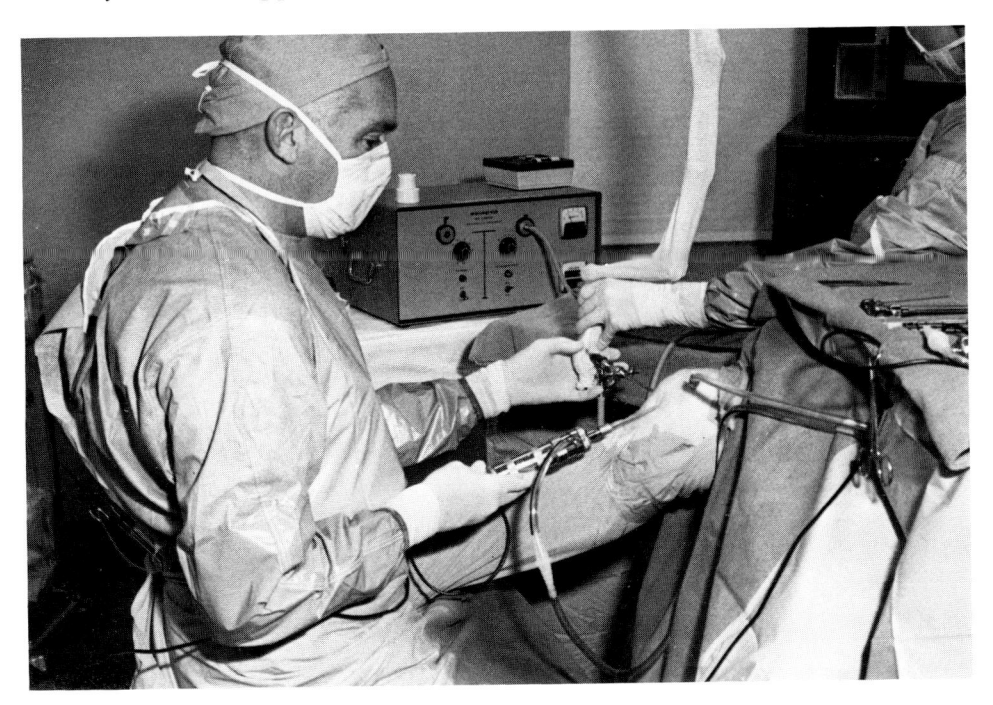

FIG. 15-43. Comprehensive arthroscopic surgical position facilitates patellar shaving from below. Interchangeability of cannula and surgical instruments is also possible.

After completion of shaving from one direction, the arthroscope is then shifted medially and the instrumentation brought in from the lateral side, and completion of the intra-articular shave and/or femoral debridement can be accomplished. The interchangeability of the arthroscope with the Intra-articular Shaver System facilitates surgical manipulation from multiple portals.

Posteromedial approach

In some instances it is necessary to use a posteromedial approach. Visualization can be from the anterolateral direction by a modified Gillquist technique. By viewing with the 70° scope, the instruments can be located first by a No. 18 spinal needle percutaneously via a posteromedial approach, followed by the cannula system and/or forceps for removal of loose bodies.

In some instances viewing from a posteromedial location via the intercondylar notch can show the posterior attachment of the meniscus better than one can see from the front. Release of the posterior horn of the medial meniscus may be accomplished by a transcutaneous posteromedial approach, viewing from the intercondylar notch.

Another method that has been used for some time is the posteromedial approach with both the arthroscope and the instrumentation in the same compartment. This is best achieved with maximal distension of the knee and with the knee in flexion. When the surgeon plans to place instrumentation in the same compartment, I recommend direct viewing with the Needlescope, since it occupies less space than a large-diameter scope. Sectioning the posterior meniscal horn and/or removing loose bodies may be accomplished in this way. Another method demonstrates the posteromedial compartment from the posteromedial puncture, and instruments gain access to the compartment from an anterolateral portal via the cannula system.

Posterolateral compartment

A separate transcutaneous puncture for instrumentation has not been necessary in the posterolateral compartment. It has been possible, by either palpation or manipulation and the use of suction, to bring materials and/or meniscus forward for surgical treatment. The specific use of these techniques has applied to conditions such as osteochondritis dissecans and torn menisci, which are discussed in subsequent chapters.

SUMMARY

There is no substitute for an adequately prepared and trained surgeon and a cooperating operative team. The best surgical equipment must be available without any deletion in the system to ensure success.

Every available portal and access route must be considered. Flexibility in surgical imagination will greatly assist in accomplishing these surgical maneuvers.

Finally, there is no substitute for experience, and I believe that is why it is still referred to as the "practice" of medicine and orthopedic surgery.

Chapter 16

Meniscal surgery

Meniscectomy
Surgical principles of arthroscopic meniscectomy
Types of tears
    Medial meniscus tears
    Lateral meniscus tears
Postoperative management
    Complications
Case reports

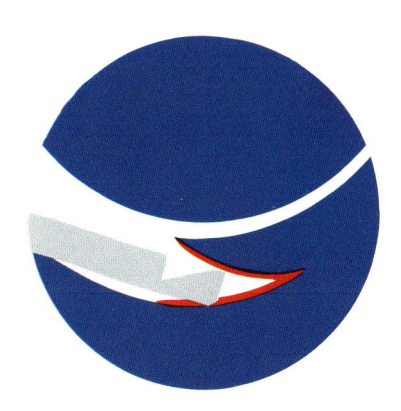

MENISCECTOMY

The meniscus has long been a focus of attention for orthopedic surgeons. It is a tissue that is commonly diseased or altered, and it is amenable to surgical removal or meniscectomy.

Years ago, opinions were divided as to whether the meniscus should be removed. Some reported that symptoms of a torn meniscus would gradually resolve without surgical intervention. Of course, the exact clinical diagnosis could not be certain, since arthrography and arthroscopy had not been developed. Others advocated arthrotomy and meniscus removal for the same type of symptoms. The longer torn cartilage was present, the greater the incidence of degenerative arthritis. Results after meniscectomy for a torn meniscus were better if the meniscus was removed soon after the injury and without multiple episodes of locking or reinjury.[9]

Furthermore, there was evidence that a normal knee had a 6% to 10% chance of developing osteoarthritis, and a knee that underwent a partial or total meniscectomy had a 40% chance of degenerative arthritis.[6,7,9] There was no long-term follow-up on the chance of degenerative arthritis in the presence of an untreated torn meniscus.

The opinions of those who agreed meniscectomy should be performed could be divided on the type of incision and the amount of tissue to be excised. Some advocated a short, single, oblique incision; others a transverse incision; and some a parapatellar incision. Cave[4] advocated the oblique incision with an optional posterior view. Tapper and Hoover[18] recommended a posterior view through a Cave or Henderson incision to remove the posterior horn. A transverse medial incision with a vertical anterior and posterior arthrotomy facilitated a more complete resection of the meniscus. Bruser[2] advocated a transverse incision following the fibers of the iliotibial band to allow complete meniscectomy on the lateral side of the knee.

Another consideration in meniscectomy was how much material should be removed. Smillie[17] advocated a total meniscectomy to the level of the synovium. Tapper and Hoover[18] and Cargill and Jackson[3] suggested there was some advantage to removing only the bucket handle when that type of tear existed. They indicated that there was less degenerative change with a long-term follow-up.

Tapper and Hoover suggested, as did Smillie, that the posterior horn should be excised; and if it were not excised, it could lead to a less satisfactory result. Meniscectomy has been used to produce degenerative arthritis in experimental animals.[11]

In 1954 it was reported that there were better results from a partial meniscectomy when performed by open methods.[1] McGinty[12] made a similar report 20 years later. Both authors used arthrotomy and indicated that there was less morbidity and less resulting degenerative change. It also should be noted that, when a partial meniscectomy could be performed, there was also less injury to the knee to start with as opposed to a patient who tore the complete meniscus, requiring total meniscectomy. Also, there was no report of second-look arthroscopy to demonstrate the actual appearance of these knees that had partial resection of the meniscus.

In my 12 years in practice I performed meniscectomies on the medial side through a transverse incision and short, anterior and posteromedial vertical arthrotomies. Technically, these were subtotal meniscectomies with approximately ⅛-inch rim left in the area of the tibial collateral ligament, balanced into the remainder of the tissues with incomplete resection of the posterior horn tissue. Follow-up arthroscopic examinations, as much as 10 years later, have shown a small regenerated and fibrous rim with good articular surfaces (Fig. 16-1).

Arthroscopy provides a means of further study of the meniscus, both before and after conventional surgical removal. Many patients have been observed to have a so-called retained or regrown posterior rim that is completely asymptomatic, even to palpation under local anesthesia. If the posterior horn is large, irregular in shape, or abnormally mobile, then it may be symptom pro-

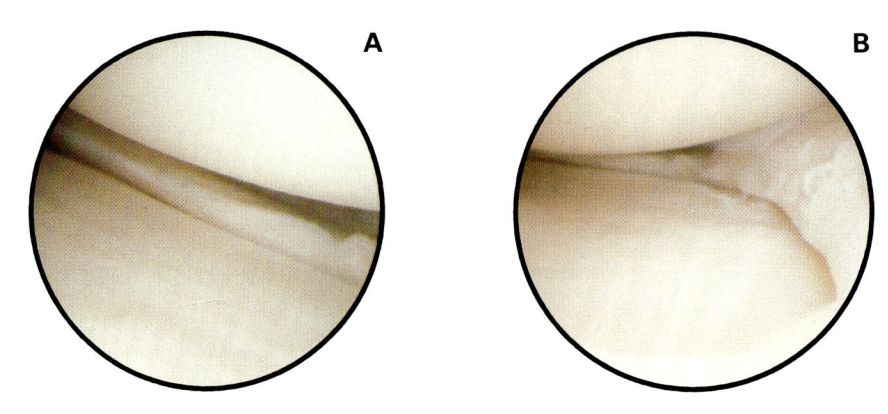

FIG. 16-1

A Arthroscopic view of medial meniscus 10 years after open subtotal meniscectomy. There is no degenerative arthritis.
B Arthroscopic view of same patient with medial meniscus near tibial collateral ligament.

ducing. This is especially exacerbated if there is a coexisting ligamentous instability. Prior to the time of arthroscopy, these situations alerted orthopedists, including myself, to the symptomatic posterior horn lesions and encouraged the complete resection of that posterior horn during meniscectomy.

A concept of partial meniscectomy by arthrotomy was difficult to accept. Knowing that the view to the posterior compartment from an anterior arthrotomy was severely limited and that the potential for an inadequate excision seemed likely, it seemed better to err on the side of a more complete meniscectomy, utilizing the posterior incision and resection, than to leave behind any nonvisualized potential meniscal tears.

My clinical experience with symptomatic, inadequate partial resections reinforced my position. In retrospect, it is obvious that these remaining or retained menisci were deformed—abnormal in size, shape, or mobility.

In addition, inspection of tissue removed in cases of bucket-handle tears showed a degeneration of the tissue within the handle and rim. It was virtually impossible to tell the difference between the two histologically. Therefore it was assumed that the degenerative tissue with microseparations would be vulnerable to future tears and subsequent morbidity and surgery.[17]

The technique of arthroscopy lent itself to better joint inspection and also the possibility of transcutaneous removal of a portion of the meniscus. Some Japanese authors reported a few cases of partial meniscus resection by arthroscopic techniques.[19] O'Connor[14] advocated subtotal arthroscopic meniscectomy by transcutaneous methods.

Jackson and Dandy[8] showed a photographic follow-up in a superficial meniscal removal. Metcalf[13] reported his experience in 600 cases. Both O'Connor[14] and Metcalf[13] presented a few postoperative photographs demonstrating healing of the meniscus in the exact area where a partial meniscus was resected.

In 1978 I set out to duplicate their experience. At that time I considered it an experiment. All our patients' lesions and the arthroscopic surgical removal of the menisci were recorded on videotape. This provided a visual data pool to compare preoperative and postoperative results. The healing of the meniscal tissue in various types of subtotal arthroscopic resection was observed by second-look arthroscopy. Healing of the meniscal tissue was substantiated by a biopsy from 2 to 6 months following arthroscopic surgery.

Still, the general concept of meniscectomy was not well defined. There are still many approaches, both open and closed. Because the amount of meniscal tissue to be removed was not established and the follow-up inspections were infrequent, the pathophysiologic basis for meniscal healing was not clear. Still, the question exists, what is meant by *meniscectomy?*

As I reviewed the videotapes, predominantly to study technique, it was apparent that the *ideal subtotal meniscectomy should include removal of all the abnormal meniscal tissue and all the abnormally mobile meniscal tissue.* By the methods to be outlined later, it was possible to determine normal and abnormal mobility. It was also possible to determine abnormal meniscal tissue and resect it. I do not believe that this was possible in any of the previous efforts on partial meniscectomy by open arthrotomy. This is not to say that the concept of partial meniscectomy is incorrect. The concept was correct, but the methods available did not solve the question of the extent of meniscal resection.

At the present time the ideal meniscectomy should be performed by arthroscopic means. This prevents the various types of arthrotomies and their attendant morbidity. By the methods described here it is possible to completely visualize and evaluate the meniscus. Other tissues within the joint that might cause clinical symptoms, such as loose bodies, degenerative arthritis, and chondromalacia, are amenable to this form of treatment. A ligamentous injury or patellar instability is not overlooked.

It is possible, by the instrumentation and the techniques outlined here, to perform a resection of all the abnormal meniscal tissue and the abnormally mobile meniscal tissue. By these microsurgical techniques the surgeon can reshape the meniscus. This has been called a *selective meniscectomy* by Shneider.[16] Follow-up clinical and second-look arthroscopic inspections, up to 2 years in our patients and longer in those of O'Connor and Metcalf, have demonstrated that this type of selective meniscectomy is successful.

Therefore the arguments over whether a person has a torn meniscus are settled by direct visual evidence of the arthroscopic inspection. The variance of opinions about what type of arthrotomy is to be performed has been somewhat settled by the transcutaneous puncture wound method. The concept of an *adequate* meniscectomy has stilled the arguments for partial, subtotal, and total meniscectomy. Adequate resection indicates that all the abnormal and abnormally mobile meniscal tissue was selectively removed. It is certain that no other lesions were overlooked or left untreated by these methods. The knowledge of the healing process by contributions of the synovium,[10] the meniscal vascularity,[15] and the meniscal tissue itself, has proved that this type of resection is the method of choice. (See Chapter 8.) Arthroscopy has provided a means of documenting and treating the lesion as well as providing the ease of access to postoperative inspection and pathologic study.

SURGICAL PRINCIPLES OF ARTHROSCOPIC MENISCECTOMY

The comprehensive surgical technique is used for all primary meniscal and combined pathologic conditions. (See Chapter 15.) The various techniques used in removing selective portions of the meniscal tissue are outlined for the different types of meniscal tears.

It is my objective to excise only abnormally diseased meniscal tissue and the abnormally mobile meniscal tissue. This sometimes requires complete resection of the posterior horn of the meniscus and only a small rim of meniscal tissue near the tibial collateral ligament similar to the subtotal meniscectomy that had been my practice by previous open methods. On other occasions, only the simple excision of a degenerated flap tear and reshaping of the remaining meniscus are indicated. In cases of ligamentous instability, every attempt is made to maintain posterior meniscal tissue. It is reshaped and excised so as not to be vulnerable to abnormal mobility and/or further tears.

Abnormal meniscal tissue can be selectively excised readily by the Intra-articular Cutter, which spares the normal cartilage. Determination of the amount to be resected is made both by palpation and visualization.

The meniscus has normal mobility. The medial meniscus, anterior horn, and medial portion displace peripherally with distension of the joint, about 1 cm. The posteromedial meniscus has some mobility but is generally stable to passive flexion and extension; also, it is stable on palpation with a probe and decompression suction. Both probing and decompression are important in making these determinations.

The lateral meniscus is highly mobile. With varus strain the meniscus lifts off the tibial plateau. It moves inward more than 1 cm with decompression suction. The posterior horn has considerable mobility with a hinge developing in the area of the popliteus tendon when decompression suction is applied. (See Fig. 15-34.) With distension the meniscus returns to a more normal position. Palpation demonstrates a fenestration under the meniscus at the popliteus sheath. There is a similar opening of the popliteal sheath above the meniscus. These must be differentiated from tears. This is best accomplished by probing.

Finally, the evaluation of the meniscus is accomplished by flexion and extension of the knee to see if the meniscus tear is abrading any particular defect and producing joint damage.

Under local anesthesia the meniscus itself can be excised without pain. Of course, either a tug or a cut at the periphery of the meniscus attachment produces discomfort. The femoral condyles are not sensitive, except to firm pressure or drilling.

After excision of the abnormal meniscal tissue and the abnormally mobile meniscus, the remaining rim is inspected. At that time the rim is balanced as advocated by Jackson.[7] This removes any sharp incongruities to the remaining rim. It is possible to leave a considerable amount of the anterior rim after almost complete excision of the posterior rim. I do not purposely perform this as Carson routinely advocates. I believe it is unnecessary and, in fact, contraindicated. Whenever possible, meniscal tissue and capsular tissue can remain. Reshaping has produced the best postoperative clinical results and has been supported by second-look arthroscopies (Fig. 16-2). I recommend inspecting the anterior horn with flexion and extension at the close of the procedure to make sure that it is not moving abnormally and not injuring an area of the femoral condyle superiorly, causing erosion; otherwise it needs to be resected.

There is no single routine for selective meniscal removal. The selective resection preserves and reshapes the meniscal rim. There are many technical details that are only learned by experience. Adequate exposure is possible with distension, excellent illlumination, and mechanical openings facilitated by the Surgical Assistant. Occasionally the synovial tissue or fringe of the fat pad may obscure the view to the meniscus. Adequate exposure may be facilitated by using the Intra-articular Shaver to remove the synovium that is blocking the view. The fat pad resection should not be routine, and, if it is performed, it should be minimal. The synovial resection can result in bleeding that further obscures the view. Second, an extensive resection of the fat pad can result in

Arthroscopic surgery of the knee

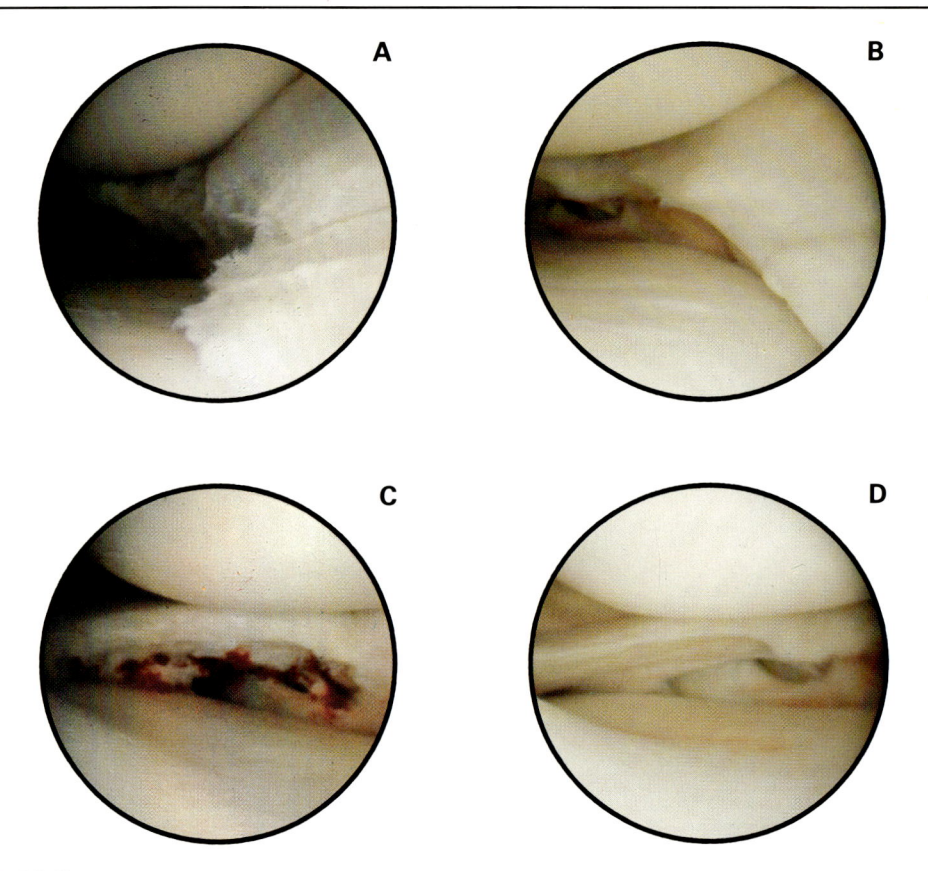

FIG. 16-2

A Immediately after subtotal arthroscopic resection of medial meniscus.
B Same area seen 6 months later.
C Posterior horn of medial meniscus after selective meniscectomy. Tourniquet has been released to bring in blood supply.
D Same area as in **C**. Posterior horn and medial meniscus 6 months following selective resection. Patient is asymptomatic.

fibrosis and postoperative pain and discomfort in that area. Sectioning of the alar ligament off the femur gives more exposure.

Exposure can be further facilitated by placing the arthroscope superior to the fat pad over the membranous ligament, and then with slight angulation the fat pad and the anterior chamber are retracted. Better visualization is achieved in this manner. A 30° inclined arthroscope position expedites this type of move. Also, the arthroscope itself is moved from the exact position of resection and allows more room for the instrumentation.

The Intra-articular Shaver System provides an unparalleled advantage for arthroscopic surgery. The multiple portals, through cannulas, reduce the amount of trauma, saline spillage, and potential contamination. The power system has interchangeable heads for meniscal, condylar, and synovial tissues, plus drilling. Using knife blades, graspers, resecters, and probes through the same cannula system can reduce the amount of tissue damage that can occur when multiple passes are made without a cannula.

FIG. 16-3. Arthroscopic view of posterior horn of medial meniscus showing fishmouth effect after resected matrix of posterior horn. This requires resection of inferior portion of the fishmouth.

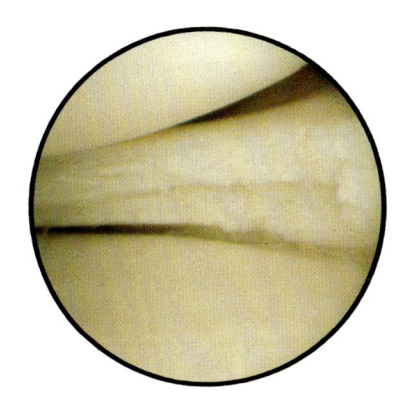

All cutting with manual or powered instrumentation should be done with the tip of the instrument in view. This is a general principle of surgery and should not be violated in arthroscopic surgery.

Inspection of the meniscus, as just outlined, dictates the subsequent surgical approach. For instance, if there is a floppy anterior horn that blocks the view to the posterior compartment, it should be resected prior to resecting the posterior horn. In most cases though, the anterior horn, if not blocking vision, should be left intact for grasping during any resection of the posterior horn.

Certain meniscal lesions are easier to manage than others. Therefore, with experience, more complex lesions can be converted to a simpler type of lesion that is more easily managed. For example, the posterior horn tear can be converted to a bucket-handle tear with a knife blade and then removed as though it were a bucket handle by mechanical means. It is not necessary to wait until after resection of the posterior lesion with the Intra-articular Cutter or basket forceps. On the other hand, soft and fragmented meniscal lesions with multiple bucket handles that are difficult to grasp mechanically can be easily removed with the suction provided by the Intra-articular Cutter. Mechanical grasping just pushes them away from the hand instrument.

I have indicated that the meniscus cutter will resect the degenerative meniscal tissue. Posterior horizontal clefts develop after meniscal matrix is resected, and they expose the fibrous collagenous transverse fibers of the meniscus. In this situation the inferior fibrous portion is resected and the anterior ledge balanced (Fig. 16-3).

The Beaver knife blade should be used judiciously. It can be of considerable advantage, but care should be taken not to create an angulatory or rotational stress. It is possible to fracture the blade, and its retrieval can be complicated and prolong the procedure; therefore IM blades are favored. In addition, care must be taken when cutting is done near the tibial collateral ligament or the anterior or posterior cruciate ligamentous tissue. Arthroscopic perspective of the tibial collateral ligament can be somewhat distorted. A cut that goes from anterior to posterior should not proceed directly posterior, but rather move around the horn of the meniscus. Otherwise, the deep fibers of the tibial collateral ligament can be lacerated. The knife blade tip should be carefully visualized, and motion should be well controlled away from the ligamentous or articular surfaces.

The surgical principle of tissue being cut under tension certainly applies for arthroscopic surgery. This is achieved either by the suction flow of the Intra-articular Shaver or by manual traction and subsequent incision. There are two special situations in which it is possible to maintain tension on the tissue to be resected. For instance, if there is an incomplete tear of the posterior horn of the meniscus halfway back on the medial meniscus, a limb should be developed first adjacent to the tibial spine, and then the excision can be completed through the cleavage line of the tear toward the tibial collateral ligament and then curving anterior. If it is freed first by the tibial collateral ligament, then it is not possible to get any tension from the anterior portal to cut the more extreme posterior limb.

A second instance concerns a bucket-handle tear of the meniscus. It should be sectioned anteriorly. When it is grasped by a clamp and pulled anteriorly, it is important to enlarge the transcutaneous incision through the capsule enough so that the entire meniscus could move through it when released. If this is not done, the clamp pulls the anterior portion of the meniscus up against the joint wall, and the posterior horn is not placed on traction for cutting or even pulled forward. The rotation of the meniscus, even without cutting the capsule, may do this; but that enlarges the bulk of the meniscal tissue, and the view of the posterior horn is somewhat compromised. When the percutaneous exit hole for the meniscus is enlarged, the tension is excellent and the posterior horn is drawn more anterior. When the incision is sharp, the anterior cruciate ligament is avoided and delivery of the meniscal tissue is facilitated. The 747 IM blade is used for the posterior horn.

Finally, the meniscus is reappraised and its posterior horn is reshaped by removing the inferior portion of any fish-mouth lesion. This is pathologically sound in that the blood supply comes up from the inferior meniscal surface, as demonstrated by injection studies[15] (Fig. 16-4). The meniscus is reappraised, both medially and anteriorly, the rim is balanced, and the final move is to debride any meniscal or articular abrasions or degenerative changes with the original Intra-articular Shaver head.

In some situations the routine of having the arthroscope entry to the side opposite the lesion may be reversed. This is especially so on the lateral side when the tear is cut up into the anterior portion. The angle approach can be improved for resection if the arthroscope is switched laterally to the side of the tear and the instruments brought in from the medial portal. This allows ease of resection of the anterior horn by the angle of the knife blade and/or of the meniscus cutter to balance off the anterior horn. This is true to some extent on the medial side (Fig. 16-5).

The approach to the anterior horn is compromised because the surgeon is not able to manipulate the instruments from the ipsilateral side. Therefore, especially when using the Intra-articular Shaver System or Cutter, viewing from the ipsilateral side of the lesion and resecting the anterior horn from the opposite side allows easier removal.

A retrievable lost fragment of meniscus is brought up into position with the constant suction of the Intra-articular Shaver System.

Meniscal surgery: medial meniscus tears

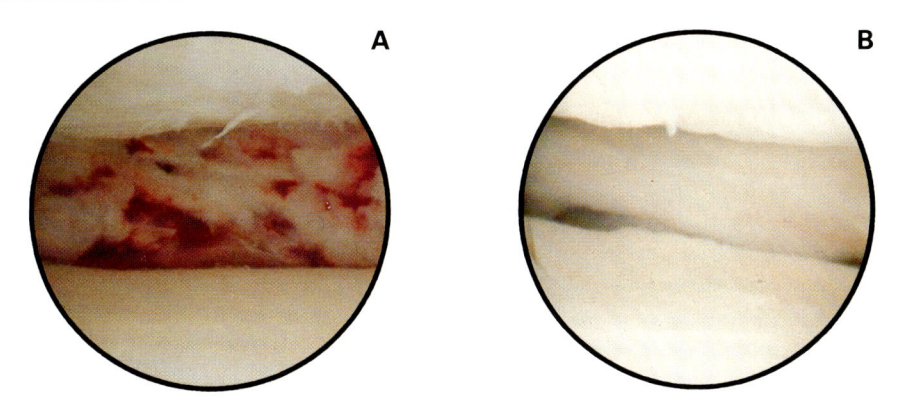

FIG. 16-4

A Immediately following lateral meniscectomy with resection back into meniscus, tourniquet is released and blood supply perfuses midportion of meniscus.
B Arthroscopic view of same patient 3 months after arthroscopic meniscectomy.

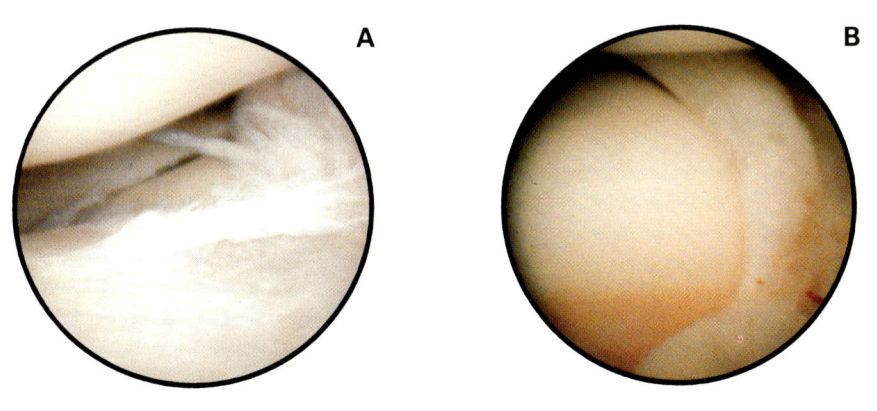

FIG. 16-5

A Extreme anterior horn tear of lateral meniscus.
B Peripheral anterior horn detachment of medial meniscus.

TYPES OF TEARS

There are various types of tears in the menisci, and they can be either medial or lateral (Fig. 16-6). The most simple and recognizable tear is a *parrot-beak tear*. One portion, usually in the middle or anterior part of the meniscus, moves or elevates itself away from the body of the meniscus and has a sharp point on it; hence the term *parrot beak*. A *flap tear* has moved away in a similar fashion, but it is rounded off and may be degenerative; the surface may be somewhat smooth and encapsulated. A *transverse tear* usually occurs in the middle portion of the body of the lateral meniscus anterior to the popliteus tendon. These occur less frequently on the medial side. A *horizontal tear* is most common in the posterior portion of the medial meniscus. It is within the substance of the meniscus, and the plane of the tear runs parallel to the tibial plateau. A *vertical tear* is a separation of the meniscus from its superior to inferior surface. The medial and lateral incidence is equal, usually on the

Arthroscopic surgery of the knee

posterior horn. On some occasions it is incomplete and is only identified by palpation. The vertical tear may become separated either anteriorly or posteriorly or in its middle; then it is recognized as a flap tear. A *bucket-handle tear* is a vertical tear that has completely separated and has, on many occasions, displaced itself over into the intercondylar notch. The incidence is more frequent on the medial than on the lateral side. A *peripheral tear* of the meniscus occurs most commonly on the medial portion and posterior. It often accompanies an anterior cruciate ligament tear. This type of patient is a good candidate for reanastomosis. A *complex tear* is a combination of these other types of tears and can include horizontal, transverse, and vertical components.

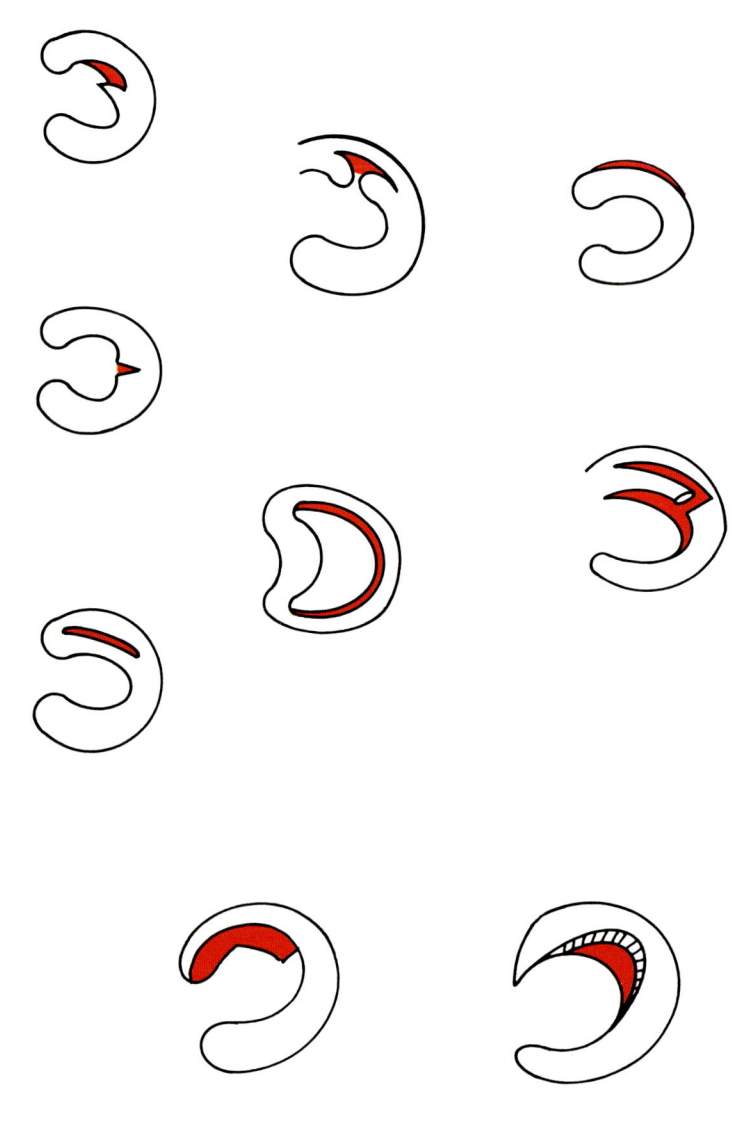

FIG. 16-6. Various types of meniscal tears.

Medial meniscus tears

Location: Medial
Type of tear: Parrot beak, medial
Arthroscope placement: Lateral, anterior, inferior
Instrumentation portal: Medial, anterior, inferior
Palpation: Needle or probe
Instruments: Knife and forceps
Resection: This type of tear is often mentioned as a sole lesion for partial meniscectomy by arthrotomy; in fact, it is included in a high percentage in this series. With the advantage of arthroscopy it can be seen that this tear is only the anterior portion of a more complex tear in the posterior part that was probably overlooked by arthrotomy at the time of the open partial meniscectomy. It does occur, however, and is usually at the middle or anterior portion of the medial meniscus. It is easily sectioned simply with a knife blade and removed with forceps.

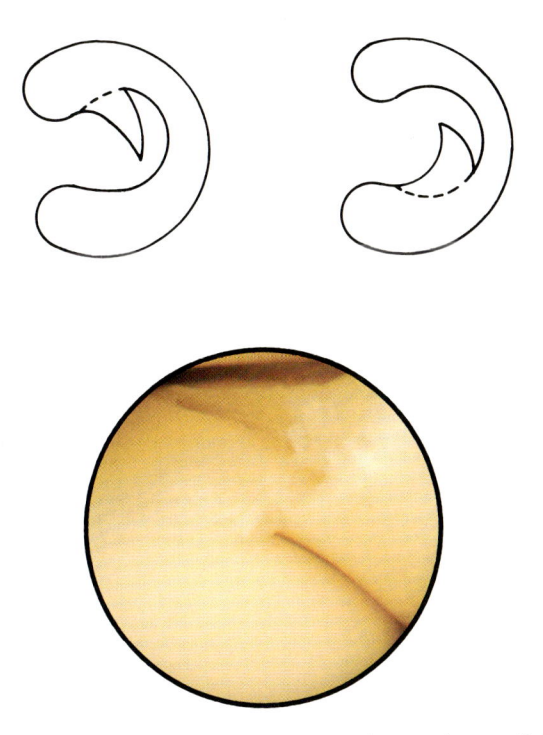

FIG. 16-7. Arthroscopic view of parrot-beak tear in medial meniscus.

Arthroscopic surgery of the knee

Location: Medial
Type of tear: Transverse
Arthroscope placement: Lateral, anterior, inferior
Instrumentation portal: Medial, anterior, inferior
Palpation: Needle or probe
Instruments: Knife blade and meniscus cutter-trimmer for clean-up
Resection: This tear is more common in the lateral meniscus. It is best managed by simple knife blade excision and PAS cutter clean-up. The anterior portion is cut first.

The transverse tear is not as common on the medial side as on the lateral side. It can be resected. The anterior horn can usually be excised by placing the knife blade at the base of the tear and drawing it anteriorly. There may be a horizontal component to the posterior portion of these transverse tears that should not be overlooked. The posterior flap is then incised with the knife blade and the meniscus cutter. The arthroscope accomplishes clean-up.

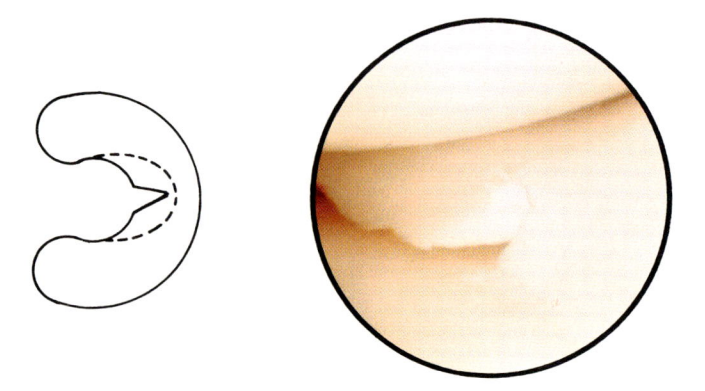

FIG. 16-8. Transverse tear of medial meniscus.

Meniscal surgery: medial meniscus tears

Location: Medial
Type of tear: Vertical
Arthroscope placement: Lateral, anterior, inferior
Instrumentation portal: Medial, anterior, inferior
Palpation: Needle or probe
Instruments: Knife blade, Cutter, basket forceps
Resection: The vertical tear can be incomplete or complete. When incomplete, it can only be identified by palpation and not by arthroscopic inspection alone. Often the superior surface is intact on the vertical-posterior horn tear and can only be visualized by palpation from the undersurface.

It is best managed by placing a No. 761 knife blade in the substance of the tear and moving the blade from the midportion of the tear toward the extreme posterior horn. The cut is then made with some traction. The second move is to come back into the tear and draw the knife blade medial and anterior, balancing the anterior rim. This can be done if the posterior horn is free because the tissue can be brought under tension with downward pressure. This is not possible if the procedure is reversed. Do not free the medial-anterior portion first, since it is then difficult to push away from the body to cut the posterior horn free. When this fragment is free, it can be removed either with grasping forceps or the Cutter. After it is removed, the rim is balanced with the use of the Cutter (occasionally the basket forceps are necessary). If the anterior portion is not well smoothed off into the anterior rim, it may be necessary to bring a knife blade into this more smooth juncture.

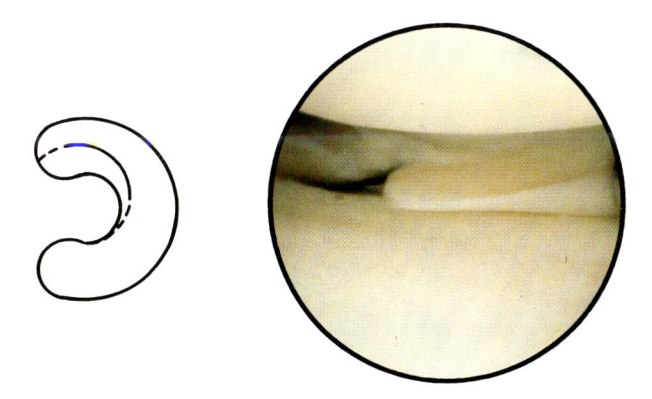

FIG. 16-9. Vertical tear of medial meniscus.

Arthroscopic surgery of the knee

Location: Medial
Type of tear: Flap tear
Arthroscope placement: Lateral, anterior, inferior
Instrumentation portal: Anterior, inferior
Palpation: Needle or probe
Instruments: Intra-articular Cutter, knife blade
Resection: The flap tear can be either based medially or at the posterior horn. On some occasions it is based both medially and laterally. Often these are vertical tears that develop a transverse component, resulting in the flap. Frequently the flap is rounded off, and these are degenerated. They can be simply excised at their base with a knife blade or by resection of the more mobile degenerative flap with the use of the Cutter. The combination of freeing with the knife blade and removing with forceps or the Cutter is also possible. The base of the meniscus should then be inspected for any transverse or complex components to not only balance the rim anteriorly, but also to reshape the posterior horn of the meniscus.

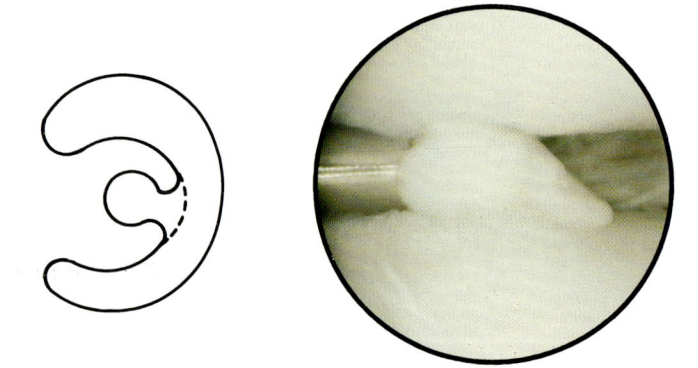

FIG. 16-10. Flap tear of medial meniscus with Intra-articular Cutter starting to resect.

Meniscal surgery: medial meniscus tears

Location: Medial
Type of tear: Peripheral
Arthroscope placement: Medial, lateral, inferior (also might use 70° scope for posteromedial inspection)
Instrumentation portal: Medial, anterior, inferior
Alternate portal: Posteromedial
Palpation: Needle or probe
Instruments: Knife blade, forceps, grasper
Resection: A peripheral tear of the meniscus, especially in the presence of a torn ligament in a young person, may indicate the need for meniscoresis (resuturing of the peripheral rim).

Arthroscopic removal is best accomplished by converting the posterior or posteromedial peripheral tear to a bucket-handle tear and then following the procedure for a bucket-handle tear. Inspect through the notch, after a modified Gillquist technique, and use knife blades by a separate posteromedial portal; or, if the tear goes over toward the medial side of the joint far enough, the connecting cut can be made from the anteromedial portal as well.

At any rate, it is best not to cut this into pieces but to keep it as a major piece and convert it to a bucket-handle tear for easy removal.

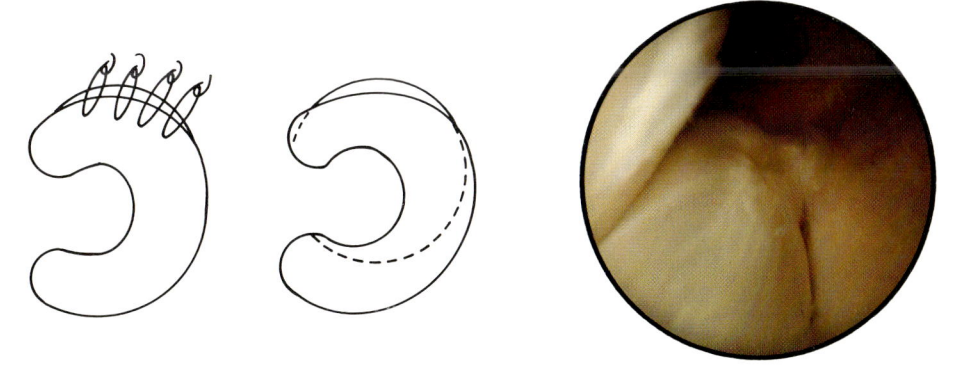

FIG. 16-11. Peripheral tear of medial meniscus from posteromedial view.

Arthroscopic surgery of the knee

Location: Medial
Type of tear: Complex combination
Arthroscope placement: Lateral, anterior, inferior
Instrumentation portal: Medial, anterior, inferior
Palpation: Needle or probe
Instruments: Intra-articular cutter, knife blades, graspers, basket forceps, scissors
Resection: This complex tear is quite common. It creates difficulty in visualizing the extent of the entire meniscus abnormality. In some cases complete resection of the torn tissue will result in virtually total resection of meniscal tissue.

It is generally approached by resecting the easily available mobile tissue with the meniscus cutter to better visualize the irregular, more firm base of any vertical, horizontal, or flap tears it comprises.

After the anterior portion of the tissue affected by synovitis is debrided, the most mobile tissue is removed; then a knife blade in the posterior portion, with scissors and/or basket forceps, can mobilize and reshape the tissue. Every attempt should be made to maintain the superior rim of meniscus posteriorly and balance that around into the anterior rim. At first this type of tear seems difficult to manage; but with the exposure afforded by the Surgical Assistant, by the resection of the very mobile, loose components, and by converting and resecting that tissue to a rather well-visualized base of the meniscal irregularities, completion of the reshaping of the meniscus is then possible.

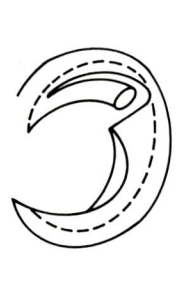

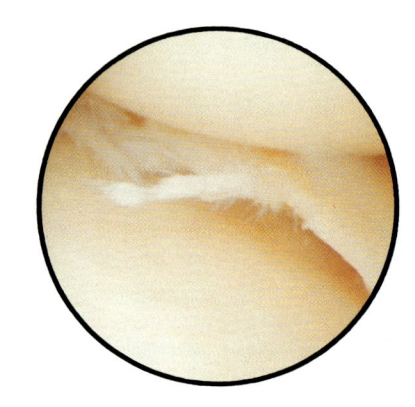

FIG. 16-12. Complex tear of medial meniscus.

Location: Medial
Type of tear: Bucket-handle
Arthroscope placement: Lateral, anterior, inferior, superior 70°
Instrumentation portal: Forceps from medial, anterior, inferior; knife from anterior, lateral, and inferior
Palpation: Needle or probe
Instruments: IM knives, forceps, Intra-articular Cutter
Resection: The bucket-handle tear is a classic meniscal tear, most common on the medial side. Probing confirms the mobility and the extent of the lesion.

Step 1: The anterior horn is incised and separated with the knife blade from the anteromedial portal.

Step 2: The meniscus is grasped from anteromedial and placed on traction. This places the tissue under tension for excision and draws the posterior horn anterior for sectioning.

Step 3: The transcutaneous approach is made with a No. 18 spinal needle from the lateral or medial side of the joint inferior to the placement of the arthroscope. When the needle enters a course to the posterior horn, the cannula is placed and then replaced with a 747 IM blade for posterior horn cutting.

Step 4: It is important to cut the capsular tissues adjacent to this exit point with a No. 15 blade. This allows the meniscus to start to move out of the joint, since it is not blocked by the capsule.

Step 5: Use a 747 IM blade to carefully excise the posterior horn of the meniscus while avoiding the anterior cruciate ligament; this should be done under direct visualization. At the moment the posterior horn is released, the meniscus will exit the joint because the portal was large enough to have it slide out. (See Step 3.)

The clean-up is accomplished with an Intra-articular Shaver System—first the Cutter and then the Trimmer. Often there is a small fragment of posterior horn or a second bucket-handle tear that can be seen and resected after the larger tear is removed.

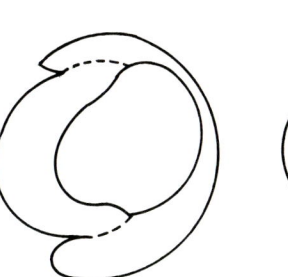

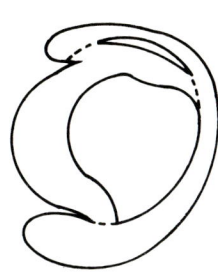

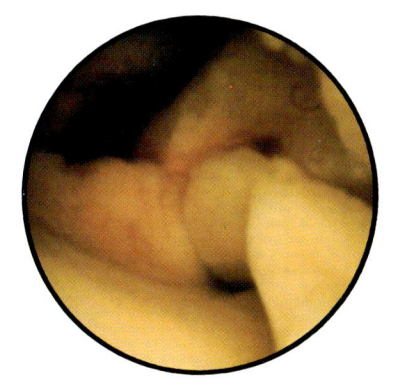

FIG. 16-13. Bucket-handle tear of medial meniscus.

Lateral meniscus tears

Lateral meniscus tears are not as common as medial meniscal tears but are more frequently diagnosed by arthroscopic inspection. With a torn anterior cruciate ligament there is approximately a 50% incidence of accompanying lateral meniscus tear. When a medial meniscal tear has been identified, it is important to search for a torn lateral meniscus.

The posterior longitudinal tear is the most common; the transverse and complex tears are next most frequent. Bucket-handle tears and discoid meniscus with fragmentation are less frequent.

The main technical detail of lateral meniscal resection is that there should be every attempt made to leave a bridge of meniscal tissue in front of the popliteus tendon as a framework for regeneration around that posterior corner. I have observed that, when this tissue has been removed, there has been a high incidence of degenerative arthritis at the posterior corner on the tibial plateau.

Generally, the arthroscope is placed medial and the resecting instruments enter via a lateral portal. The extreme posterior and anterior horns of the lateral meniscus are more easily resected with the arthroscope lateral and the instrument angled from medial. This is especially so when using the Intra-articular Cutter, which requires a 45° angle approach to tissue for optimal resection.

A posterior peripheral tear does not lend itself to resuturing because of the difficult posterolateral approach.

A torn lateral meniscus resection in the presence of a torn anterior cruciate ligament and rotary instability requires holding the patient's leg in varus position and exerting an external rotational force; otherwise, the exposure is lost due to the shift of the surfaces.

Location: Lateral
Type of tear: Transverse
Arthroscope placement: Anterior, medial, inferior
Instrumentation portal: Lateral, anterior, inferior
Palpation: Needle or probe
Instruments: Knife blade and Intra-articular Shaver System
Resection: The lateral meniscus is normally quite circular. The most common tear is in the central portion of the meniscus. This tear is transverse, and it occurs approximately 1 cm anterior to the popliteus tendon. This lesion is best managed by excising it with a knife blade and balancing its anterior horn. Then the meniscus cutter trims off the anterior horn and adjacent area affected by synovitis. This allows excellent visualization of the posterior portion of the tear. Again, the knife blade comes into position and balances out the posterior rim, leaving a small bridge anterior to the popliteus sheath for continuity of the meniscus. The meniscus cutter is then brought into the lesion to excise any degenerative tissue. Exposure and resection of any clefts that might go back into the meniscus tissue are done with a meniscus cutter.

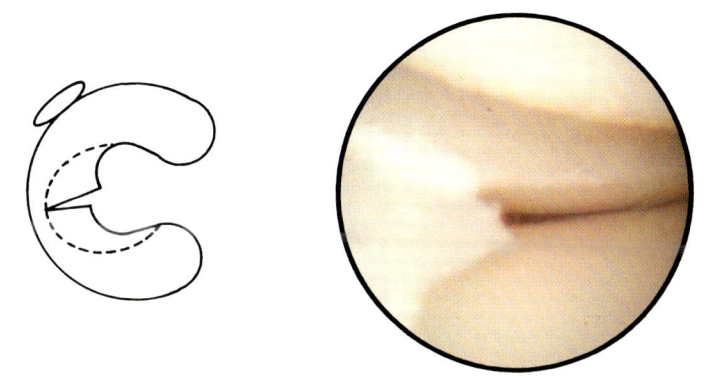

FIG. 16-14. Transverse tear of lateral meniscus.

Location: Lateral
Type of tear: Lateral meniscal, discoid
Arthroscope placement: Medial
Instrumentation portal: Lateral
Palpation: Probe and suction
Instruments: Knife blade and meniscus cutter
Resection: The discoid meniscus is sometimes difficult to diagnose because it occupies the entire compartment and can be interpreted as just being the tibial plateau. There may be difficulty in locating the meniscus, but backing away from that compartment (as viewed from the medial side) will allow one to determine the extent of the lesion. This lesion can be excised in the central portion and rebalanced into a meniscus readily duplicating the size and shape of the normal meniscus. It should be noted that the resection has to be extensive enough to remove all the clefts and also the degenerative tissue. Often a discoid meniscus will have a central area of degeneration not visualized from its exterior surfaces. (See Fig. 9-5, *B*.) The resection needs to be adequate; I have experienced a recurrent tear in a discoid meniscus that was less than adequately resected.

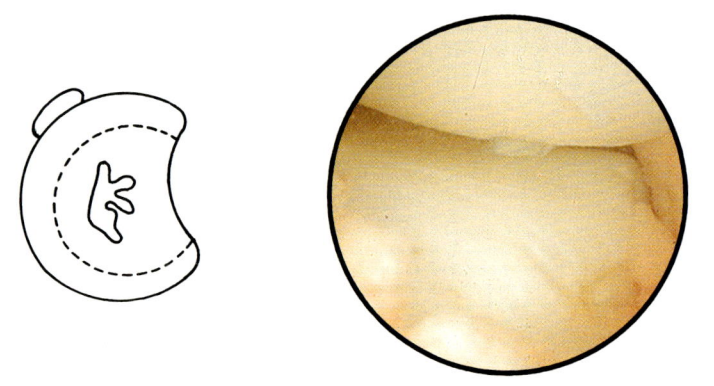

FIG. 16-15. Discoid meniscus.

Meniscal surgery: lateral meniscus tears

Location: Lateral
Type of tear: Incomplete posterior horn tear, vertical
Arthroscope placement: Medial
Instrumentation portal: Lateral
Palpation: Probe and suction
Instruments: Knife blade and Intra-articular Shaver System
Resection: If the posterior horn tear is approximately halfway back on the horn but not free from either edge, then the easiest mode of removal is to place the 761 IM blade in the cleft from the superior surface, angling posteriorly and inferiorly. A cut is made toward the intercondylar notch or the most extreme posterior horn. If the anterior portion is cut, it is more difficult to cut the area near the intercondylar notch because the attachment near the tibial collateral ligament has been released. As in all surgery, tissue should be cut under tension. First, release the tissue toward the intercondylar notch. Second, remove the knife blade from its base near the tibial collateral ligament, and with a single, slow move balance it up into the anterior rim. The tissue is removed percutaneously. A clean-up is performed with the Cutter and the Trimmer.

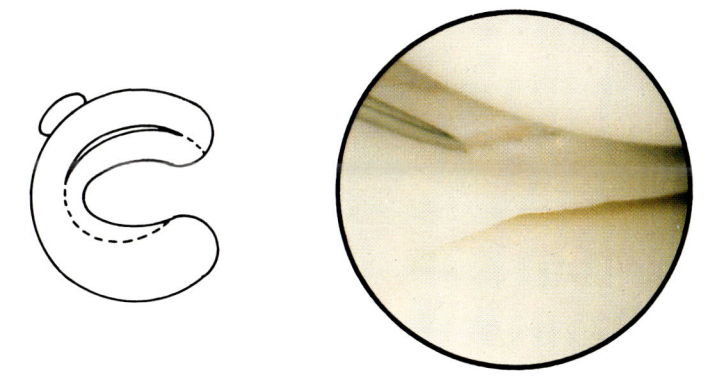

FIG. 16-16. Vertical tear of posterior horn in lateral meniscus.

Arthroscopic surgery of the knee

Location: Lateral
Type of tear: Degenerative flap tear
Arthroscope placement: Anterior, medial, inferior
Instrumentation portal: Lateral, anterior, inferior
Palpation: Needle or probe
Instruments: Knife blade and Intra-articular Shaver System
Resection: These tears occur in three positions. One is the free edge toward the tibial collateral ligament; another is the free edge toward the intercondylar notch; the third is based at each end. If the free edge is toward the tibial collateral ligament, then an incision can be made with the knife blade obliquely toward the intercondylar notch, and the piece can easily be removed percutaneously by mechanical means.

If the free edge is toward the intercondylar notch, the incision is even more easily done by placing the 761 IM blade in the slot posteriorly and drawing it up toward the anterior rim with a single, slow move, slightly rotating the knife as it comes toward the anterior horn to balance and shape the meniscus. Again, the piece is removed transcutaneously with forceps if it is small enough. The meniscus cutter is then used to debride the remaining fragments of the abnormal and abnormally mobile meniscal tissue.

The degenerative flap tear is not as common on the lateral side. It is easily completely resected with the Intra-articular Cutter.

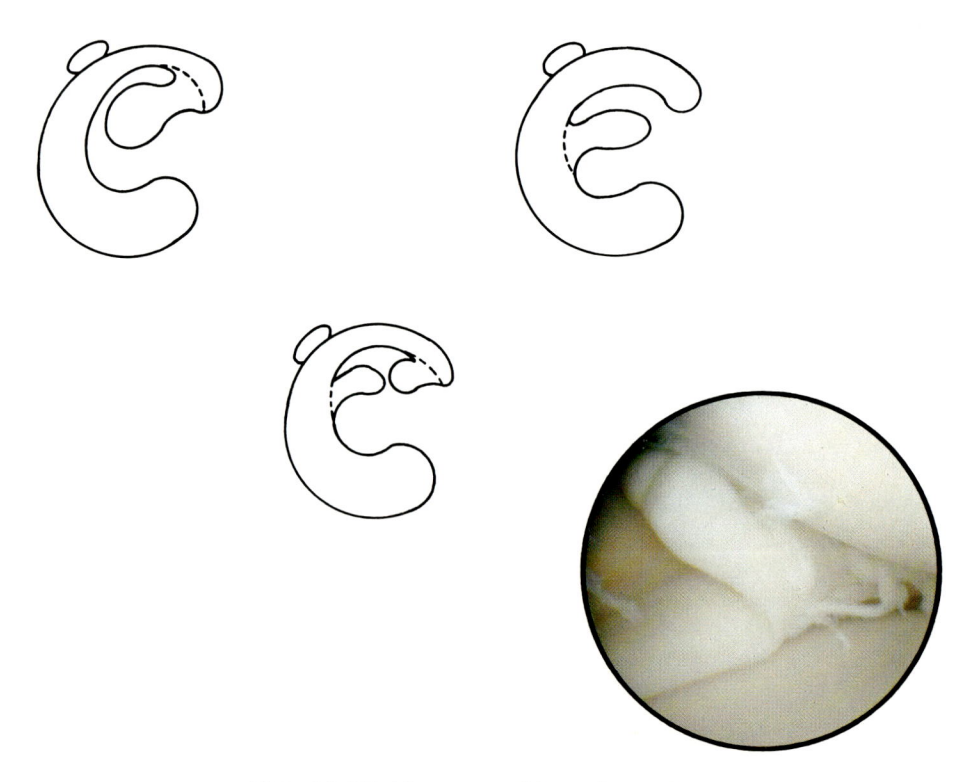

FIG. 16-17. Flap tear of lateral meniscus.

Meniscal surgery: lateral meniscus tears

Location: Lateral
Type of tear: Posterior horn tear from periphery
Arthroscope placement: Medial
Instrumentation portal: Lateral
Palpation: Probe and suction
Instruments: Knife blade and Intra-articular Shaver System
Resection: This lesion is identified either through the intercondylar notch or through a separate posteromedial puncture approach. In most cases it is possible, with valgus strain and external rotation, to place a probe back into that notch and determine the potential for placing the knife blade in that same position and completing the incision up to the anterior compartment. Basically, the surgeon hopes to convert the large posterior horn into a bucket-handle tear and then remove it in the same manner as for a bucket-handle tear. Meniscoresis would be technically difficult.

Viewing is either from the intercondylar notch or a separate posterior puncture. The knife blade is brought in from the anterior and medial sides. It is the best time to bring the cannula in without the knife blade protruding. Then the knife blade protrudes from the cannula for the cutting. In rare instances it may be necessary to place the knife blade percutaneously by a posterolateral puncture to complete the cutting. This is somewhat difficult to achieve technically early in one's experience. It is best performed with a small percutaneous IM blade. One should not completely release the posterior horn attachment at the intercondylar notch first. This will release the tension.

After this lesion has been converted to a bucket-handle tear and the large fragment has been removed transcutaneously via a lateral portal, the Intra-articular Shaver System with its various cutter heads is used to trim and balance up the entire rim. In some instances the posterior horn tear is of such magnitude that the procedure can be accomplished entirely by a knife blade. This is then a simple technical maneuver.

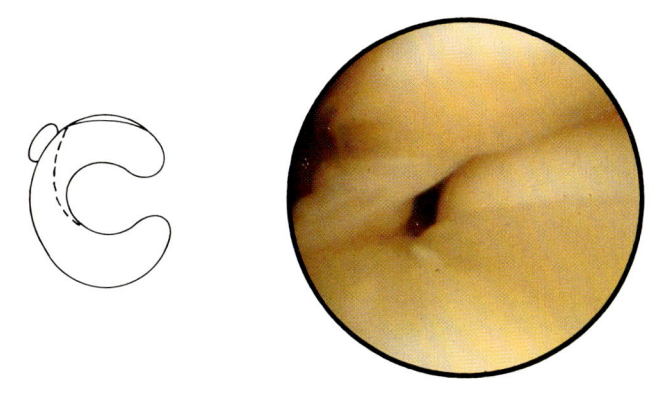

FIG. 16-18. Peripheral tear of lateral meniscus.

Arthroscopic surgery of the knee

Location: Lateral
Type of tear: Complex tears
Arthroscope placement: Medial
Instrumentation portal: Lateral
Palpation: Probe and suction
Instruments: Knife blade and Intra-articular Shaver System
Resection: Complex tears are less common on the lateral than on the medial side. They still occur and are often associated with loss of meniscal substance and degenerative change on both the femoral and the tibial sides. The most common area for loss of articular tissue is immediately anterior to the popliteus tendon on the tibial side. Debridement is usually accomplished with the Intra-articular Shaver System Cutter head. Debridement of the entire meniscal rim and articular surfaces is accomplished with the trimmer and/or shaver. Also, localized synovectomy can be carried out above and below the meniscal attachment as well as in the anterior compartment.

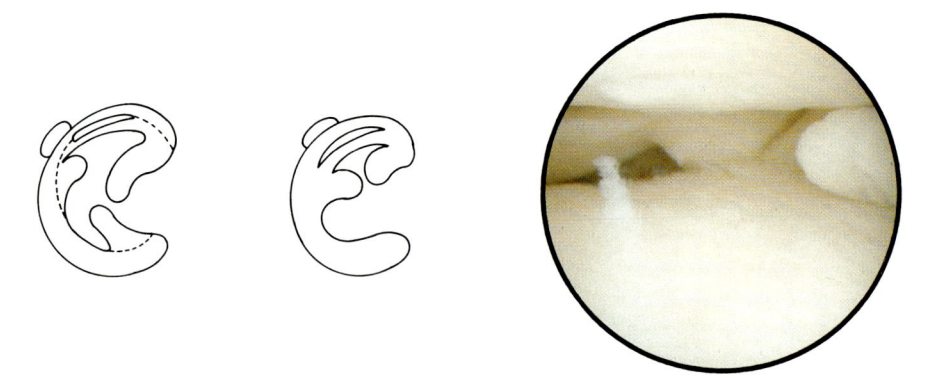

FIG. 16-19. Complex tears of lateral meniscus.

Location: Lateral
Type of tear: Bucket-handle tear
Arthroscope placement: Medial
Instrumentation portal: Lateral, viewing from medial, entry point on lateral side determined by placement of needle
Palpation: Probe and suction
Instruments: Knife blade and Intra-articular Shaver System
Resection: It is usually easy to resect the bucket-handle tear on the lateral side with just a knife blade and no traction. The posterior portion can be incised first; then the anterior portion is excised. The knife blade is removed; the meniscus cutter is brought into place, and the lesion is resected. An alternate method is to remove the lesion transcutaneously with forceps. A small lesion is amenable to resection with the Intra-articular Cutter.

An alternate method is to incise either the anterior or posterior horn. In that situation, the bucket handle has been converted to either an anterior or posterior flap tear. Resected as a flap tear, all the abnormal and abnormally mobile meniscal tissue is removed.

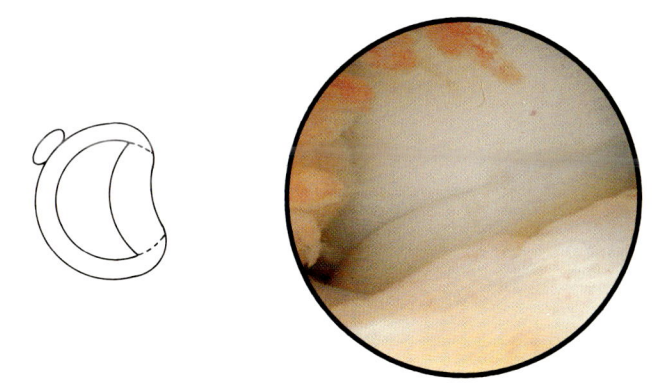

FIG. 16-20. Bucket-handle tear of lateral meniscus.

POST OPERATIVE PATIENT INFORMATION
ARTHROSCOPIC MENISECTOMY

Your operation was performed by arthroscopic methods. The interior of your joint was visualized with a small telescope. The diagnosis was established and the appropriate surgery was performed with special micro-instruments.

DRESSING: A soft dressing has been applied to your knee. This compression dressing should be confortable and absorb any leakage of fluid and/or blood. Although the dressing may become moist or blood stained, this is not usually a cause for alarm. We have not experience any hemorrhage or excessive bleeding in our patients.

The dressing may be removed safely at anytime. Routinely, the dressing is removed the day after surgery, and the appropriate number of bandaids are applied. The bandaids may be utilized over the next several days.

PAIN: Upon discharge you should secure a prescription for pain medication. Usually this will be an analgesic with **codiene**. Please inform us of any known drug allergy. **Codiene** may produce nausea and/or a fine skin rash. In that case, the medication should be discontinued and our office contacted for an alternate medication. The application of an ice pac to the knee will decrease swelling and discomfort in the first 48 hours. Please do not use aspirin, as it may increase bleeding in the first few days.

WOUNDS: The small points of entry may be sore and develop bruising over the next several days. This bruising will eventually disappear and does not require any special care.

BATHING: The sensation of "splashing" of fluid in the joint is not a cause for concern. It represents residual fluids from surgery, and they will absorb. It will be safe to shower 48 hours following surgery. Bathing or soaking should be delayed for several days. Cleansing of the skin adjacent to the small wounds with soap and water may be performed with the first dressing change.

ACTIVITY: Crutches may be necessary for comfort in the first week following surgery. You may step upon your surgical leg when comfortable. Active motion and tightening of quadricep muscles (the muscles on front of the thigh) should start the day of surgery. A twice a day activity (10-15 min.) for motion and muscle contraction should continue through three weeks.

Swimming and bicycling are permissable as tolerated. Jogging, running, or stop and go sports should be deferred for 6 or 8 weeks. Heavy weight lifting should be delayed for 4 months.

RESULTS: Preliminary reports as well as our experience have shown arthroscopic surgery produces results equal to, if not better than surgery performed by open, conventional methods. The benefits are in less discomfort, risk, and scarring for the patient.

We frequently remind patients that although the external incisions are small, they still have had an operative procedure inside their joint. Experience has shown that internal healing takes several weeks. In fact, complete healing to mature tissue may take three months. If an arthritic condition also exists, then the convalescence may be lengthened.

PRECAUTIONS: If you develop any fever ($101°$ F or above), unexpected pain, redness, or swelling in your legs, please contact our office for consultation or examination.
TELEPHONE (517) 351-7450.

Thank you,
Lanny L. Johnson, M.D.

FIG. 16-21. Patient information sheet. (Color code: blue; see p. 245.)

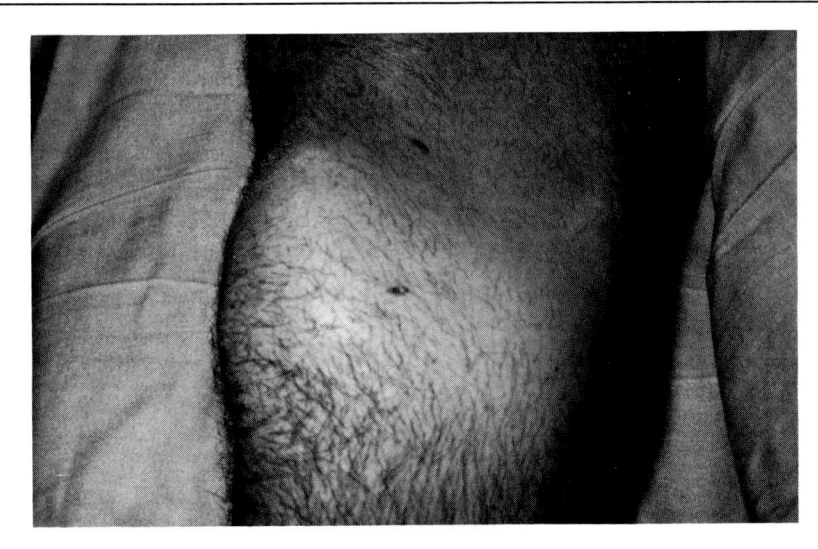

FIG. 16-22. Wounds require no sutures by this method, heal readily, and are cosmetically satisfactory.

POSTOPERATIVE MANAGEMENT

Postoperative atrophy has been minimal because of the minimal morbidity. At the conclusion of the operative treatment the tourniquet is released, dressings are applied, and the patient is given the postoperative patient information sheet (Fig. 16-21). The pathology specimen is obtained from the collection bag. The wounds require no sutures, so healing is cosmetically satisfactory (Fig. 16-22). Patients return for office visits periodically.

Complications

To my knowledge no patient has developed infection or thrombophlebitis. There have been two instances of sudden postoperative bleeding at 7 to 10 days following surgery. This patient had very little initial morbidity, was without crutches, was weight bearing fully, and was physically active at that time. I presume there was a sudden rupture of a small blood vessel. Aspiration within the joint and conservative measures resolved the problem. There were no incidences of hemorrhage or aneurysm.

There were two instances of significant effusion, one that lasted for 3 months and another that lasted for 6 months. Both patients remained physically active after surgery, and both had a lateral meniscectomy. One was a male and one a female. They eventually recovered after repeat arthroscopic aspiration and debridement. Degenerative change set in, and both had a virtually total lateral meniscectomy on the basis of their type of tear. One elective total meniscectomy by arthroscopic means was carried out at the beginning of this series. I do not recommend a total lateral meniscectomy, except when necessitated by the type of tear.

Arthroscopic surgery of the knee

CASE REPORTS

Case 1

A 32-year-old white man who was a long-distance runner for 20 years, including up to 10 miles a day, had persistent pain and swelling with tenderness along the lateral side of his knee. The physical examination showed some mild catching along the medial joint line, and the x-ray examination results were within normal limits. The patient was admitted for arthroscopy and arthroscopic surgery. He had a torn lateral meniscus of the complex type. Fig. 16-23 shows the arthroscopic operative procedure used.

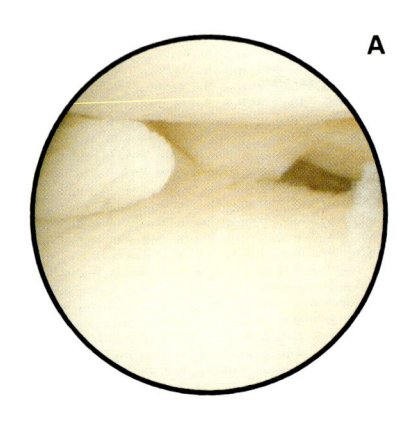

FIG. 16-23

A Arthroscopic view of complex tear of lateral meniscus.
B Intra-articular Shaver System with Cutter commences resection of anterior flap.
C Further resection of anterior flap.
D Complete resection of degenerative flap.
E Knife blade comes through cannula to balance off anterior horn.

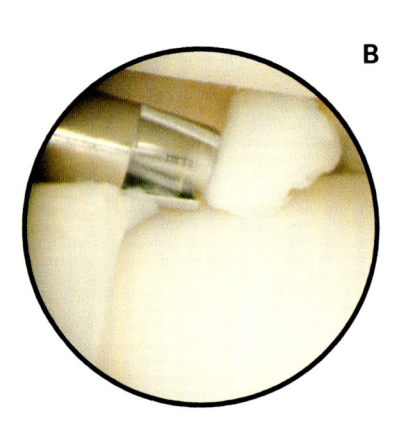

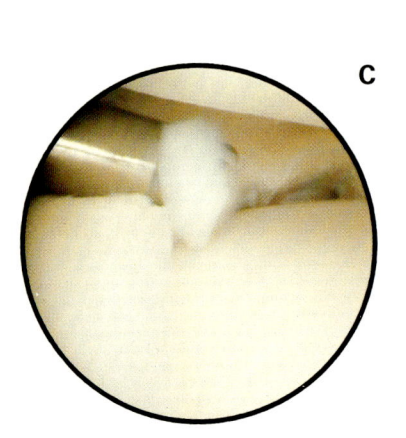

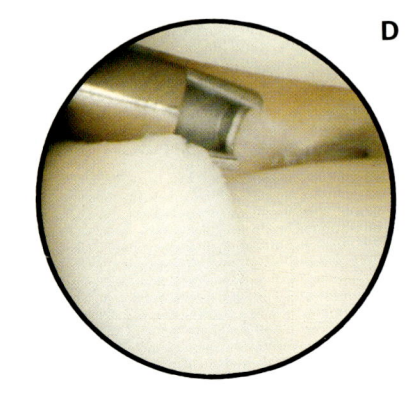

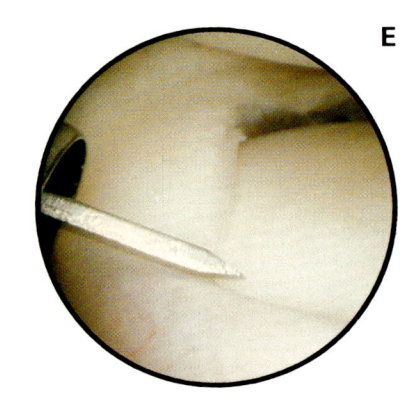

Meniscal surgery

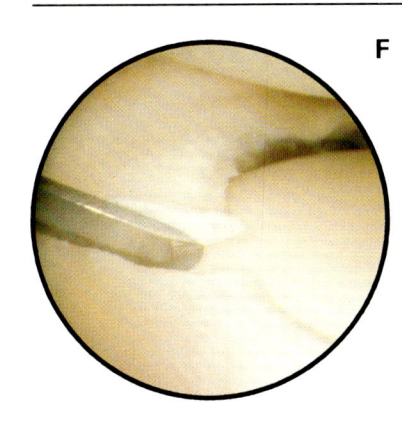

F FIG. 16-23, cont'd

F Knife cut moves from anterior to posterior.
G Knife cut is near completion, and piece is subsequently removed.
H Probing of posterior horn indicates flap tear.
I Scissors resect posterior flap tear.
J Basket forceps further remove posterior horn tear.
K Final clean-up is performed with Trimmer of Intra-articular Shaver System.
L Immediate postoperative inspection. After 3 months patient was completely asymptomatic and submitted to repeat arthroscopic examination for academic purposes.

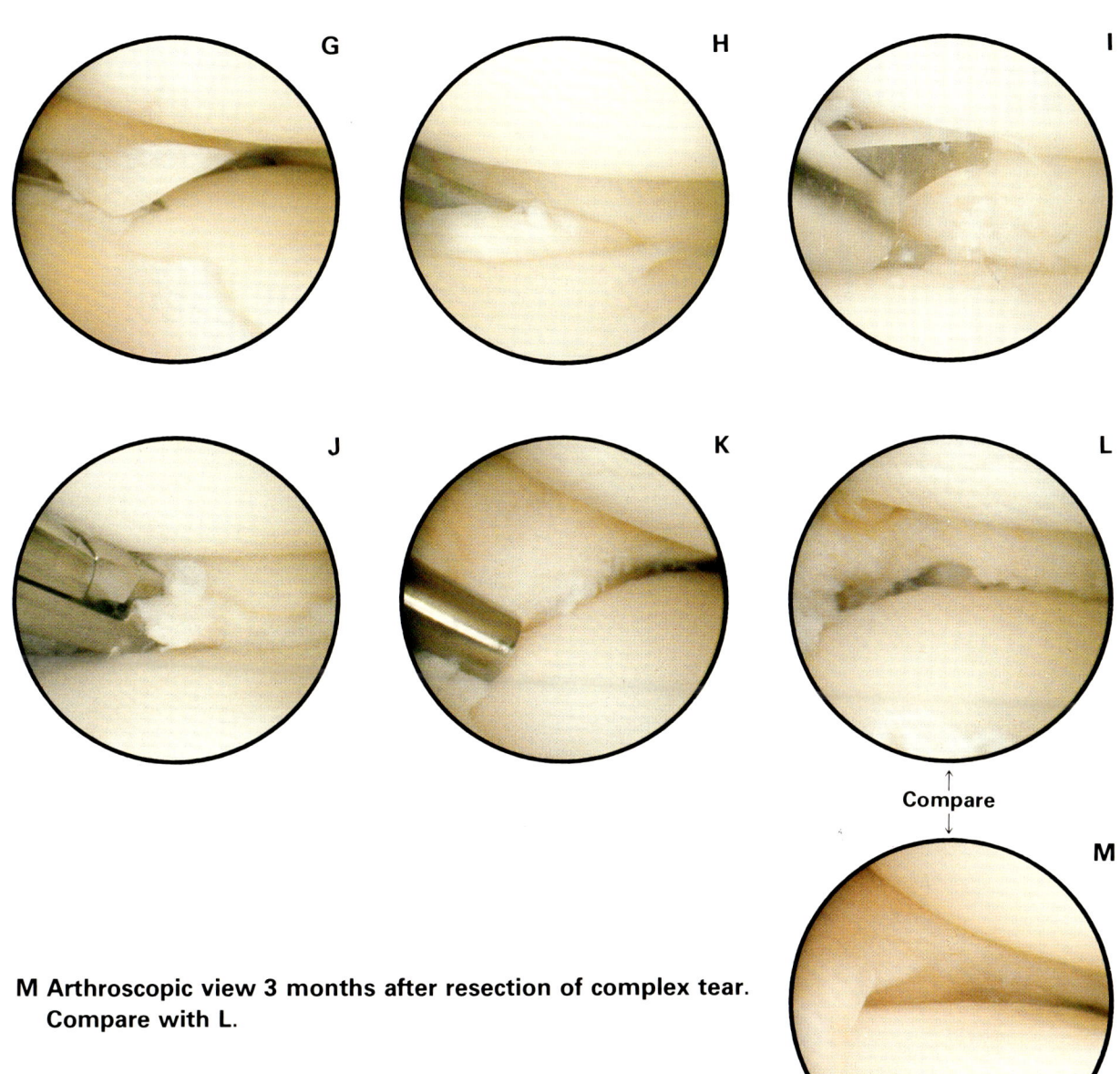

Compare

M Arthroscopic view 3 months after resection of complex tear. Compare with L.

313

Arthroscopic surgery of the knee

Case 2
A 15-year-old white girl sustained an acute injury to her knee approximately 8 months prior to arthroscopic inspection and surgery. She had persistent locking and catching in her knee without remission of symptoms in spite of physiotherapy. (See Fig. 16-24.) Release of bucket handle on medial side can be achieved by knife blade resection of the anterior horn, grasping either through anterior medial portal with forceps or anterior lateral portal and bringing in knife blade from opposite portal for resection. It is a matter of which portal gives best opportunity for excising posterior horn with knife blade without injury to anterior cruciate ligament. The remaining rim is then cleaned up.

FIG. 16-24

A Bucket-handle tear is locked in notch medially.
B Bucket-handle tear has been reduced with probe.
C Knife blade commences resection on anterior horn.

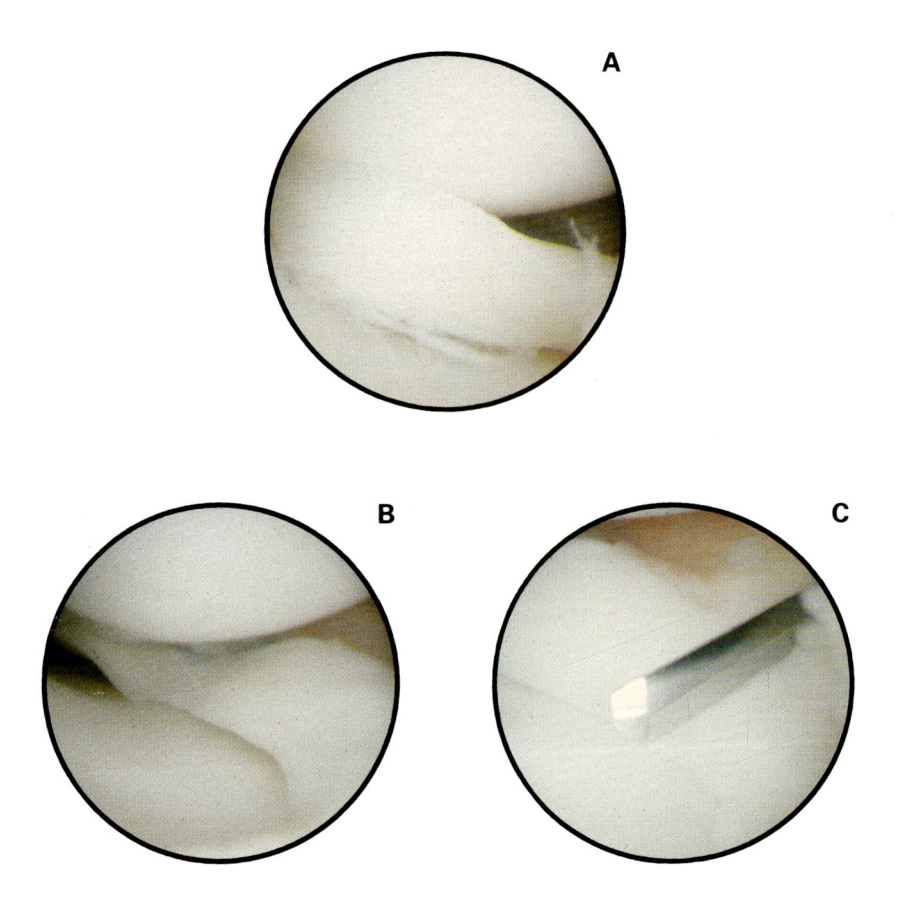

Meniscal surgery

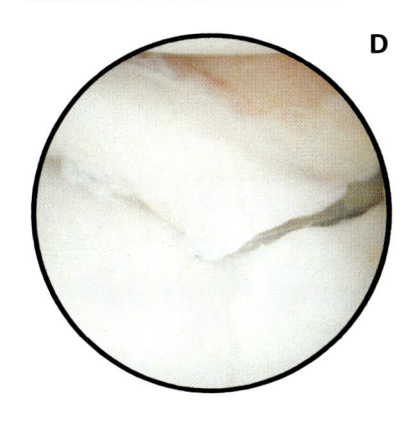

FIG. 16-24, cont'd

D Completion of anterior horn resection is achieved.
E Forceps reach in from anterior medial portal.
F Knife blade is passed along course of cannula system from lateral and inferior to arthroscope. A 747 IM blade is now preferred.
G Small posterior horn remnant after bucket-handle fragment excision.
H A 3.5-mm Cutter is often necessary to reach the most extreme posterior horn tag.
I Arthroscopic resection of bucket-handle tear is completed, and Intra-articular Shaver System Trimmer cleans up rim of meniscus.

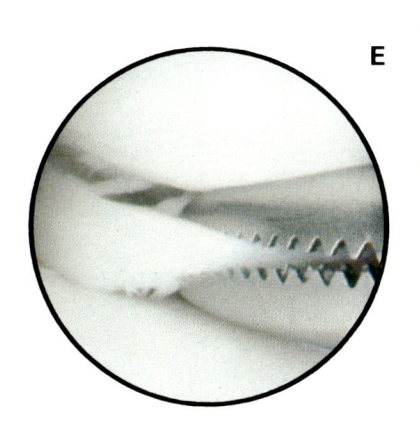

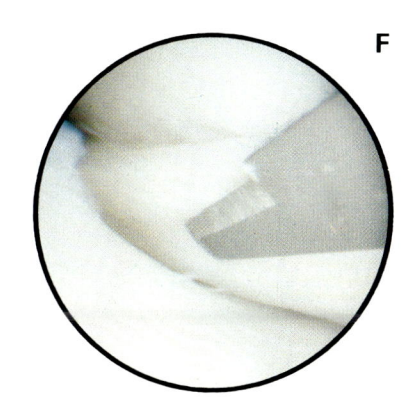

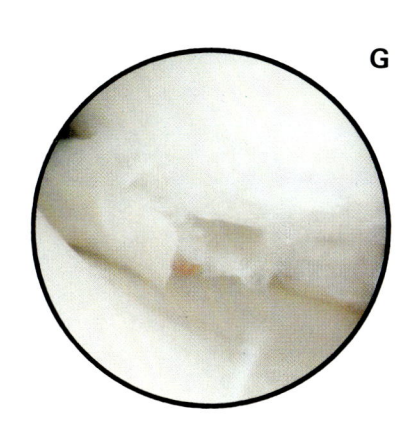

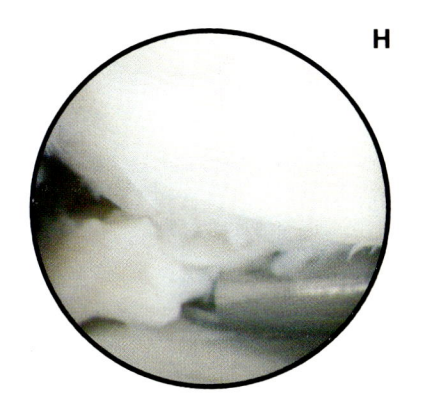

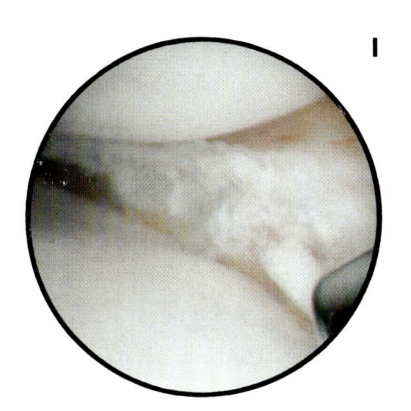

Arthroscopic surgery of the knee

REFERENCES

1. Arstrand, T.: Treatment of meniscal rupture of the knee joint, Acta Chir. Scand. **107**:145, 1954.
2. Bruser, D. M.: A direct lateral approach to the lateral compartment of the knee joint, J. Bone Joint Surg. (Br.) **42**:348, 1960.
3. Cargill, O. R., and Jackson, J. P.: Bucket handle tear of the medial meniscus, J. Bone Joint Surg. (Am.) **58**:248, 1976.
4. Cave, E. F.: Combined anterior-posterior approach to the knee joint, J. Bone Joint Surg. (Am.) **17**:427, 1935.
5. Dandy, D. J.: Early results of closed partial meniscectomy, Br. Med. J. **1**:1099, 1978.
6. Fairbanks, T. J.: Knee joint changes after meniscectomy, J. Bone Joint Surg. (Br.) **30**:664, 1948.
7. Jackson, J. P.: Degenerative changes in the knee after meniscectomy, Br. Med. J. **2**:525, 1968.
8. Jackson, R. W., and Dandy, D. J.: Arthroscopy of the knee, New York, 1976, Grune & Stratton, Inc.
9. Johnson, R. M., Kettlekamp, D. B., Clark, W., and Leaverton, P.: Factors affecting late results after meniscectomy, J. Bone Joint Surg. (Am.) **56**:719, 1974.
10. King, D.: The healing of semilunar cartilage, J. Bone Joint Surg. (Br.) **18**:333, 1936.
11. Lutfi, A. M.: Morphological changes in the articular cartilage after meniscectomy, J. Bone Joint Surg. (Br.) **57**:525, 1975.
12. McGinty, J. B., Geuss, L. F., and Marvin, P. S.: Partial or total meniscectomy, J. Bone Joint Surg. (Br.) **59**:763, 1977.
13. Metcalf, R. W., Personal communication, 1978.
14. O'Connor, R., Arthroscopy, Philadelphia, 1977, J. B. Lippincott Co.
15. Scapenelli, R.: Studies of the vasculature of the human knee joint, Acta Anat. **70**:305, 1968.
16. Shneider, D., Personal communication, 1979.
17. Smillie, I. S.: Injuries of the knee joint, ed. 4, Edinburgh, 1970, Churchill Livingstone.
18. Tapper, E. M., and Hoover, N. W.: Late results after meniscectomy, J. Bone Joint Surg. (Am.) **51**:517, 1969.
19. Watanabe, M., and Takeda, I.: Atlas of arthroscopy, ed. 2, Berlin, 1969, Springer-Verlag.

Chapter 17

Patellar surgery

Standard procedures
Intra-articular shaving
    Complications of the procedure
    Results
    Adequacy of resection
    Patellofemoral degeneration
    Postoperative management
Lateral release
    Postoperative management
    Complications

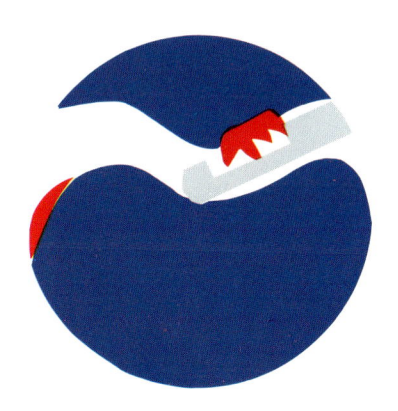

STANDARD PROCEDURES

The most common conventional surgical procedures performed for pathologic conditions of the patella are probably quadriceps realignment,[6] treatment of displaced fractures, and patellectomy.[3,7] On rare occasions a patient develops osteochondritis dissecans or severe localized chondromalacia of the patella that necessitates arthrotomy and surgical treatment. The osteochondritic lesions are removed and the edges sharply excised at an angle perpendicular to the articular surface (Fig. 17-1). Curettage down to bone produces some hemorrhage and fibrosis and ultimately satisfactory results.[4] The same is true in selective cases of severe chondromalacia patellae.

The open shaving of articular cartilage for severe chondromalacia patellae or in traumatic articular injuries related to direct trauma and/or dislocation of the patella at times does not produce clinically satisfactory results[3,7] (Fig. 17-2).

In particular cartilage lesions of the patella, clefts developed, especially in cases of dislocation. I have had experience drilling down in these minute clefts with 1-mm drill bits (Fig. 17-3). This brought the blood supply in and sealed the lesions. Second-look arthroscopic inspections as much as a year later showed that these articular lesions had healed.

In the past, more severe cases were treated by open chondrectomy. Shaving with or without drilling has been advocated.[3,4,7] Other operations have been directed toward malalignment; also, elevation of the tibial tubercle to reduce compression has been performed.[2] Even a patellectomy has been recommended.[3,7] These procedures all necessitated an arthrotomy and its attendant morbidity.

Arthroscopic surgery of the knee

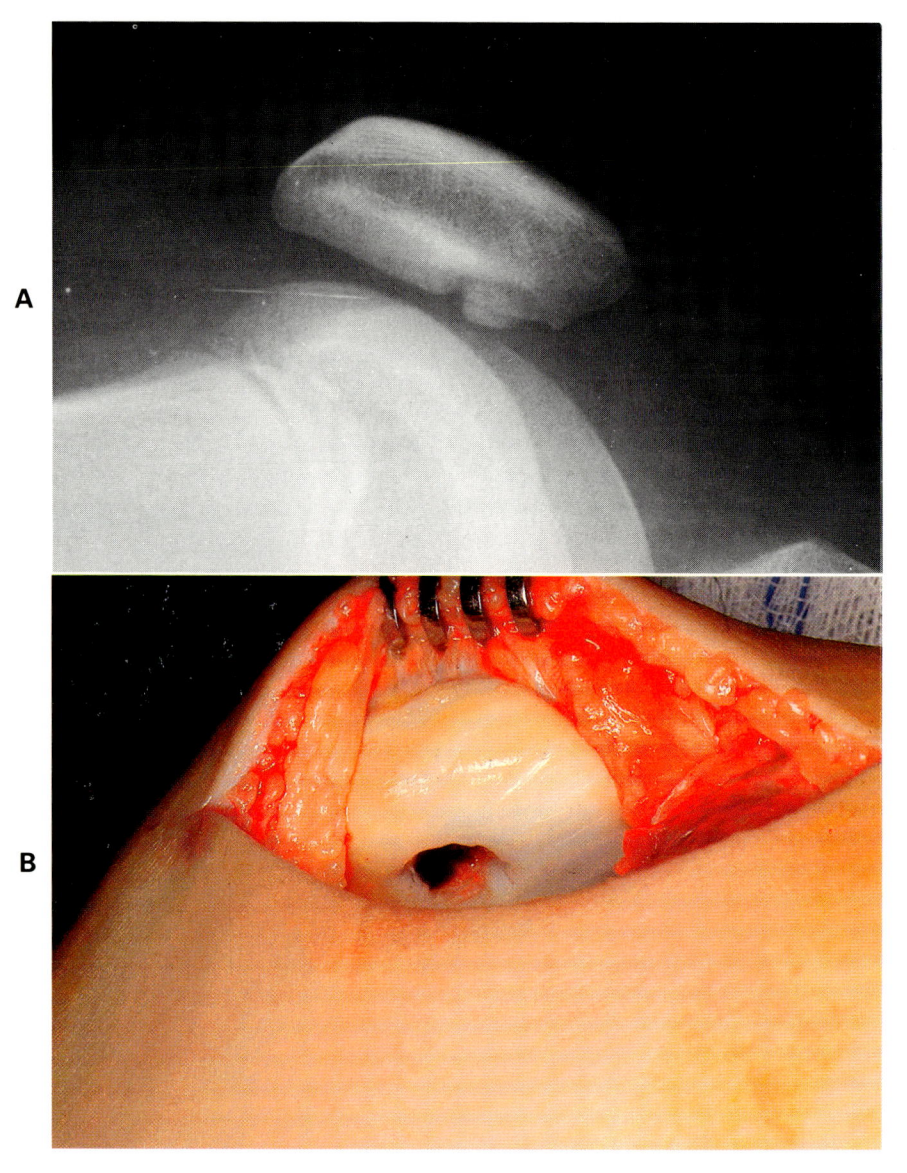

FIG. 17-1. **A,** X-ray film of osteochondritis dissecans patellae. **B,** Excision of patellar lesion with sharp clean margins perpendicular to articular surface is acceptable former method.

Patellar surgery

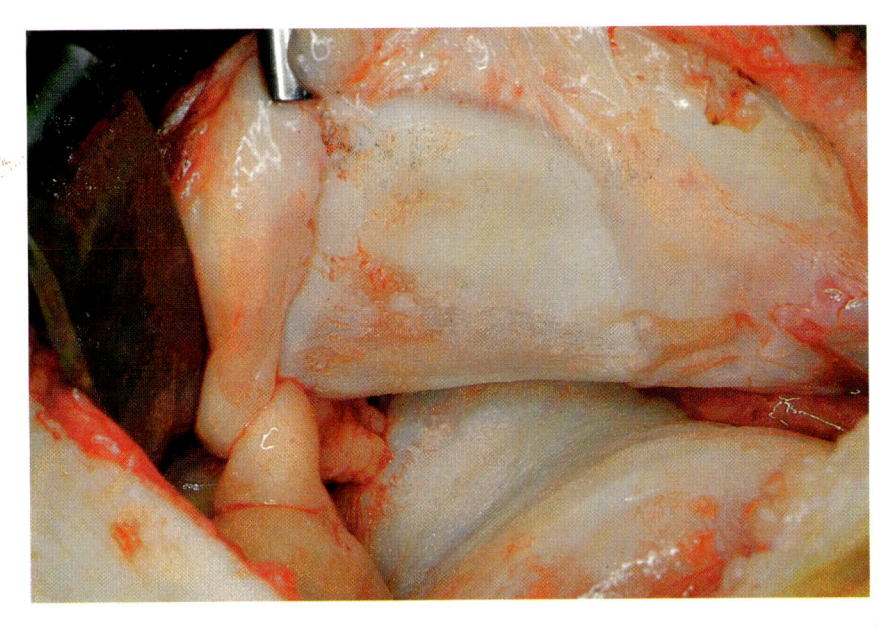

FIG. 17-2. Patellofemoral surface 4 years after open shave of patella. There is subsequent degenerative change and complete alteration of patellofemoral contour and articulation.

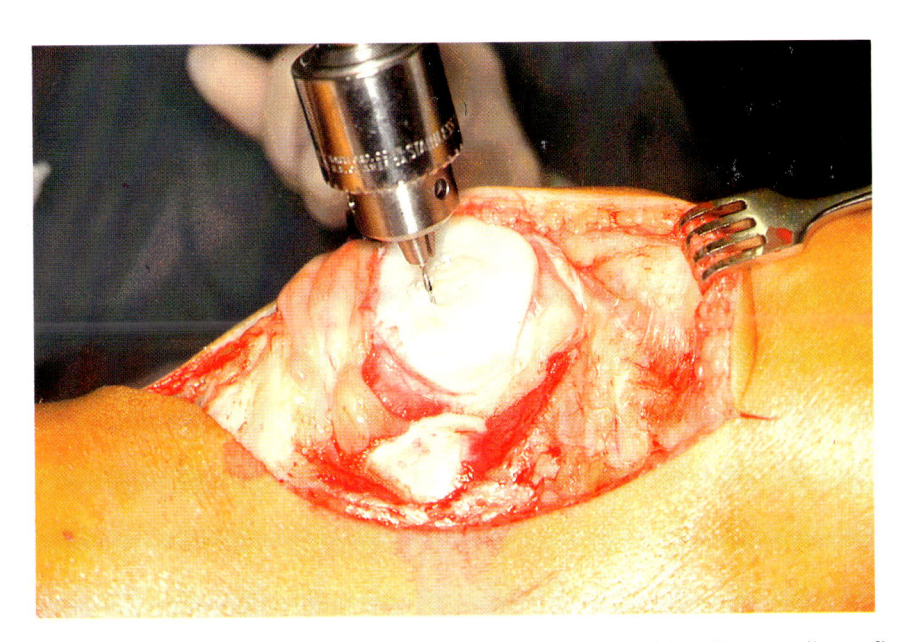

FIG. 17-3. Drilling 1-mm holes into clefts between normal hyaline cartilage fissures brings in the blood supply and fibrocartilaginous healing.

Arthroscopic surgery of the knee

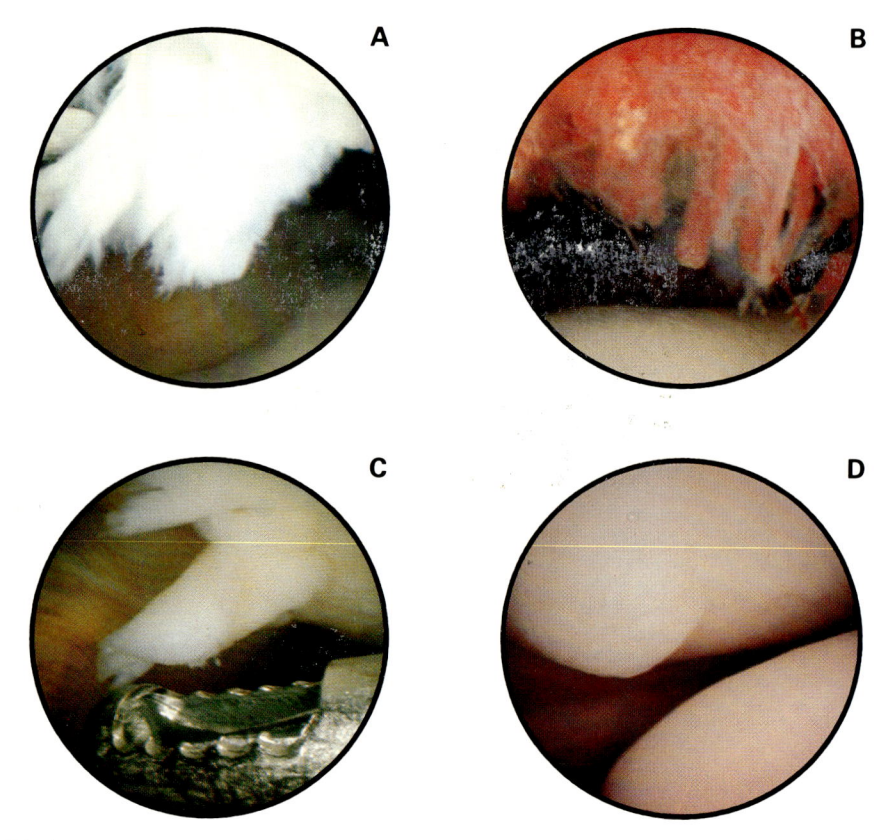

FIG. 17-4

A Arthroscopic view of severe chondromalacia of patella.
B Marked peripatellar synovitis.
C Intra-articular Shaver resecting area affected by chondromalacia.
D Fifteen-month follow-up showing healed articular surfaces.

INTRA-ARTICULAR SHAVING

The earliest application of arthroscopy in the treatment of chondromalacia was to identify it diagnostically and to wash the joint free of articular debris. (See Figs. 10-2 and 10-3.) It has been my experience that this can render a joint asymptomatic, but in the severe cases recurrent debris occurs in the joint, and the patient again has symptoms usually within about 1 year. The patient then returns for some form of treatment. The initial treatment of chondromalacia patellae is always conservative.

I now have 4 years of experience (with an excess of 200 cases) in the treatment of severe chondromalacia of the patella with the Intra-articular Shaver System. This experience has eliminated the necessity for arthrotomy, drilling, or curetting into the patella, and the dramatic improvement in clinical symptoms is supported by second-look arthroscopy with photography and histologic studies (Fig. 17-4).

My initial report included 72 patients with chondromalacia patellae. These patients were seen in an active private orthopedic practice with a special concentration in knee problems. Also, many patients were referred by orthopedic surgeons specifically for this treatment. A single knee was involved in 56 patients, 21 left knees and 34 right. In 16 patients both knees were treated, for a total of 89 knees in 72 patients. Forty-four of the patients were women and 28 were men. The women's ages ranged from 14 to 64 years, with an average age of 31.6 years. The men's ages ranged from 15 to 55, with an average age of 30.4 years. The age range of all patients was 14 to 64, and the average age of all patients was 29.4 years.

Patients complained of pain, swelling, and crepitus. Often they had trouble climbing stairs and getting up out of chairs after sitting for a while. They all had had previous conservative surgical treatment that failed. These complaints were confirmed by physical examination, but the actual severe chondromalacia was identified by direct visualization during the comprehensive arthroscopic examination.

Some patients' complaints suggested severe chondramalacia, but these were not confirmed by the arthroscopic viewing and were deleted from this series. Also in the original series, patients had chondromalacia plus other pathologic findings; for instance, degenerative change opposite the femoral condyle or one of the other compartments was eliminated.

These were patients who had not responded to conservative methods of treatment for up to 15 years, including physiotherapy, anti-inflammatory medication, cortisone injections, and even diagnostic arthroscopy with lavage of loose bodies in two instances.

There are many contributing factors to the chondromalacia in this group. Fifteen patients had a history of direct trauma to the patella, including one with a previous fracture. Two patients had a partial torn cruciate ligament at the time of the arthroscopic examination but no clinical instability.

Many of the patients had undergone previous operative procedures. Nine had had meniscectomies: seven were medial, one was lateral, and one had both a medial and a lateral meniscectomy. Eleven patients had had a patella malalignment procedure. An open patella shave was performed in four of the patients having the alignment procedures. Two of the people with realignment procedures had an eventual patella baja as a result of the tibial tubercle transplant.

Five patients had had an open lateral release for dislocation of the patella. Three patients in this group had an open patellar shave via arthrotomy. One patient had an open shave performed twice. In all, 11 of the 72 patients had a previous patellar shave by open knife blade methods.

There were 12 patients with untreated subluxation of the patella. Five patients had untreated dislocation of the patella. There were only eight patients in whom there was no identifiable contributing factor in chondromalacia of the patella.

Most of the patients had changes of the patella visible on x-ray examination (Fig. 17-5). Scalloping under the patella was seen in the lateral view. Many of the older patients had osteophytes around their patellar surface. Those with

Arthroscopic surgery of the knee

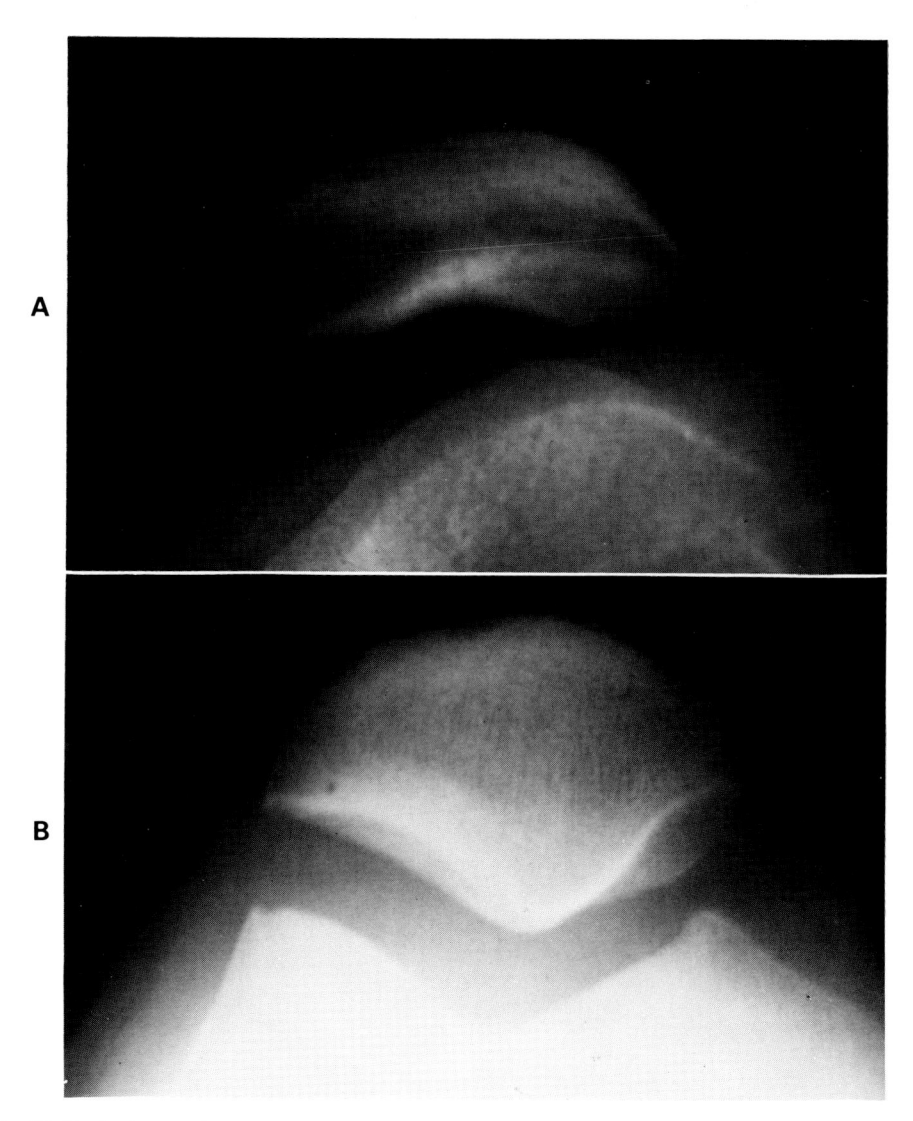

FIG. 17-5. A, Lateral x-ray view of patella showing common scalloped bony changes. **B,** Skyline view of patella with minimal osteoarthritic changes, which are common.

Patellar surgery

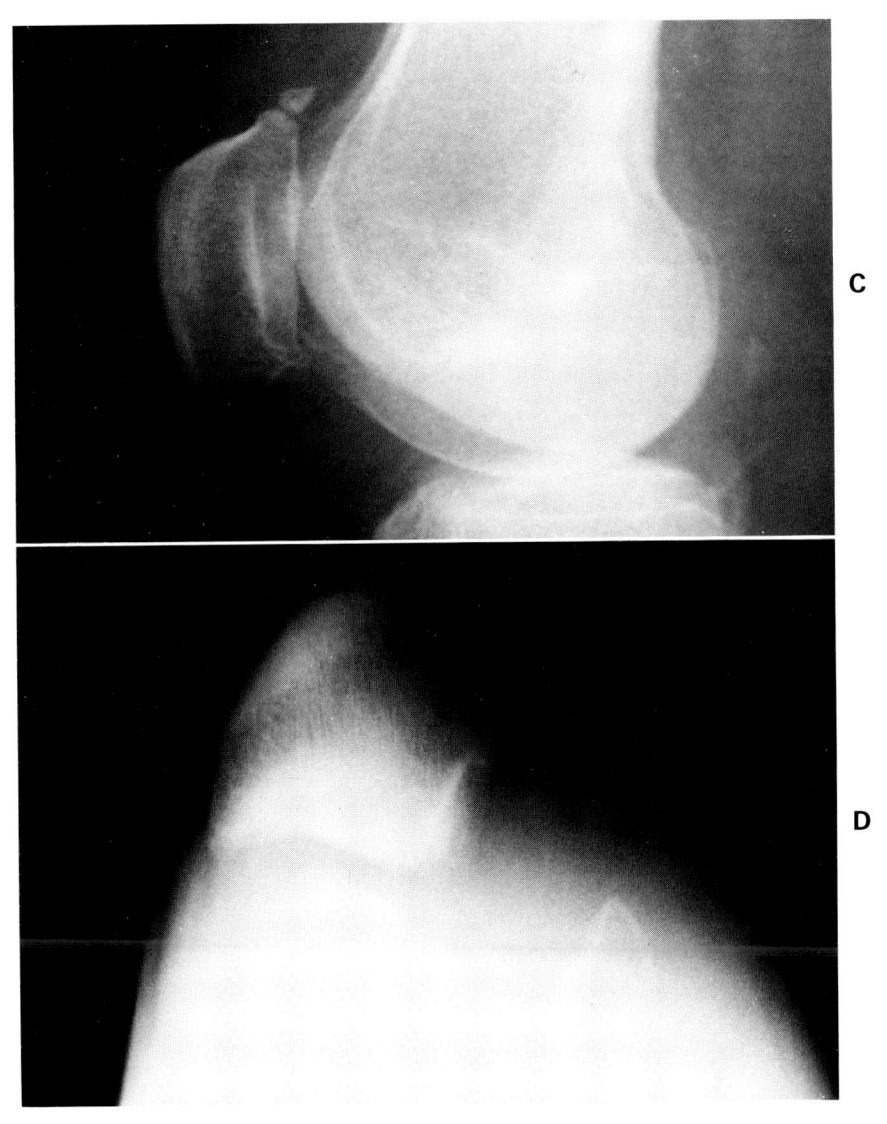

FIG. 17-5, cont'd. C, Increased osteoarthritic changes and bone spurs. **D,** Skyline view of patella showing lateral compression syndrome and marked changes in older person.

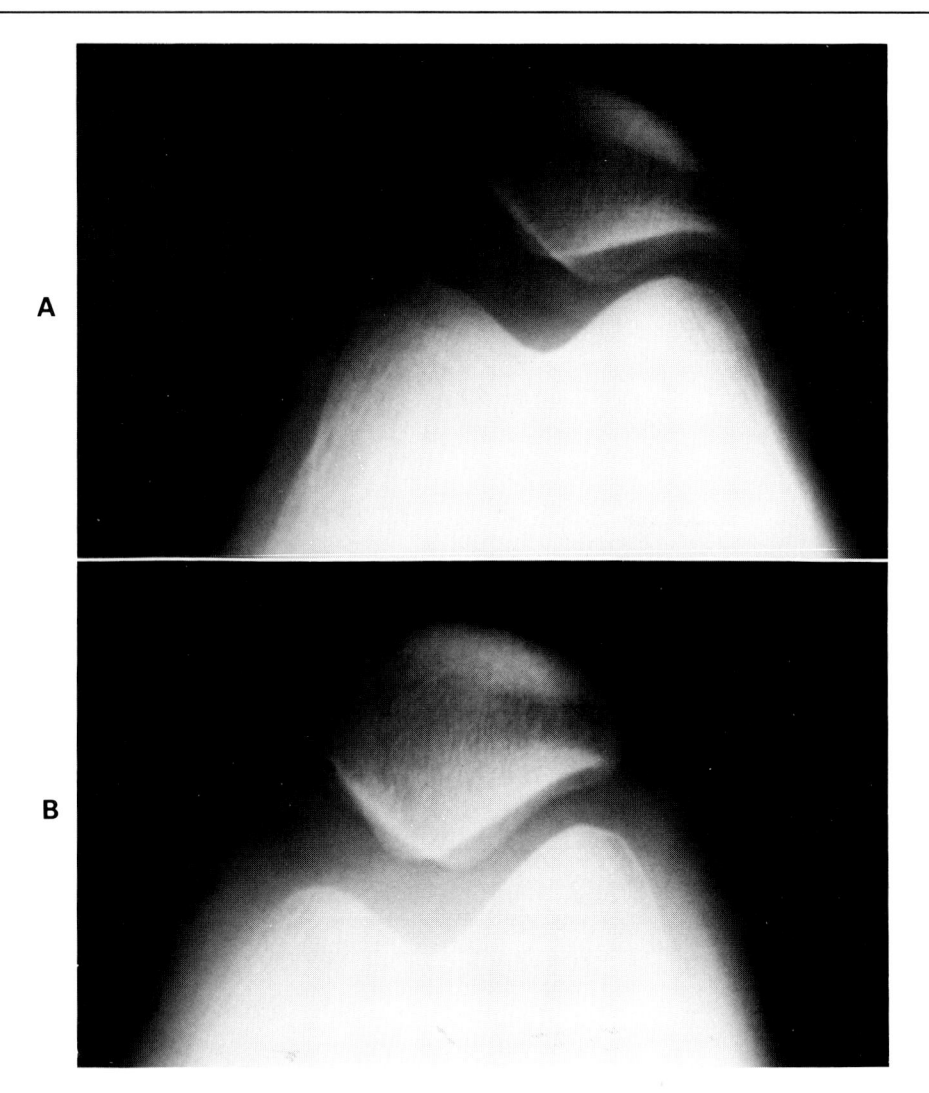

FIG. 17-6. A, Preoperative lateral release x-ray findings. **B,** After lateral release. Skyline view shows reduction of patella in groove in younger person.

subluxation and dislocation frequently had a lateral sitting patella seen in the skyline view (Fig. 17-6, *A*).

A medical history and physical examination were required for all patients, as well as routine x-ray examinations of the knee, including the skyline view (Fig. 17-6, *B*). No patient had an arthrogram. The arthroscopy either preceded or accompanied the surgical procedure.

Local anesthesia was used in 25 patients and general anesthesia in the remaining number. The local anesthetic used was directly infiltrated 1% plain lidocaine at the area of the arthroscopic or instrument portal. Those patients who had a lateral release were given 0.25% marcaine injected along the course of the anticipated lateral release.

Under local anesthesia I was unable to duplicate the typical clinical symptoms or feelings of chondromalacia of the patella. Neither cutting the articular cartilage of the patella nor pressure or manipulation of the patella reproduced those symptoms. The fat pad was anesthetic, as was the parapatellar synovium.

Patients frequently noticed what they described as a cold cut or a clipped feeling during the cutting of the synovium or the patellar surface. Even though it is extremely painful when the synovium of the suprapatellar pouch or the walls of the joint are incised, I could not evoke this sensation.

It is possible what the patient senses may be related to crepitus and a visceral type of deep proprioceptive pain, rather than a type of pain produced by pressure separation of tissues. Recently, palpation of the femoral side has more closely duplicated the symptoms.

Commonly, patients have a click or crepitus under their patella, discomfort with distal push, or fixation of the patella with contraction of the quadriceps and yet have a normal arthroscopic finding of their patellar surface.

Also, the common physical examination test that includes subluxating the patella and palpating either under the lateral or medial facet of the patella may not be diagnostic. Discomfort probably results from direct pressure on the skin or capsule and not the intra-articular tissue. We know now that tissues in the patella and parapatellar area are insensitive to cutting. Therefore this test does not seem to be reliable for diagnosis of chondromalacia of the patella or synovitis.

Complications of the procedure

The technical details of intra-articular shaving of the patella are described in Chapter 15. It should be noted that problems may occur with the apparatus. On several occasions during manipulation the Intra-articular Shaver has accidently hit against the arthroscope, resulting in a fracture or abrasion of the lens covering the arthroscope. This is a costly complication and necessitates either repolishing or replacement of the telescopic lens.

An early prototype failed to rotate in one direction, which did not compromise the result but did prolong the procedure. The first production model of the shaver was made of a softer type of metal, and deformation of the outer cannula was possible, causing tissue to catch between the inner rotating tube and the outer tube. This has been substantially eliminated by improved metallurgy in the present models.

Occasionally the shaver has hit or bitten a small nick in the metallic cannula sheath of the arthroscope. Damage is done to the shaver blades as well as to the arthroscope.

It should be noted that the blades of the original Intra-articular Shaver were purposely not sharpened and were dull. They could therefore be used for more than 200 or 300 cases before necessitating replacement.

The main technical problems of the patellar shaver are those common to arthroscopy—loss of distension and lack of visualization due to poor illumination. Distension can be solved by intermittent clamping of the outflow tract. Illumination can be improved by frequent changes of the light bulb and having fresh, clean light cables.

One patient after intra-articular shave developed a painful catching synovial tag at the lateral inflow site (see Fig. 17-14). It was confirmed and excised under local anesthesia.

Results

In the original group 55% of the patients were asymptomatic and considered to have shown excellent results, that is, they had no awareness of pain, swelling, and crepitus. They were able to maintain their normal full activities.

Thirty-six percent of the patients had no pain or effusion but had some awareness of patellar crepitus, although lessened. They maintained their full activities but complained of some discomfort during vigorous activities. Medication was unnecessary, and the result was considered good.

There were six patients who were unchanged and therefore considered to have shown poor results. They still complained of occasional pain, crepitus, or an effusion with activity. However, no patient was made worse by the procedure. Therefore 91% of the patients had good or excellent results.

One patient complained of occasional swelling after vigorous activities, but this was managed by anti-inflammatory medication. Only three patients had occasional pain. No patient in the "excellent" group recognized any crepitus, but a fine crepitus or a click could occasionally be demonstrated to the patient. The most common reason for failure to show excellent results was crepitus recognizable by the patient. However, they were improved over their preoperative status, and crepitus was not troublesome. Patellar crepitus persisted in 32% of all patients, although no patient's condition at the time of operation worsened.

Ewing and Gradisar[5] have demonstrated the benefits of this type of surgery by clinical studies correlating arthroscopic evaluations and knee sound recordings (Fig. 17-7).

It was possible to evaluate the healing of the articular surface and adjacent synovial tissues by repeat arthroscopic examination in 11 patients. The earliest inspection was at 2 months, and the longest follow-up now is 3½ years (Fig. 17-8).

The articular surface shows fibrous cartilage coalescence as early as 2 months. In fact, some areas with loose blocks of hyaline cartilage showed coalescence to adjacent areas at 2 months. This occurred without excision or drilling to bleeding bone. Patients over 50 years of age with previous malalignment problems or multiple surgeries frequently showed small areas of fibular degeneration around the patella. The major area of articular shave was smooth and rounded off when seen arthroscopically. When articular cartilage was lost and bone exposed, resurfacing of bone did not occur. This is true for the patella but not for femoral or tibial condyles.

The second-look arthroscopies have shown only one patient to have developed any changes on the femoral side opposite the patella when the femoral side had previously been normal (Fig. 17-9). In this case, a 17-year-old white boy, who had a direct blow to his patella with severe chondromalacia as a result, underwent an intra-articular shave. He ignored my preoperative instructions and initiated quadriceps exercises immediately. He had an effusion that persisted and an intra-articular fracture of the metacarpal, which necessitated open reduction. At the time of the open reduction the patient permitted a second-look arthroscopy. At that time there was marked synovitis. The

Patellar surgery

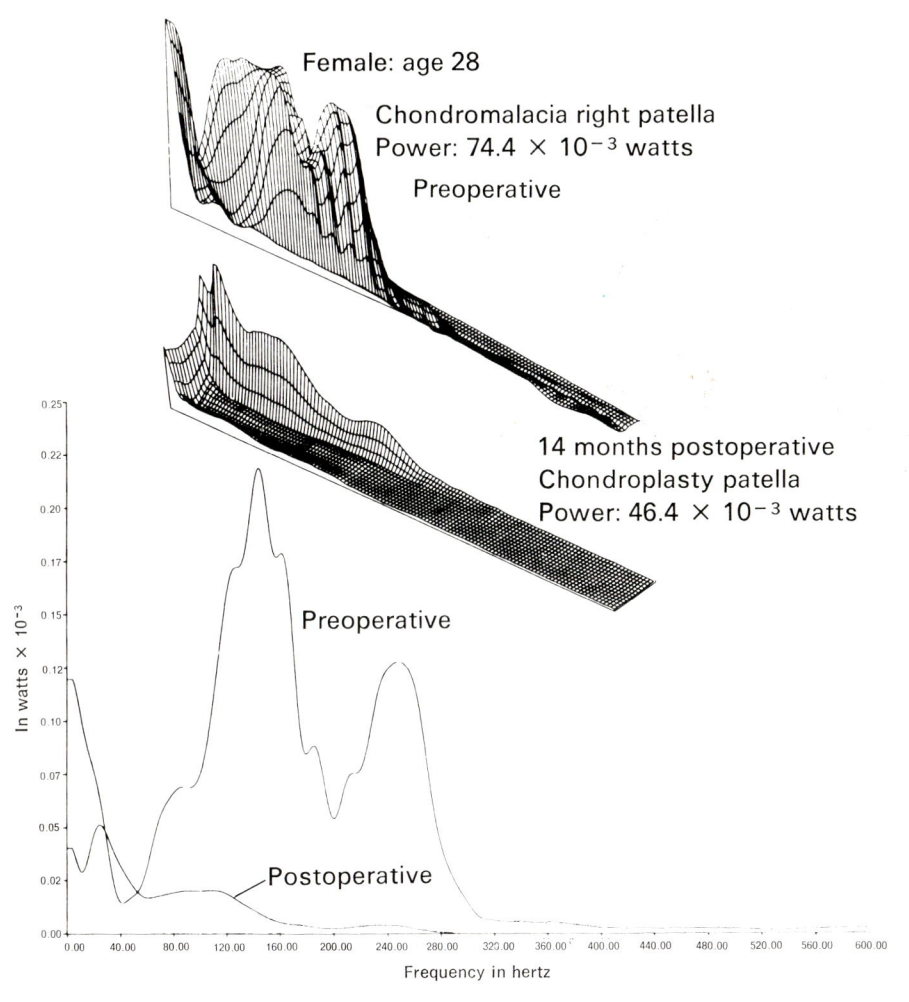

FIG. 17-7. Gradishar's results 1 year after intra-articular shave of patella show before and after computerized reduction and noise spectrum of crepitus.

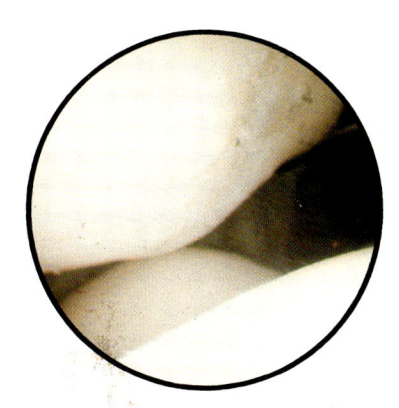

FIG. 17-8. Arthroscopic view of 2½-year follow-up second look after intra-articular shave of patella showing healed defects superior (2 o'clock) and no changes on remainder of patella or femoral condyle.

Arthroscopic surgery of the knee

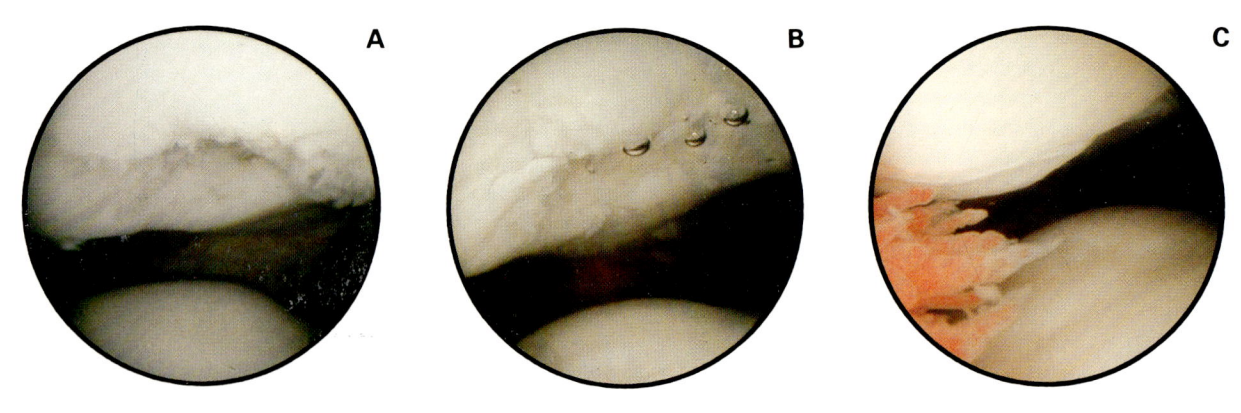

FIG. 17-9

A Arthroscopic view immediately following patellar shave after resection of tissue up into patella.
B Same arthroscopic view 3 months later, showing depression and defect healing in.
C Same patient, showing synovitis and alterations of femoral side. Patient refused to wait for articular healing and was doing vigorous quadriceps exercises.

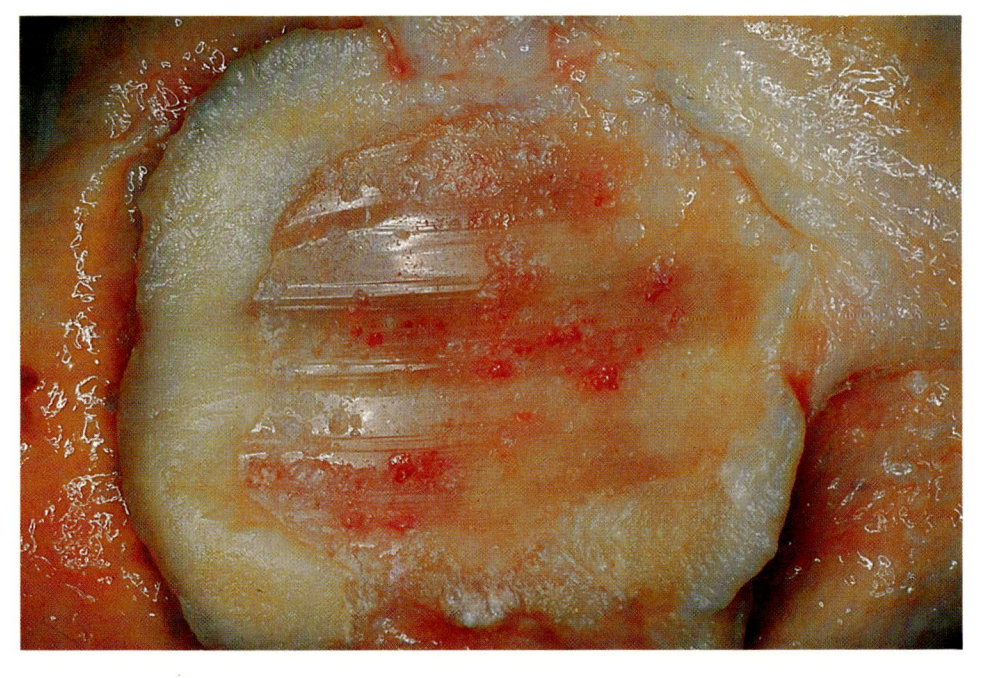

FIG. 17-10. Gross anatomic view of patella 5 years after open patellar shave at time of patellectomy.

patellar surface was well healed with adjacent superficial abrasions of the articular surface of the femur (Fig. 17-9, B and C).

Open shave of the patella that markedly altered the patellar surface has resulted in subsequent degenerative changes on the opposite femoral side, even in young people.[2] The greater the resection of patellar cartilage, the poorer the result (Fig. 17-10).

There seem to be two ways to prevent subsequent femoral side changes. One is to carry out a limited shave with the Intra-articular Shaver; the second is to allow healing of the patellar surface for approximately 2 months before initiating vigorous activities.

Adequacy of resection

In early cases, the patellar shaver seemed to be inadequate in its aggressiveness. Therefore in 13 of my first 72 cases I used the knife blade as an additional method to develop articular surfaces. It should be noted that those patients did not improve as much as those in whom the knife blade was not used, and crepitus persisted. Second-look arthroscopies did show the articular surfaces had healed at about 2 months, but the knife caused greater damage to the contour of the patella than did the disease. Once knife blade cutting starts on any patellar lesion, it is difficult not to injure the adjacent normal articular hyaline cartilage. Continuing the resection until the patellar surfaces are altered, as by open shaving methods, is contraindicated. In fact, two of 11 patients in whom a knife blade plus shave were used had poor results.

Second-look arthroscopies have demonstrated that, even in the early cases, the Intra-articular Shaver has been remarkably efficient in producing uniformly satisfactory results, even in inexperienced hands.

The question of how long to continue the shaving is difficult to determine in any one case. In general, the articular shaving will probably seem inadequate. It was not designed to cut deep down into patellar surfaces. All the material that can be removed by both curetting and oscillating motion should be taken out. Also, the patellar lesion ought to be shaved from at least two different portals. Parapatellar synovium should also be resected.

At the present time I have some reservations about using even the cutter on the patella. It may be too aggressive and resect more deeply into patellar surfaces and normal hyaline cartilage than is necessary. I use it carefully to trim sharp edges.

There is a question of whether lavage of loose bodies and conservative measures would be just as effective in severe chondromalacia. Prior to the advent of the Intra-articular Shaver, I used lavage of loose bodies in two patients who returned a year later with recurrent synovitis and symptoms. Both these patients underwent an intra-articular shave of the patella and have had complete remission of symptoms since that time.

It has been suggested that chondromalacia of the patella occurs with compression syndrome and/or malalignment. If those problems are addressed surgically, then there is remission of the symptoms of the chondromalacia and no need for intra-articular shaving or debridement of the patella. But this has not been true in my experience.

Arthroscopic surgery of the knee

Three patients in my initial series had subluxation of the patella and were candidates for an intra-articular shave of the patella, plus a lateral release. The patients refused the lateral release because of the increased chance of it producing morbidity over the patellar shave alone. Those three patients had excellent results, yet their malalignment was not treated surgically.

A 16-year-old white girl had subluxation of the patella with some fissures seen in the patellar surface at the time of surgery. Only a lateral release was performed because the patellar surface had some small fissures and no tissue was available for intra-articular shave (Fig. 17-11, A and B). The patient had no further symptoms of subluxation. Four months later there was marked crepitus, effusion, and discomfort in the patella. A second-look arthroscopy demonstrated severe chondromalacia of the patella with a crab-meat appearance (Fig. 17-11, C and D). She underwent local anesthesia and intra-articular shave of the patella, which resulted in marked diminution of her crepitus and pain and reduced her symptoms.

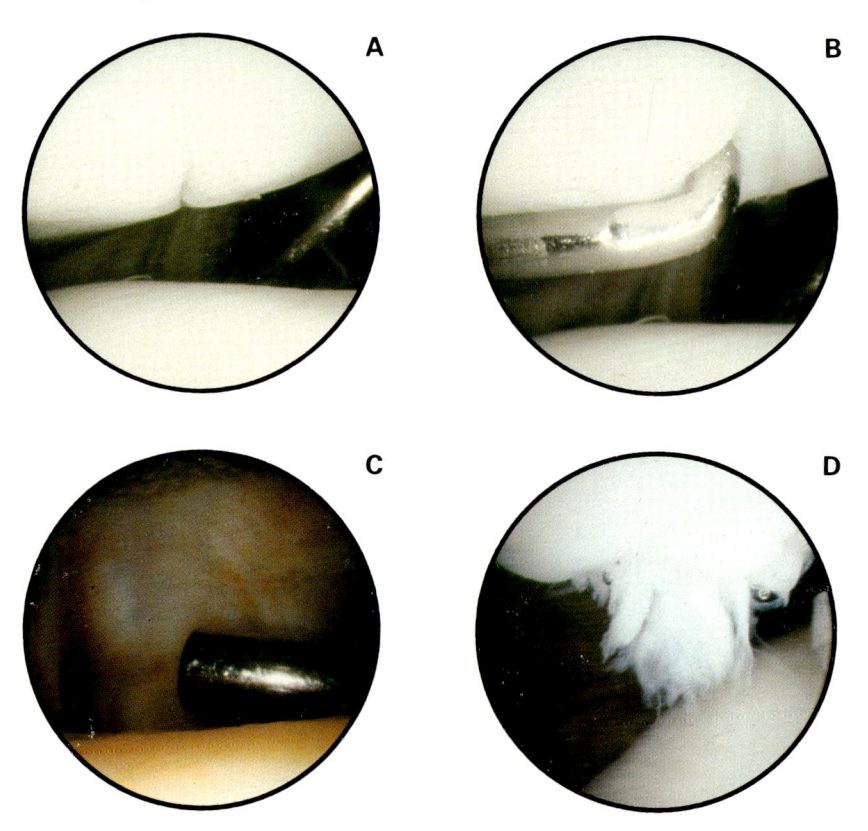

FIG. 17-11

A Small crack or defect in articular cartilage in patient with subluxation at time of lateral release.
B Probe palpation of small defects in articular cartilage. Patellar shave was not performed.
C Repeat arthroscopic view at 4 months showing healed defect of lateral release.
D Subsequent severe chondromalacia of patella, symptomatic even after lateral release. The fissures progressed to gross degeneration in 4 months, even though the patella was realigned.

Patellar surgery

Dislocation of the patella is different. We had one patient who had dislocation of the patella and three subsequent dislocations within a year. I misinterpreted the initial diagnosis and did only a patellar shave. In spite of the fact that he sustained three subsequent known dislocations, which occurred on a trampoline, the last of which became clinically and easily recognizable, there was no further injury to the patellar surface. At that time the patient chose to have treatment by conventional methods, and a realignment procedure was performed (Fig. 17-12).

Many patients in the series had only open realignment surgery. Therefore it seems that realignment procedures alone without treating the patellar abnormality are not sufficient. The loose debris should be removed to reduce the patient's symptoms and promote healing. Although not recommended, treatment of the patellar surface alone in lateral compression syndrome removed symptoms in three patients.

I believe that the dislocated patella should have whatever realignment procedure is necessary, as well as a patellar shave.

There were 13 patients in my original series who had a previous open shave of the patella by arthrotomy. Their orthopedist referred them for intra-articular shave. Eleven of those 13 patients were improved by debridement of the parapatellar area affected by synovitis and the fibrosis and scar about the joint and the removal of whatever debris there was on the patellar surface. None of these patients has had any abnormality of the femoral surface as yet.

Two of the original 13 patients were not improved and therefore considered in the poor result group. They did not worsen, and neither required a patellectomy.

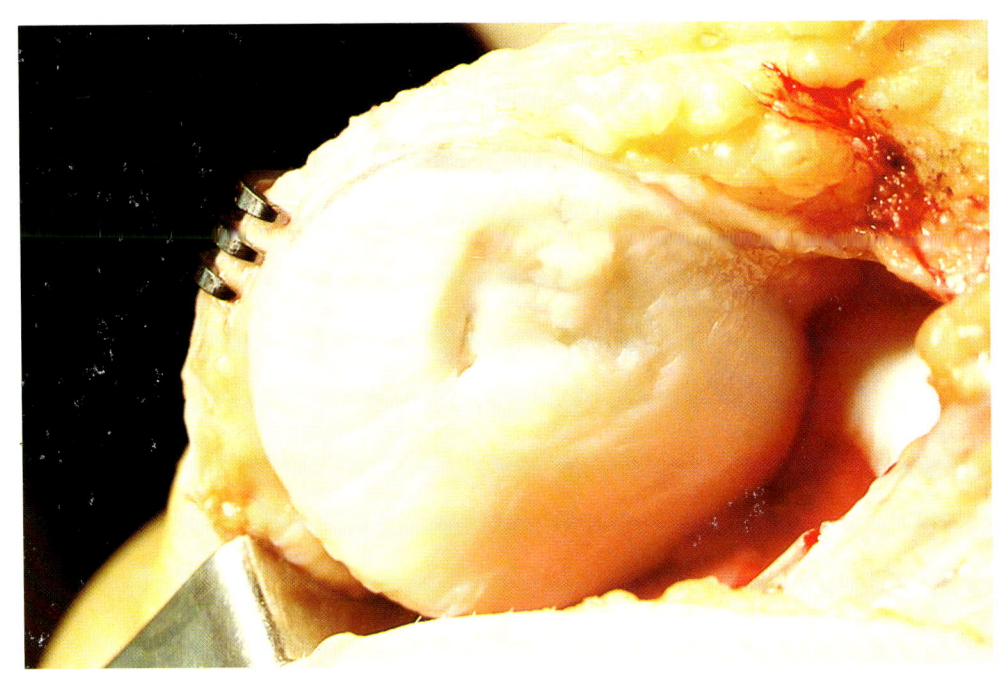

FIG. 17-12. Gross anatomic specimen at time of conventional realignment procedure. Patella shows healed defect 11 months following intra-articular shave of patella.

Arthroscopic surgery of the knee

POST OPERATIVE PATIENT INFORMATION
INTRAARTICULAR SHAVING CHONDROPLASTY

Your operation was performed by arthroscopic methods. The interior of your joint was visualized with a small telescope. The diagnosis was established and the appropriate surgery was performed with special micro-instruments.

DRESSING: A soft dressing has been applied to your knee. This compression dressing should be confortable and absorb any leakage of fluid and/or blood. Although the dressing may become moist or blood stained, this is not usually a cause for alarm. We have not experience any hemorrhage or excessive bleeding in our patients.

The dressing may be removed safely at anytime. Routinely, the dressing is removed the day after surgery, and the appropriate number of bandaids are applied. The bandaids may be utilized over the next several days.

PAIN: Upon discharge you should secure a prescription for pain medication. Usually this will be an analgesic with **codiene**. Please inform us of any known drug allergy. **Codiene** may produce nausea and/or a fine skin rash. In that case, the medication should be discontinued and our office contacted for an alternate medication. The application of an ice pac to the knee will decrease swelling and discomfort in the first 48 hours. Please do not use aspirin, as it may increase bleeding in the first few days.

WOUNDS: The small points of entry may be sore and develop bruising over the next several days. This bruising will eventually disappear and does not require any special care.

BATHING: The sensation of "splashing" of fluid in the joint is not a cause for concern. It represents residual fluids from surgery, and they will absorb. It will be safe to shower 48 hours following surgery. Bathing or soaking should be delayed for several days. Cleansing of the skin adjacent to the small wounds with soap and water may be performed with the first dressing change.

ACTIVITY: Crutches may be necessary for comfort in the first week following surgery. You may step upon your surgical leg when comfortable. Active motion and tightening of quadricep muscles (the muscles on front of the thigh) should start the day of surgery. A twice a day activity (10-15 min.) for motion and muscle contraction should continue through three weeks.

Swimming and bicycling are permissable as tolerated. Jogging, running, or stop and go sports should be deferred for 6 or 8 weeks. Heavy weight lifting should be delayed for 4 months.

If a severe arthritic condition exists, then crutch use will be longer and activity modification recommended.

RESULTS: Preliminary reports as well as our experience have shown arthroscopic surgery produces results equal to, if not better than surgery performed by open, conventional methods. The benefits are in less discomfort, risk, and scarring for the patient.

We frequently remind patients that although the external incisions are small, they still have had an operative procedure inside their joint. Experience has shown that internal healing takes several weeks. In fact, complete healing to mature tissue may take three months. At that time, most patients have a decrease in pain and swelling.

PRECAUTIONS: If you develop any fever ($101°$ F or above), unexpected pain, redness, or swelling in your legs, please contact our office for consultation or examination.
TELEPHONE (517) 351-7450.

Thank you,
Lanny L. Johnson, M.D.

FIG. 17-13. Patient information sheet. (Color code: green; see p. 245.)

Patellar surgery

The success of the Intra-articular Shaver is based on several principles. The natural history of chondromalacia has been compressed into 20 or 30 minutes of surgical time. Any loose or articular debris is vacuumed from the joint; any potential debris is excised from the patella. The resulting synovitis is eliminated, the reactive parapatellar synovitis is excised, and the contour of the patella is not altered beyond that which the disease has already produced. This procedure eliminates the morbidity possible with an arthrotomy. The articular surface heals with fibrocartilage. The rehabilitation of the quadriceps musculature is enhanced.

Patellofemoral degeneration

When there is degenerative change on the patellofemoral joint at its articulation, the prognosis is worse and the patient should be so informed. These patients usually complain not only of crepitus but also of a pain deep to their patellar tendon. Flexion and extension produce greater crepitus than when there are patellar alterations alone. These may be seen in patients who have had patellar compression syndromes. When the patient has just patellar changes and no compartmental alterations, I can perform intra-articular shaves. It does necessitate resecting a considerble part of the tongue of the fat pad to see the femoral side. The meniscus cutter is used to debride the femoral side because there is more tenacious articular surface along the edges.

These patients' conditions can be improved, but the results are not as satisfactory as in patients who have only patellar abnormalities. My follow-up has not been adequate enough to classify these patients.

Postoperative management

Following an intra-articular shave, the patient is given the postoperative patient instruction sheet (Fig. 17-13). Morbidity is minimal.

My earliest postoperative second-look arthroscopy has been at 1 month. It showed excellent healing and regeneration of articular cartilage from articular cartilage to fibrocartilage. This may occur, of course, prior to 1 month after surgery. These patients generally have a remarkable relief from pain, crepitus,

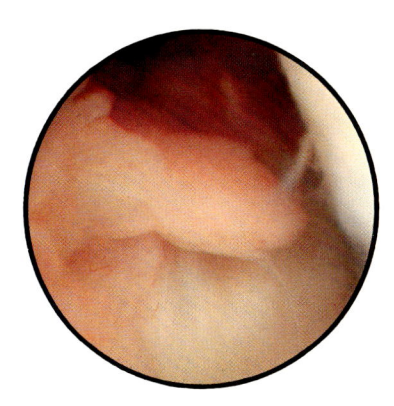

FIG. 17-14. Arthroscopic view of synovial tag adjacent to lateral inflow tract site. It was painful and catching and was resected under local anesthesia.

and effusion. I have been restricting vigorous sports for approximately 2 months until there is complete healing. Most patients can return to bicycling or swimming and less vigorous activities within a week. We certainly have recommended that they stay away from progressive weight lifting until at least 3 months and maybe longer, depending on the severity of the lesion. One patient had a synovial tag at the inflow cannula site that required resection (Fig. 17-14).

LATERAL RELEASE

The present indication for a lateral release is a clinically identifiable subluxation of the patella, including a "grimace" sign; clinical symptomatology with x-ray evidence of a lateral sitting patella or a lateral compression syndrome; acute single traumatic dislocation of the patella; and recurrent dislocation of the patella in selected patients.

I have not routinely recommended arthroscopic lateral release in patients who are over 30 years of age or who have patella alta, recurrent congenital dislocation, or fixed degenerative changes in the patella and femoral articulation. Patients with knee pain but no positive clinical, x-ray, or arthroscopic findings should not have this procedure.

The ideal patient has subluxation of the patella without clinical or x-ray evidence of dislocation, with or without chondromalacia. If chondromalacia exists, I combine the patellar shave and the lateral release. Approximately half the patients with lateral sitting patellas shown on x-ray examination have undergone lateral release. In younger patients the patella has returned to the correct position, as shown on the x-ray film (Fig. 17-16). However, there are those whose symptoms have improved but show no improvement radiographically. Therefore I hesitate to do a lateral release in patients who are in the older age groups or those who already have evidence of loss of patellofemoral articulation with degenerative changes, in spite of the fact that they do have subluxation.

For those patients with recurrent congenital dislocation of the patella I advise that lateral release could provide relief from their recurrent dislocations. They must understand that a conventional realignment procedure may be necessary and that the arthroscopic surgery should not be considered the final treatment in that particular condition.

Although lateral release may remove the chance of any further dislocation, there is a sense of insecurity in the absence of the medial repair. Patients must understand that there is a risk of less than total satisfaction. They run the risk of recurrent dislocation. If they understand that, then we can proceed with lateral release as the initial treatment.

Postoperative management

Patients who have had a lateral release are given a yellow postoperative information sheet to instruct them of possible morbidity. Every effort is made to reduce their discomfort. The preincision injection of 0.25% marcaine, intermittent tourniquet release, ice bags, compression dressing, splinting, and narcotic prescription all are directed toward that purpose. (See Chapter 15.)

Patellar surgery

No effort has been made to reduce the hematoma or swelling by electrocoagulation or suction drainage. The persistent effusion may have some benefit. It distracts the edges of the lateral release while the area is resurfaced with synovium. This occurs prior to 2 months after surgery, as confirmed by arthroscopy.

At 3 weeks after surgery the swelling diminishes and activity of flexion and extension is easier. By 6 weeks the swelling is greatly diminished, but the return to normalcy usually takes about 3 months.

This procedure produces no palpable defects or synovial herniations. Care should be taken not to violate the subcutaneous tissue. Although performed through small puncture wounds, this is still a 4- to 6-inch arthrotomy. The patient should be advised that the swelling and edema are greater than those which accompany open surgery. Because of this I do not recommend bilateral lateral releases.

Complications

There has been no incidence of infection or thrombophlebitis in my patients. There have been a number of patients with a significant hematoma (Fig. 17-15). One even had subcutaneous extravasation of blood with inflammation, but this subsided with rest and time. No antibiotics were necessary. There were no patients with restriction of motion. It is interesting that three patients with subluxation became dislocators after lateral release and required open medial imbrication.

Fig. 17-16 illustrates a case history of reconstructive procedures for dislocation of the patella, severe injury to the articular surface, and marked changes on the patellofemoral joint.

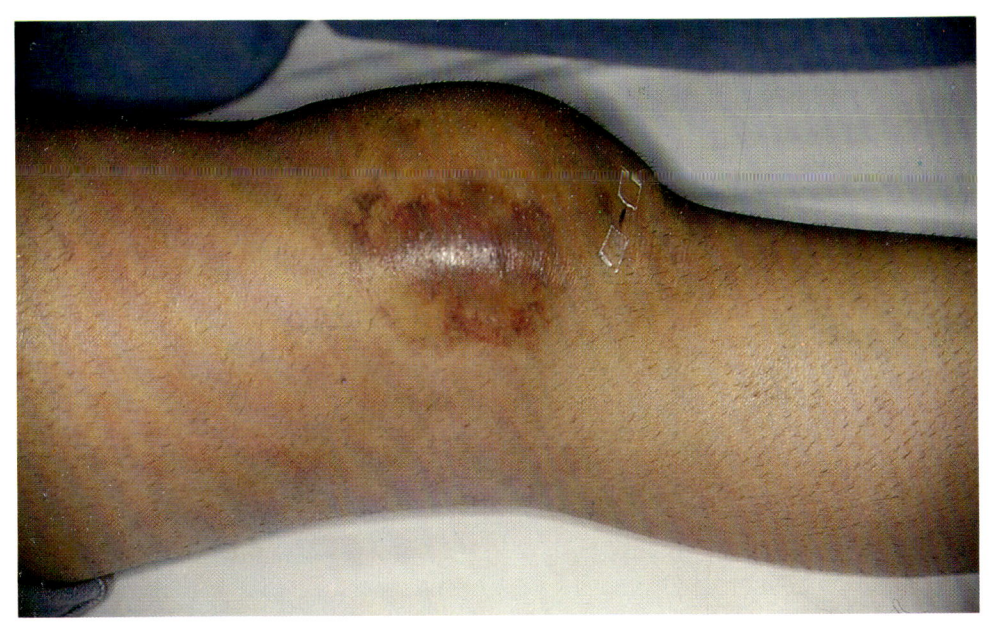

FIG. 17-15. One week after lateral release with large area hematoma and erythema. Worst of postoperative swelling in our series subsided with rest and time.

Arthroscopic surgery of the knee

CASE REPORT

A 26-year-old white man had pain, swelling, and marked crepitus following a conventional reconstructive procedure for dislocation of the patella. Severe patellofemoral changes then developed. Arthroscopic chondroplasty was performed. The femoral involvement worsened the prognosis, but the patient was greatly improved.

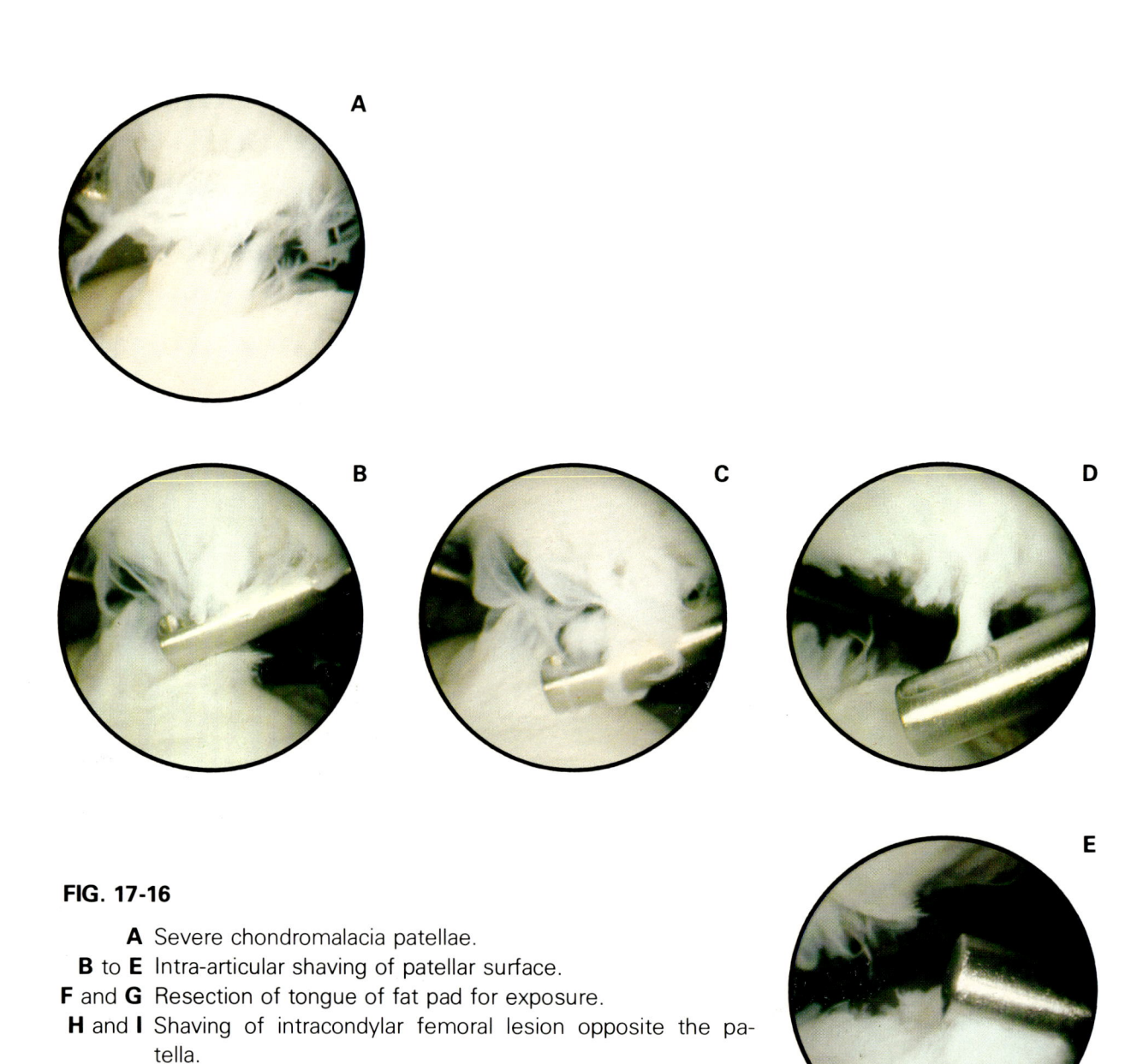

FIG. 17-16

- **A** Severe chondromalacia patellae.
- **B to E** Intra-articular shaving of patellar surface.
- **F and G** Resection of tongue of fat pad for exposure.
- **H and I** Shaving of intracondylar femoral lesion opposite the patella.
- **J and K** View of patellofemoral surface after arthroscopic shave.

← Completed resection →

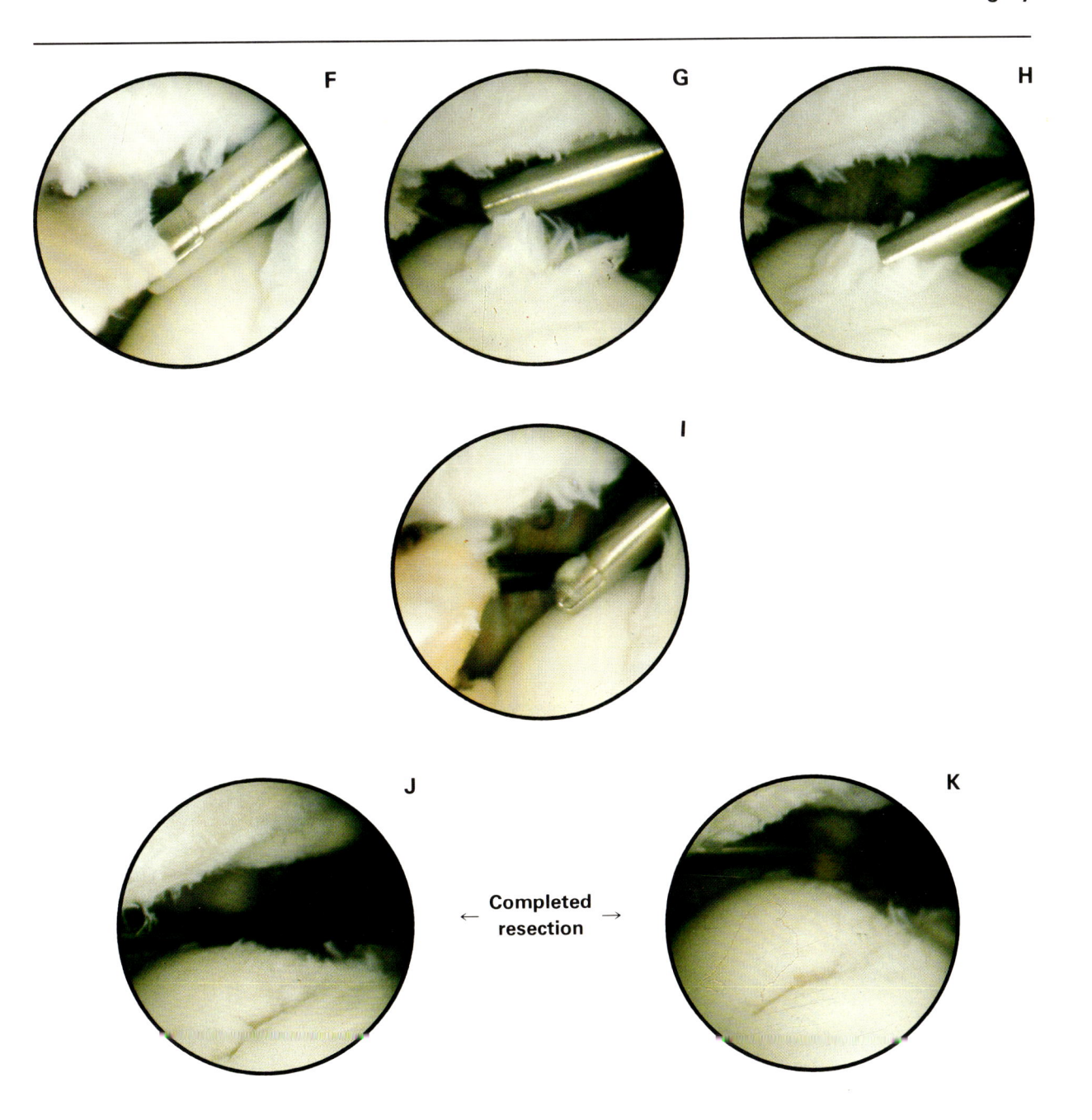

REFERENCES

1. Abernathy, P. J., Townsend, R. R., Rose, R. M., and Rudin, E. L.: Is chondromalacia patellae a separate clinical entity? J. Bone Joint Surg. (Br.) **60**:205, 1978.
2. Bandi, W., and Brennwald, J.: The significance of femoropatellar pressure in the pathogenesis and treatment of chondromalacia patellae and femoropatellar arthrosis. In Ingwersen, O. S., et al., editors: The knee joint, New York, 1974, American Elsevier Publishers, Inc.
3. Bently, G.: Chondromalacia patellae, J. Bone Joint Surg. (Am.) **52**:221, 1970.
4. Ficat, R. P., and Hungerford, D. S.: Disorders of the patellofemoral joint, Baltimore, 1977, The Williams & Wilkins Co.
5. Gradisar, I. A., Jr.: Personal communication, 1979.
6. Insall, J.: Chondromalacia patellae: patellar malalignment syndrome, Orthop. Clin. North Am. **10**:117, 1979.
7. Wiles, P., Andrews, P. S., and Devas, M. B.: Chondromalacia patellae, J. Bone Joint Surg. (Br.) **38**:95, 1976.

Chapter 18

Chondral conditions

Indications for treatment
Loose bodies
Osteochondritis dissecans
Condylar defects
Chondronecrosis
Degenerative arthritis with compartmental loss and deformity
All-compartment shave

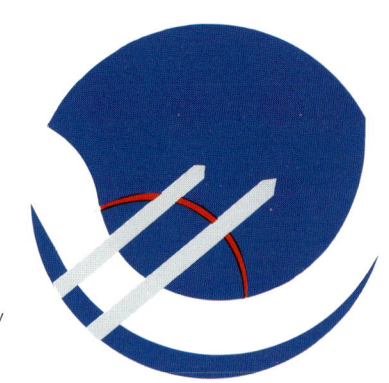

For the most part, chondral conditions such as degenerative arthritis, chondronecrosis, traumatic arthritis, and osteochondritis dissecans were generally ignored in knee joint surgery except as an explanation for less than optimal results. Prior to the development of arthroscopy it was possible to clinically palpate large osteophytes and to see smaller ones by x-ray examination. These changes represented a rather significant long-term alteration in the articular surface. The view of the articular cartilage at the time of meniscectomy was limited to the side of the arthrotomy and virtually ignored on the opposite side. Because of limited visualization possibilities, many patients, following arthrotomy, carried effusion even after "clean" meniscectomy. This was due to overlooked or subsequent articular changes. If the degenerative changes in compartmental alterations were severe enough, patients underwent a high tibial osteotomy. Empirical conclusions were drawn that the lateral compartment was adequate, after examination of standing AP x-ray films. Others have undergone so-called total-knee replacements for "severe degenerative changes." These decisions were made without the benefit of arthroscopy.

INDICATIONS FOR TREATMENT

The technique of arthroscopy has greatly increased the awareness and respect for articular cartilage changes on the condylar surfaces. Because of the microscopic view, it is possible to see even the most early alterations of the skin of the articular surfaces. A more specific prognostic sign or specific diagnosis can be rendered and a more conservative rehabilitation program instituted for the benefit of the patient. Arthroscopy provides a way of monitoring severe articular defects that have been either curetted or drilled, as previously advocated, until there is sufficient healing to allow increased weight bearing and activity. It is possible, also, to monitor arthroscopically the healing of osteochondritis dissecans or even remove transcutaneous loose pieces. Loose bodies associated with degenerative change can either be vacuumed or removed by forceps under local anesthesia by transcutaneous arthroscopic control.

Experience with the Intra-articular Shaver on the condylar surface of the

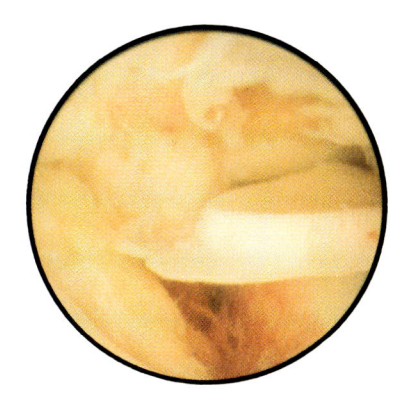

FIG. 18-1. Full-thickness defect not down into bone.

femur and the tibia with severe chondromalacia has shown similar benefits on a patella.

Articular injury may be overlooked at conventional arthrotomy. The palpating finger under the patella or a cursory look to the lateral compartment does not compare with comprehensive arthroscopy. Partially detached articular cartilage, even loose bodies, can be shaved or vacuumed from a joint at the time of arthroscopic surgery (Fig. 18-1). This eliminates the necessity of removal by synovial mechanisms, and therefore less synovitis and postoperative morbidity can be expected.

Articular abrasion or even full-thickness loss of articular cartilage accompanies most types of meniscal tears, especially those with anterior cruciate ligament injury. Acute dislocation of the patella often traumatizes the patella and leaves a loose body off the lateral femoral condyle. Direct trauma to the patella or femoral condyles may crack or avulse articular cartilage. The lesions vary in location, depth, and size.

The articular surfaces are best inspected by arthroscopy. The lesions can be shaved or even repaired by arthroscopic surgery. No longer should a primary diagnosis be accepted without a complete search and treatment of any and all coexisting articular cartilage injuries.

Second-look arthroscopy and clinical evaluation have revealed healing after treatment of these superficial lesions in younger people by intra-articular shave without drilling to bleeding surface. This somewhat dismisses the need for violation of the osseous tissue to bring in the blood supply. In fact, when the osseous tissue is drilled or curetted, second-look arthroscopy has demonstrated a rather pliable, irregular base and retarded healing. (See Fig. 11-3, D.) In some instances multiple drill holes into the femoral condyles of a younger person have caused them to remain symptomatic for over a year. Radioisotope uptake studies of the knee demonstrated increased vascularity in the area of drilling. The increased activity is indicative of the unnecessary overdrilling and reparative process.

At this time, I do not advocate deep drilling curetting into the osseous tissue for degeneration of fibrocartilage. Hyaline cartilage injuries treated only by intra-articular shaving on the condyles will heal except in elderly people who have marked sclerotic changes with compartmental loss. Even those patients may be rendered clinically asymptomatic through abrading the exposed bone. Cartilaginous resurfacing occurs within 2 months.

If one chooses to drill on the femoral condyle or tibial plateau, the drilling need not be more than 1 mm to bring vascularity to that area. In fact, it should not be deeper, since it produces trauma to the subchondral bone, subsequent microscopic fractures, and increased morbidity. The application of this same technique to injured articular surfaces has produced microscopic evidence of vascularity. This readily occurs in a resurfaced, healing, full-thickness lesion. It also occurs in partial-thickness lesions. This suggests (in vivo) that there is subchondral penetration of vascularity in articular cartilage injury and even in partial-thickness or healing lesions.

It certainly is not necessary to drill or curette deep defects down into the condyles; in fact, it is contraindicated except in cases of osteonecrosis when the defect is being removed or drilling across an osteochondritic lesion.

LOOSE BODIES

Loose bodies can be radiopaque and radiolucent. Both radiopaque and radiolucent loose bodies can exist in the same patient. They can be removed arthroscopically. Therefore any patient who has x-ray evidence of a radiopaque loose body at the time of arthroscopy should have a search made for other loose bodies that may not have been radiopaque. Loose bodies are most often found in the lateral sulcus and in the posterolateral compartment. In addition, other occult areas are under either menisci or along the medial sulcus of the suprapatellar pouch.

It is important to have a sterile loose body instrument set available in the operating room. (See Appendix.) The size of some of the loose bodies necessitates significant arthrotomy to remove the material. The large loose bodies are grasped preferably with the large Jaws forceps. This may be performed under local anesthesia. Infiltration of the removal area is necessary. A No. 15 knife blade widens the skin and the capsule as tension is applied to extract the loose body. Usually a loose body can be removed through an incision smaller than the size of the loose body itself (Fig. 18-2). Still, some will require a capsular suture or subcutaneous suture with paper tape. The small percutaneous puncture wounds for cannulas do not require suturing.

The technique of removal of loose bodies is to deliver the material to a space where it is easily manipulated and removed from the joint. Second, it is important to remove the smaller loose bodies first to reduce any leakage from the larger arthrotomy that would result in loss of distension during attempts to retrieve the smaller pieces.

Loose bodies can be manipulated manually from the posterolateral compartment into the anterior compartment or from one of the other sulci, up into the suprapatellar pouch, or preferably into the intercondylar notch area, and removed one after another.

Small loose bodies may be removed by just vacuuming or suctioning from the joint, even with the arthroscope in place (Fig. 18-3). Larger ones can be

Chondral conditions

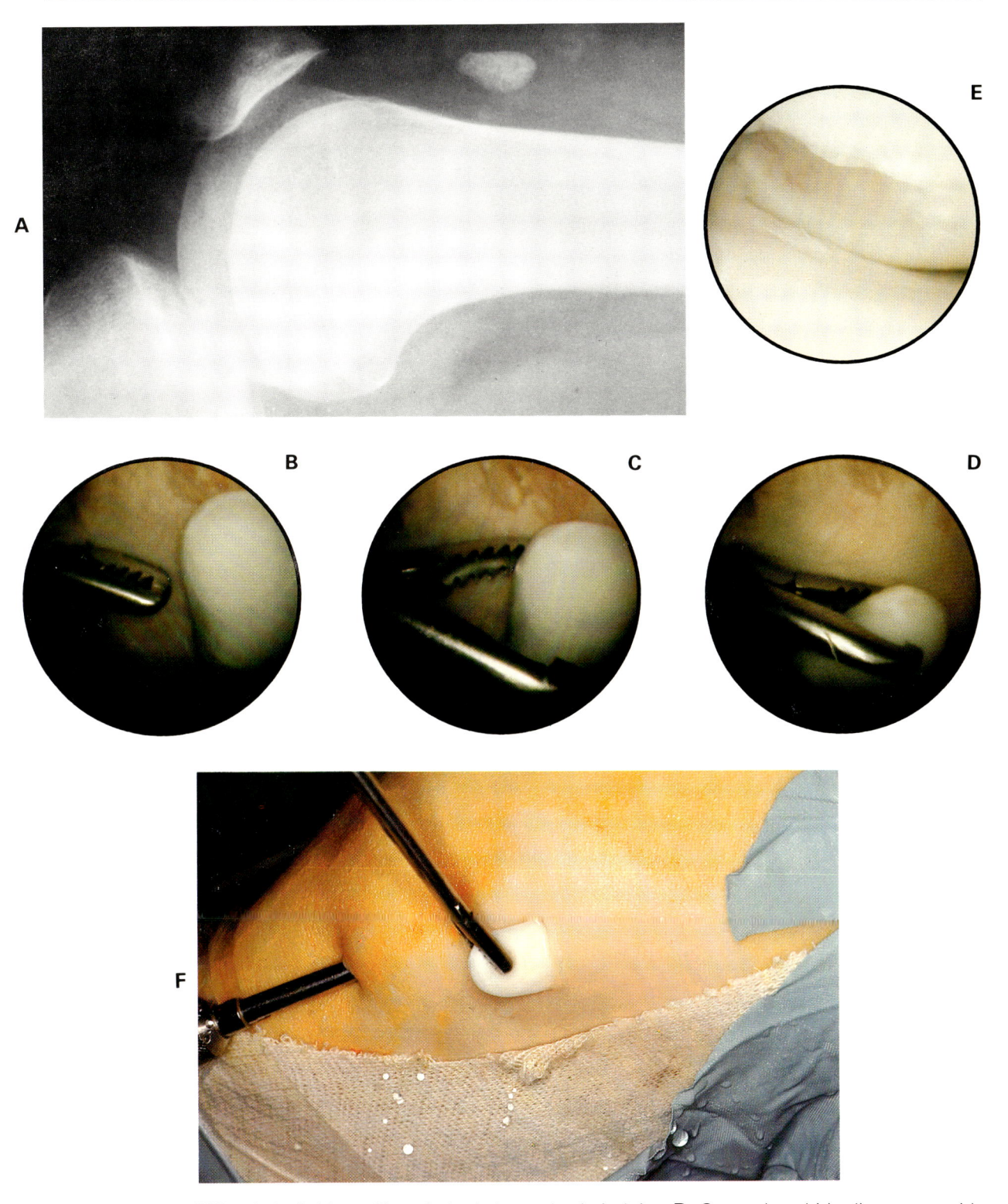

FIG. 18-2. A, X-ray film of single loose body in joint. **B,** Osteochondritis dissecans with healing, probably after more than 3 months since there is no vascularity in bed. **C,** Forceps approaching loose body. **D,** Forceps grasping loose body. **E,** Removal of loose body. **F,** Transcutaneous removal of loose body through incision smaller than mass of loose body.

Arthroscopic surgery of the knee

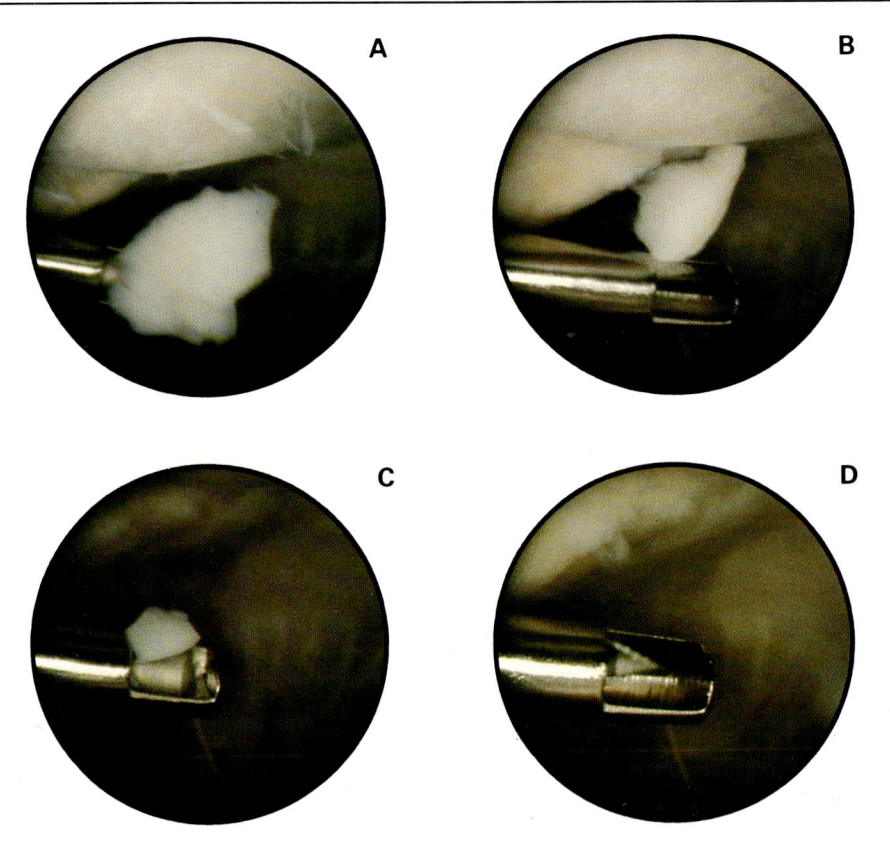

FIG. 18-3

A Loose body being attracted by suction of Intra-articular Shaver.
B Resection initiated by Intra-articular Shaver System.
C Most of loose body has been resected and is sucked from joint.
D Loose body completely removed.

vacuumed from the joint through the arthroscopic cannula. Others that are soft but larger can be removed by the Intra-articular Shaver or Cutter, which reduces their size and clears them away by resection (Fig. 18-3, *A* and *B*). The loose body is tethered by suction in front of the window of the Intra-articular Shaver and Cutter, which subsequently remove it without difficulty. The Intra-articular Shaver's blunt head, with the sucker at the side, is good for passing under and over the menisci and into the posterior compartment to remove loose bodies that cannot be grasped with forceps.

One of the problems in using forceps to grab loose bodies is that it is very much like squeezing a watermelon seed. The loose body can move away if there is no suction; hence the preference for Intra-articular Shaver removal of the smaller and more viable loose bodies.

Loose bodies that are somewhat large or remote, for example, in the posterolateral compartment, can be manipulated into the anterior compartment by external pressure on the knee. Manipulation forward permits placing either a needle into the loose body or "spooning" with a curette. The forceps are applied after the loose body is in the anterior chamber.

In some patients, loose bodies have been attached to the synovium adja-

Chondral conditions

cent to the femoral condyles and/or the patella, necessitating sectioning prior to resection and removal. A large loose body may be broken prior to removal.

I have treated two patients with multiple loose bodies, or rice bodies, not related to rheumatoid or traumatic arthritis. My suspicion was that the patient had a form of osteochondromatosis, but that could not be identified. Arthroscopic lavage of loose bodies in two separate incidences, 1 year apart, rendered the patient asymptomatic. The presence of hundreds of loose bodies increases the suspicion of synovial osteochondromatosis, which would necessitate further synovial resection as well. This may be performed arthroscopically.

With a Needlescope I have visualized a posterolateral loose body that could not be moved to the anterior compartment. I saw that it was attached and not movable in the anterior compartment operating and moving from posterolateral. The loose body was grasped with the forceps, and the arthroscope was then removed. An incision was made into the posterolateral compartment transcutaneously, following the course of the forceps to procure and deliver the loose body.

In another instance a patient had a loose body in the posterolateral compartment. It was visualized in the popliteus sheath with the Needlescope. With the patient under local anesthesia I then changed to the larger diameter rodlens scope to see if it could be retrieved through the scope itself, but it was not possible to suck the loose body out of the popliteus sheath. At that time I elected, with the patient's permission, to retract the telescope a few millimeters up the cannula. This caught the loose body in the popliteus sheath with the cannula. While I was viewing the loose body, it was pushed out of the popliteus sheath into the popliteus musculature. Thus I avoided a rather large arthrotomy to retrieve the loose body. Some loose bodies naturally become extrasynovial and asymptomatic, as in this patient.

OSTEOCHONDRITIS DISSECANS

Osteochondritis dissecans is not necessarily limited to persons under age 20. I have treated several patients over 20. Osteochondritis dissecans can be treated arthroscopically. Every attempt should be made to reconstitute the joint, especially near the weight-bearing surface in young people. Guhl[3] has more experience than others, and he has advocated drilling by transcutaneous methods, including curettage of the subchondral granulation tissue and subchondral bone grafts. My experience is limited to the fixation and drilling of osteochondritic defects (Fig. 18-4). There have been some situations in which it has been impossible to accomplish anything but removal. The management of the osteochondritic lesion is based on its clinical appearance.

A patient who has an osteochondritic lesion with accompanying symptoms should be inspected arthroscopically. If there is no alteration of the articular surface and there is no looseness of the articular defect on palpation, then drilling a few 2-mm diameter holes in the defect just barely crossing its depth is all that is necessary. I do not immobilize these patients. They have been allowed weight bearing but no vigorous sport activities. Generally, healing evi-

Arthroscopic surgery of the knee

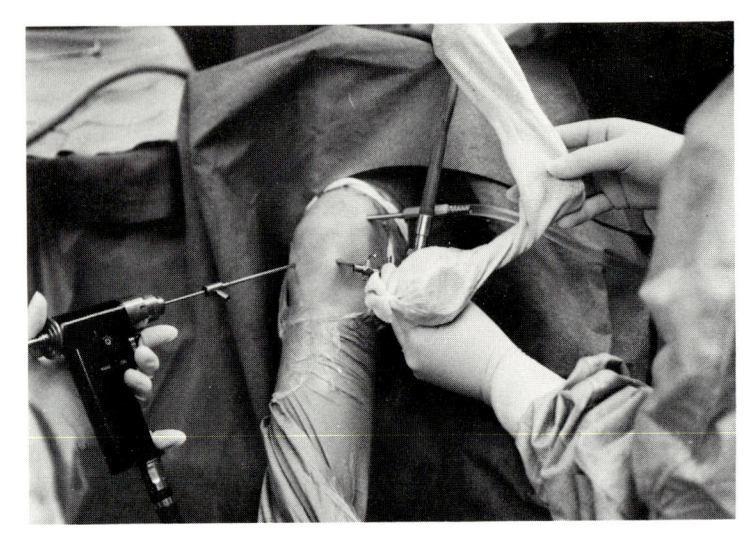

FIG. 18-4. Drilling of osteochondritic defect by arthroscopic control, and video monitoring via stockinette-covered articulated viewing device.

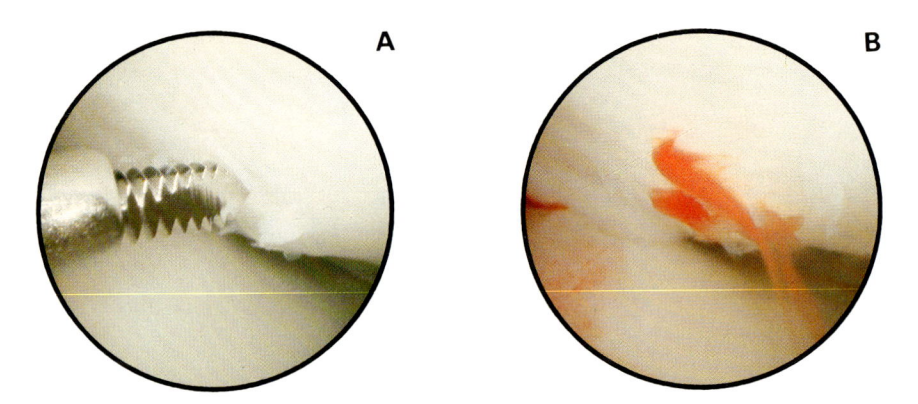

FIG. 18-5. Arthroscopic view of drilling of articular defects. **A,** Threaded pin for fixation. **B,** Tourniquet down and bleeding after multiple drilling.

dent on x-ray examination occurs between 3 and 6 months, even though the patient is asymptomatic prior to that (Fig. 18-5).

For a patient with symptomatic osteochondritic defect that at the time of visualization feels loose on palpation, I use a transfixation threaded wire brought out through the medial femoral condyle. The lesion is reduced with a 2.7-mm cannula, and pressure is applied with the cannula. The threaded Kirschner wire is placed across the defect. When the wire comes out of the skin medially, it is retrograded while the surgeon arthroscopically watches the pin disappear immediately beneath the articular surface so as not to abrade the tibia. Then four or more drill holes are placed in the articular defect to bring in the blood supply. The tourniquet can be removed at this stage, the inflow cut off, and the vacuum applied to the arthroscope to demonstrate the suction effect of drawing the vascularity into that area to confirm adequate depth of drilling. Again, the depth of drilling need not be much beyond the calculated depth of the defect itself (Fig. 18-6).

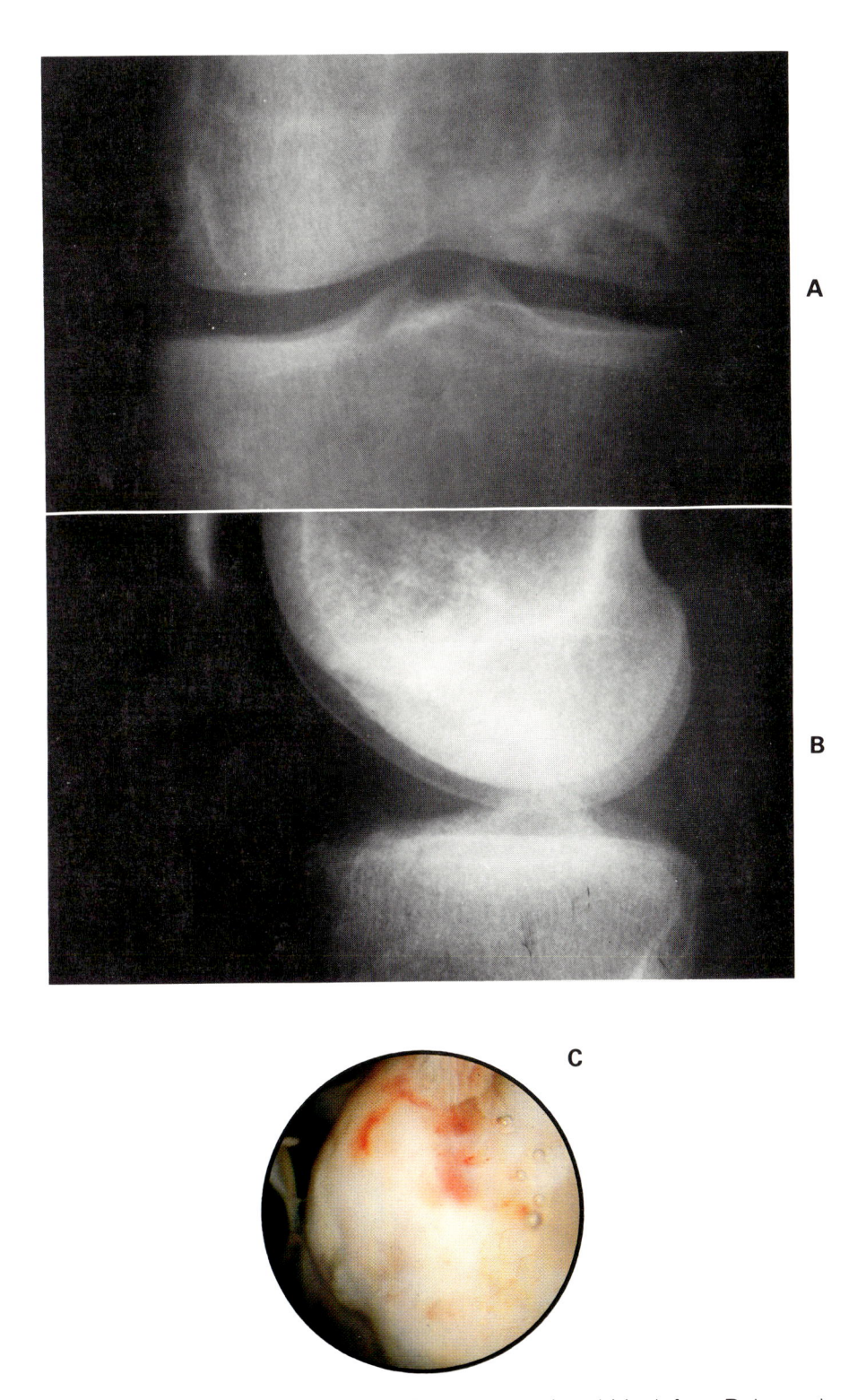

FIG. 18-6. A, Anteroposterior x-ray view of large osteochondritic defect. **B,** Lateral x-ray view of large osteochondritic defect. **C,** Six weeks after drilling and pin fixation. Revascularization and drill holes are visible.

For those patients who have an elevated and loose articular piece and who have had a defect along the edge of the articular cartilage, a similar method is used. In addition, it has been necessary to level or shave the edge of articular cartilage when reduction has not been exactly anatomic. After their transfixation, these patients are casted. After 6 weeks they return for the removal of the cast and pin and repeat arthroscopy and palpation. So far, even in large lesions, the defect has united at 6 weeks. I have had 2 patients who, although a cast was applied, have broken their cast in playing sports and then broken their pin (Fig. 18-7). In 1 patient I had to remove both fragments of the pin at 6 weeks. At that time the articular defect was completely healed, since bone removal was necessary to retrieve the pin deep in the femoral condyle.

In a second patient the pin broke at the osteochondritic portion, but the portion of the wire in the femur was sufficiently deep to the articular surface, and healing was excellent. In this patient the superficial wire was removed, and a debridement was carried out because the irregular articular and fibrocartilage healing had occurred. The patient has remained asymptomatic but is still under my observation.

I have not had experience with a completely loose articular piece that was replaced arthroscopically. I would remove those pieces which were loose with no bone on the loose piece, since they could not have resulted in any union. For technical reasons I would replace this through a small arthrotomy rather than the apparent, more laborious, task arthroscopically. The same is true for grafting. It is my opinion that just because arthroscopy is available, it should not make the cases more difficult. If the case can be done more effectively by conventional methods, then they should be chosen.

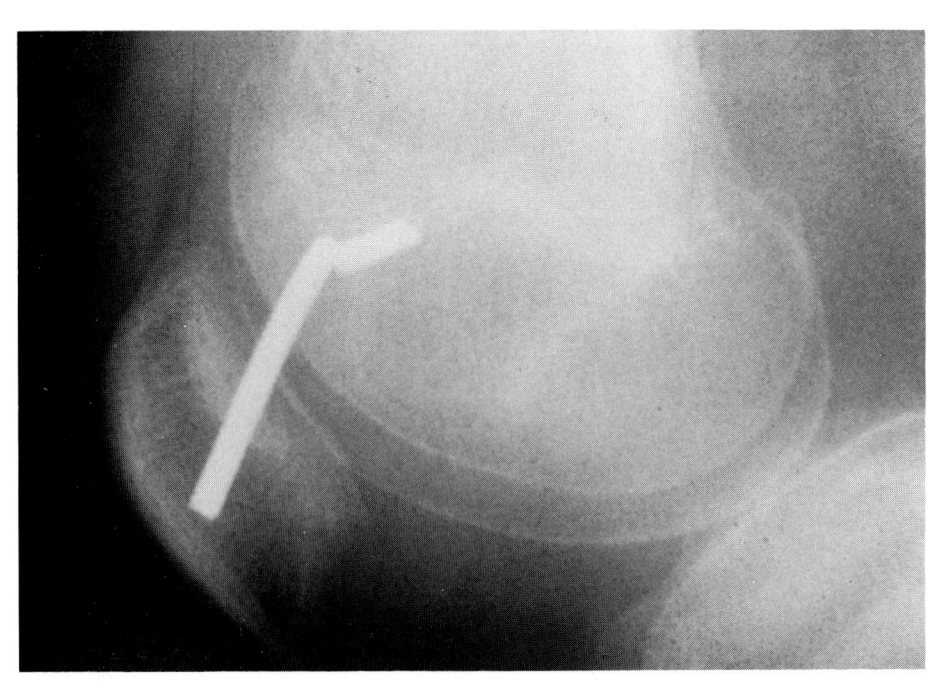

FIG. 18-7. X-ray film of fractured pin at 6 weeks, in spite of cast immobilization. It was removed.

Chondral conditions

CONDYLAR DEFECTS

Defects on the femoral condyle accompany many meniscal lesions. Condylar defects should be superficially debrided with the Intra-articular Shaver and Trimmer at the time of a meniscectomy without violating the surface deeply, but removing debris that is loose and would cause problems in the postoperative period.

I have seen a number of patients who have symptoms of a torn cartilage but actually have only articular cartilage abrasions of various sizes and shapes. The depth is partial thickness. It usually occurs only with some severe trauma or ligamentous injury (Fig. 18-8). These patients have catching and popping in their joints. They are tender along their joint line, and there is no meniscal abnormality on inspection and palpation. I have performed intra-articular shaves to debride these articular defects.

Although these patients have decreased effusion and inflammation around the knee, the symptoms of catching or popping can exist for several months.[1]

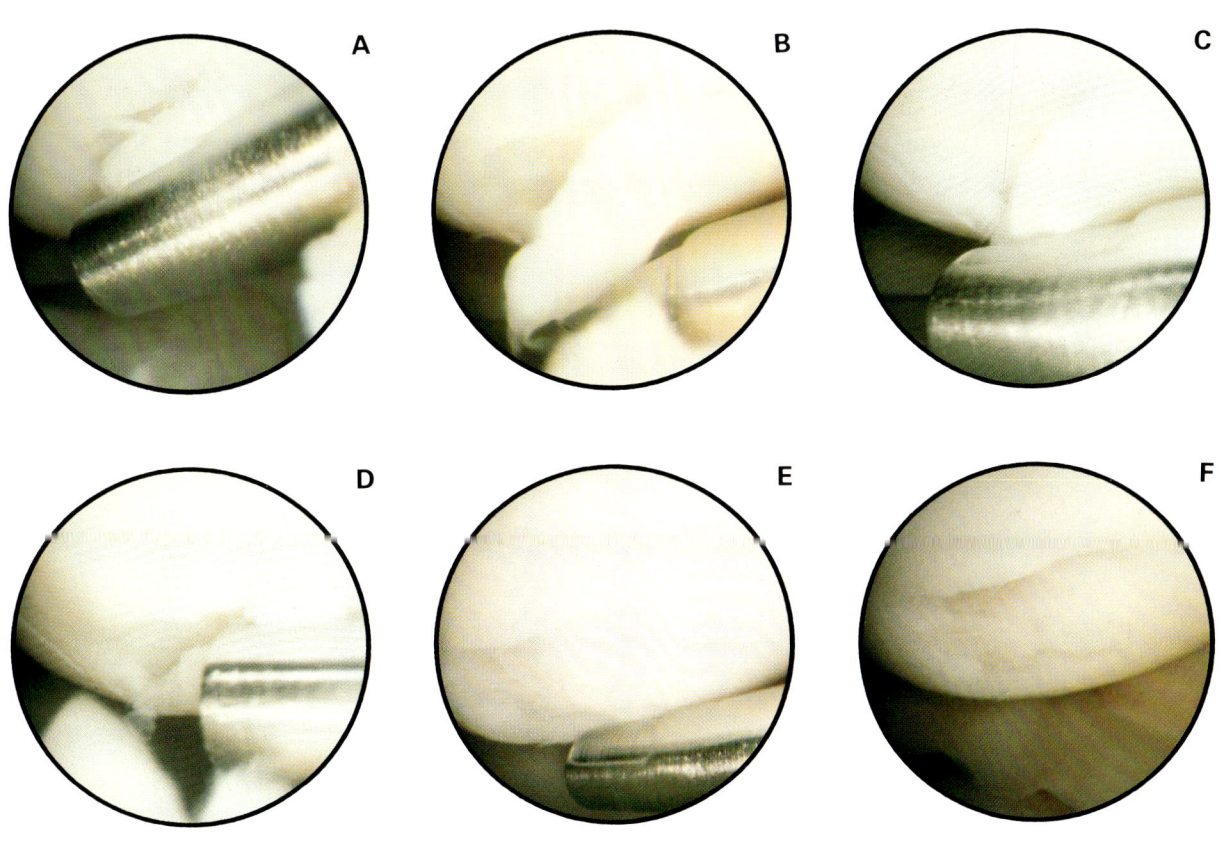

FIG. 18-8

- **A** Arthroscopic view of lesion of articular surface and Intra-articular Shaver.
- **B and C** Resection of articular cartilage with Intra-articular Shaver.
- **D** Resection near completion.
- **E** Cleaning up with Intra-articular Trimmer.
- **F** Debrided defect at finish of procedure.

Arthroscopic surgery of the knee

When I see that type of lesion, my recommendation for postoperative management is no or partial weight bearing for approximately 2 months, whether it accompanies a torn meniscus or exists independently.

The large partial-thickness articular injury has a poor prognosis. After arthroscopic shaving it may take 6 months for reduction of symptoms. The patient may complain of catching, popping, and pain with weight-bearing. It usually does not produce effusion. Second-look arthroscopy has shown a healed surface as early as 2 months, and no breakdown later. The radioactive uptake may be increased in that compartment for 4 to 6 months.

CHONDRONECROSIS

There is another type of articular cartilage abnormality, which I have termed *chondronecrosis* (Fig. 18-9). It is a superficial necrosis or chondrolysis of the articular surface, usually in the femoral condyle in an adult. It is not related to trauma, is considerably painful, has adjacent synovitis, and can mimic a torn cartilage. It is not the type of articular abnormality that occurs with a torn cartilage, and it is seen in the absence of meniscal injury. An Intra-articular Shaver debridement of the femoral condyle removes the cheese-like appearance of the superficial articular cartilage. The morbidity can be considerable.

One patient (a physician) with a mild tibia vara had immediate relief for about 2 months, but with weight bearing there was increased pain. Although he was in his 40s and had only minimal tibia vara, he was unable to work without crutches. A high tibial valgus-producing osteotomy rendered this patient asymptomatic. A second-look arthroscopy has not been carried out, and it has only been a year since his surgery. Generally, I would not have considered this type of patient an ideal candidate for high tibial osteotomy, and it would seem somewhat premature, but it was the only procedure that allowed a return to work.

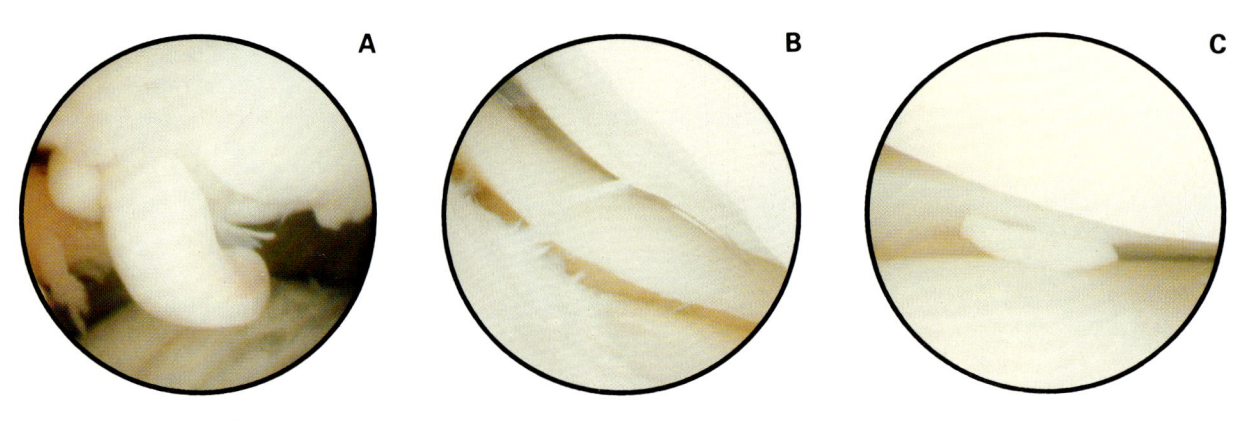

FIG. 18-9

A Severe chondronecrosis on patella and all compartments.
B Chondronecrosis on femoral condyle and tibial plateau.
C Loose body and chondronecrosis in 16-year-old boy.

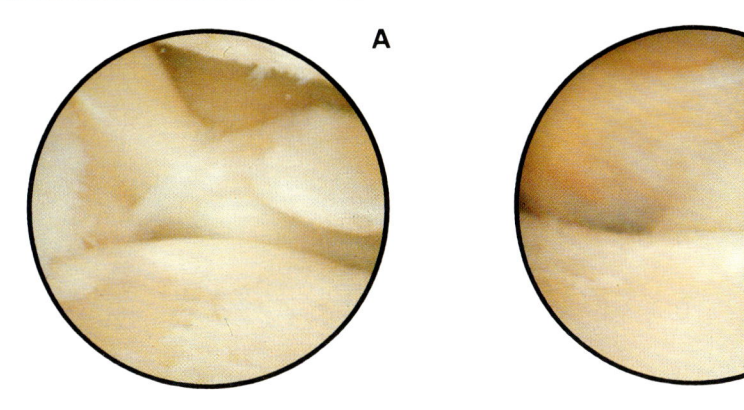

FIG. 18-10

A Right knee, lateral compartment. Complete loss of meniscus without surgery. Articular loss to bone on tibia and femoral side.

B Arthroscopic view of left knee in same patient with genu valgus. Notice relation to popliteus tendon.

DEGENERATIVE ARTHRITIS WITH COMPARTMENTAL LOSS AND DEFORMITY

I have treated a group of patients who had degenerative changes throughout either the medial or lateral compartment (Fig. 18-10) with accompanying tibia vara or associated valgus. These patients had considerable symptoms relating to the involved compartment. They had pseudo-opening of that compartment, and loss of compartmental space was seen on standing AP x-ray films.

I have performed a number of debridements, especially in the medial compartment, with a subtotal meniscectomy and selective synovectomy in that compartment both under and above the meniscus, as well as debridement of the femoral condyles. Patients have been placed on partial weight bearing from 4 to 8 weeks postoperatively. Recovery can take 6 months.

If an older patient has an erosion or loss of articular cartilage down to bone, the results have not been as satisfying as those in which debridement can be carried out with preservation of articular cartilage.[2] I have deferred high tibial osteotomy in a number of patients by intra-articular shaving and debridement of isolated compartments in this manner.

ALL-COMPARTMENT SHAVE

There are two groups of patients who have severe degenerative arthritis in all compartments of the joint. One type has only mild articular debris and mild synovitis. The second group displays diffuse reactive synovitis plus the multiple compartment degenerative change and loose bodies. The latter group does poorly with intra-articular shave; in fact, I have not had a patient yet benefit from it. When I see reactive synovitis, I advise the patient that inactivity or not working may be necessary for 6 months, and even open synovectomy and debridement may be necessary. Still, the prognosis is poor.

Patients who have multiple compartment degeneration with osteophyte formation, but no marked synovitis, have improved by multiple compartmental

Arthroscopic surgery of the knee

shaves—patellar, femoral, medial, lateral, and tibial, subtotal meniscectomies, or, in those who have already had their menisci removed, debridement of that compartment and removal of loose bodies as well. Also, it has been possible by transcutaneous methods to resect large osteophytes along the rims of the tibia to the femur. This frequently can be done with a small hand-set rongeur (Fig. 18-11). A motorized burr can help.

I have several patients with severe degenerative arthritis and multiple types of capsular transarticular ligamentous repairs who have had as many as eight knee operations and still have knee pain and effusion. The salvage procedure, an all-compartment intra-articular shave, has benefited a number of these patients by rendering them rapidly asymptomatic and allowing them to return to work and/or activities.

The long-term value of these salvage procedures with the intra-articular shave has not been determined. It is a way to avoid the trauma of multiple surgical procedures. The salvage procedure is gaining popularity with referring orthopedic surgeons, even those who have little interest in arthroscopy. They see this as a means to avoid another arthrotomy.

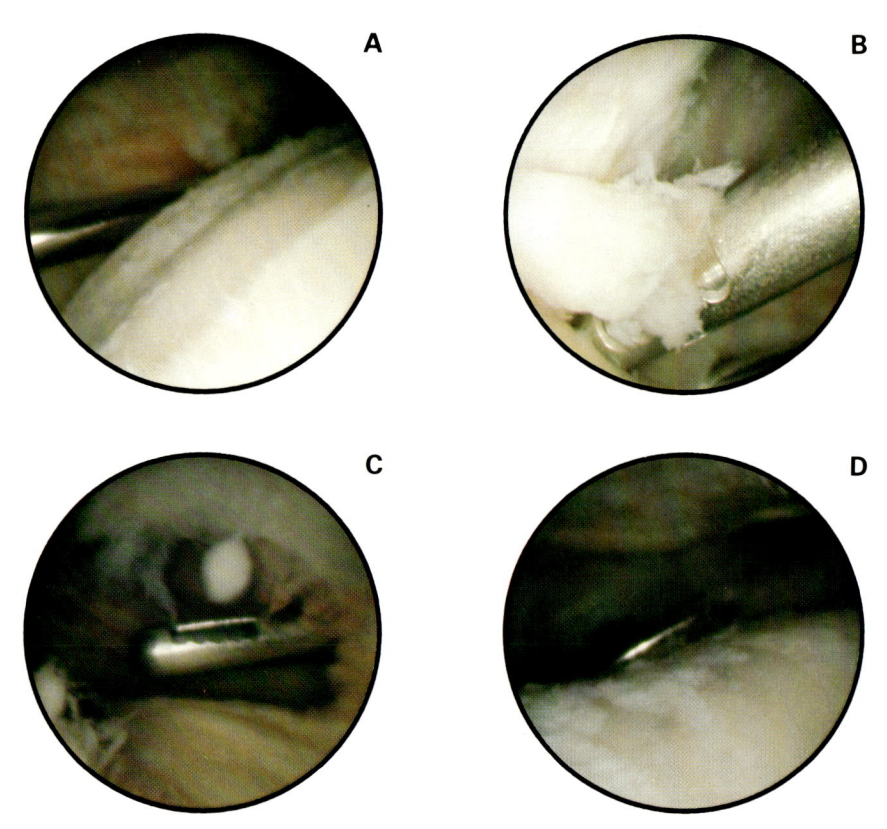

FIG. 18-11

A Arthroscopic view showing loss of articular cartilage to bone on distal femur.
B Debridement of large cartilaginous lesion of patella.
C Resection with Intra-articular Shaver System of area affected by synovitis and articular debris.
D Completion of debridement of patellofemoral joint, viewed from opposite side.

REFERENCES

1. Campbell, C. J.: The healing of cartilage defects, Clin. Orthop. **64**:45, 1969.
2. Fujisawa, Y., Marsuhara, K., and Shiomi, S.: The effect of high tibial osteotomy in osteoarthritis of the knee, Surg. Clin. North Am. **10**:585, 1979.
3. Guhl, J. F.: Arthroscopic treatment of osteochondritis dissecans—preliminary report, Orthop. Clin. North Am. July, 1979, p. 671.

Chapter 19

Extrasynovial disease

Acute tear of the anterior cruciate ligament
Chronic instabilities
Cysts
Ankylosis
Extra ossicles
Osteophytes

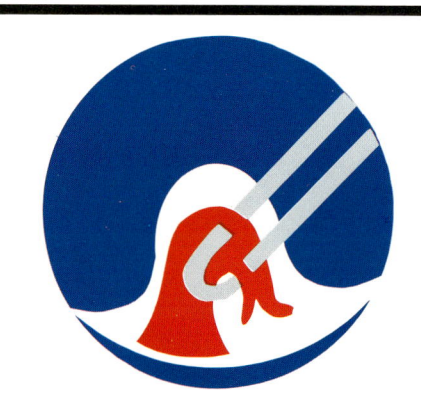

Arthroscopic surgical techniques offer no treatment at this time for ligamentous injuries or instabilities. They are limited to reducing unnecessary arthrotomy by arthroscopic meniscectomy and chondroplasty. They usually immediately precede the repair or reconstructive surgery. Of course, if the meniscectomy could more easily be performed at the time of open repair, then the arthroscopic methods should be abandoned. *Arthroscopic surgery is not a substitute for carefully planned and executed reconstructive procedures within and around the knee.*

Inspecting a joint with a torn cruciate ligament and resecting it and then implying that the patient will never require any further reconstructive surgery is certainly misleading. If the patient tears the anterior cruciate ligament, there is a 70% chance of a torn meniscus, even after arthroscopic surgery has rendered the patient symptom free. A stable knee to even the most discerning clinical examiner could sustain repeated injury, ligamentous laxity, or even a subsequent meniscus injury and require reconstructive surgery in the future. Increased skills in arthroscopic surgery certainly do not replace clinical judgment and advice in the management of instability of the knee joint.

It also should be mentioned that there are certain loose bodies which are either so large or placed extra-articularly that no attempt at arthroscopic removal should even be considered (Fig. 19-1). It does not make sense to perform a procedure by arthroscopic means that could more easily be performed by an arthrotomy, which would be required anyway to remove a mass of that size. The same holds true for cystic structures.

ACUTE TEAR OF THE ANTERIOR CRUCIATE LIGAMENT

It has been my experience that a tear of the anterior cruciate ligament, when seen arthroscopically, will be a so-called isolated lesion about 20% of the time. There may be some mild capsular hemorrhage, but no gross instability or meniscal or articular injury. When that is the case, the anterior cruciate ligament may be torn either completely or partially. Occasionally a portion of the anterior cruciate ligament will lay out into the lateral compartment or even posterior and produce catching and popping in the joint. When this is the case, a simple resection of the torn portion may be performed with the Intra-articular

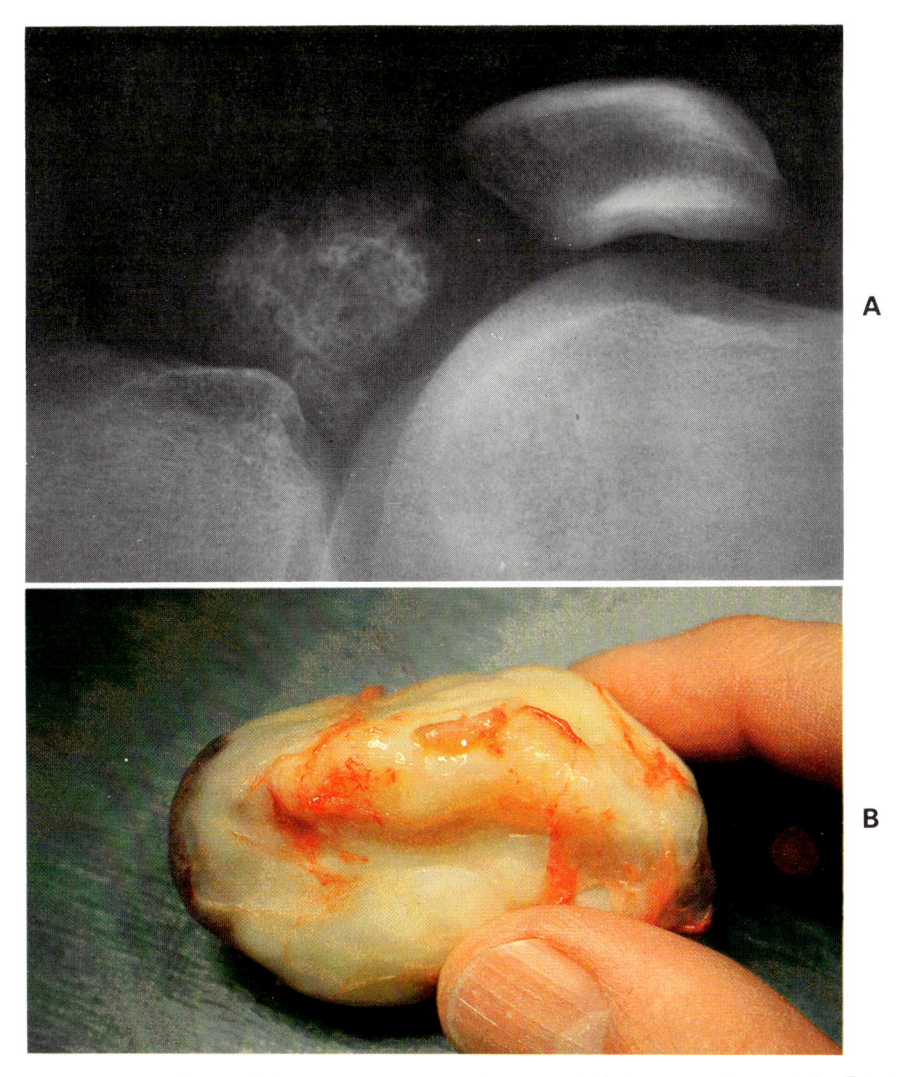

FIG. 19-1. A, X-ray view of large loose body in area of intercondylar notch. **B,** Large loose body specimen was outside joint and could not be removed arthroscopically.

Shaver (Fig. 19-2). In some instances the anterior cruciate ligament, when completely torn, may form a large fibrous ball on the tibial surface, and the resulting mass can produce pain, especially with extension of the knee (Fig. 19-3, *A*). Then a simple resection of tissue that is not amenable to repair can be considered.

Further attention must be given to the possibility of a torn meniscus, usually in the posterior compartment. Visualization of that posterior aspect is either by a separate posterior medial puncture or by modified Gillquist technique.

The subtotal selective reshaping of the meniscus preserves the capsular integrity and lends stability to the joint. This is especially true when the posterior cruciate ligament is partially torn, yet clinical rotary instability is minimal. Functional stability could exist if a complete meniscal resection were performed, whether open or closed.

Arthroscopic surgery of the knee

FIG. 19-2

A Partial tear of anterior cruciate ligament.
B Medial compartment. Comprehensive examination (front and back) showed only abrasion of medial femoral condyle.
C Intra-articular Shaver System in joint.
D Trimmer smooths injured elevated half of cruciate ligament injury to femoral condyle.
E Intra-articular Shaver System with Cutter resecting loose half of nonrepairable anterior cruciate ligament.
F Careful resection preserves integrity of remaining cruciate ligament.
G Completion of anterior cruciate ligament subtotal resection.
H Immediate postoperative view of lesion of medial femoral condyle.

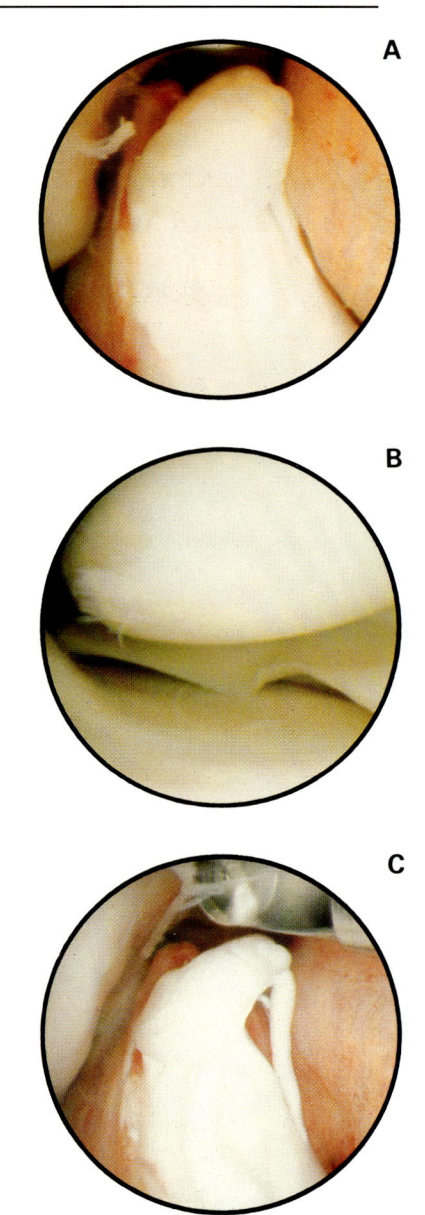

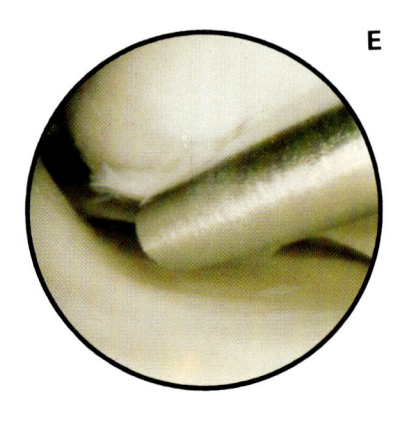

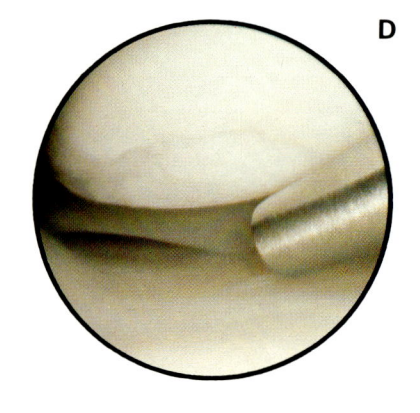

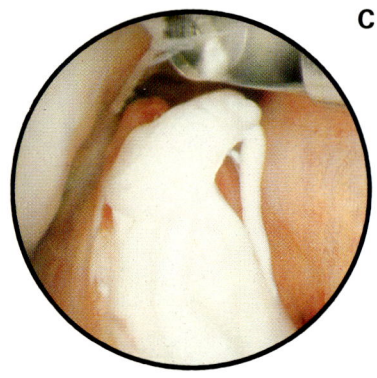

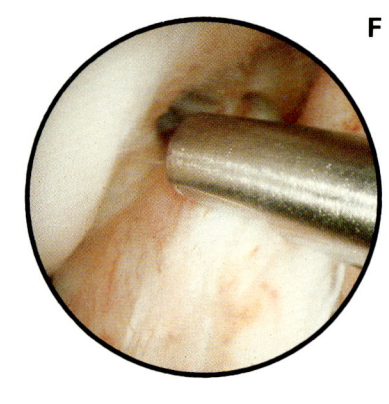

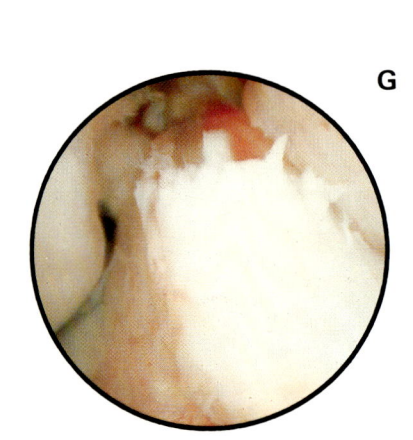

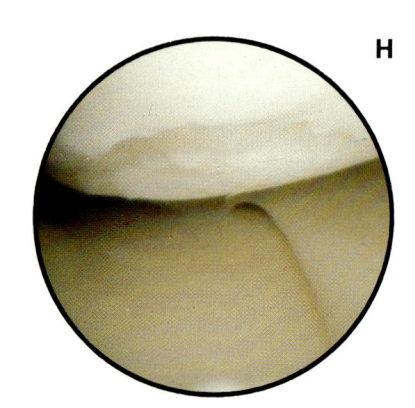

Extrasynovial disease

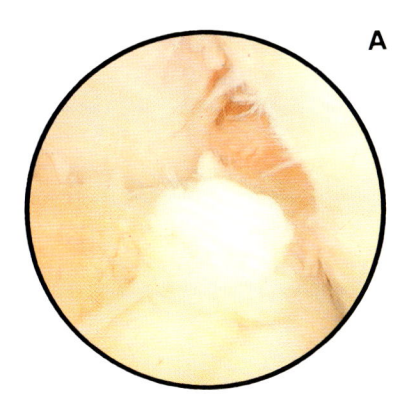

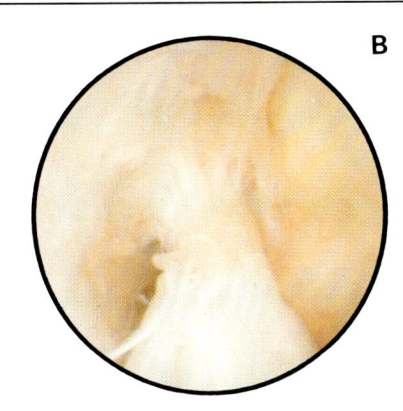

FIG. 19-3

A Old torn anterior cruciate ligament beyond repair.
B Five-year follow-up repair of anterior cruciate ligament to femur.

Adolescent participation in competitive sports has produced a number of major cruciate ligament injuries including torn menisci, usually medial and lateral and often in girls. In these patients, because their epiphyses are still open, I have performed arthroscopic surgery with subtotal meniscectomy. The patients have been advised to modify their activities for approximately 1 year, use a Lenox Hill brace, and be reevaluated at intervals until skeletal maturity. At that time reconstructive surgery might be considered.

My early experience has been that all except the most devastating injuries have resulted in surprisingly stable knees throughout the first year of following this form of treatment. Therefore it has been difficult to restrain these individuals from sports, even as early as 3 months following their injury. This type of patient and the accompanying parents find it difficult to understand that the knee joint is probably more important than the immediate gratification of competition.

In adults this same situation with a partial cruciate ligament tear without capsular stretch or injury has provided an opportunity for selective resection and reshaping of meniscal tears without resulting instability. At this time, it is my impression that in a knee with cruciate ligament injury without major capsular disruption, every attempt should be made to preserve and reshape the remaining meniscal rim. Early results have been satisfying.

In a patient with massive ligamentous and capsular destruction the tissue disruption may not require arthroscopy. The surgical exposure necessary for a complete repair allows total inspection of the knee. Arthroscopy is contraindicated perhaps because of the possible massive extravasation of saline through the capsular disruption. If an arthroscopy is performed, care should be taken not to have a large inflow tract pressure of saline, which can cause potential vascular compression in the popliteal space or one of the compartments of the leg.

CHRONIC INSTABILITIES

In a patient with chronic instability and multiple surgeries, diagnostic arthroscopy can be of considerable benefit prior to the day of surgery. This

Arthroscopic surgery of the knee

establishes the condition of the articular surfaces, the menisci, and any intra-articular debris. The patient's expectations can be better addressed and the prognosis established. More important, they can have an effect on the surgical design.

The arthroscopic surgery can either follow or immediately precede the reconstructive surgery. It may be possible, by these transcutaneous methods, to perform an intra-articular chondroplastic shave on the patellar or femoral condyles, remove a loose body, or resect the abnormal meniscal or abnormally mobile meniscal tissue. These procedures can eliminate the surgical dissection and the morbidity, and, as a result, perhaps hasten the rehabilitation.

A common circumstance is a torn anterior cruciate ligament with resultant lateral rotary instability, as evidenced by a lateral pivot shift. There is minimal instability in the neutral and in the drawer sign and no anteromedial or anterolateral Slocum-Larson sign.

Arthroscopic surgery is performed on the torn posterior horn of the medial meniscus and for debridement of the abraded articular surfaces, including

FIG. 19-4

A Posteromedial view of posterior cruciate ligament at rest.
B Same patient with posterior drawer sign and opening of joint with posterior displacement.

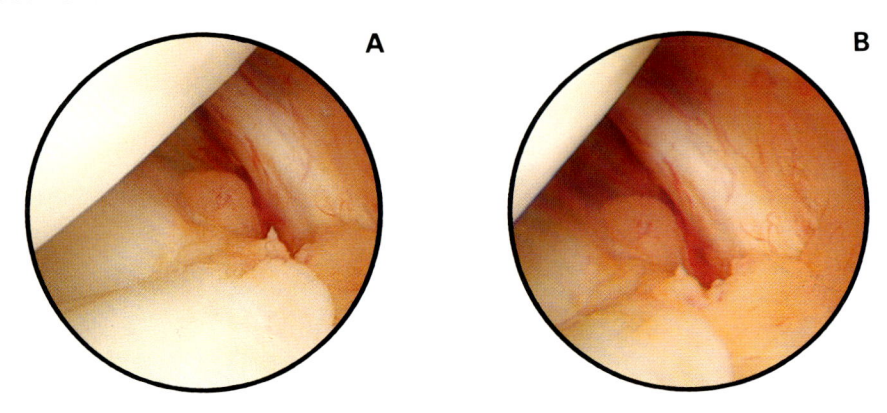

C Posteromedial view with complete disruption of posterior cruciate ligament.
D Posteromedial view 1 year after repair of acute posterior cruciate ligament injury with medial meniscus.

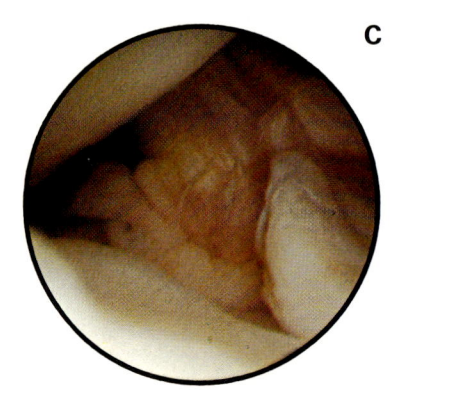

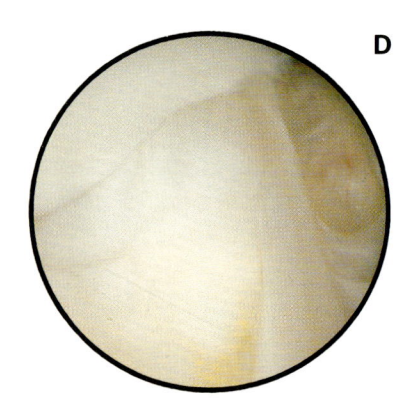

even the subtotal lateral meniscectomy and perhaps removal of loose bodies. The conventional surgical exposure is limited to the lateral capsular structures. No lesion is untreated, and the posterior capsule–meniscal attachments with the reshaped meniscus are maintained with a minimum of dissection.

Posterior cruciate ligament evaluation at the time of arthroscopic surgery can determine the status of the ligament (Fig. 19-4, A to C). Care for the lateral compartment problem arthroscopically reduces the dissection necessary for tendinous or ligamentous advancements. Reconstruction of the posterior cruciate ligament is extensive enough. The placement and size of the incisions, therefore, are exact, eliminating unnecessary dissection and morbidity.

A patient who has had multiple previous surgeries (medial and lateral capsular, transcondylar, or over-the-top) may still have ankylosis and/or catching or popping in the joint. That same patient may have had a reasonable restoration established in his knee, and yet his symptoms exist.

The arthroscopic surgery provides a means of smoothing any condylar surfaces that have been abraded, removing any loose bodies and doing a so-called all-compartment shave and a "housecleaning" of ankylosis, bands, synovitis, and degenerated-regenerated menisci. This all-compartment, intra-articular chondroplasty and debridement has proved very beneficial in a number of patients who have had as many as six arthrotomies. It does not set them back in their rehabilitative process.

CYSTS

Cystic structures can occur in many sites around the knee joint. They can come off tendinous tissues, including the quadriceps, or accompany semimembranosis, or are seen commonly in association with degenerative tears of the lateral meniscus. Occasionally they attach to the medial meniscus.

In the past I have had the opportunity, when examining degenerative lesions that showed no intra-articular tear of the meniscus, to see that resection of the cyst alone has been beneficial in some patients. Cystic degeneration can continue, and subsequent meniscectomy might be necessary.

More recently, the selective resection by arthroscopy of the abnormal meniscal tissue has resulted in decompressing the meniscal cyst. In one case I actually passed the Intra-articular Shaver into the cyst and debrided the cystic lining. I have now had 4 patients over the past year who have not had recurrence of their symptoms or the cystic mass. This eliminated the need for an arthrotomy and specifically the wide resection of capsular structures necessary by conventional means.

ANKYLOSIS

Ankylosis can occur in patients who have had severe injuries or multiple surgeries around the knee joint. Extra-articular causes can be ruled out clinically. On the other hand, arthroscopy may demonstrate multiple intra-articular fibrous bands. These are most commonly seen after major reconstructive surgery, especially quadriceps realignment procedures with the lateral release. I have seen fibrous bands that have crossed the condyles and have also bridged

Arthroscopic surgery of the knee

from femur to tibia and from femur to patellar articular surfaces. Arthroscopic resection of these fibrous bands has not only reduced patients' pain but has also increased their range of motion.

At this time I recommend preceding any major surgical exploration for ankylosis with arthroscopic surgery and intracapsular resection of fibrous tissue. This may eliminate the need for extensive surgery and quadricepsplasty that may have been considered.

EXTRA OSSICLES

Extra ossicles, loose bodies, or major bone prominences around the knee can be located arthroscopically. In cases of Osgood-Schlatter disease I have done arthroscopic inspection to make sure that no intra-articular lesion was overlooked at the time of resecting a painful extra ossicle nonunion in previous treatment for Osgood-Schlatter disease. To date I have not found any intra-articular disease accompanying that lesion, even in older patients.

If the juxta-articular loose body or prominent bone spur is intra-articular, it can be managed arthroscopically. On one occasion surgery was performed for a large loose body in the intercondylar space of a patient with a 30-year-old injury, sustained during combat. At the time of surgery it was apparent that this was an avulsion of the tibial attachment of the anterior cruciate ligament, and over the years it had reformed articular surface over the elevated piece of bone as well as the bed. This was removed by transcutaneous methods and the use of the Intra-articular Cutter. Resection of the flap exposed cancellous bone. The bed it was lifted from was debrided of fibrous tissue, exposing bleeding

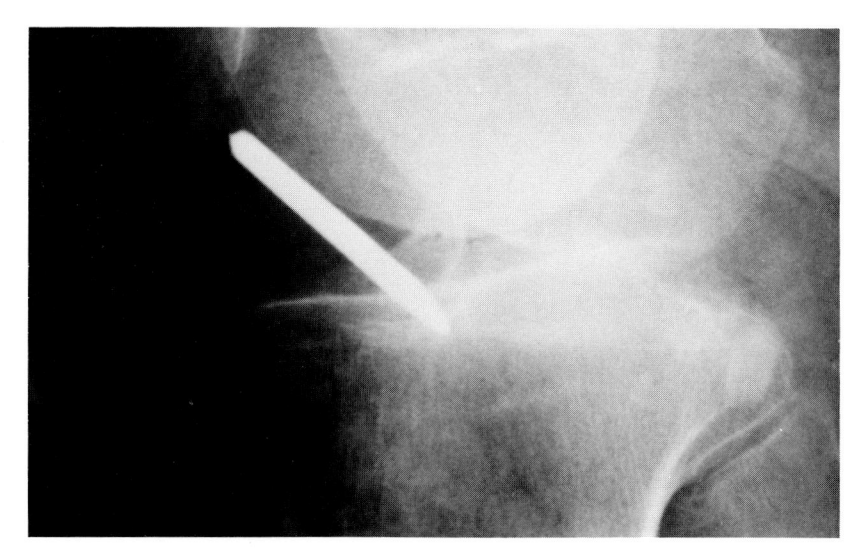

FIG. 19-5. What appeared to be loose body in preoperative films was arthroscopically demonstrated as avulsion of 30 years' duration of anterior cruciate ligament and bony attachment to tibia. Area was denuded arthroscopically, and transcutaneous wire fixation by arthroscopic means reduced the bony fragment and held it for potential healing. Resection would have resulted in gross instability of joint because it was connected to entire anterior cruciate ligament attachment.

cancellous bone. This anterior cruciate ligament maintained its integrity as the elevated bony flap remained somewhat intact. A transcutaneous reduction and wire fixation were carried out (Fig. 19-5).

If this so-called loose body had been resected, the patient would have had increased symptoms due to the instability of completely freeing the cruciate ligament.

OSTEOPHYTES

In patients who have permanent osteophytes that are palpable and irritating in the synovium, it is possible to perform arthroscopic surgery and chondroplasty by the shaving methods on the articular surfaces and care for any abnormal menisci. At the close of the procedure, through an incision less than ½ inch, and using a small osteotome or even a curved rongeur, the surgeon should resect those osteophytes. Doing this at the end of the procedure prevents the considerable leakage of fluid that would interfere with visualization and/or shaving or meniscal procedures.

Many patients have x-ray evidence of juxta-articular prominences, hypertrophic bone, and/or possible loose bodies that prove to be extra-articular. One patient had considerable abnormalities of his patella, old osteochondritis dissecans, and apparently, a small ossicle. The arthroscopy demonstrated no intra-articular abnormality. In fact, inspection of the articular surface was normal, as was palpation of those surfaces; therefore no arthroscopic surgery was even considered.

Chapter 20

Synovial surgery

Synovial folds
Medial shelf
Lateral plicae
Plica resection technique
Synovial adhesions
Localized synovial lesions
Synovitis
Arthroscopic synovectomy technique
Pigmented villonodular synovitis
Osteochondromatosis
Synovitis plus chondral abnormalities
    Peripatellar synovitis
    Juxta-articular synovitis
Foreign body
Infection

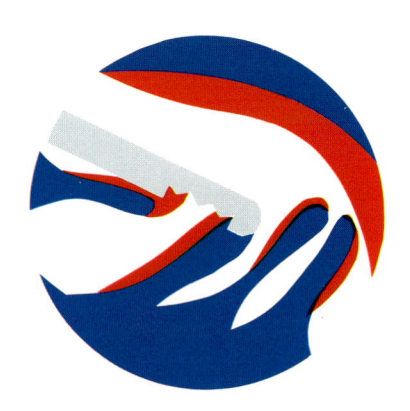

Arthroscopic surgery has benefited many patients with abnormalities of the synovial lining.[1-6] Procedures range from simple incising of the medial shelf to the all-compartment synovectomy in a rheumatoid arthritic patient. The use of multiple portals and exact positioning is essential. Synovectomy is perhaps the most tedious and demanding of all transarthroscopic surgical procedures. The Dyonics synovectomy set shortens the procedure.

SYNOVIAL FOLDS

The normal synovial folds include the suprapatellar plica, the medial shelf or medial plica, and a normal U-shaped fold in the lateral sulcus. (See Fig. 20-3.) I have seen three lateral shelves or lateral plicae that were asymptomatic. I have also seen a dome-shaped plica in one patient's suprapatellar pouch.[3] Patel[6] has an excellent review of this anatomy.

Normal synovial folds may become symptomatic in some patients. It has been estimated that they exist in approximately 60% to 80% of normals. My experience, with patients under local anesthesia, is that virtually every patient's plica is asymptomatic when probed. When viewing under local anesthesia without intra-articular anesthetic, it is possible to probe, pull, or catch the plica. The patient feels that sensation, and it is only the rare patient who can identify it as a feeling ever experienced before.

When I treat a patient who is clinically suspected to have a plica that is symptomatic, the anesthesia of choice is local. This allows exact correlation of the plica with the patient's symptoms. If the patient has no other intra-articular abnormality and indicates, by direct correlation of intra-articular viewing and grasping, that this is the symptom-producing problem, then resection or sec-

Synovial surgery

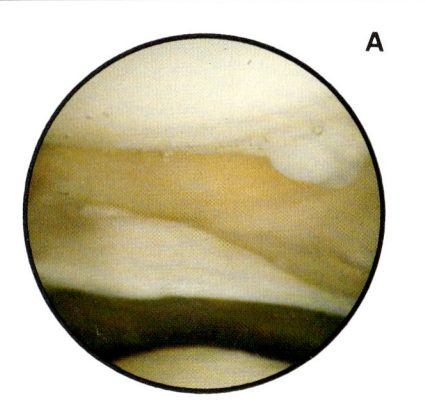

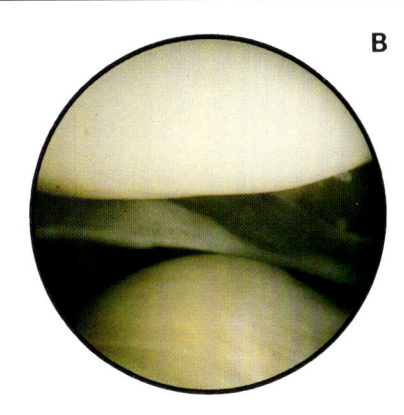

FIG. 20-1

A View of medial shelf from lateral with knee in extension and maximal distension. Plica is elevated off femoral condyle.

B With decompression of knee joint, saline infusion, and slight flexion the plica rests against the medial femoral condyle.

tioning is indicated. This can be accomplished under local anesthesia; for a more sensitive patient, standby anesthesia is available for general administration. Flexion-extension, distension, and decompression help measure the potential for femoral condylar contact (point of abrasion) (Fig. 20-1).

The suprapatellar plica is virtually never asymptomatic. I have had occasion to see one patient whose very large suprapatellar plica came down and was caught between the patella and the femur during flexion and extension, producing symptoms of chondromalacia. Resection of that plica relieved the patient's symptoms.

The routine observation or presence of the plica is not an indication for its resection. I do not routinely resect the plica during arthroscopic surgery. It is a normal structure and is rarely the cause of symptoms. Resection leaves a fibrous scar.

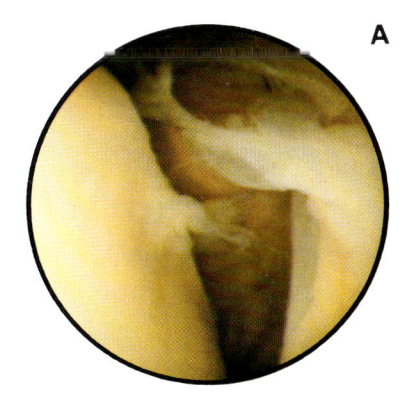

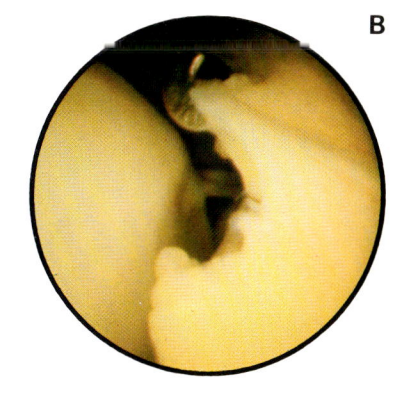

FIG. 20-2

A Medial shelf opposite erosion on medial femoral condyle seen from lateral with knee in slight flexion.

B Intra-articular Shaver resection of medial shelf.

MEDIAL SHELF

The medial shelf can be symptom producing. The patient may feel catching, popping, or even a rolling or palpable mass on the medial femoral condyle. The arthroscopic evidence of it being the cause of the problem is best determined under local anesthesia. In addition, the patient may have thickening or even a tear of the medial shelf that can be symptomatic. In the symptomatic patient there will frequently be an abrasion of the femoral condyle or increased pannus formation, even with pedunculation where the thickened medial plica rolls across the medial femoral condyle (Fig. 20-2, A). In this case the section or resection can be performed (Fig. 20-2, B).

LATERAL PLICAE

I have seen three lateral shelves that were asymptomatic in patients who were under local anesthesia for diagnostic purposes. I have never known the synovial fold in the lateral sulcus to be symptom producing (Fig. 20-3). These have not necessitated any treatment.

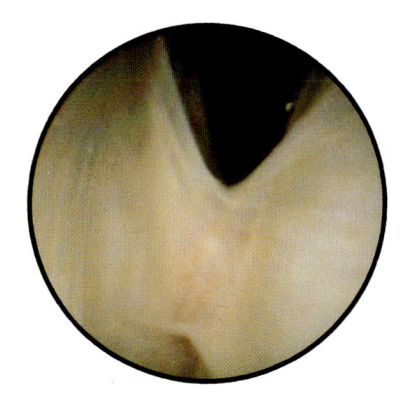

FIG. 20-3. Normal lateral synovial fold.

PLICA RESECTION TECHNIQUE

The technique for suprapatellar plica resection can be done through various portals. The suprapatellar plica is easily incised and then resected back to its synovial wall with an Intra-articular Shaver or Cutter. This preliminary incision of the plica facilitates the resection.

A simple incision of the plica, even under local anesthesia, has rendered a number of patients asymptomatic. I have not had a chance for a second-look arthroscopy in any of those patients.

The medial shelf is best viewed from a lateral portal either inferior or superior to the patella. The instrumentation for resection best approaches the patella from the lateral aspect as well. It is possible to interchange cannulas and carry out some of the resection from anteromedial, inferior, or through the inflow cannula sites superior and medial to the patella. Resection might even require multiple portals.

Synovial surgery

The resection of the medial shelf back widely into synovium has produced a wide band of fibrous tissue in that area. I have seen that on three occasions by second-look arthroscopy. There were no symptoms in any patient, but there was a marked adhesion in each (Fig. 20-4).

During wide resection of the plica with the Intra-articular Cutter the fibrous band is seen to continue posteriorly. Continued resection shows this fibrous band all the way down to the meniscus near the tibial collateral ligament area. It is my opinion that this extensive resection is not necessary and can be avoided (Fig. 20-5). Therefore at this time I recommend simple incision of the plica where it crosses the femoral condyle. Cut to the synovial wall band and then resect proximal and distal to that incision site without widely resecting the plica.

Debridement can also be carried out with the Intra-articular Shaver of the abraded or irregular surface or the pannus of synovium on the femoral condyle as well (Fig. 20-5, *F*). Gradishar and Ewing[2] have shown dramatic audiogram follow-up studies after plica resection (Fig. 20-6).

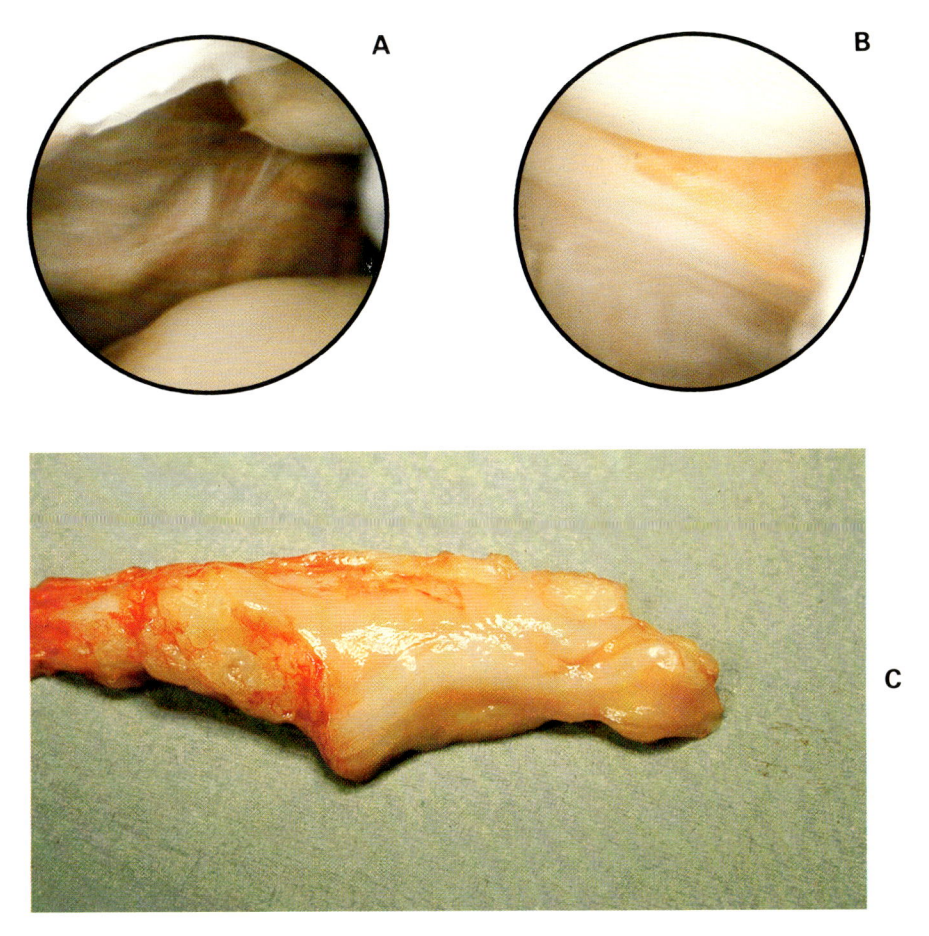

FIG. 20-4. A, Four months after plica resection fibrous band on medial joint wall is visible. **B,** Eleven months after medial shelf resection shows mature fibrous band. **C,** Gross anatomic specimen from same patient.

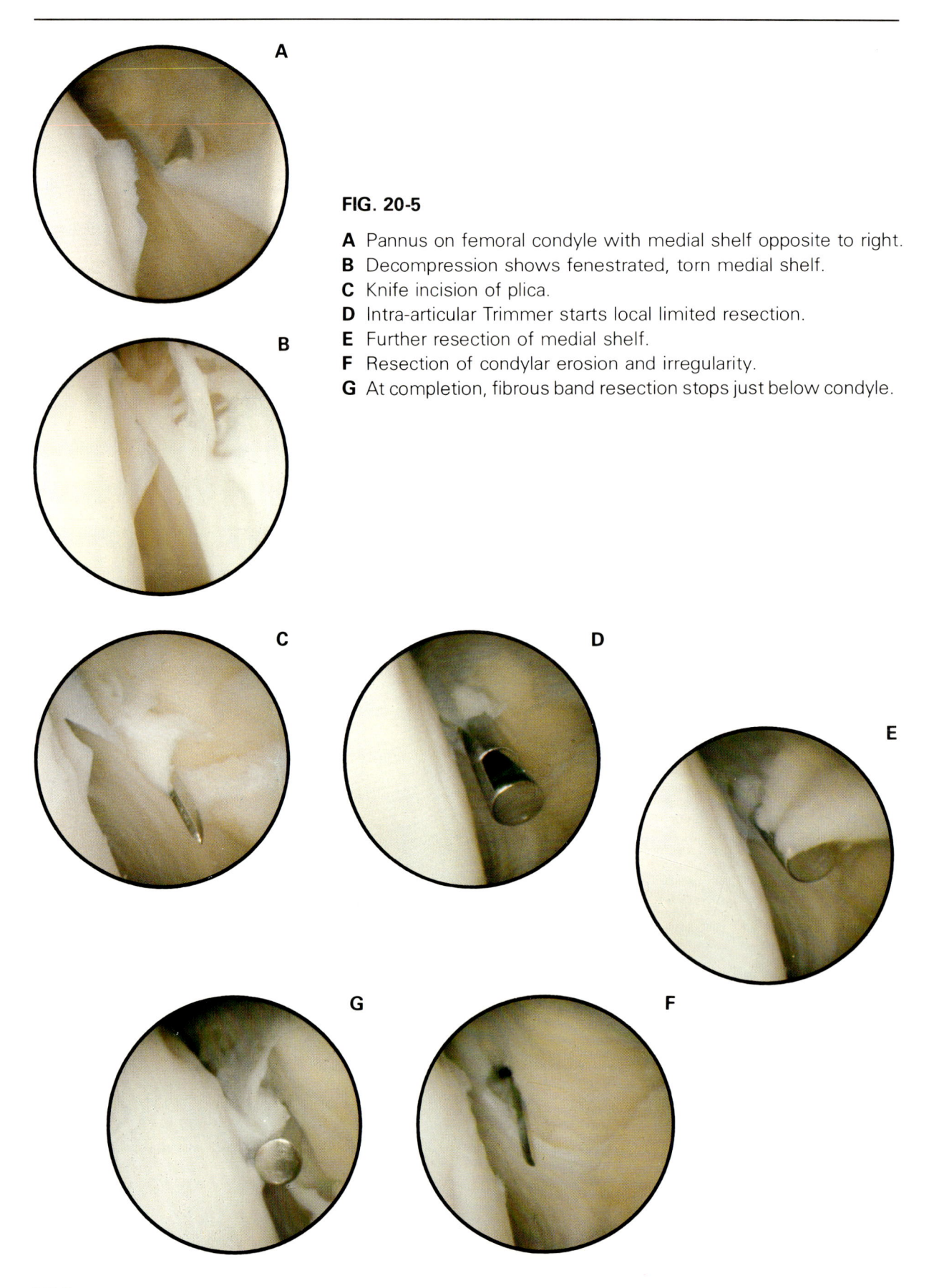

Arthroscopic surgery of the knee

FIG. 20-5

A Pannus on femoral condyle with medial shelf opposite to right.
B Decompression shows fenestrated, torn medial shelf.
C Knife incision of plica.
D Intra-articular Trimmer starts local limited resection.
E Further resection of medial shelf.
F Resection of condylar erosion and irregularity.
G At completion, fibrous band resection stops just below condyle.

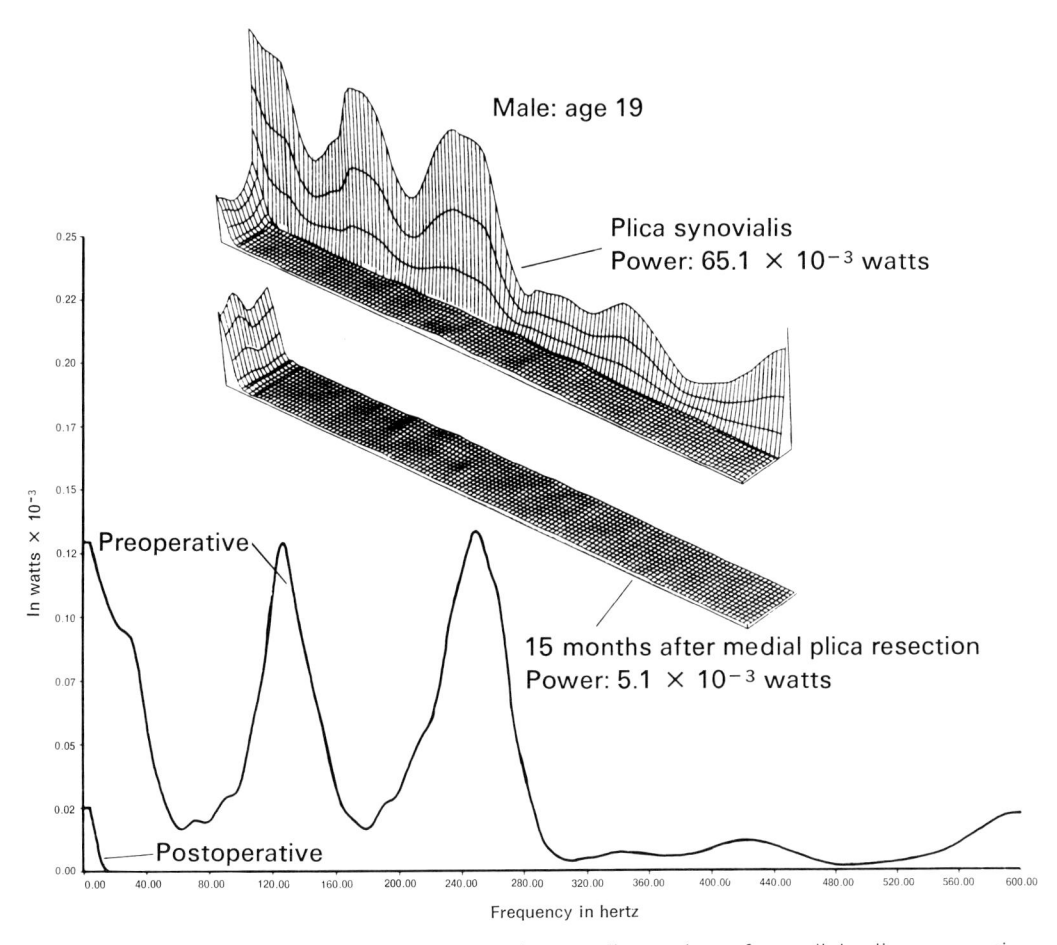

FIG. 20-6. Preoperative and postoperative audiographs of medial plica resection. (Courtesy Dr. Ivan Gradishar.)

SYNOVIAL ADHESIONS

Synovial adhesions occur following reconstructive procedures, especially those involving lateral release. I have seen fibrous adhesions following even arthroscopic lateral release. There was a fibrous band from the inferior capsular margin across the lateral femoral condyle. I have seen fibrous adhesions that cross from tibia to femur and from femur to patella as well as from articular surfaces to adjacent synovial surfaces. The Intra-articular Shaver and/or Cutter, or simple section of these bands, can reduce symptoms, reduce pain, and also improve range of motion.

LOCALIZED SYNOVIAL LESIONS

Localized pigmented villonodular synovitis has been observed. Treatment consists of simple section of its pedunculated base and forceps removal. It can also be removed through the Intra-articular Shaver. This does not produce quite as acceptable a pathologic specimen (Fig. 20-7).

One of my patients had a clear-cut episode of tearing along the medial joint line and had pedunculated synovitis adjacent to what was probably a ruptured medial shelf. In another patient I have seen localized synovitis, adjacent to a

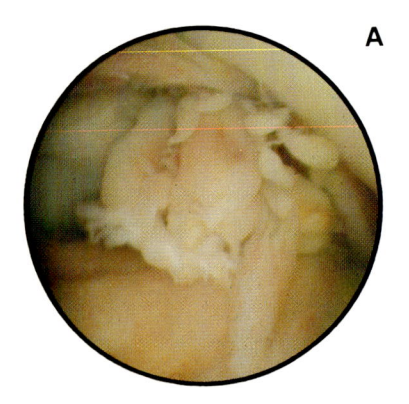

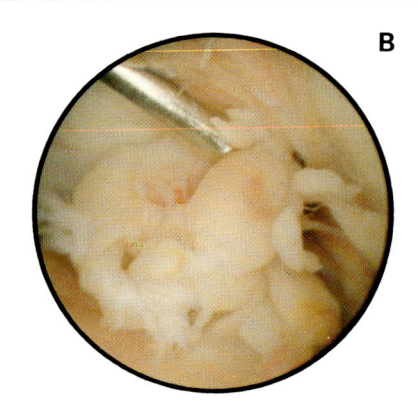

FIG. 20-7

A Localized nodular synovitis.
B Intra-articular Shaver starts resection.

plica and secondary to multiple cortisone injections. When examined under local anesthesia, it demonstrated that the localized synovitis was the symptomatic area and not the adjacent plica. A localized synovectomy rendered the patient asymptomatic.

SYNOVITIS

The most common cause of synovitis, of course, is rheumatoid problems. The conditions of rheumatoid arthritis with synovitis are amenable to arthroscopic synovectomy. These procedures are performed through multiple portals, which greatly minimizes the morbidity. The edema is gone in approximately 3 weeks, and the rehabilitation process is facilitated. The effect of this type of synovectomy has lasted approximately 2 years.

The loose-jointed rheumatoid knee with boggy, loose capsular tissue does not do as well after arthroscopic synovectomy. There are some patients, because of the nature of the bogginess of their joint, in whom a conventional synovectomy produces capsular adhesions that decompress the joint in a way better than the simple resection of villi would by a transarthroscopic method.

Both gout and pseudogout can produce symptomatic joints and acute localized synovitis. These respond just to irrigation by arthroscopic means without transcutaneous instrumentation.

ARTHROSCOPIC SYNOVECTOMY TECHNIQUE

The comprehensive arthroscopic surgical position is used with the Surgical Assistant and the articular viewing device (Fig. 20-8). Multiple portals are necessary to complete the synovectomy. This technical procedure, by arthroscopic means, is tedious and laborious. It takes at least 90 minutes to accomplish. The Intra-articular Shaver, with its larger opening, has been the attachment of choice for this procedure.

Arthroscopic synovectomy resects the villi but not the base synovium. The villous projections on the end of the fat pad and adjacent to the articular

Synovial surgery

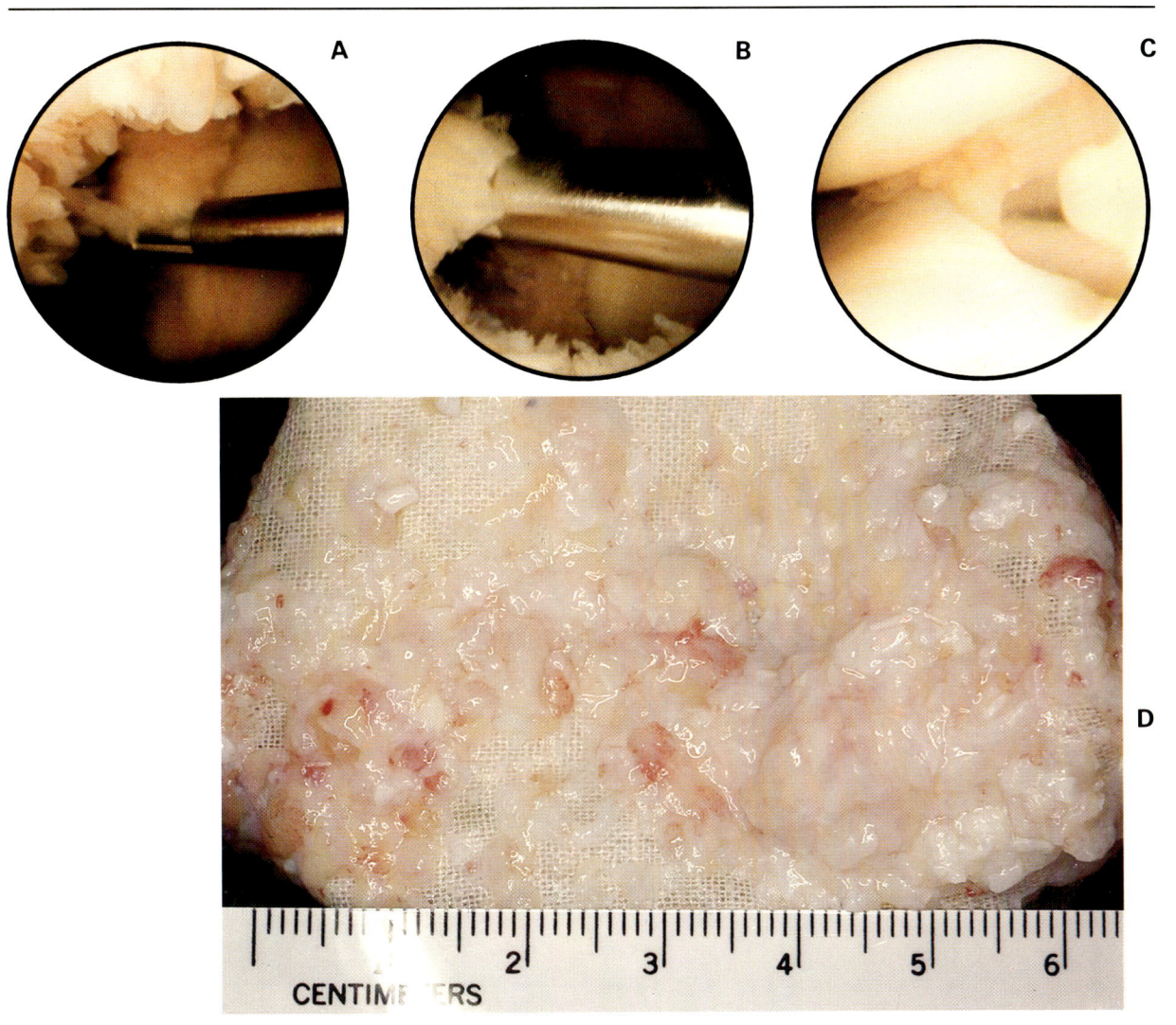

FIG. 20-8. A, Intra-articular Shaver resecting synovium in suprapatellar pouch of rheumatoid knee. **B,** Synovial villi are resected from lateral suprapatellar pouch. **C,** Synovium above and below meniscus is removed without violating meniscus. **D,** Gross anatomic specimen caught in "tobacco bag" trap.

surfaces can be debrided, as can the synovial polyp adjacent to the normal synovial folds.

The arthroscopic synovectomy is most effective in the areas adjacent to the intercondylar notch and especially posterior compartments that can just be reached into with the safe Intra-articular Shaver head. It is also possible to go under and above the menisci and along the walls of both the medial and lateral sulci using the multiple portal method. It also is not necessary to remove the meniscus to achieve the resection of synovial tissue above and below it. These areas are frequently very difficult to reach by open surgery. Second-look arthroscopy has shown only minimal recurrence at 18 months in 1 patient.

A patient undergoing arthroscopic synovectomy is given a special patient information form (Fig. 20-9).

> **POST OPERATIVE PATIENT INFORMATION**
> **SYNOVECTOMY**
>
> Your operation was performed by arthroscopic methods. The interior of your joint was visualized with a small telescope. The diagnosis was established and the appropriate surgery was performed with special micro-instruments.
>
> DRESSING: A soft dressing has been applied to your knee. This compression dressing should be comfortable and absorb any leakage of fluid and/or blood. Although the dressing may become moist or blood stained, this is not usually a cause for alarm. We have not experienced any hemorrhage or excessive bleeding in our patients.
> The dressing may be removed after surgery, and the appropriate number of bandaids are applied. The bandaids may be utilized over the next several days.
>
> PAIN: Upon discharge you should secure a prescription for pain medication. Usually this will be an analgesic with **codiene**. Please inform us of any known drug allergy. **Codiene** may produce nausea and/or a fine skin rash. In that case the medication should be discontinued and our office contacted for an alternate medication. The application of an ice pac to the knee will decrease swelling and discomfort in the first 48 hours. Please do not use aspirin, as it may increase bleeding in the first few days.
>
> WOUNDS: The small points of entry may be sore and develop bruising over the next several days. This bruising will eventually disappear and does not require any special care.
>
> BATHING: The sensation of "splashing" of fluid in the joint is not a cause for concern. It represents residual fluids from surgery, and they will absorb. It will be safe to shower 48 hours following surgery. Bathing or soaking should be delayed for several days. Cleansing of the skin adjacent to the small wounds with soap and water may be performed with the first dressing change.
>
> ACTIVITY: You may walk on the leg with/or without crutches. Muscle tightening exercises will "milk" swelling out of the extremity and assist healing. Bending of the knee should commence at one week. It will go slow at first.
> Swimming and bicycling may be possible after three to six weeks. Expect three months to return to more vigorous sports.
>
> RESULTS: Preliminary reports as well as our experience have shown arthroscopic surgery produces results equal to, if not better than surgery performed by open, conventional methods. The benefits are in less discomfort, risk, and scarring for the patient.
> We frequently remind patients that although the external incisions are small, they still have had an operative procedure inside their joint. Experience has shown that internal healing takes several weeks. In fact, complete healing to mature tissue may take three months.
>
> PRECAUTIONS: If you develop any fever (101 F° or above), unexpected pain, redness, or swelling in your legs, please contact our office for consultation or examination. TELEPHONE (517) 351-7450.
>
> Thank you,
>
> Lanny L. Johnson, M.D.

FIG. 20-9. Patient information sheet. (Color code: pink; see p. 245.)

PIGMENTED VILLONODULAR SYNOVITIS

Pigmented villonodular synovitis that has undergone surgery many times has been especially amenable to arthroscopic surgery. In those patients who have had a wide synovectomy, the lesion has been removed in the suprapatellar pouch and some of the anterior chambers, but areas adjacent to the menisci and also in the intercondylar notch have not been resected. This area on the cruciate ligament is especially amenable to arthroscopic methods and prevents multiple arthrotomies in patients with this type of problem. My results have been encouraging. Also, chondroplasty is possible on areas where the synovium has invaded the articular surfaces.

OSTEOCHONDROMATOSIS

Arthroscopic surgery allows selective synovectomy of tissues that are producing the cartilaginous bodies in the suprapatellar pouch, intercondylar notch, and even the posterior compartments. Not only are the loose bodies removed, but also those synovial tissues which are created by metaplasia.

It was beneficial in one instance in a patient who had previous open synovectomy; a considerable amount of synovial metaplasia recurred around the intercondylar notch and posterior compartments. The patient had minimal morbidity and a rapid return to a full range of motion and function following this arthroscopic procedure.

SYNOVITIS PLUS CHONDRAL ABNORMALITIES
Peripatellar synovitis

In severe chondromalacia patellae, it is not uncommon to see adjacent synovial proliferation. In the normal healing process of an articular defect adjacent to the synovial reflection the synovial tissue with its vascularity folds into that articular defect. In addition, even where there is not a peripheral lesion around the patella, it is common to see a very shaggy synovium hanging about the articular surface. This is also seen in patients who have had previous open shaves around the patella. Both can benefit by peripatellar synovial resection even though the patellar surfaces have been greatly altered.

Juxta-articular synovitis
Juxtachondral synovitis

There is juxtachondral synovitis adjacent to or opposite most lesions of the articular surface. There may be a torn meniscus and adjacent articular defect that have existed for some time. A tongue of reactive synovitis usually appears opposite the chondral defect on the synovial wall. The resection of that inflamed synovium gives immediate removal of symptoms. The chondral lesion itself may produce a catching or popping feeling, but the pain production is related to the synovitis on the opposite wall of the joint. This lesion should be looked for during all chondral surgery. A localized synovectomy with the Intra-articular Shaver is indicated.

Synovitis and degenerative arthritis

The synovitis that accompanies severe degenerative arthritis is amenable to intra-articular shaving unless it is chronic, degenerative arthritis with acute inflammatory synovitis. If there is considerable injection in the synovial tissue, then the prognosis is poor. In fact, intra-articular shaving has not rendered these patients asymptomatic.

Because my early experience has been discouraging, I treat patients who have all-compartment degenerative change accompanying inflammatory synovitis with medications and up to 6 months of rest. Some I treat simply by open synovectomy. In chronic, degenerative, noninflammatory synovitis a chondroplasty with accompanying synovectomy has been very beneficial.

FOREIGN BODY

Foreign body, whether glass or wood splinters, can cause localized synovitis in the joint. The foreign body may have even been removed prior to the arthroscopic surgery, yet the area of localized trauma still can cause the inflammation inside the joint. This is amenable to transcutaneous arthroscopic resection.

INFECTION

The infections that I have seen have been infrequent and chronic. Acute infections have been reported to be treated by arthroscopic means. Chronic fibrosis from infection can be treated by transarthroscopic synovectomy with considerable benefit after the acute process has been completed.

REFERENCES

1. Aritomi, H., and Yamamoto, M.: A method of arthroscopic surgery: clinical evaluation of synovectomy with the electric resectoscope and removal of loose bodies in the knee joint, Orthop. Clin. North Am. **10**:565, 1979.
2. Gradishar, I.: Personal communication, 1979.
3. Johnson, L. L.: Arthroscopic anatomy and how to see it. In The American Academy of Orthopaedic Surgeons: Instructional course lectures, vol. 27, St. Louis, 1978, The C. V. Mosby Co.
4. Klein, W., Schultz, K. P., and Huth, F., Die "Plica-Krankheit" des Kniegelenks, Dtsch. Med. Wochenschr. **104**:1261, 1979.
5. Mital, M. A., and Hayden, J.: Pain in the knee in children: the medial plica shelf syndrome, Orthop. Clin. North Am. **10**:713, 1979.
6. Patel, D.: Arthroscopy of the plicae—synovial folds and their significance, Am. J. Sports Med. **6**(5):217, 1978.

PART THREE

DIAGNOSTIC AND SURGICAL ARTHROSCOPY: OTHER JOINTS

Little attention has been given to arthroscopy of joints other than the knee.[2-4] Potentially, any synovial joint lends itself to arthroscopic inspection. Scattered reports still have not brought many arthroscopists to explore the various synovial joints. By the summer of 1978 it was estimated that only 6% of members of the American Academy of Orthopaedic Surgeons had ever explored a joint other than the knee by arthroscopic methods.[1]

The same principles used in arthroscopy of the knee are applicable to the other joints. (See Chapter 3.) Palpation, pistoning, scanning, distension, and visualization with a good light source are all necessary for success in the smaller joint arthroscopy. Initially, these joints are best explored under general anesthesia and with a small endoscope. Later, with experience, it is possible to enter some of these joints with a larger diameter endoscope, but only following some experience with the smaller scopes. Last, with increased experience and skills, it is possible to perform many of these procedures under local anesthesia.

The following chapters reflect my experience to date. Arthroscopy of each joint is discussed according to its clinical applications, techniques for accomplishment, and illustrations of findings. In addition, surgical techniques and experience under development are outlined.

Because it is possible to inspect these joints arthroscopically, a better understanding of their anatomy and function is essential. Experience with these joints certainly should parallel that with the knee. Arthroscopy of the knee joint has increased the physician's diagnostic abilities and afforded teaching and research potential never before realized. More important, it has afforded better patient care. The same should be true for every one of these other synovial joints.

REFERENCES
1. American Academy of Orthopaedic Surgeons, Second membership questionnaire, 1978.
2. Chen, Y.-C.: Arthroscopy of the wrist and finger joints, Orthop. Clin. North Am. **10**:723, 1979.
3. Watanabe, M., Takeda, S., and Ikeuchi, H.: Atlas of arthroscopy, ed. 3, Berlin, 1979, Springer-Verlag.
4. Wiley, A. M., and Older, J.: Shoulder arthroscopy; investigation with a fiberoptic instrument, Paper presented at the American Orthopaedic Society for Sports Medicine Annual Meeting, Dallas, Texas, 1978.

Chapter 21

Temporomandibular joint

Technique
Distension
Arthroscopic landmarks
Indications
Normal findings
Pathologic findings
Postoperative developments
Complications

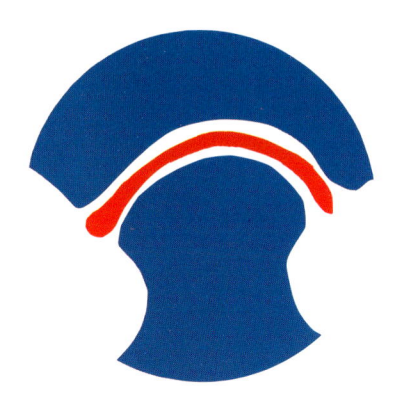

The temporomandibular joint (TMJ) is of considerable interest to otolaryngologists and oral surgeons. An orthopedist infrequently sees a patient with a TMJ problem except on a referral basis. I have had four opportunities for arthroscopic inspection. Pain and subluxation syndromes related to this joint would undoubtedly be better defined by someone more knowledgeable about this anatomic region. The description that follows is not intended to reflect any deep understanding of the problems with the TMJ but rather to outline the technique and observations I have made with my limited experience or to serve as a point of reference from which others may further explore the area.

TECHNIQUE

Anesthesia of choice is general. The patient is positioned supine.

Point of entry is anterior and slightly lateral to the TMJ on the surface of the patient's cheek (Fig. 21-1). The direction from that point is posterior and angled 15° toward the joint. The jaw should be passively open at the point of entry and allowed to come into a closed position after capsular penetration. A No. 21, 1½-inch hypodermic needle establishes the original course and enters the anterior portion of the joint. This space is widened with the mouth passively open.

The procedure is best performed under x-ray control or with image intensification. With a No. 21 needle passed transcutaneously toward the anterior portion of the joint, the exact site of entry can be located. There is still great demand for palpation skills because it is very easy to slide deep to the joint and into the area of the oral cavity. An x-ray film taken at the time of the needle passage can determine the exact entry site into the anterior portion of the TMJ for the novice arthroscopist.

Care should be taken to make only a minimal puncture with the No. 11 blade in the skin. A puncture deep into the subcutaneous tissue might lacerate portions of the facial nerve. The angle of penetration should be superficial enough to avoid penetrating deep into the TMJ. It is a common surgical practice to approach the TMJ from posterior. This approach has been more difficult

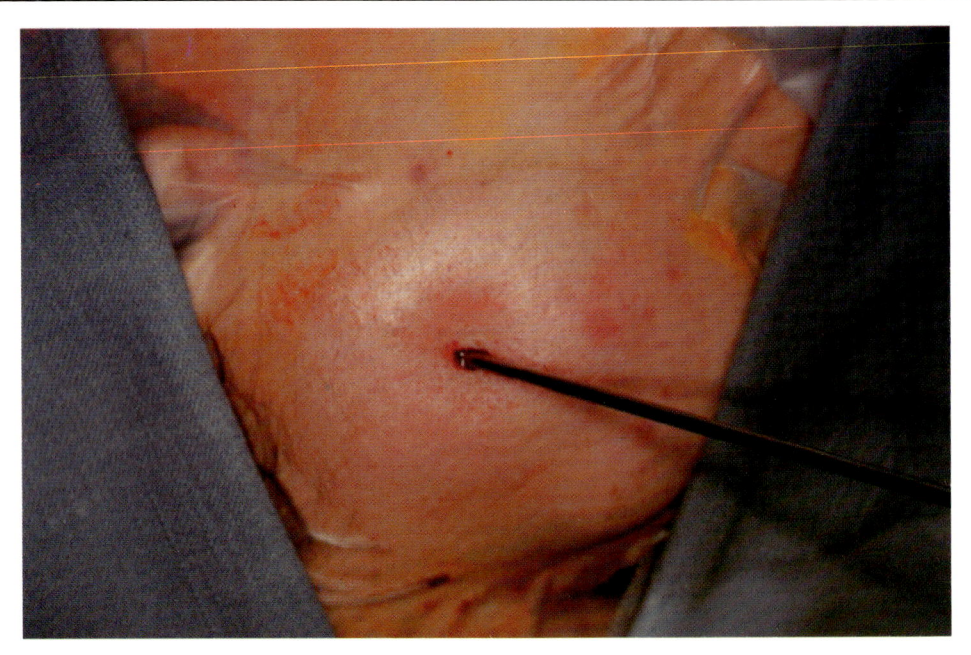

Diagnostic and surgical arthroscopy: other joints

FIG. 21-1. Needlescope in TM joint from anterior cheek. Notice edema with leak of saline around puncture. This subsided readily.

for transcutaneous arthroscopy. The anterior approach, by opening the mouth, enables a wider capsular target.

DISTENSION

The joint is distended with saline by a No. 21 needle; the needle is then removed and the cannula system follows the same course. Confirmation of entry could be by x-ray examination but is best established by the palpation.

Inspection of the joint confirms the entry. The extravasation of saline from the joint is minimal and not a useful sign of entry in the knee.

ARTHROSCOPIC LANDMARKS

Passive opening and closing of the mandible will provide orientation for the arthroscopist. Within the temporomeniscal joint space, movement of the jaw shows no motion inferior. The meniscomandibular space shows the condyle moving inferior to the meniscus (Fig. 21-2, *A*).

INDICATIONS

Unexplained TMJ pain, subluxation of the TMJ, degenerative arthritis, torn temporomandibular meniscus, and tumor are indications for arthroscopic examination.

NORMAL FINDINGS

There is fine vascularity throughout the entire normal temporomandibular synovium (Fig. 21-2, *B*). The meniscal surface, whether superior or inferior, is smooth with little vascularity. The articular surface of the temporal bone is rather small and poorly defined and flows right into the synovium.

Temporomandibular joint

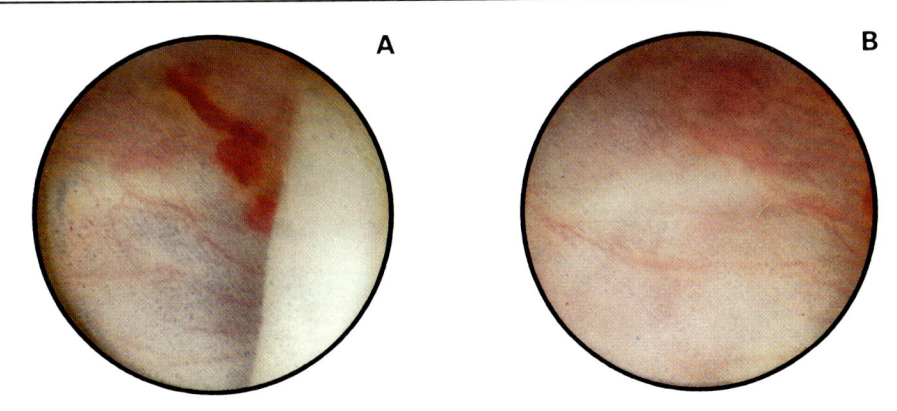

FIG. 21-2

A Posterior aspect of mandible and posterior wall of TM joint.
B TM joint with normal synovial patterns.

The condyle of the mandible is more easily defined as articular cartilage similar to that in the knee. It should be noted that the synovial space goes down 1 cm around the neck of the mandible, inferior to the condyle. A puncture in the inferior portion of that joint can actually show bone of the neck of the mandible; by moving up, the reflection of the articular surface can be seen.

PATHOLOGIC FINDINGS

Patients with subluxation have abrasions of the meniscal surface as well as fibrous bands across the joint. A fibrinoid type of exudate was seen in 2 patients. My youngest patient was a 5-year-old boy who was being inspected 6 weeks after resection of a hemangioma that went down to the level of the joint. The purpose of the arthroscopy was to rule out intra-articular hemangioma. The ENT surgeon did not want to resect the joint unnecessarily. Arthroscopy confirmed that there was no hemangioma in the joint itself; therefore further resection was neither indicated nor performed.

POSTOPERATIVE DEVELOPMENTS

Each patient had considerable swelling and extravasation of saline around the joint following the procedure. Their cases were taken over by the otolaryngologist or oral surgeon. Postoperative swelling around the TMJ resolved within a day. There were no infections, and the puncture wound for the 2-mm cannula left only a minimal scar.

COMPLICATIONS

None of my patients has experienced any complications.

Chapter 22

Shoulder joint

Indications
Technique
Identifiable lesions
    Congenital problems
    Rotator cuff injury
    Subluxation or dislocation of the shoulder
    Loose bodies
    Degenerative arthritis
    Ruptured biceps tendon
    Frozen shoulder
    Avulsed and displaced anterior labrum
Postoperative evaluations
Rheumatoid arthritis
Operative arthroscopy

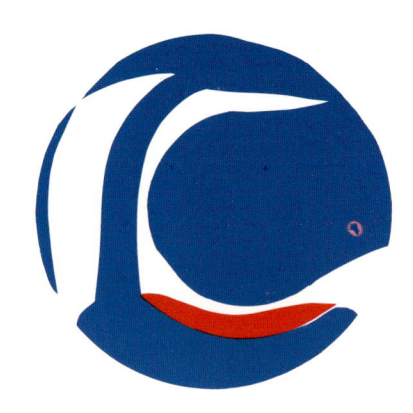

The shoulder is a frequent site of complaint. Shoulder symptoms could be related to cervical arthritis or neural compression, but there are many abnormalities of the shoulder that go undiagnosed or are placed empirically in various diagnostic groupings, such as bursitis, tendinitis, and rotator cuff degeneration. In my experience with inspection of the shoulder joint, arthroscopy has solved diagnostic problems for many patients with shoulder complaints.

INDICATIONS

Shoulder pain, catching, popping, locking, crepitus, subluxation of the shoulder that has never been recorded by x-ray examination or documented by an experienced examiner, an old dislocation (and ruled-out loose body), synovitis, frozen shoulder, possible rotator cuff tear, or biceps tendon rupture indicates a need for arthroscopy.

TECHNIQUE

Local or general anesthesia can be employed. The patient is placed in the lateral decubitus position (Fig. 22-1). The surgeon assumes a position posterior, and the first assistant is anterior. The second assistant stands over the patient's lower extremities to apply traction to the upper extremity. The equipment (including the light source) is positioned at the front of the patient or anterior.

Drape the shoulder with the same surgical barrier drapes as for the knee (Fig. 22-2). It is important in the draping to seal off the shoulder from any unsterile area. Especially important is a plastic drape that adheres to the skin on the arm as well as the drape so that, with continued traction throughout the procedure, the sterile drape on the upper extremity is not pulled down over the elbow, exposing unprepared areas of skin.

Shoulder joint

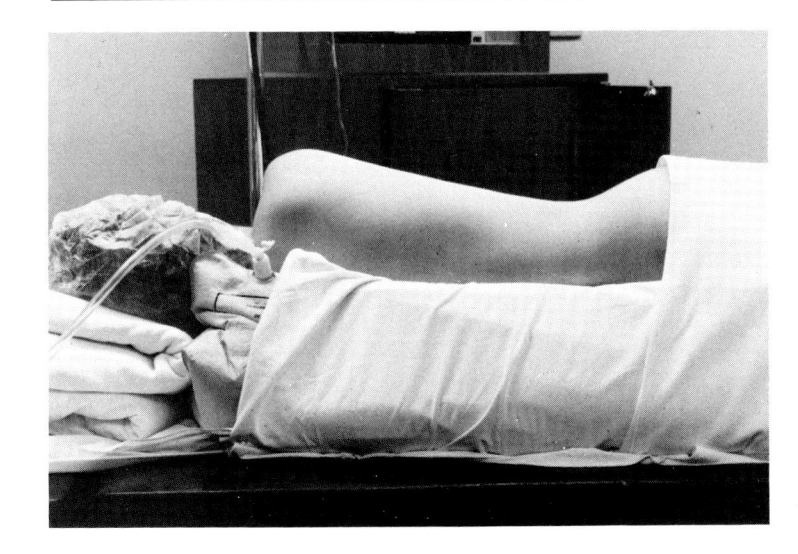

FIG. 22-1. Patient in lateral decubitus position.

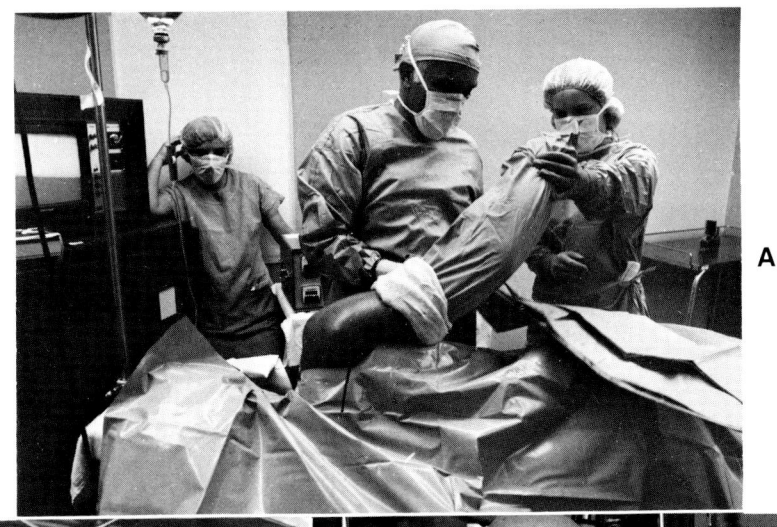

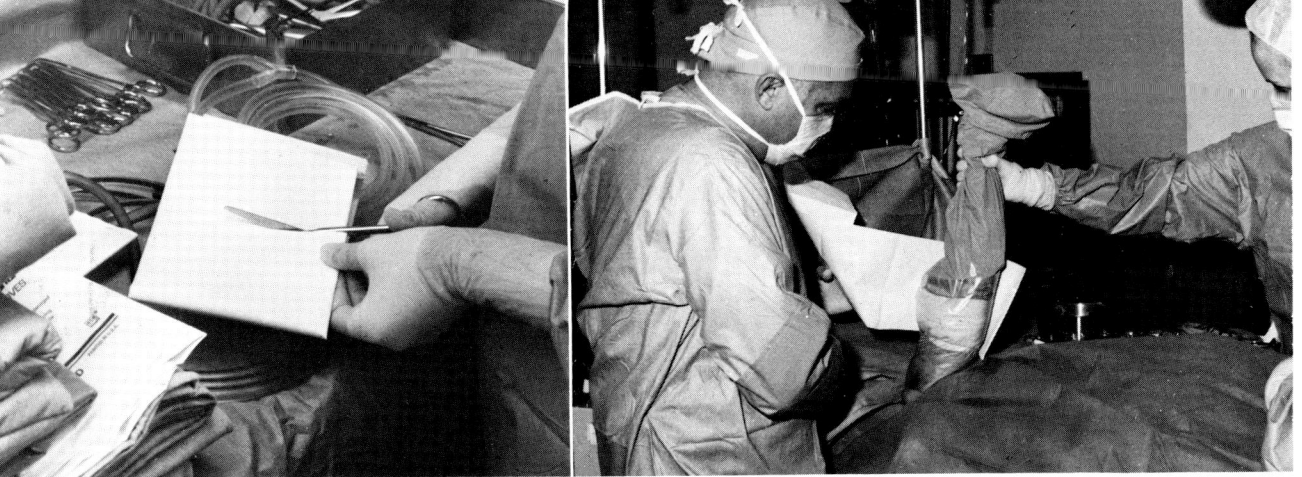

FIG. 22-2. A, Plastic barrier draping of patient for shoulder arthroscopy. **B,** Cutting 4-inch strip of adhesive plastic drape. **C,** Plastic strip holds upper extremity drape to skin and eliminates contamination; traction might pull it down.

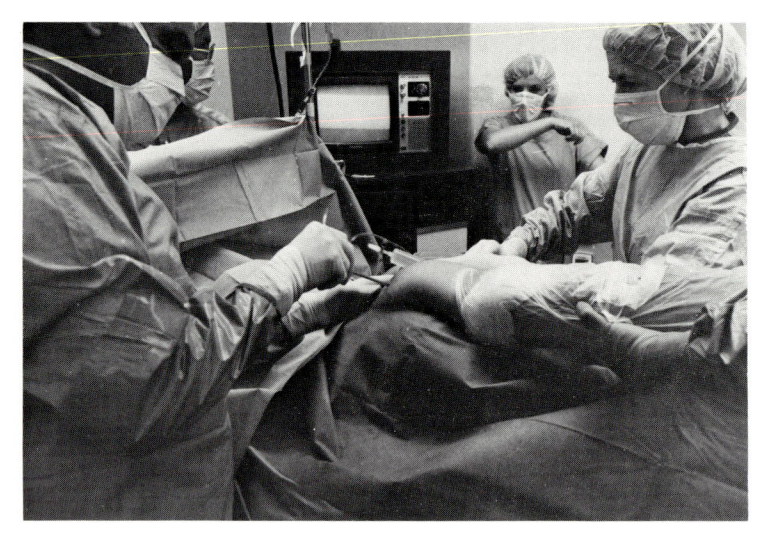

Diagnostic and surgical arthroscopy: other joints

FIG. 22-3. Posterior approach is favored in shoulder arthroscopy.

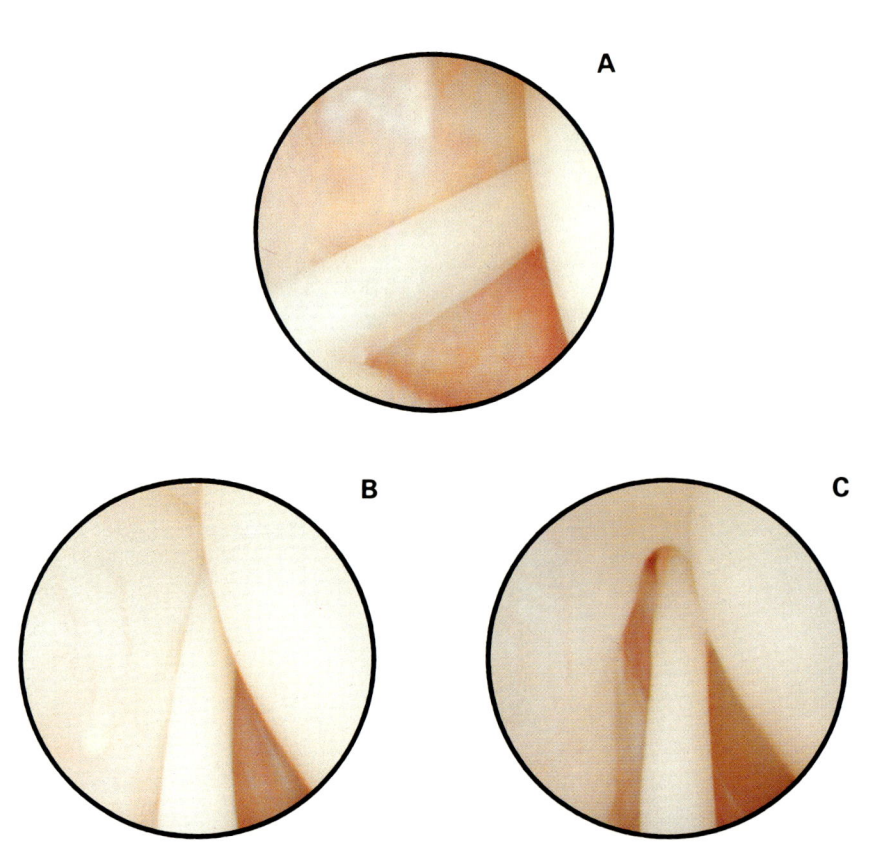

FIG. 22-4. Normal biceps tendon.

A Right shoulder joint from posterior. Notice biceps tendon and humeral head.
B Right shoulder. With external rotation of humerus, more of tendon is seen.
C Right shoulder with external rotation and elevation, and penetration of arthroscope. Biceps brachia is followed to bicipital groove.

Shoulder joint

A posterior site of entry is favored over an anterior approach. The posterior route traverses less tissue and does not require external and internal rotation for joint entry. A comprehensive examination can be achieved from posterior.

Distend the joint with saline. A No. 18 1½-inch needle and syringe deliver saline prior to the arthroscopic entry. Gentle distraction of the glenohumeral joint facilitates entry. This is accomplished by the second assistant.

The point of entry is inferior and slightly medial to the posterior corner of the acromion (Fig. 22-3). There is a small sulcus in that area which is easily palpable, and the needle traverses horizontal to the floor and perpendicular to the long axis of the patient. A sharp trocar carries the cannula through the capsule; a blunt trocar enters the joint as in other arthroscopy. Again, basic arthroscopic skills of placement and palpation and a sense of entry in the joint are important.

Inspection via the posterior approach will show the biceps tendon at its junction with the glenoid (Fig. 22-4, A). External rotation permits coursing along the biceps tendon to its outlet from the shoulder joint in the bicipital groove (Fig. 22-4, B and C). Elevation and external rotation of the arm facilitate this examination.

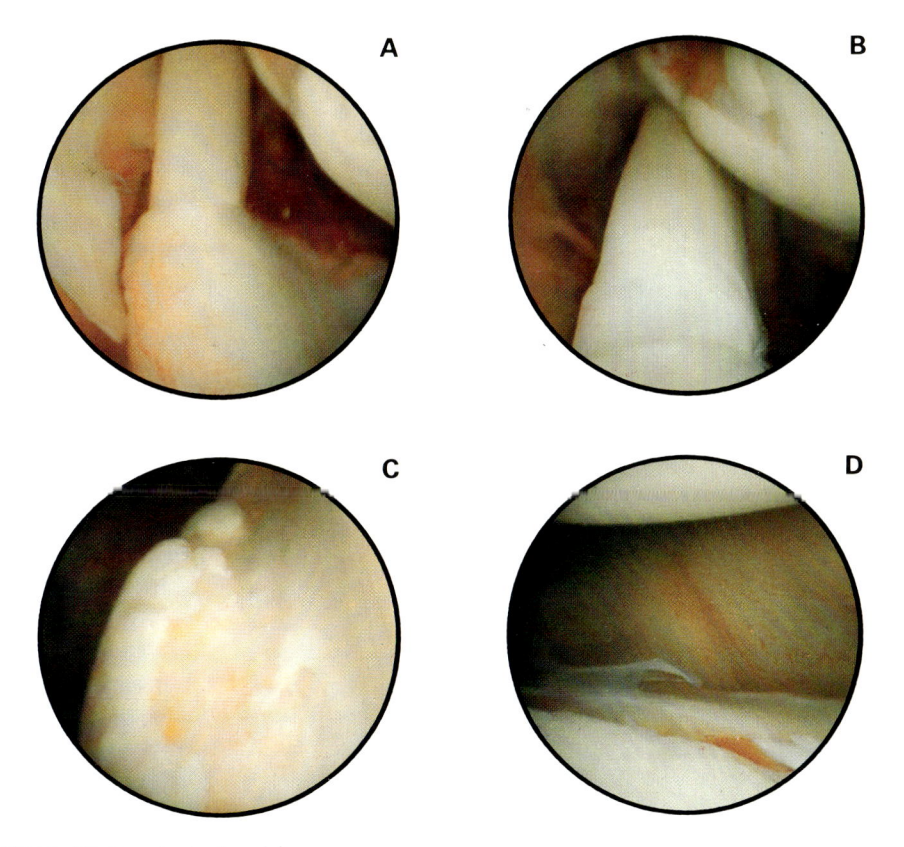

FIG. 22-5. Dislocated shoulder.

A Right shoulder from posterior. Notice biceps attachment at superior glenoid.
B Biceps with Hill-Sach lesion of head of humerus.
C Hill-Sach lesion (compression fracture) of right humeral head.
D Anterior labrum separated off glenoid with hemorrhage at margin.

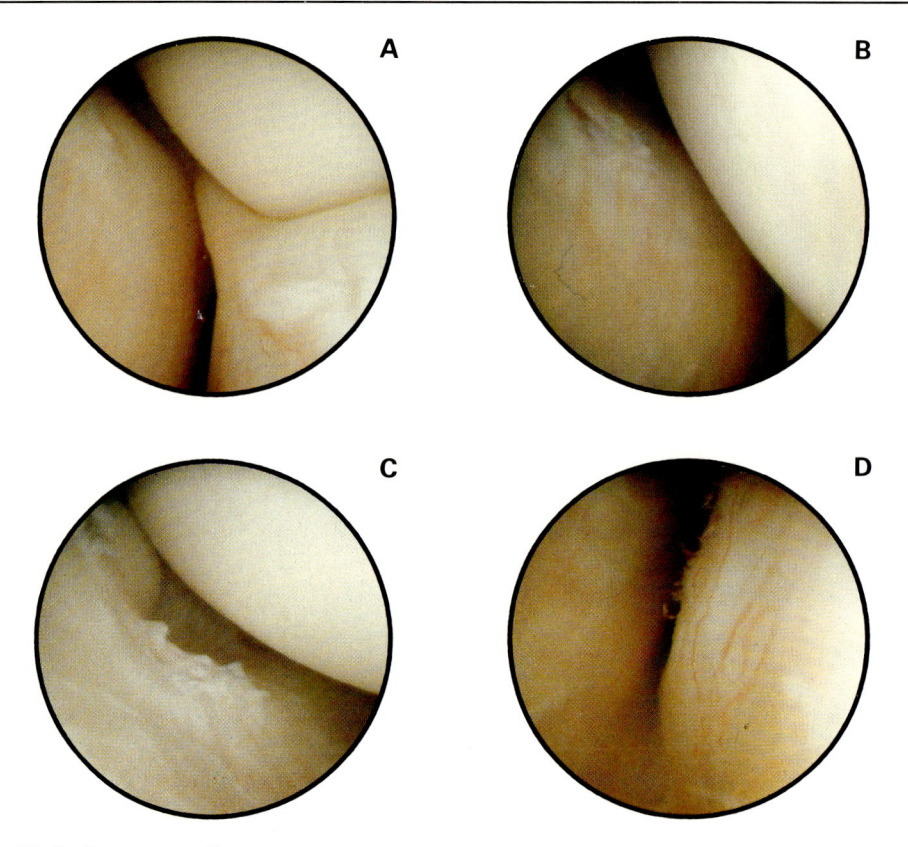

Diagnostic and surgical arthroscopy: other joints

FIG. 22-6. Rotator cuff tear.

A Right shoulder arthroscopy from posterior. Notice humeral head above and to right and glenoid below rotator cuff area to left.
B Humeral head to right. Rotator cuff with small tear to left.
C Humeral head above and to right. Rotator cuff separation to left.
D Sulcus above glenoid to right and rotator cuff to left. Notice normal vascularity of patella.

With distraction and elevation it is possible to withdraw the arthroscope and see the glenohumeral joint as well as the anterior rim in subluxations (Fig. 22-5). With external rotation and slight withdrawal a Hill-Sach lesion can be identified (Fig. 22-5, *B* and *C*).

With the arm in this neutral position it is possible to move up the glenoid past the biceps. Slightly retract the scope and visualize the rotator cuff area thoroughly (Fig. 22-6). With slight flexion and elevation it is possible to penetrate past the biceps tendon and see the anterior wall in the glenohumeral ligament traversing that area (Fig. 22-7).

With rotation of the endoscope an oblique view of the posterior humeral head is possible. The synovial reflection is sharply marked from the hyaline cartilage cap of the humerus (Fig. 22-8).

Arthroscopy of the shoulder is easier than one might expect. After a few experiences, confidence can be gained in the normal anatomy. It is possible to perform this procedure under local anesthesia without great difficulty.

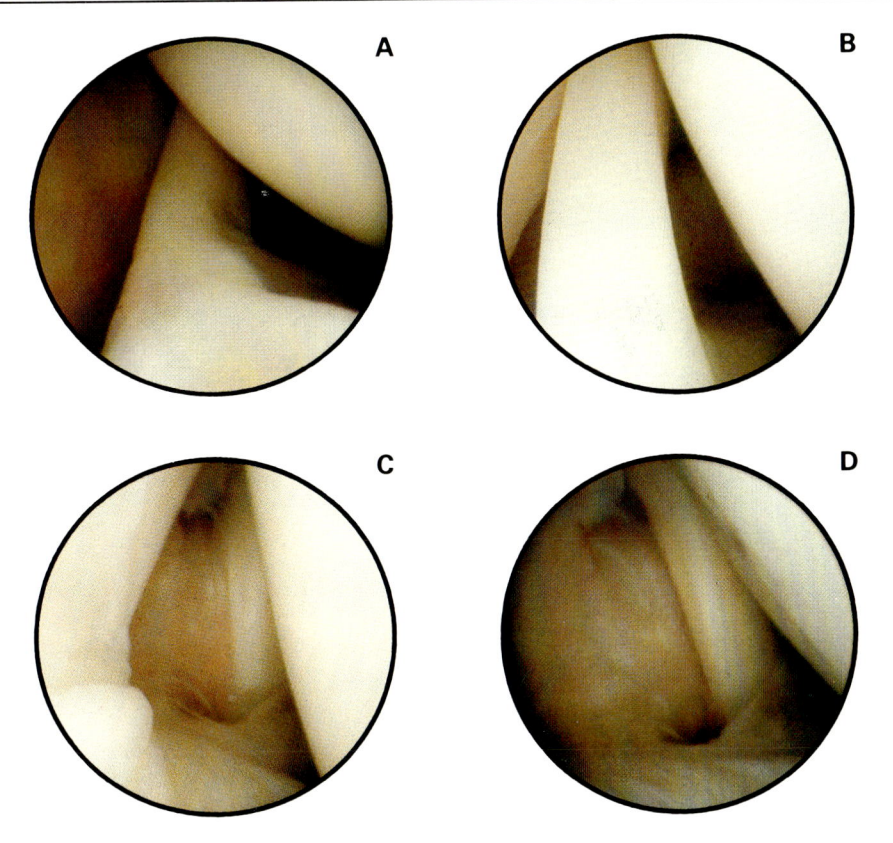

FIG. 22-7. Glenohumeral ligament (superior).

A Right shoulder from posterior with biceps tendon at superior glenoid attachment.
B Close-up of humeral head.
C Passing between biceps and humeral head to anterior wall of joint, glenohumeral ligament is seen deep in view.
D Glenohumeral ligament adjacent to opening to sulcus capsularis bursae.

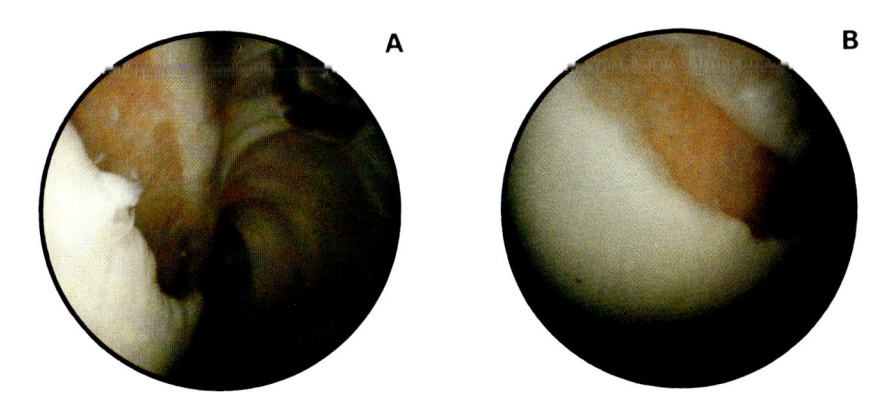

FIG. 22-8. Normal synovial reflection (posterior).

A Posterior tangential view of humeral head with hyaline cartilage at left and synovial reflection at right.
B Rotation of humeral head gives direct view of posterior synovial reflection.

Diagnostic and surgical arthroscopy: other joints

IDENTIFIABLE LESIONS
Congenital problems

I have observed a number of what I consider normal variations in size and shape of the different shoulder structures. Most notable was a 10-year-old girl with an actual sling, or pulley, around her biceps tendon. She had a history of locking, catching, and popping in her shoulder, and it would lock up in the abducted position. Arthroscopy revealed that loop of fascial tissue about her biceps tendon, easily explaining her symptoms.

Rotator cuff injury

Partial rotator cuff injuries that may even be old and sealed over are usually identifiable. (See Fig. 22-6.) The acute hemorrhagic change is easily identifiable, even through the synovium. I have seen areas of avulsion of the rotator cuff from the humeral head several weeks after a manipulation of the shoulder.

An older lesion that has some fibrosis or hemorrhage in the defect may not show on arthrogram but is easily identifiable arthroscopically. I have identified old rotator cuff tears with tags of the tendon hanging down in the joint, resulting in the catching, popping, locking, and pain. These have been excised arthroscopically (Fig. 22-9).

The undersurface of the rotator cuff is an area that can have irregularities in its contour, probably with adjacent microscopic tears and synovial proliferation. These produce the crepitus felt with internal and external rotation or rapid abduction and adduction of the shoulder.

Subluxation or dislocation of the shoulder

A subluxation or dislocation is easily identifiable by viewing the anterior limb of the labrum where it is separated from the bony glenoid. This can be accompanied by hemorrhage in an acute case or just fibrosis and synovial proliferation in a chronic situation. (See Fig. 22-5.)

In addition, there is an easily identifiable Hill-Sach lesion on the surface of the humerus posteriorly. (See Fig. 22-5.) Posterior labrum separation may also be identified (Fig. 22-10).

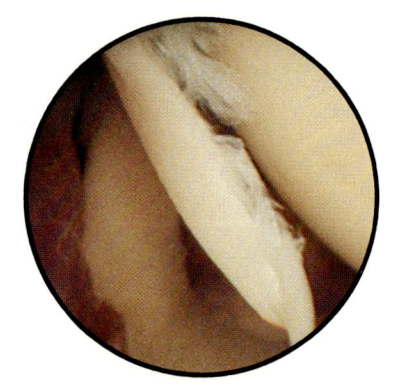

FIG. 22-9. Fragment of ruptured rotator cuff impinging on shoulder joint.

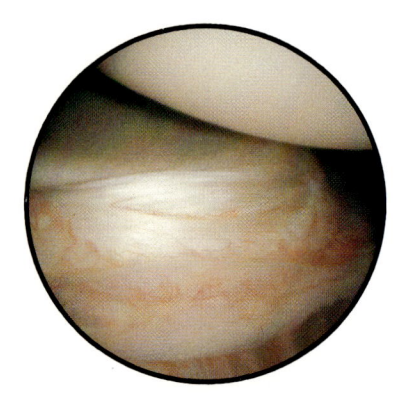

FIG. 22-10. Posterior glenoid rim tear off humerus (posterior view).

Shoulder joint

Loose bodies

Several instances of loose bodies have been identified in the shoulder accompanying either a fracture or subluxation. These are easily identified arthroscopically. They have been removed percutaneously.

Degenerative arthritis

Diffuse degenerative change can occur in an aging shoulder (Fig. 22-11). The patient may benefit from vacuuming and lavage like that performed in the knee. Of course, if the changes are to the level of bone on both sides, the prognosis is not as good.

Ruptured biceps tendon

The biceps tendon may be frayed in degenerative arthritis of the shoulder (Fig. 22-12), or a rupture might occur with a fragment catching in the joint. Also, inadequate resection following biceps stabilization in the bicipital fossae can produce the same symptoms (Fig. 22-13).

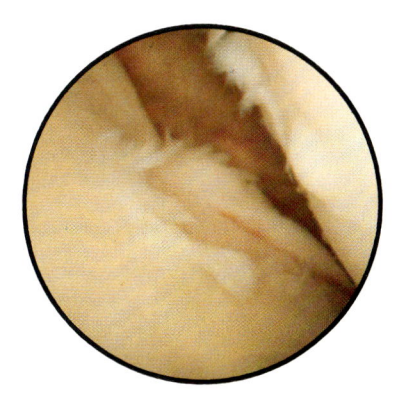

FIG. 22-11. Glenohumeral degenerative arthritis.

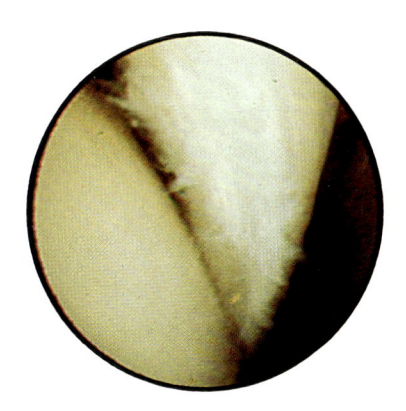

FIG. 22-12. Frayed biceps tendon in degenerative arthritis of shoulder joint.

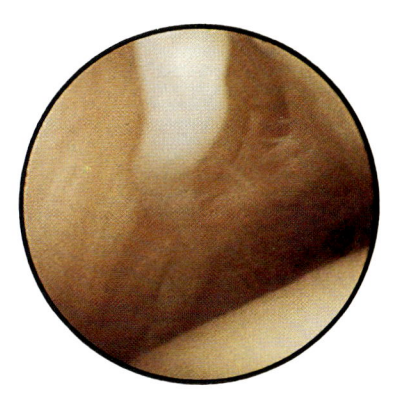

FIG. 22-13. Proximal end of ruptured biceps tendon in shoulder.

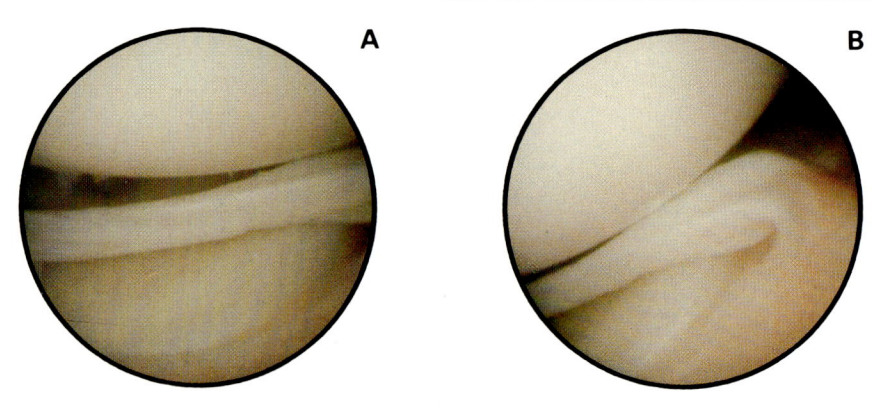

FIG. 22-14

A Posterior arthroscopic view of shoulder joint showing posteriorly displaced anterior labrum.
B Displaced rim still attached at inferior glenoid.

Frozen shoulder

There have been severe instances of an arthroscopic examination showing acute inflammatory but not rheumatoid synovitis in patients with a frozen shoulder. An arthroscopic examination and lavage of the joint plus cortisone instillation have eliminated the need for any manipulations. I have not seen so-called frozen shoulder that has any demonstrable intra-articular adhesions. Perhaps the capsular "adhesions" are a result of the synovitis. When the nonspecific synovitis has subsided, the range of motion increases. Arthroscopy eliminates the morbidity of manipulation; therefore the rehabilitation phase is started, and the natural history of the condition is shortened.

Avulsed and displaced anterior labrum

I have seen three cases of an anterior labrum that had displaced into the posterior portion of the shoulder. It produced locking, catching, and popping very much like a bucket-handle tear of the knee (Fig. 22-14). Arthroscopic resection has produced remission of symptoms.

POSTOPERATIVE EVALUATIONS

A number of patients, after shoulder injury and/or surgery, have resultant fibrosis, scarring, and even small loose bodies. Arthroscopic evaluation in the problem shoulder following surgery can delineate any intra-articular abnormality, and frequently this can be cared for either by the arthroscopy alone or by simple surgical manipulative transcutaneous methods.

RHEUMATOID ARTHRITIS

Rheumatoid arthritis conditions comprise synovitis and degenerative changes (Fig. 22-15). An assessment can be made of the exact articular and synovial changes for diagnostic purposes and therapeutic recommendations. It is possible in early rheumatoid arthritis to benefit from cortisone injections or washout of multiple loose bodies, with relief lasting from 6 to 12 months, by

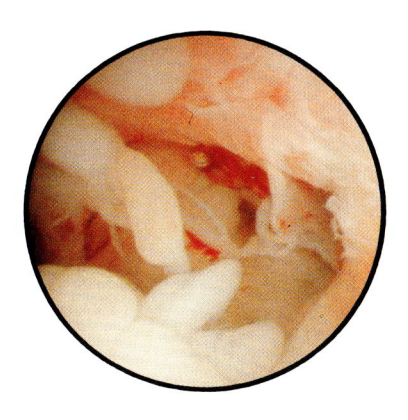

FIG. 22-15. Synovitis accompanying rheumatoid arthritis.

simple outpatient local arthroscopy and vacuuming. Synovectomy has been performed.

OPERATIVE ARTHROSCOPY

Arthroscopic surgery has provided removal of loose bodies by transcutaneous methods, the resection of a remnant of previously resected biceps tendon, fragmenting of the intra-articular rotator cuff, and synovectomy in rheumatoid diseases.

The patient is placed in the same position as for an arthroscopic examination. The procedures can be facilitated by video projection and operation. The inflow cannula can be superior (Fig. 22-16, *A*); the arthroscope is posterior (Fig. 22-16, *G*); and the manipulative instrumentation is anterior (Fig. 22-16, *O*). This creates somewhat of a problem for the surgeon by forcing him to work back toward himself rather than in the same direction. But it is difficult to insert two instruments from posterior or two from anterior, such as an arthroscope and a cannula or forceps.

The shoulder is best distended with a No. 18 needle in the midline portion and superior, immediately under the olecranon. When the shoulder is distended, the cannula that accompanies the Little Shaver can enter the joint through this area and be attached to the inflow tubing to allow continued distension and saline flow.

There should be a constant, smooth distraction to the shoulder as well. The arthroscope is inserted from posterior in an area immediately inferior and toward the midline of the posterior angle of the acromion. Inspection of the shoulder is then carried out in a routine fashion as in any shoulder arthroscopy.

I then visualize through the anterior portion of the shoulder and palpate with the opposite hand, viewing off the television monitor and visualizing the entry site with a No. 18 spinal needle. This enters the joint and the needle is moved around the humeral head in all areas of potential surgical access. Then, after I view the site and plane of the needle, it is removed, and the Little Shaver is placed into the shoulder joint. Synovectomy, resection of the biceps tendon remnants, or resection of the rotator cuff remnants is performed next.

It is important to maintain distension at all times throughout the procedure.

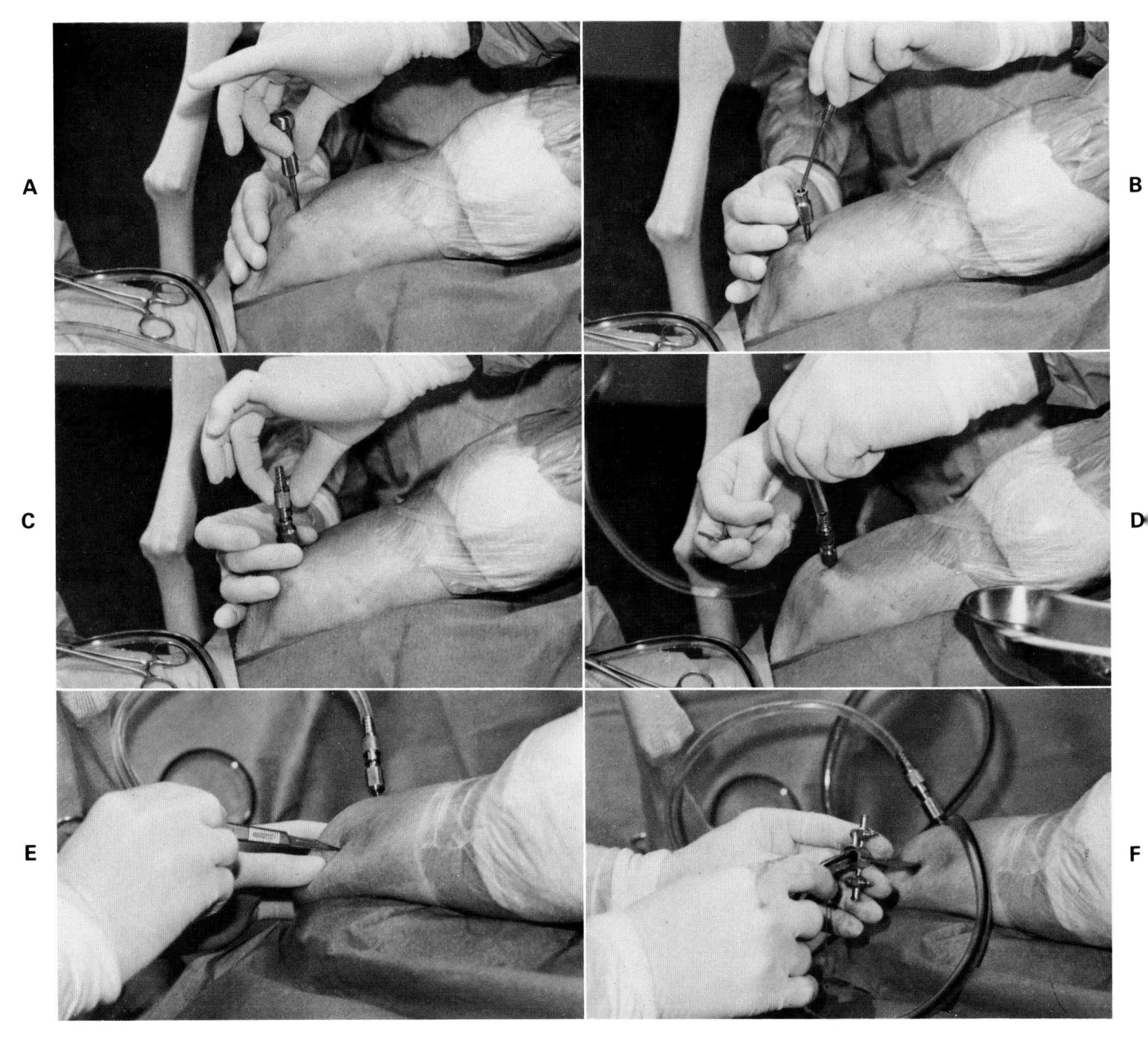

Diagnostic and surgical arthroscopy: other joints

FIG. 22-16

A Inflow cannula shown superior.
B Obturator removed.
C Adapter attachment.
D Inflow tubing attached.
E Posterior incision with No. 11 blade.
F Arthroscopic cannula in joint during vacuuming.

Shoulder joint

FIG. 22-16, cont'd

G Direct arthroscopic inspection.
H Articulated viewing device (AVD) to TV camera.
I Sterile plastic figure eight tape seals off AVD to arthroscope.
J Arthroscope in place. Viewing from television monitor.
K Surgical staff viewing television monitor.
L Arthroscopic view of shoulder. Rheumatoid synovitis.

Continued.

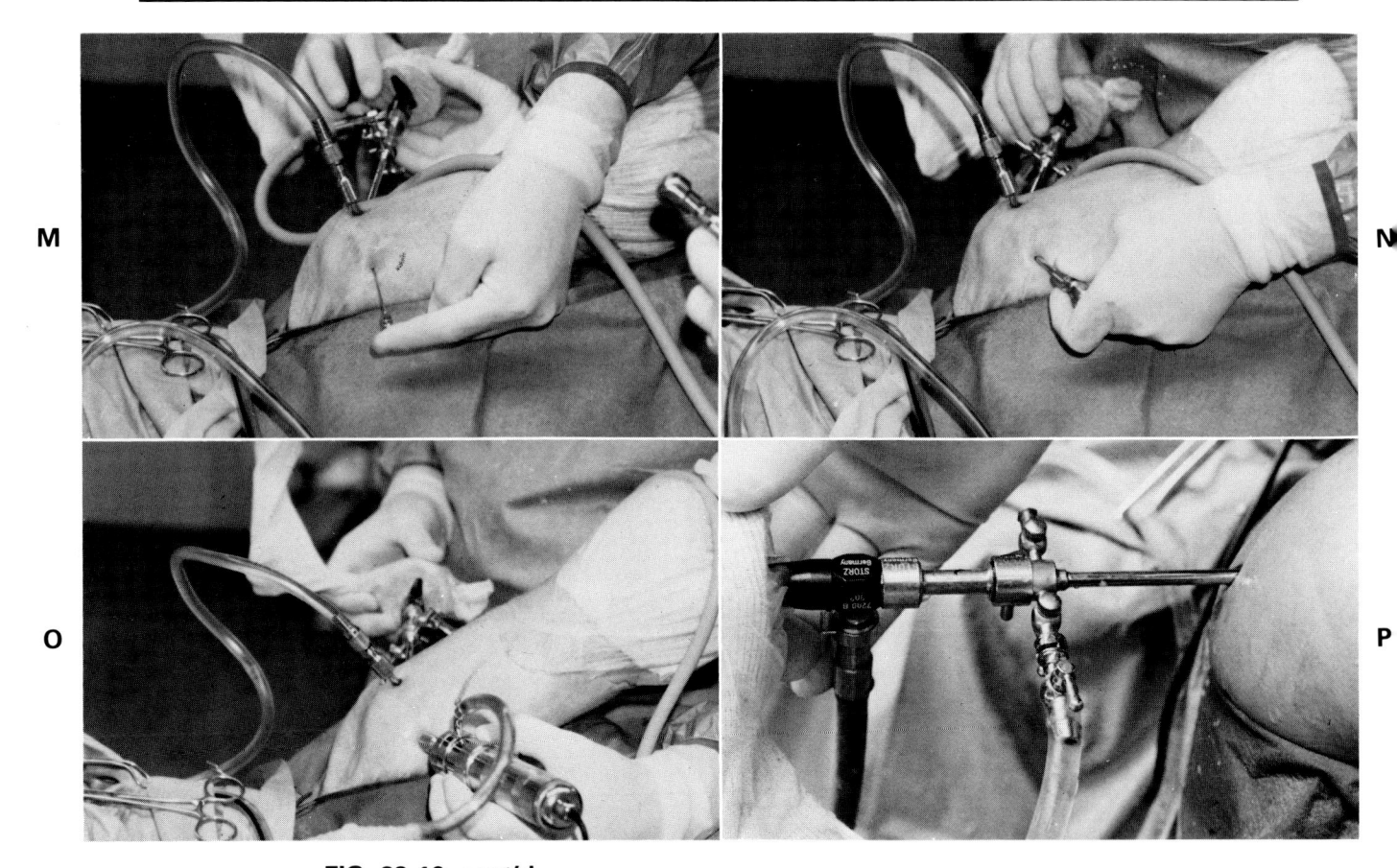

Diagnostic and surgical arthroscopy: other joints

FIG. 22-16, cont'd

M Needle for Intra-articular Shaver.
N Cannula in same tract.
O Intra-articular Shaver in shoulder.
P Inflow of saline attached to arthroscope by separate spigot that delivers sufficient inflow to small joints. Used in both ankles and shoulders. This is adequate in small joint but not knee because of need for greater volume and flow.

The organizational setup should be rapid and the surgical procedure and team well coordinated, since saline extravasation in the shoulder joint is easier than in any other I have had experience with. After saline extravasates into the adjacent tissues, swelling does not permit manipulation of the instruments or arthroscope. The shoulder joint is compressed, and the surgery is then compromised and must be terminated. This may last only about 20 minutes, so I have experienced some delays in organizational setup that necessitated aborting the surgical portion of the procedure before it ever started. Therefore practice techniques should be carried out to prevent this complication.

Shoulder joint

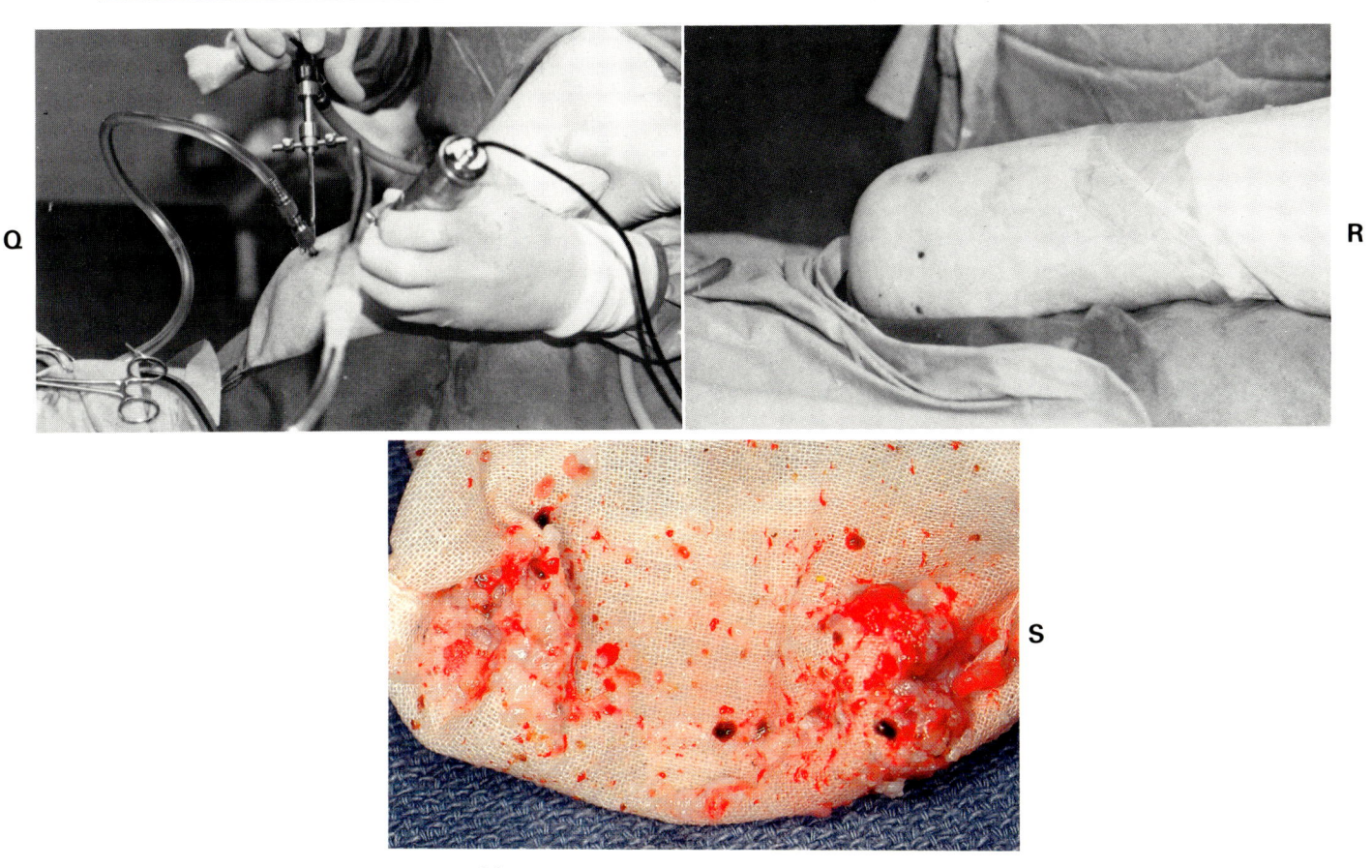

FIG. 22-16, cont'd

Q Adjusted inflow via arthroscope.
R Small puncture at end of rim.
S Anatomic specimen.

After the Little Shaver has gained access to the joint, it is possible to exchange it for the original Intra-articular Shaver and continue the debridement.

The morbidity is minimal (Fig. 22-16, Q). A pathologic specimen is retrieved in the same manner as in knee surgery (Fig. 22-16, R).

I have performed intra-articular shaves through the cannula system in patients with rheumatoid arthritis with rather remarkable results for approximately 1 year. Chondroplasty is also possible, as in the knee.

Chapter 23

Elbow joint

Technique
Normal anatomy
    Radial or lateral view
    Ulnar or medial approach
Findings or conditions
    Degenerative arthritis
    Rheumatoid arthritis
    Fracture
    Osteochondritis dissecans or Panner disease
Loose body removal
Operative arthroscopy

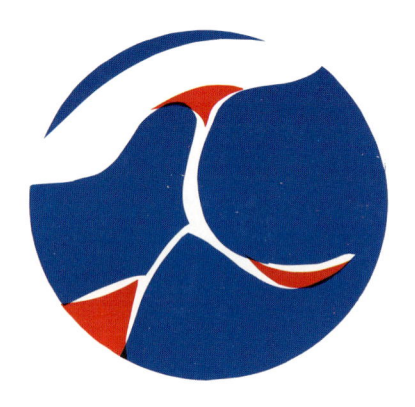

The elbow is another common site of pain and dysfunction. The clinical diagnoses of tendinitis, bursitis, and tennis elbow are not infrequent. Arthroscopy, used to its fullest extent, could further delineate these clinical diagnoses into actual pathoanatomic lesions, resulting in more specific treatment. Elbow arthroscopic experience is limited at this time. The knee joint has taken precedence in arthroscopic experience, and there are not many physicians exploring joints other than the knee.

TECHNIQUE

Anesthesia used is local, infiltrative, or IV regional (Fig. 23-1). General anesthesia is rarely employed. The patient is supine with the arm positioned on a Boyes-Parker table and suspended for surgery (Fig. 23-2). The surgeon is first on the lateral or radial side (Fig. 23-3) and then changes to the ulnar side (Fig. 23-4). The first assistant begins on the ulnar side and then changes position with the surgeon. Instruments are positioned on the Mayo stand at the end of the table. The light source is just beyond the instrument stand.

Multiple points of entry are possible in the elbow joint. Distension can be achieved first from the lateral side, a familiar site at which to enter the elbow (Fig. 23-5). This site is anterior to the lateral epicondyle and immediately superior and slightly anterior to the radial head. The radial head can be identified by palpation at the same time there is passive supination and pronation being applied to the forearm. The medial approach is immediately superior and just slightly anterior to the medial epicondyle. (See Fig. 23-11.)

The posterolateral pouch is best inspected in a maximally distended elbow (Fig. 23-6). It is possible to see and palpate a bulge between the humerus and the ulna laterally. One enters from anterior and approaches obliquely toward the posterior aspect into the olecranon fossa. A direct perpendicular puncture in this area would not provide a space large enough to enter. Therefore the

Elbow joint

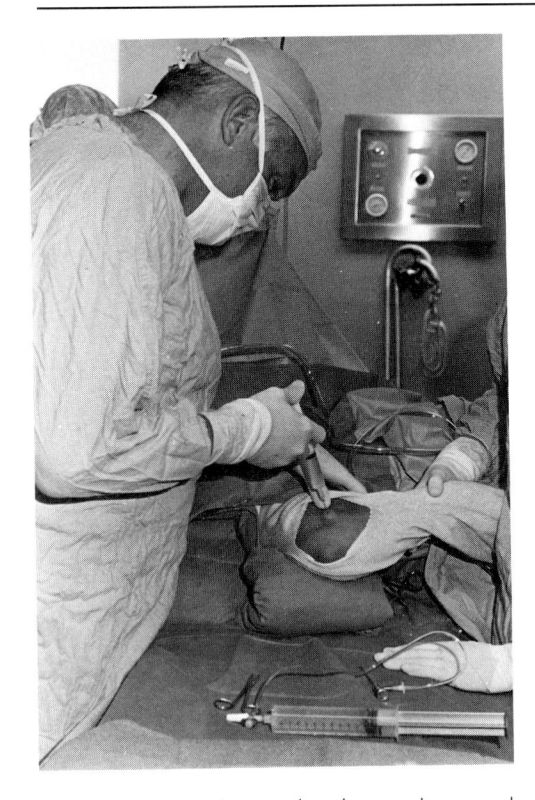

FIG. 23-1. Local anesthesia can be used for elbow joint arthroscopy.

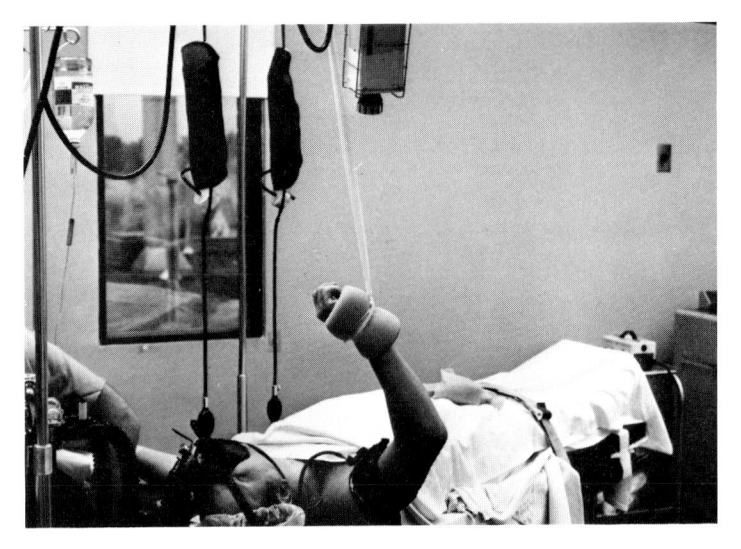

FIG. 23-2. Operative suspension. This position facilitates manipulation of instrumentation from all portals and spheres around elbow.

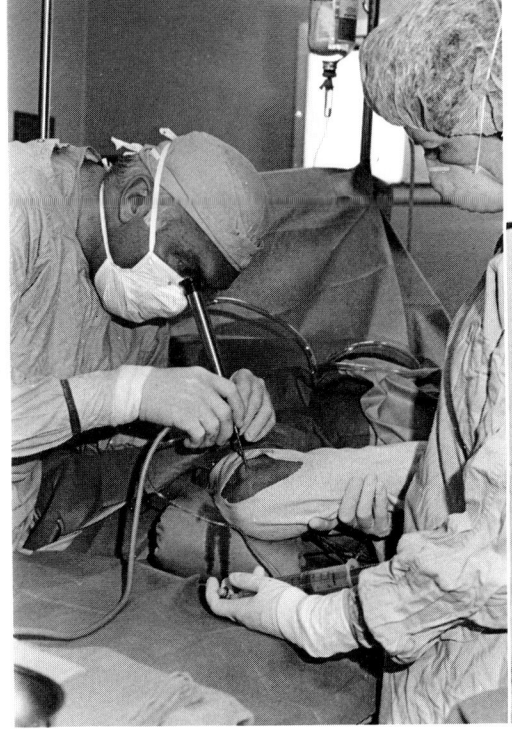

FIG. 23-3. A, Viewing elbow joint from lateral point immediately anterior to lateral epicondyle and superior to radial head. **B,** Rotation, supination, pronation, flexion, and extension help identify radial head and other landmarks in elbow.

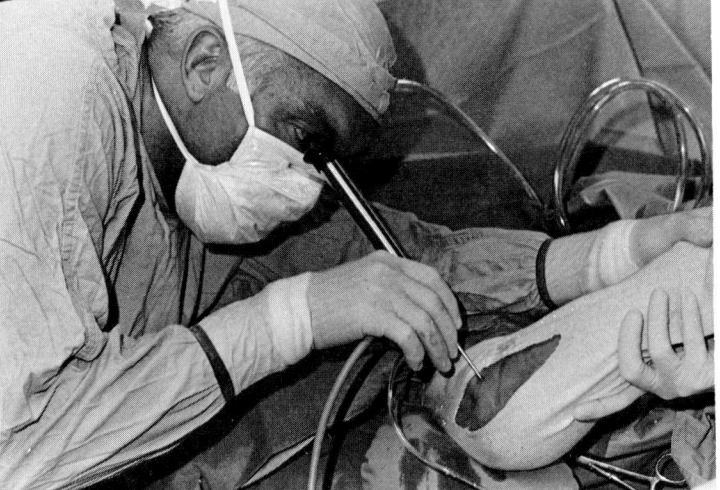

Diagnostic and surgical arthroscopy: other joints

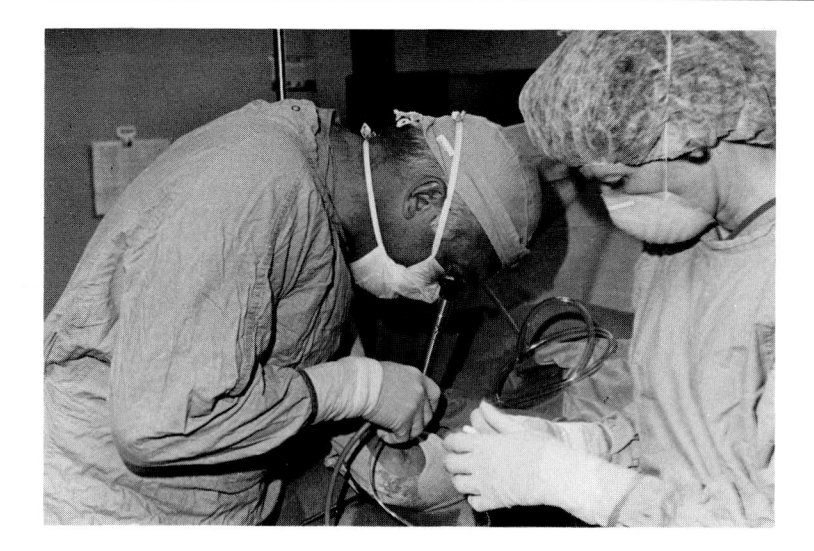

FIG. 23-4. Viewing from medial portal is done with arm in external rotation. It is better if arthroscopist and assistant change positions.

FIG. 23-5. With elbow distended, insertion can be made immediately anterior to radial head and slightly distal to epicondyle.

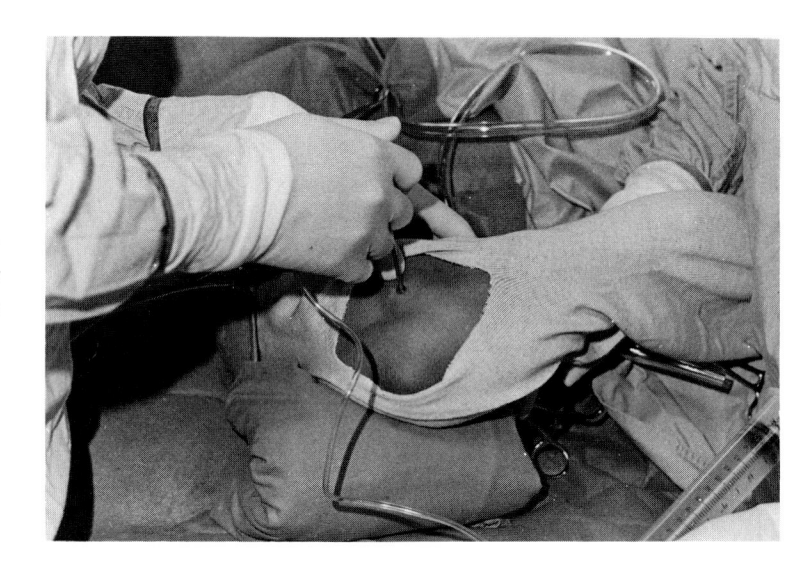

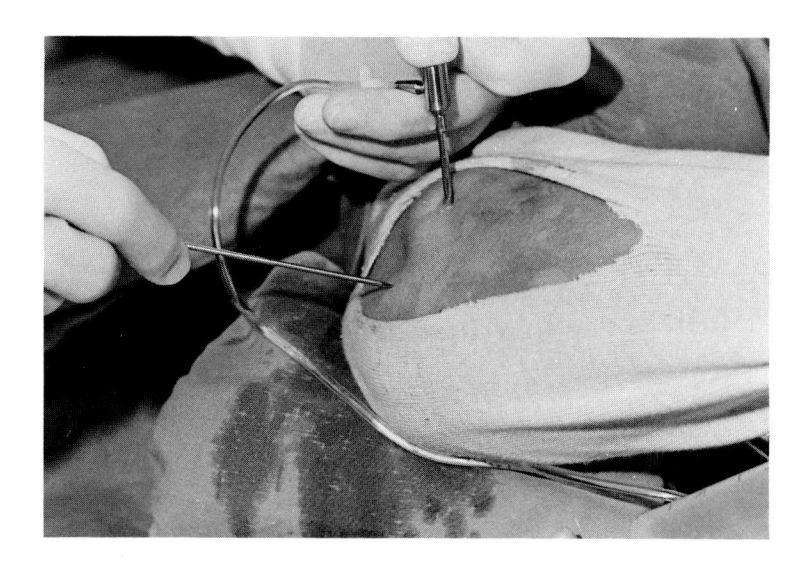

FIG. 23-6. With elbow distended through inflow cannula of anterior puncture, bulge is seen lateral at area of olecranon fossa.

Elbow joint

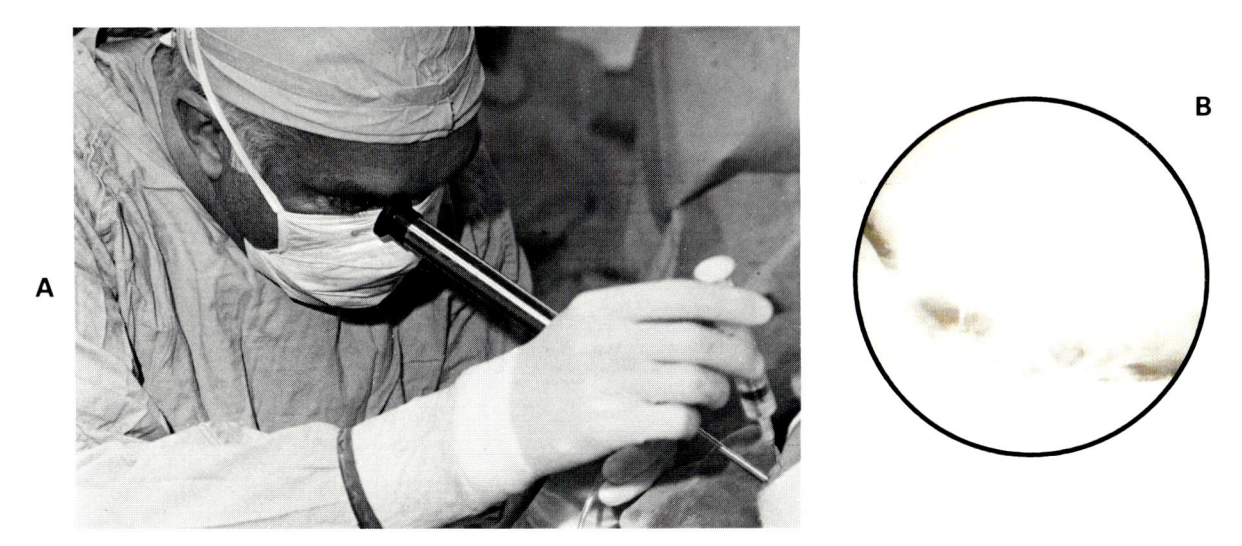

FIG. 23-7. A, Olecranon fossa can be seen. Separate needle puncture establishes entry point for triangulation techniques. **B,** Arthroscopic view of olecranon fossa with degenerative arthritic change.

sleeve created by the distension along the bony articulation of the humeral-olecranon fossa allows one to enter the joint; then, with retraction, it is possible to view the olecranon fossa (Fig. 23-7).

NORMAL ANATOMY
Radial or lateral view

The synovium of even a noninflamed elbow has rather marked synovial villae, especially on the anterior wall of the joint. From this approach it is possible to see the synovial reflection on the humerus and the coronoid process. With very gentle retraction it may be possible to even see the radial head, but that is less likely.

Ulnar or medial approach

This approach is better than the radial approach. The radial head is easily identified with supination and pronation passively applied to the forearm (Fig. 23-8, *A* to *D*). This landmark allows one to move with marked supination and pronation all the way into the joint between the humerus and the radius, and flexion and extension afford an even better examination (Fig. 23-8, *E*).

The posterolateral approach is carried out with maximal distension. It is possible to see the olecranon process, a rather large potential space in the posterior aspect of the elbow. With retraction and redirection and flexion and extension one can achieve exact two-hand manipulative positioning and can course all the way through the olecranon fossa and up to the anterior compartment of the joint. A continual maximal distension is necessary to achieve this.

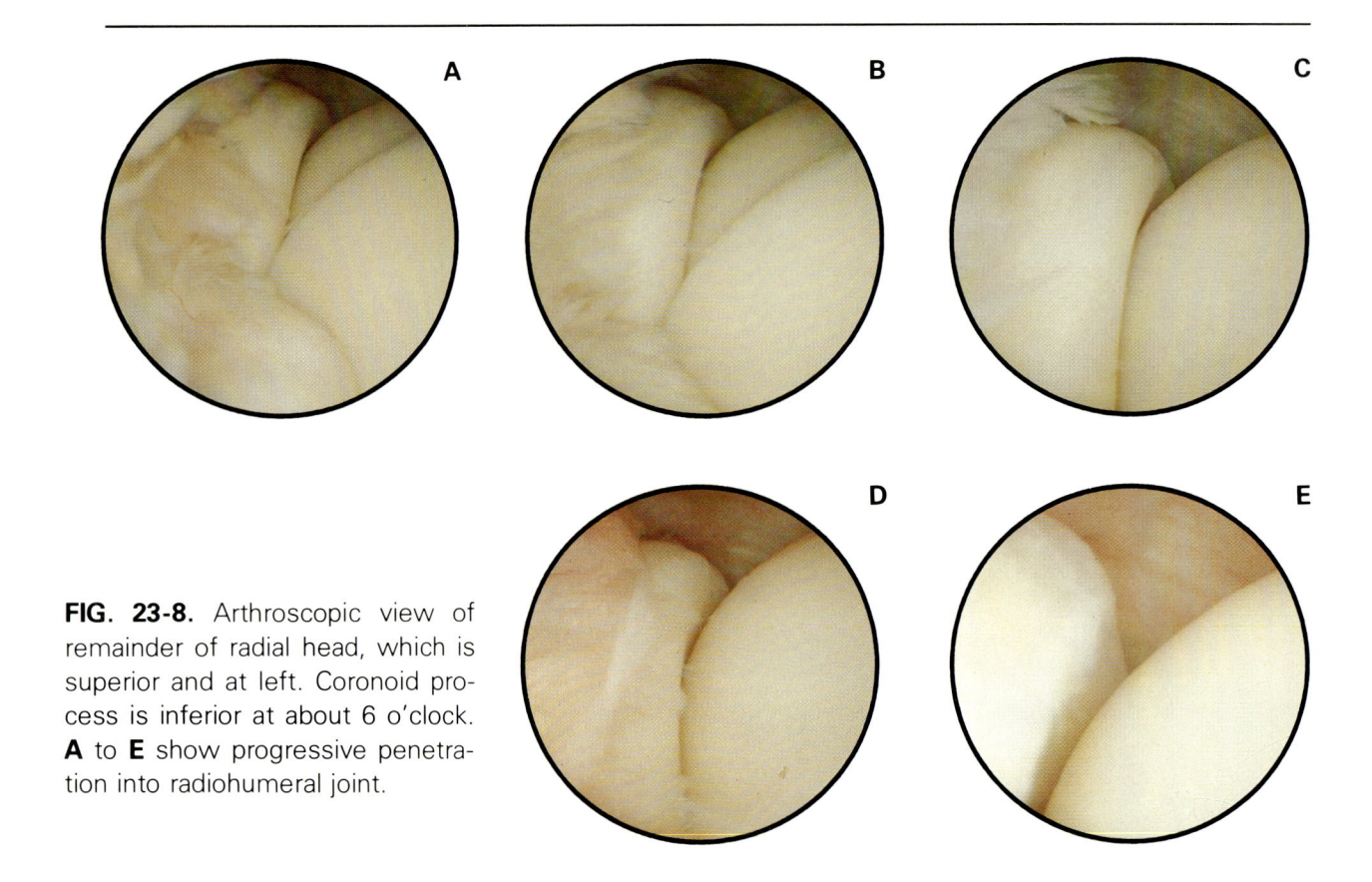

Diagnostic and surgical arthroscopy: other joints

FIG. 23-8. Arthroscopic view of remainder of radial head, which is superior and at left. Coronoid process is inferior at about 6 o'clock. **A** to **E** show progressive penetration into radiohumeral joint.

FINDINGS OR CONDITIONS

Several patients whom I have examined with refractory tendinitis or tennis elbow have had mild synovitis and even early degenerative arthritis with fine, loose articular debris. The lavage of this material has resulted in the subsiding of the tennis elbow symptoms. I have not yet seen a large inflamed synovial fold.

Degenerative arthritis

Patients with degenerative change and incongruity may have loose debris in their joint or even loose bodies recognizable on x-ray examination (Fig. 23-9). These can be lavaged or removed transcutaneously, thus avoiding the need for an arthrotomy (Fig. 23-10).

Rheumatoid arthritis

Rheumatoid arthritic synovium can be appraised and perhaps also managed by cortisone injections or partial synovectomy with removal of loose bodies by transcutaneous methods. (See Fig. 23-14.)

Fracture

Arthroscopy can make an exact assessment of the separation and/or the incongruity of the fractured surfaces and dictate the management or indication

Elbow joint

for open reduction. This has been beneficial in a few patients. I also have had a patient with a nonunion and minimal displacement of the olecranon. The arthroscopic examination determined that the articular surface had healed and there was no incongruity or step-off. Therefore the joint was not opened, and a sliding bone graft was performed on the nonunion of the ulna, resulting in healing and a good range of motion. Assessment of displacement in the radial head articular fracture may be determined arthroscopically. It is important to recognize the magnification factor in these small spaces, which is learned by experience.

Osteochondritis dissecans or Panner disease

These conditions may be evaluated and any loose piece can be removed. I have not had any experience with drilling or fixation. It would be possible to use a posterior or oblique transcutaneous portal, avoiding the antecubital fossae.

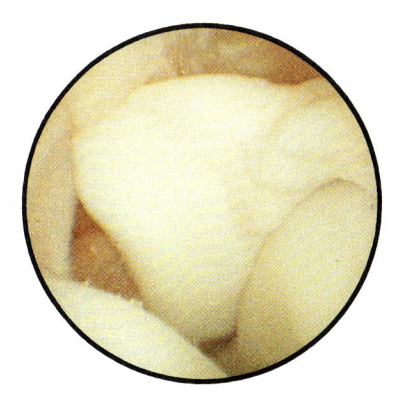

FIG. 23-9. Arthroscopic view of loose body in elbow joint.

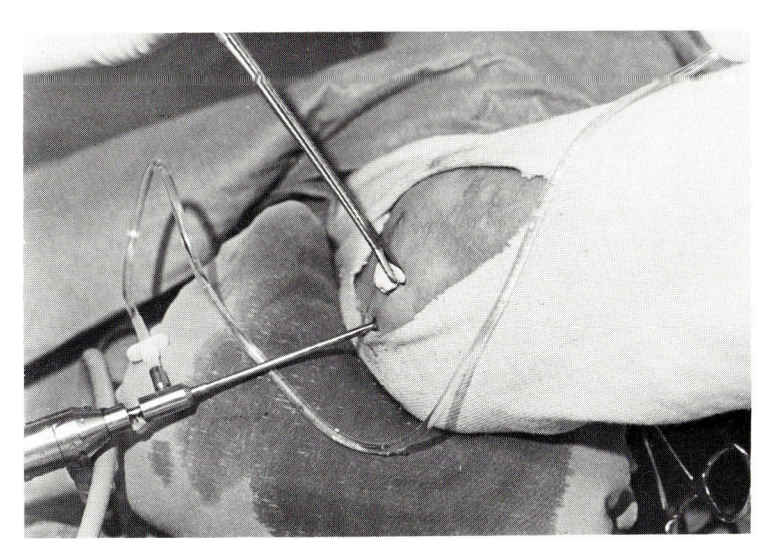

FIG. 23-10. Complete removal of loose body from olecranon fossa of elbow by arthroscopic means, thus avoiding arthrotomy.

Diagnostic and surgical arthroscopy: other joints

LOOSE BODY REMOVAL

Loose bodies in the elbow may or may not be identified by x-ray examination. Suspicion in the presence of negative x-ray evidence is an indication for arthroscopy. A small loose body or even multiple loose bodies can not only be identified but also removed by transcutaneous methods under arthroscopic control.

The first step is to perform a complete arthroscopic inspection of the joint (Fig. 23-3, *B*). Distension is maintained by compression on a 60-ml syringe attached to the arthroscopic cannula by way of a K-52 catheter. This is very much like the technique used with the Needlescope in arthroscopy of the knee.

When the loose body is identified, a separate transcutaneous puncture is made with a needle. If performed under local anesthesia, a syringe attached to the needle can infiltrate the tissue on the way in (Fig. 23-6). The skin is then lanced for placement of forceps along the same tract the needle established (perfect for triangulation) (Fig. 23-11). Forceps are placed into the joint after laceration of the skin capsule (Figs. 23-12 and 23-13). Under direct visualization the forceps grasp the loose body. After it is in the firm grasp, visualization is no longer necessary. The arthroscope can be retired momentarily and the incision made adjacent to the forceps shaft for transcutaneous delivery.

In other circumstances it can be valuable to have the arm suspended to allow viewing from one side with the arthroscope attached to either video or direct viewing equipment; then make the transcutaneous entry from the opposite side of the elbow. Viewing is usually from the lateral side and entry from the medial side. Care must be taken on medial punctures to avoid injuring the ulnar nerve. Landmarks, again, are best identified with the initial transcutaneous placement of a spinal needle, as in arthroscopic surgery of the knee.

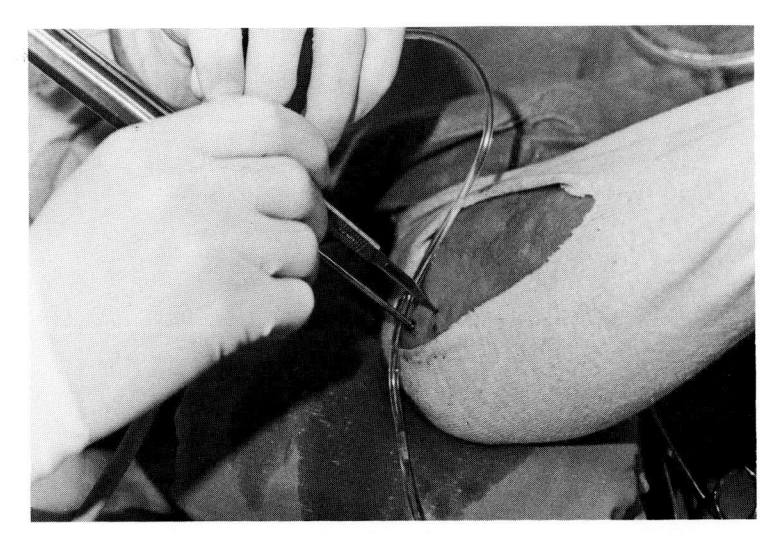

FIG. 23-11. Lateral view of olecranon fossa. Knife blade enters joint to open an area for loose body removal.

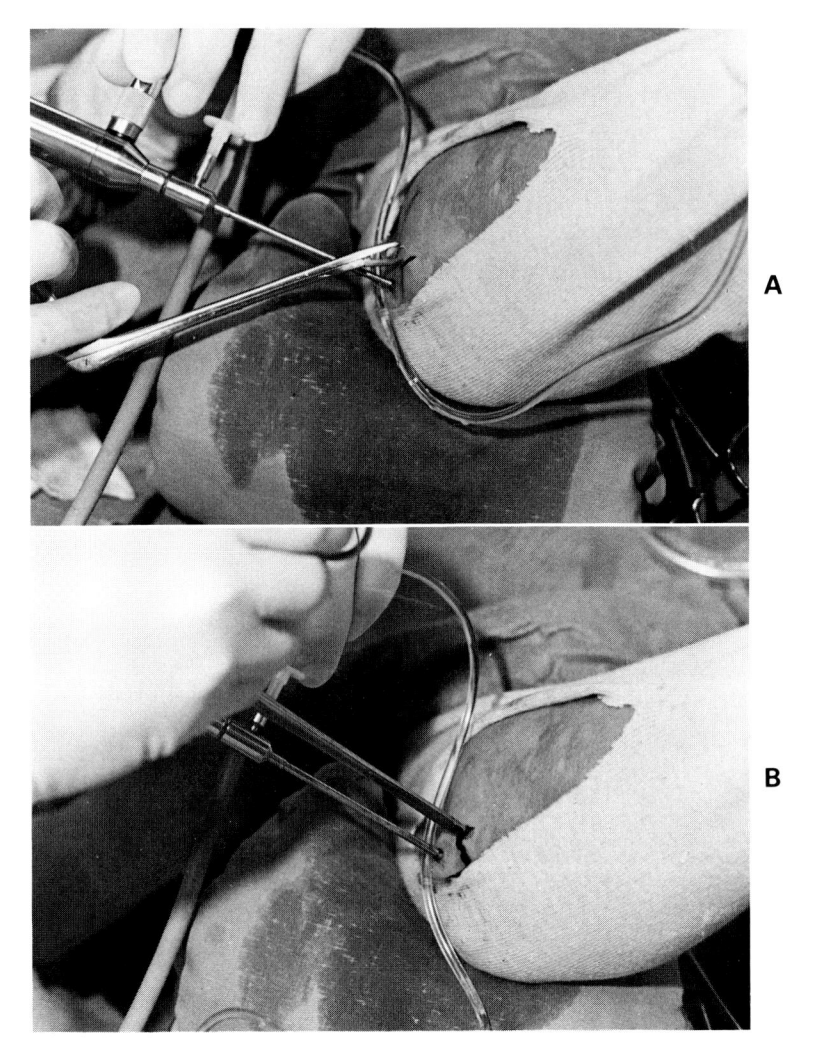

FIG. 23-12. A, Forceps approach in joint to make percutaneous entry. **B,** Forceps within joint and loose bodies visible.

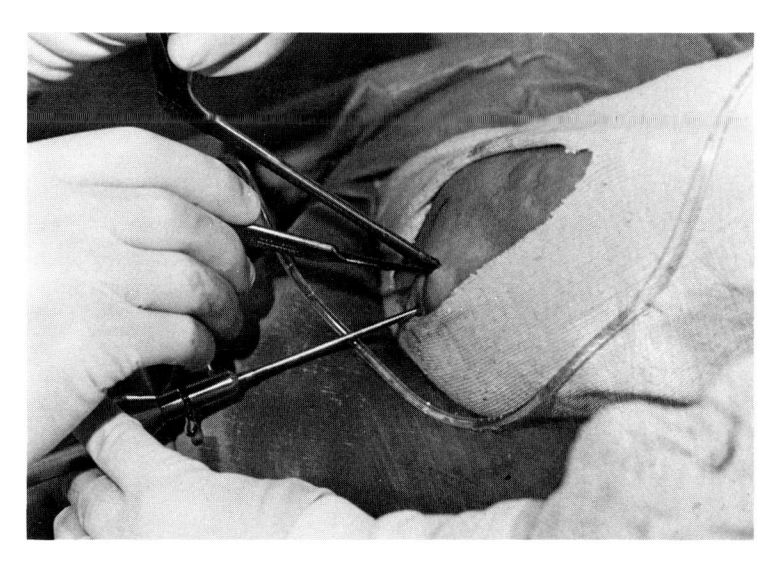

FIG. 23-13. Loose body is grasped while assistant holds arthroscope. Viewing is not taking place, and soft tissues are being released around loose body being retrieved from elbow.

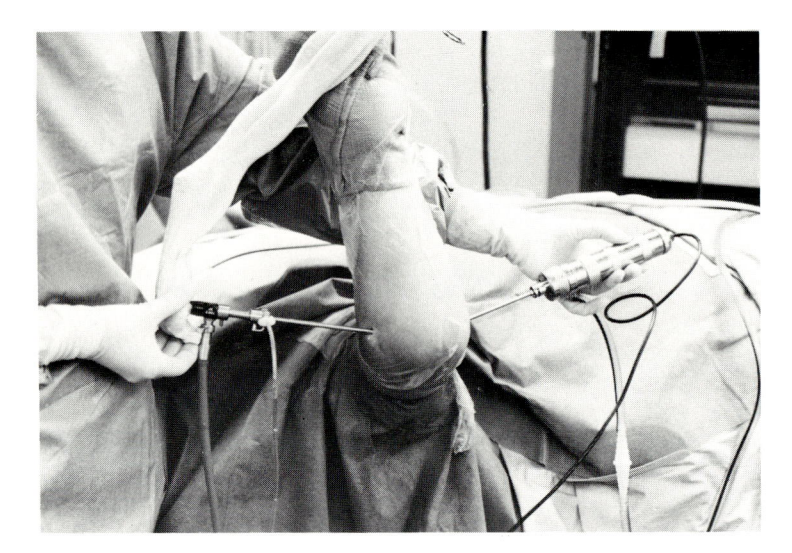

Diagnostic and surgical arthroscopy: other joints

FIG. 23-14. Arthroscopic viewing via articulated viewing device into video monitor allows manipulation from opposite side of elbow for intra-articular shaving.

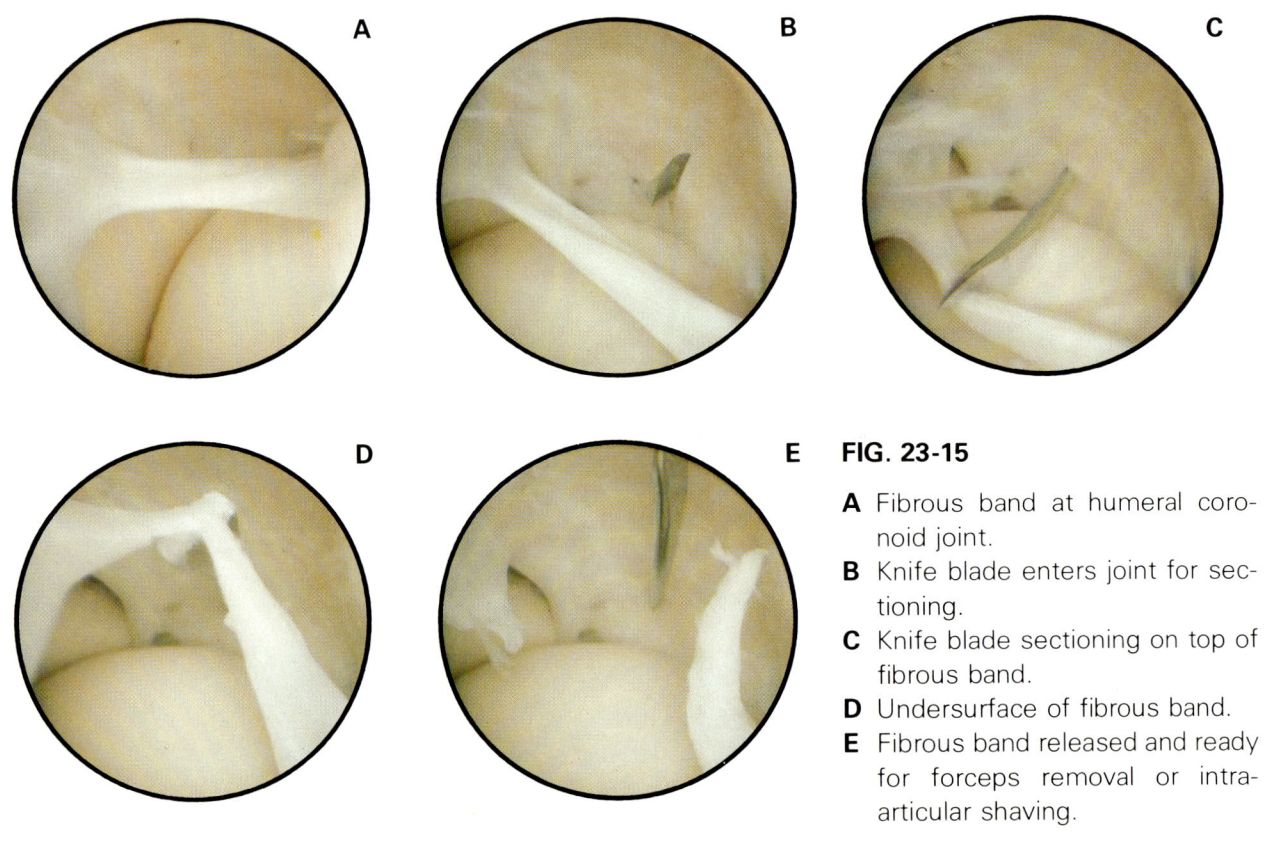

FIG. 23-15

A Fibrous band at humeral coronoid joint.
B Knife blade enters joint for sectioning.
C Knife blade sectioning on top of fibrous band.
D Undersurface of fibrous band.
E Fibrous band released and ready for forceps removal or intra-articular shaving.

OPERATIVE ARTHROSCOPY

The best position for operative arthroscopy is to suspend and drape the patient's elbow. (See Fig. 23-2.) Sometimes, because of the small joint space, compression of the saline inflow is necessary. The arthroscope approaches from one side and the Intra-articular Shaver from the opposite side for synovectomy (Fig. 23-14). The plastic drape should not cover the elbow joint entirely because it limits the amount of distension possible.

Fibrous bands can cause elbow symptoms such as popping and snapping. It is possible to care for these arthroscopically by section and/or resection with forceps, small knife blades, or the Intra-articular Shaver (Fig. 23-15).

Chapter 24

Wrist joint

Technique
Diagnostic problems
Meniscoid lesion
Synovitis
Compression articular fracture

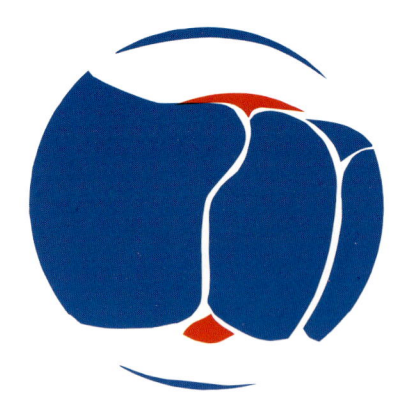

The wrist joint, surprisingly, lends itself to arthroscopic evaluation. My personal experience is limited. There are many undiagnosed wrist problems that certainly would be amenable to this type of investigation.

TECHNIQUE

Anesthesia used is either local or IV regional. The patient is supine; the surgeon stands on the radial side of the patient; the first assistant is on the ulnar side; instrumentation is located at the end of the table; the light source is beyond the end of the table.

A barrier drape is used to ensure sterility if there is saline spillage. An absorbent paper-face drape is used on a Boyes-Parker table.

The wrist may be entered from the radionavicular portal; course from distal to proximal and use palpation (Fig. 24-1). Entry should be accomplished by first placing a 22-gauge needle into the space to determine the exact direction and alignment and to distend the space prior to entering with the arthroscope (Fig. 24-2). It also may be entered from the ulnar side immediately distal

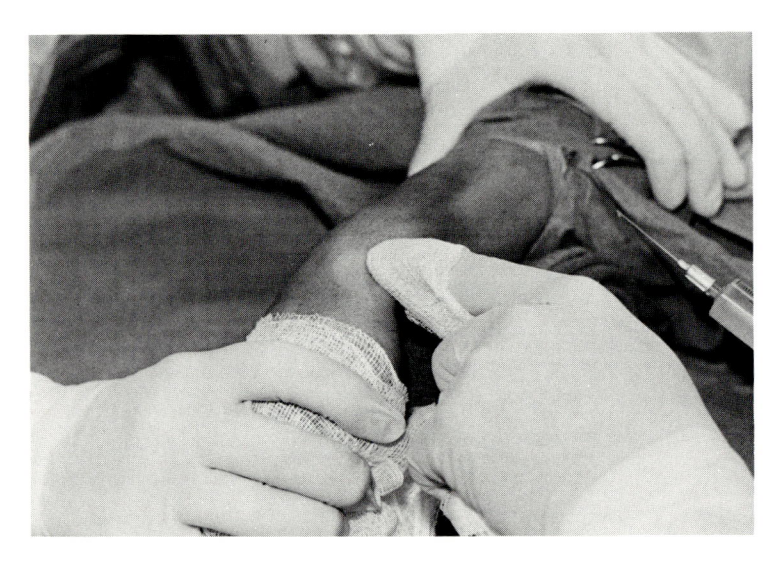

FIG. 24-1. Palpation of radiocarpal joint.

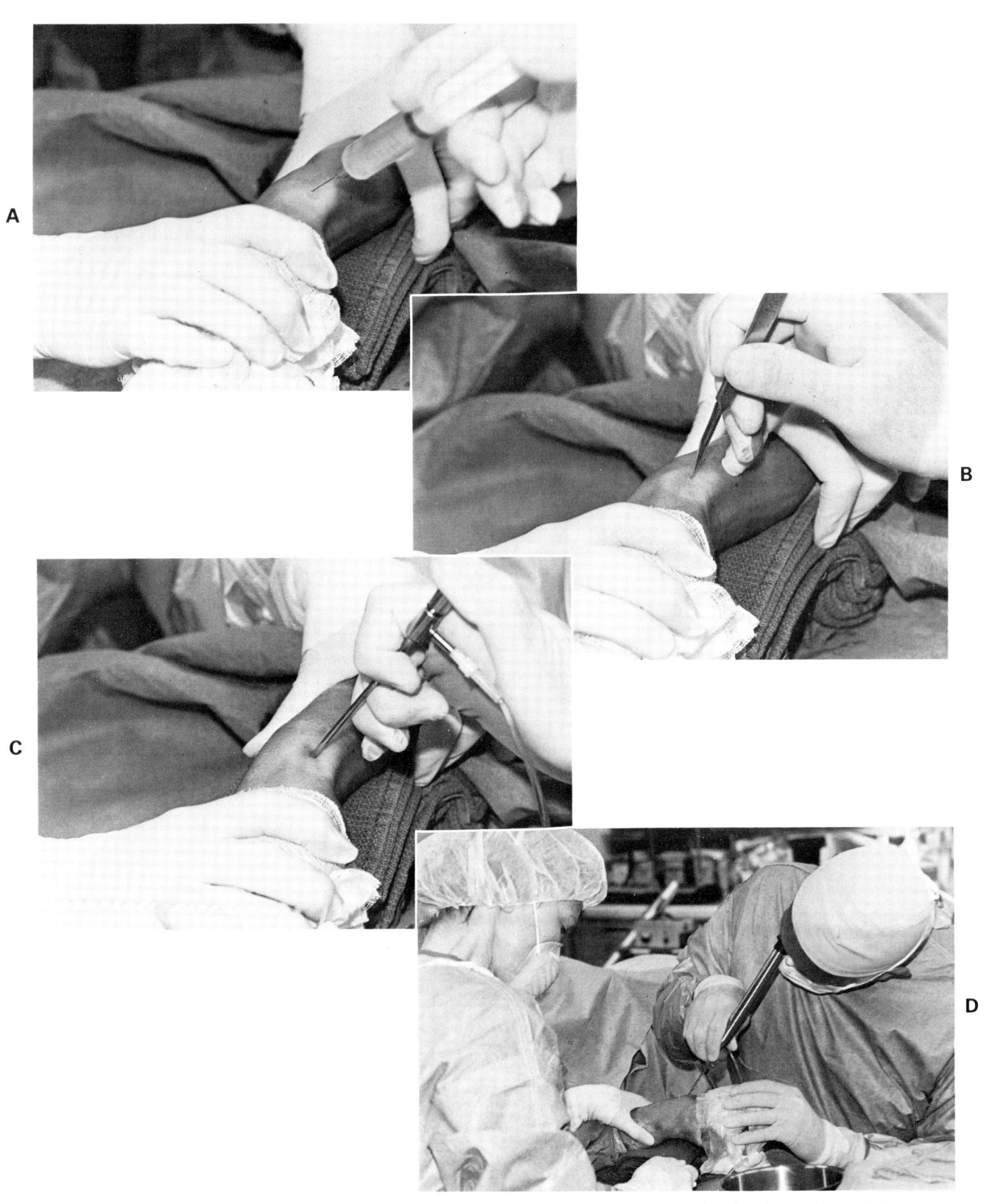

FIG. 24-2. A, Injection with No. 22 needle into radioulnar joint for distension. **B,** Laceration of skin only, avoiding superficial branch of the radial nerve, which is often palpable. **C,** Needlescope enters radioulnar joint. **D,** Arthroscopic viewing of distal radioulnar joint with Needlescope.

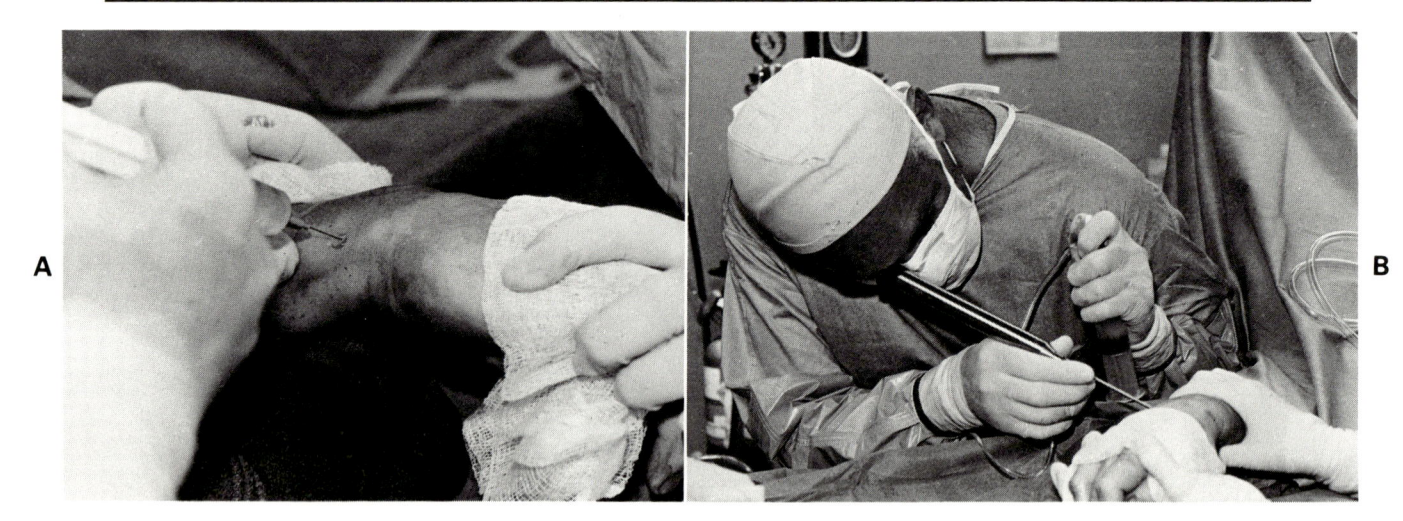

Diagnostic and surgical arthroscopy: other joints

FIG. 24-3. A, Lateral approach to wrist joint is immediately dorsal and distal to ulnar styloid. Again, distension with No. 22 needle facilitates entry. **B,** Arthroscopic inspection of lateral aspect of joint.

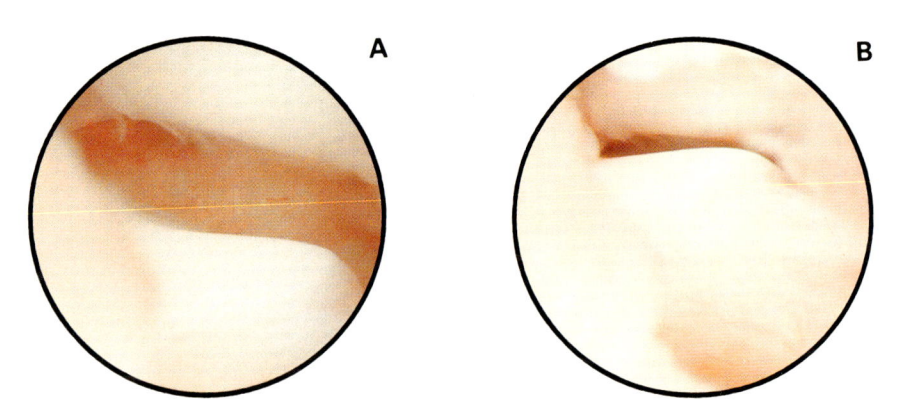

FIG. 24-4

A Arthroscopic view of intercarpal bones of lateral aspect.
B Intercarpal view above lateral aspect of triquetrum.

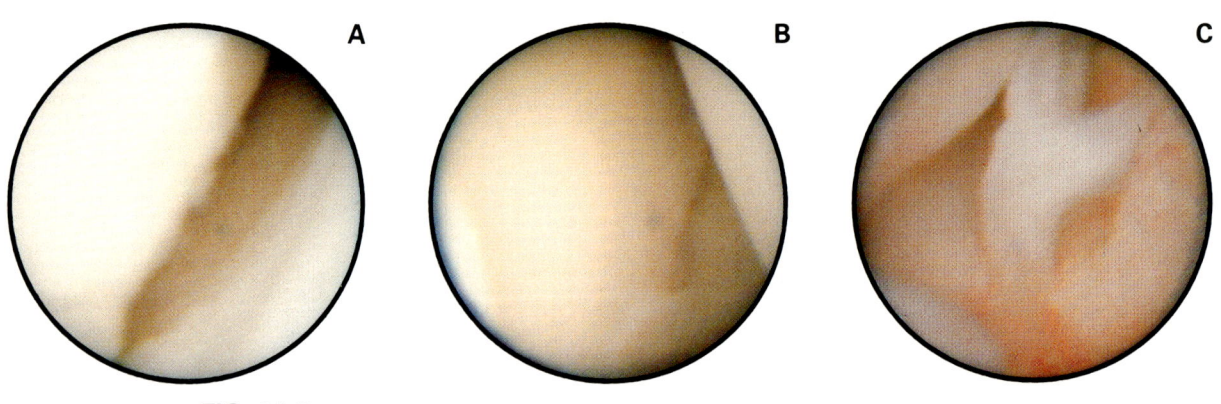

FIG. 24-5

A Distal ulna and radius at right and navicular bone at left.
B Tip of radius at right and body of navicular bone at left.
C Meniscoid lesion in distal radioulnar joint.

to the ulnar styloid (Fig. 24-3). Any wrist space can be entered. Intercarpal spaces, as well as the distal radioulnar articulation, may be visualized (Fig. 24-4).

DIAGNOSTIC PROBLEMS

Diagnostic problems are usually related to trauma. I have not had any experience with rheumatoid or degenerative changes; this is because of the nature of my practice.

MENISCOID LESION

One patient had a meniscoid type of lesion. He complained of pain during grasping. I was able to demonstrate and vividly record the lesion and its compression. I correlated palpation of the lesion (under local anesthesia) with the patient's complaints (Fig. 24-5). Subsequent excision of the lesion by arthrotomy relieved the symptoms.

SYNOVITIS

Several patients I treated had synovitis. After examining them for undiagnosed pain, I discovered rather marked nonspecific synovitis at the radioulnar articulation. Vacuuming and cortisone instillation into the joint resulted in remission of symptoms. It appeared to be a localized phenomenon, not diffuse, rheumatoid, or degenerative.

COMPRESSION ARTICULAR FRACTURE

Articular cartilage fracture has been observed following injury. The x-ray evidence was negative. The patient had chronic cracking in the dorsum of the wrist. The lesion was in the capitate surface opposite the lunate bone (Fig. 24-6).

FIG. 24-6. Articular cartilage fracture of capitate where it articulates with lunate in wrist.

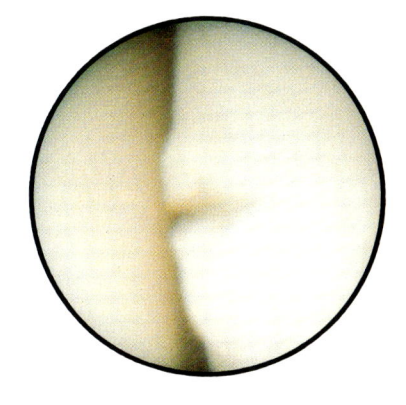

Chapter 25

Finger joint

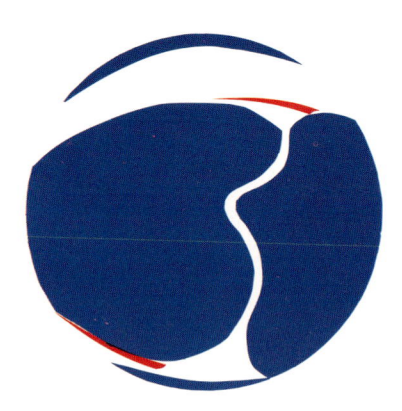

Finger joint arthroscopy can be performed under local anesthesia. The anesthetic can be applied with a No. 25 needle and carried all the way into the joint, which distends it. The needle is brought in from the lateral or medial aspect at a site adjacent and volar to the border of the extensor tendon. The placement is slightly oblique from distal to proximal. This dorsal area, under maximal distension, affords a surprising amount of space for visualization of the articular surfaces both proximal and distal (Fig. 25-1).

There is rarely an indication for arthroscopy of the finger joint. The most common indication is to determine whether an ossicle is inside or outside the joint. Also, incongruity of the articular surfaces following a traumatic episode is a valid indication for arthroscopy. It allows the surgeon to intelligently discuss and plan arthroplastic or fusion procedures with the patient.

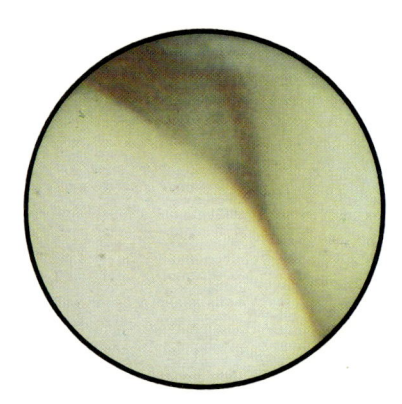

FIG. 25-1. Arthroscopic view of finger joint with 2.2-mm Needlescope. Intercondylar depression of proximal phalanx is at left and prominence of middle phalanx is at right.

Chapter 26

Hip joint

Technique
Findings
    Early degenerative arthritis
    Synovitis
    Trauma
    Osteochondritis dissecans
    Aseptic necrosis
Evaluation for reconstructive surgery

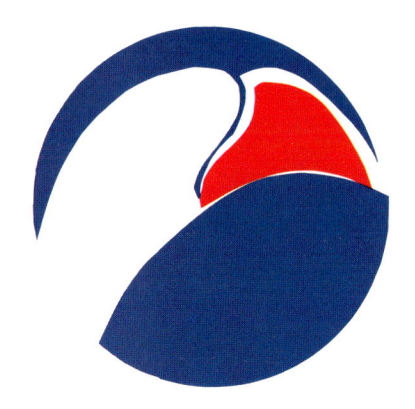

The depth of the hip joint makes clinical examination difficult. Palpation and x-ray examination, including tomograms and arthrograms, help establish the diagnosis. Over a period of time there may be hip pain in the absence of any radiologic changes. This situation lends itself well to arthroscopic evaluation.

TECHNIQUE

General anesthesia is recommended. The patient is supine on a fracture table with traction potential (Fig. 26-1). The surgeon is lateral to the patient,

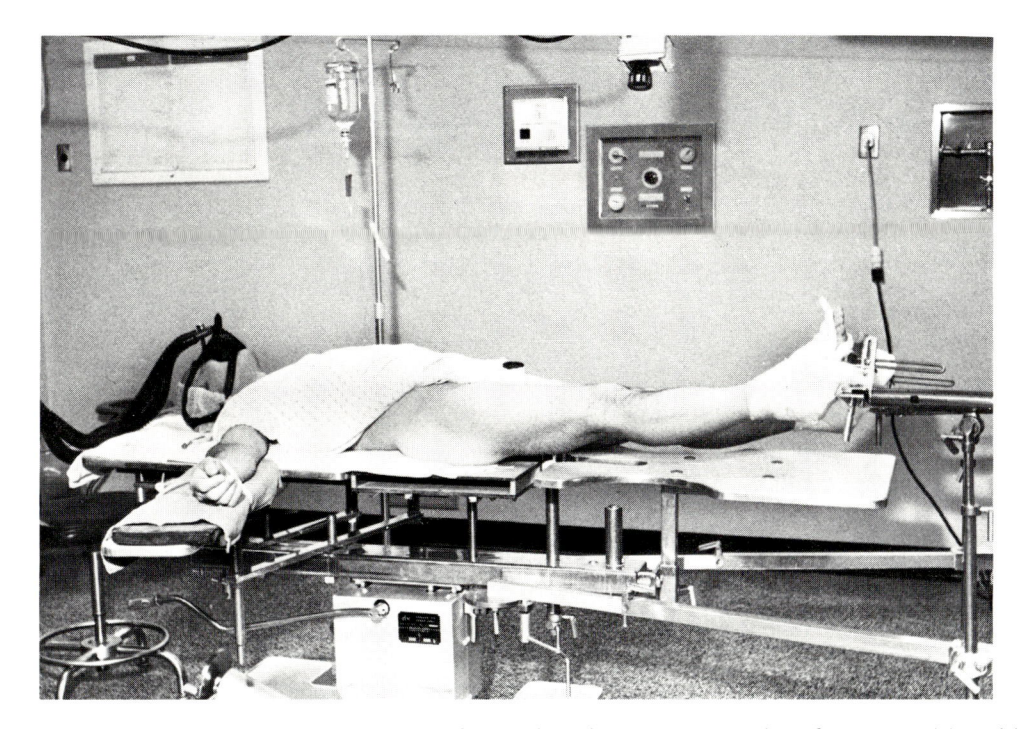

FIG. 26-1. Hip arthroscopy is best performed under x-ray control on fracture table with traction.

and the first assistant is on the opposite side of the table. Instruments are positioned on the opposite side of the table, as is the light source.

The anterolateral approach has been most serviceable (Fig. 26-2). With the hip in slight distraction, flexion, and slight abduction, there is a potential space anterior and lateral. Draw a line from the anterosuperior iliac spine. The topographic site is at a point where that line perpendicularly intersects a line drawn across from the symphysis pubis. A 6-inch spinal needle is placed at 45° inferior and then lateral 45° (Fig. 26-3). X-ray control best secures this position.

After the hip entry is confirmed by palpation and/or x-ray control, the hip is distended and will accommodate approximately 15 to 30 ml of saline. The needle is withdrawn slowly, and the surgeon continues to watch the needle's course. The skin is lanced with a No. 11 blade, and the arthroscope is passed down that same tract and into the hip, under x-ray control if necessary. It is also possible to leave the long spinal needle in for irrigation purposes and place the arthroscope adjacent to it (Fig. 26-4).

In children or thin patients a Needlescope with a 2.2-mm diameter is excellent. A 1.7-mm scope is quite malleable and difficult to manipulate through the musculature without the possibility of injury to the arthroscope. In larger patients a smaller diameter (2.7 mm) Storz scope has been used. The disadvantage is that it has a 55° field of view and also is a very malleable scope. The image becomes elliptic easily. Therefore, in large adult patients I often use the 5-mm endoscope. With care it can be placed within the hip joint.

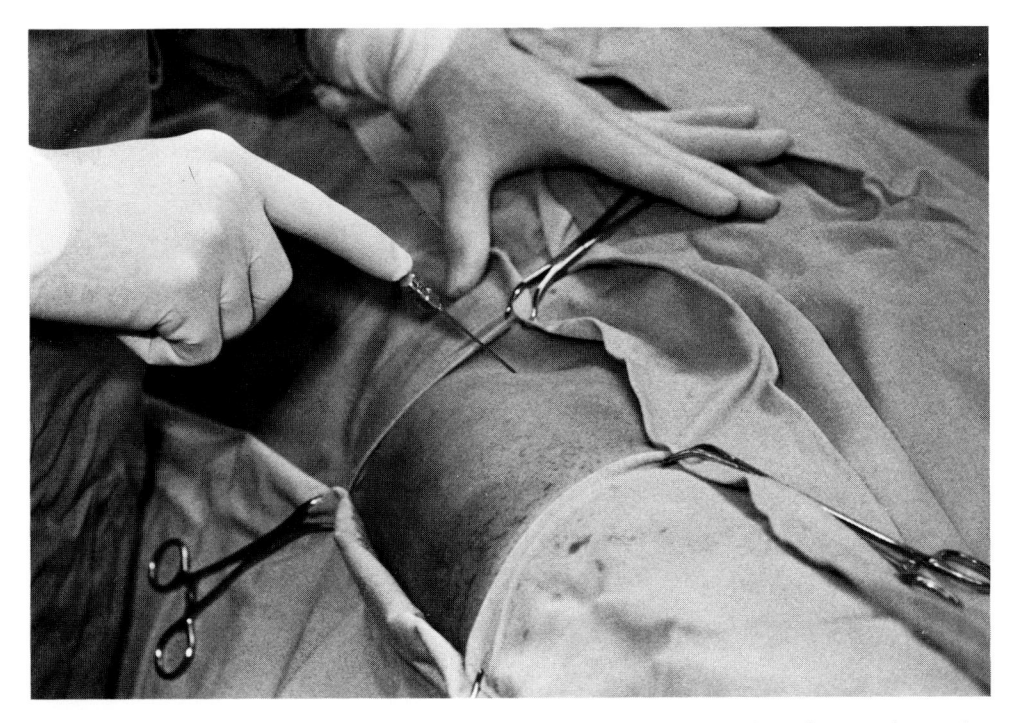

FIG. 26-2. Long spinal needle enters hip joint at point where line drawn down from anterior superior iliac spine intersects with line drawn across from pubis.

Hip joint

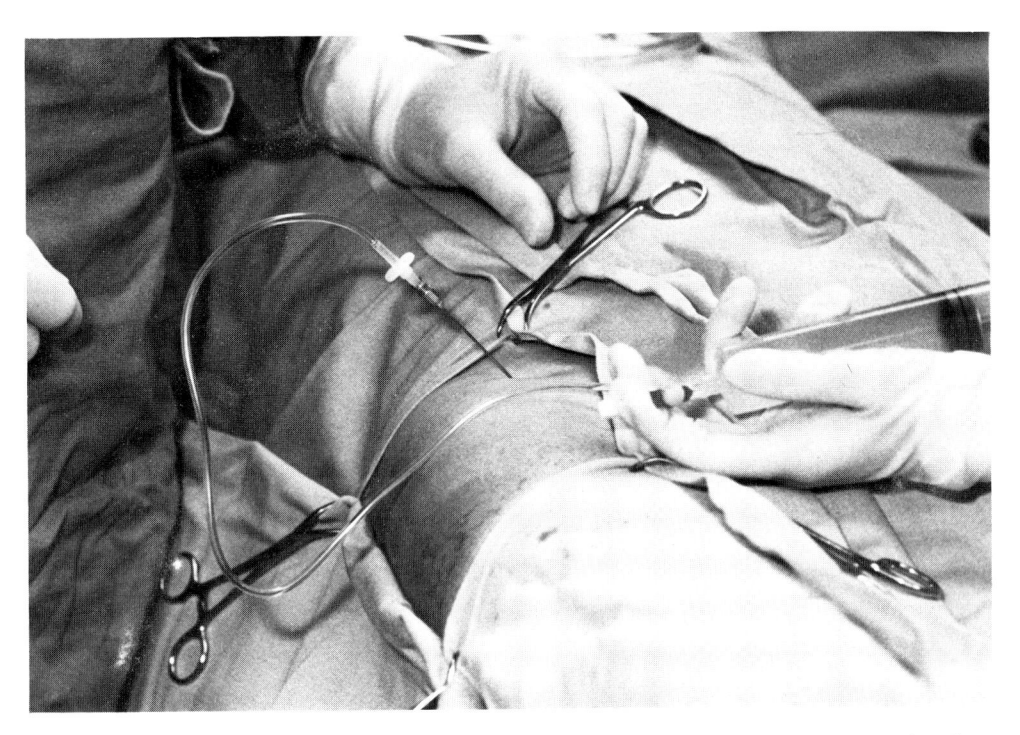

FIG. 26-3. After needle is in the joint, distension is created with infusion of saline.

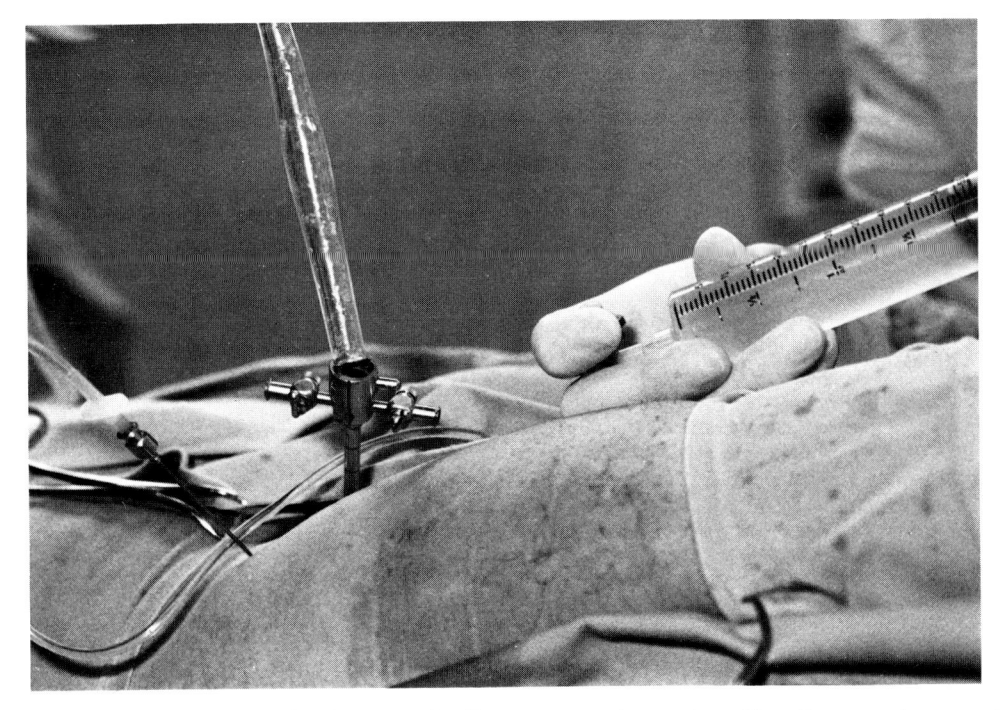

FIG. 26-4. Needle is still in place, and adjacent entry is made with arthroscopic cannula for cleansing and vacuuming of loose bodies or chips from joint.

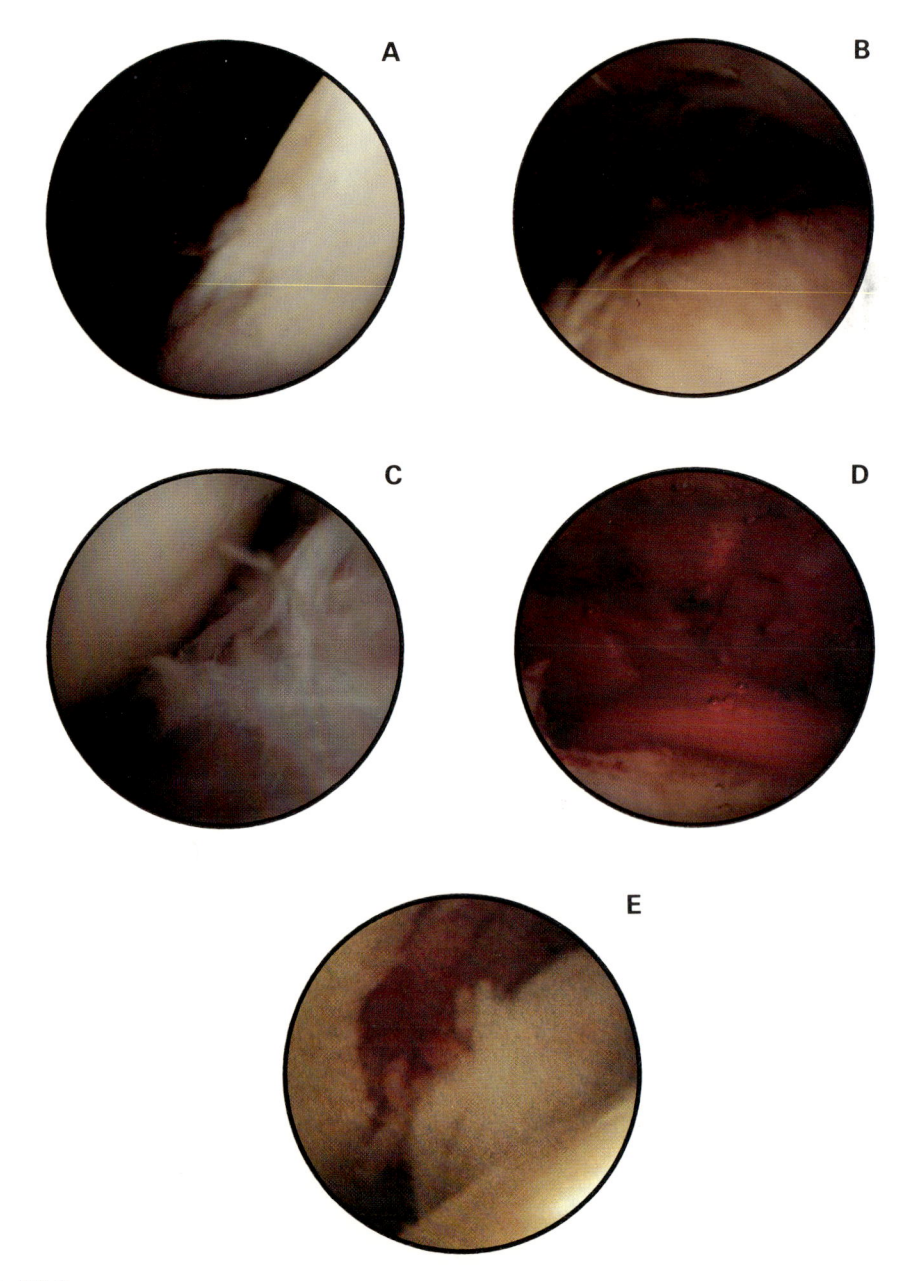

Diagnostic and surgical arthroscopy: other joints

FIG. 26-5

A Arthroscopic view of femoral head showing degenerative irregularity and chondronecrosis.
B Inflammatory change seen in fovea adjacent to denuded articular cartilage.
C Multiple loose bodies seen in the acetabular portion of hip.
D Fovea with inflammatory changes and multiple loose bodies in joint.
E With distraction, excellent view is given down into acetabulum.

Hip joint

FINDINGS
Early degenerative arthritis

I have had several patients with hip pain, without either x-ray film or tomogram evidence of change, in whom arthroscopy showed chondronecrosis with loose articular debris that was washed and vacuumed from the joint (Fig. 26-5).

One 48-year-old man had 18 months' remission of symptoms following this procedure and no longer needed his cane or anti-inflammatory medications. His symptoms did recur, and a second arthroscopy was performed (Fig. 26-6). There was some progression of the osteonecrosis, and the patient again underwent lavage, an anti-inflammatory medication regimen, and a period of nonweight bearing; he is currently in a state of remission.

Arthroscopy of the hip certainly has some diagnostic value in this situation, but it has special therapeutic value in postponing a resurfacing procedure or a total-hip replacement.

Synovitis

Both nonspecific synovitis and early rheumatoid changes have been observed. Also, one instance of pigmented villonodular synovitis has been observed by David Shneider.[2]

Trauma

Evaluation of articular surfaces following acetabular or head fractures can be accomplished arthroscopically. With internal and external rotation of the hip and distraction, a considerable amount of acetabulum can be visualized, as can the articular surfaces (Fig. 26-6, C).

Osteochondritis dissecans

The defect of osteochondritis dissecans may be evaluated arthroscopically.

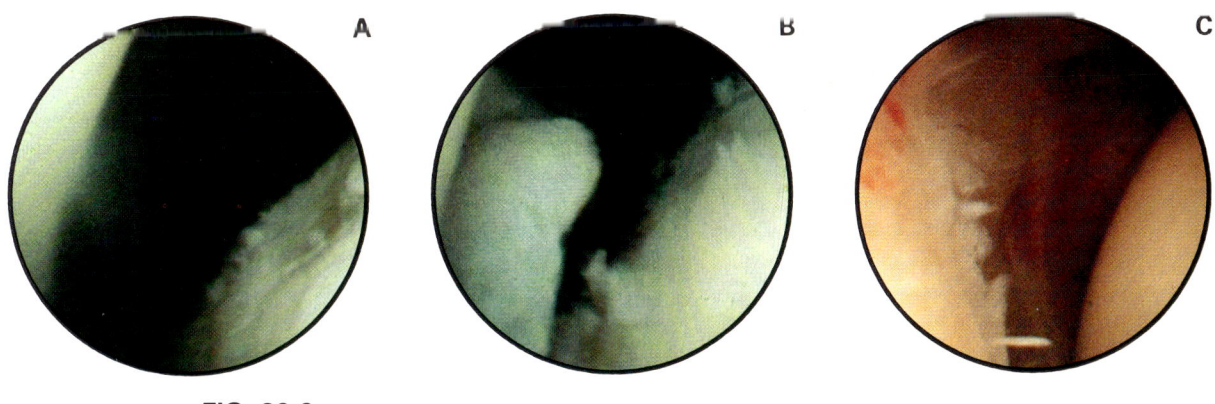

FIG. 26-6

A Oblique view showing acetabulum of femoral joint above eroded head of femur.
B Loose body on hip joint. This can be lavaged.
C After lavage, it is possible to see degenerative changes on acetabular side.

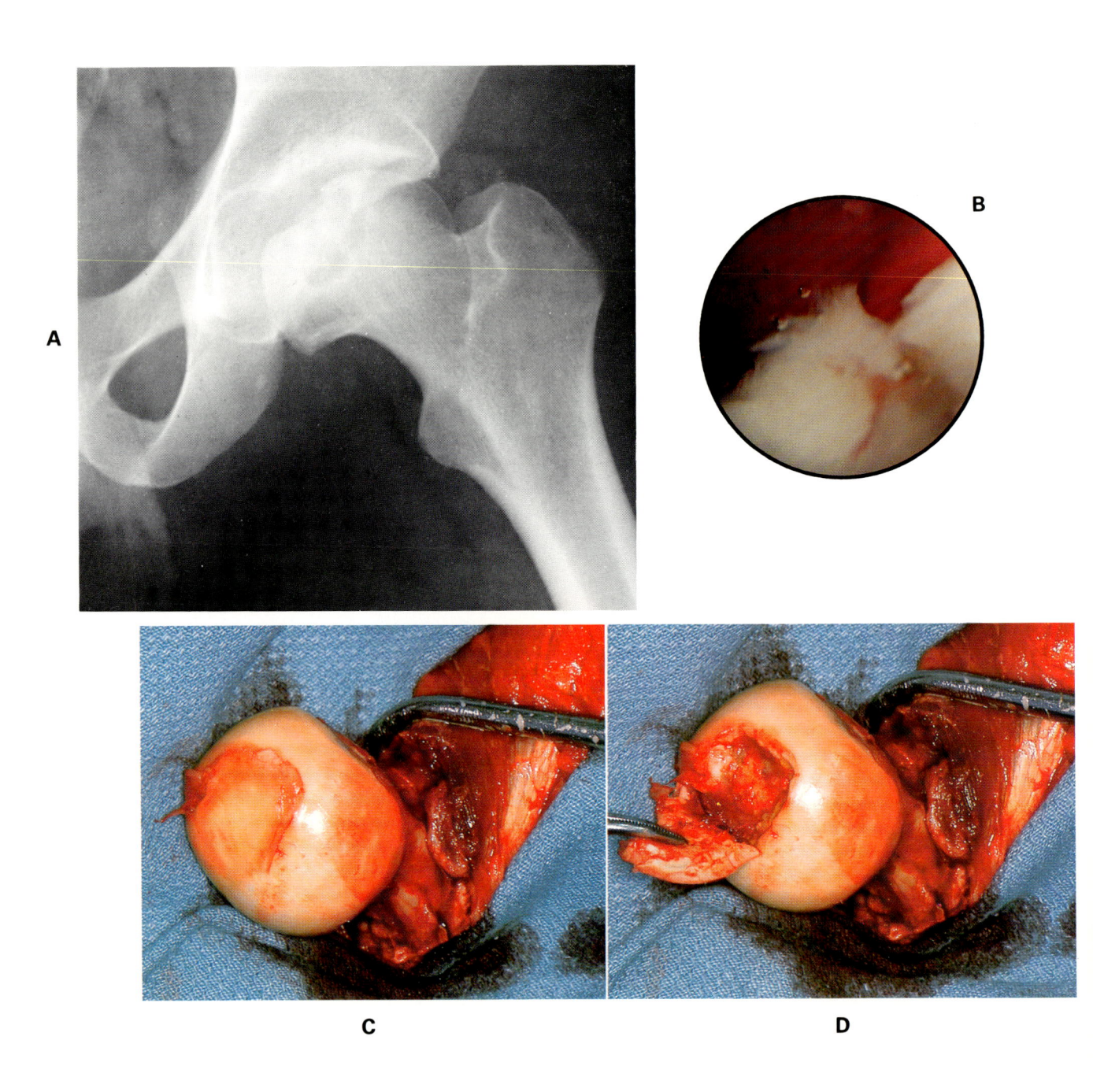

Diagnostic and surgical arthroscopy: other joints

FIG. 26-7. A, X-ray film of patient being considered for proximal femoral osteotomy or surface arthroplasty. **B,** Arthroscopic view of similar patient with elevation of articular surface. Osteotomy would probably not be successful in this case. **C,** Flap elevation off femoral head. **D,** Loose articular fragment is elevated. This patient was best suited for resurfacing arthroplasty. (Courtesy William H. Harris, Boston, Mass.)

Hip joint

Aseptic necrosis

Many patients with aseptic necrosis have separation of the articular surface that is not easily demonstrated by x-ray evaluation. Curls or incongruities of the articular surface or actual fractures or separations in that surface can be seen on arthroscopic examination.

EVALUATION FOR RECONSTRUCTIVE SURGERY

The assessment for whether osteotomy, surface replacement, or conventional total-hip replacement will be done may be assisted by arthroscopic evaluation of the articular surface of both the acetabulum and the head.

One patient had angulation or shortening of his femoral neck, and an osteotomy was being considered (Fig. 26-7, A). Determination of the exact status of the articular surface is beneficial. Arthroscopy pointed out the irregularities of the surface of the femoral head being considered for osteotomy (Fig. 26-7, B). The arthroscopy clearly demonstrated the elevated articular surface, as seen in Fig. 26-7, C and D. Therefore a surface replacement was considered.[1]

In another situation it might be possible to see considerable change around the joint that would indicate the value of conventional total-hip over conservative surface replacement.

There have been other, older patients who have had minimal changes that were evident on x-ray examination. They had been denied total-hip replacement because of lack of x-ray changes in spite of continuing symptoms. The arthroscopy demonstrated a chondronecrosis, considerable degenerative change, and loss of the articular surface. There also was synovitis. This patient then could easily meet the criteria for resurfacing or total-hip replacement on the basis of arthroscopic evaluation.

REFERENCES

1. Harris, W.: Personal communication, 1979.
2. Shneider, D.: Personal communication, 1979.

Chapter 27

Ankle joint

Technique
Findings
    Osteochondritis dissecans
    Loose bodies
    Degenerative arthritis
    Rheumatoid arthritis
    Fibrosis and fibrous adhesions
    Subluxation
    Degenerative change
Operative arthroscopy

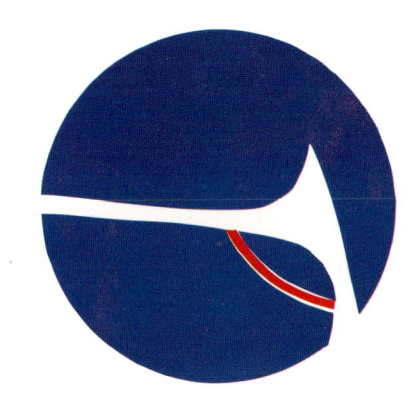

TECHNIQUE

The ankle joint is easily accessible for arthroscopic inspection (Fig. 27-1).

I recommend using a Needlescope. Occasionally a rod-lens endoscope with an anterolateral approach is possible. Local anesthesia is preferred; occasionally general is necessary or advantageous.

The patient is supine. The surgeon's position is at the end of the table. The first assistant stands at the lateral aspect of the involved part; the second assistant's position is on the side opposite the involved ankle. Instruments are placed on the same side as the involved ankle, between the first and second assistants, and the light source is at the perimeter of that area.

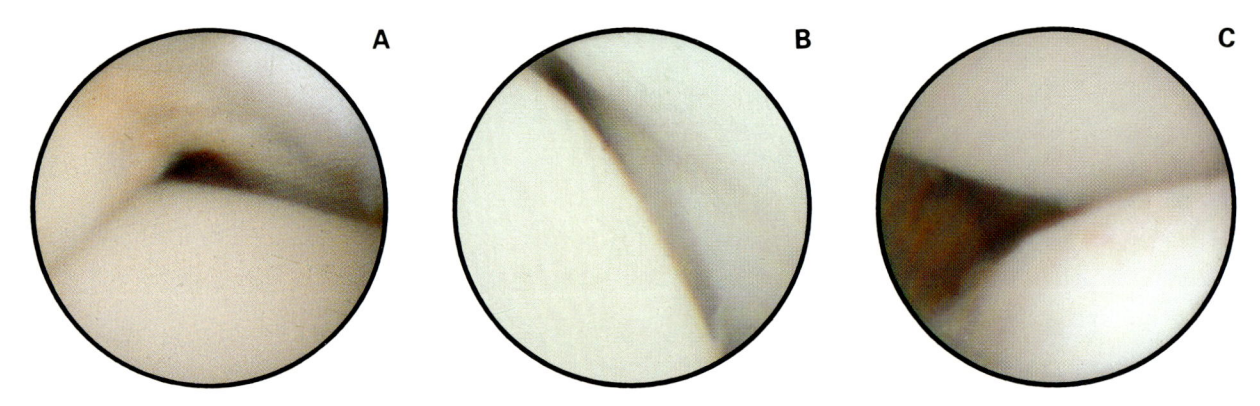

FIG. 27-1. Normal ankle arthroscopy.

A Arthroscopic view of talus and medial malleolus.
B Partial view of talus below and tibia above.
C Lateral view over dome of talus to synovium adjacent to tibia.

Ankle joint

Points of entry include direct anterior, anterolateral, anteromedial, and posterolateral approaches. Flexion and extension of the ankle plus palpation help identify the joint line. The point of entry can be easily determined at the time of injection of the anesthetic agent, which can be carried into and distend the joint. Then, with a small No. 21 needle, it is possible to determine the angle and position of entry and also achieve the distension at the same time (Fig. 27-2).

The direct anterior point of entry is used most commonly (Fig. 27-3, A and B). The anterolateral approach can be used for an oblique approach, and a larger diameter endoscope could be used for that particular area. The joint can be vacuumed of debris (Fig. 27-3, C).

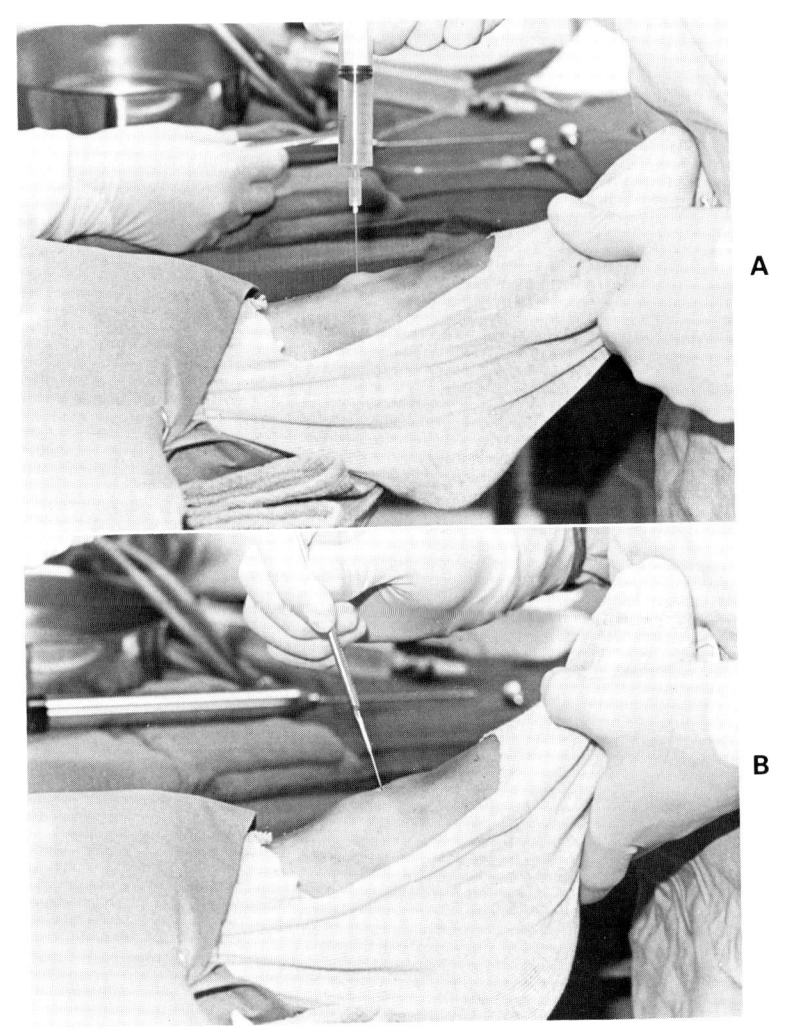

FIG. 27-2. A, Arthroscopy of ankle under local anesthesia. Plain lidocaine, 1%, is injected directly anterior. **B,** Skin laceration immediately anterior avoids dorsal cutaneous nerves of foot.

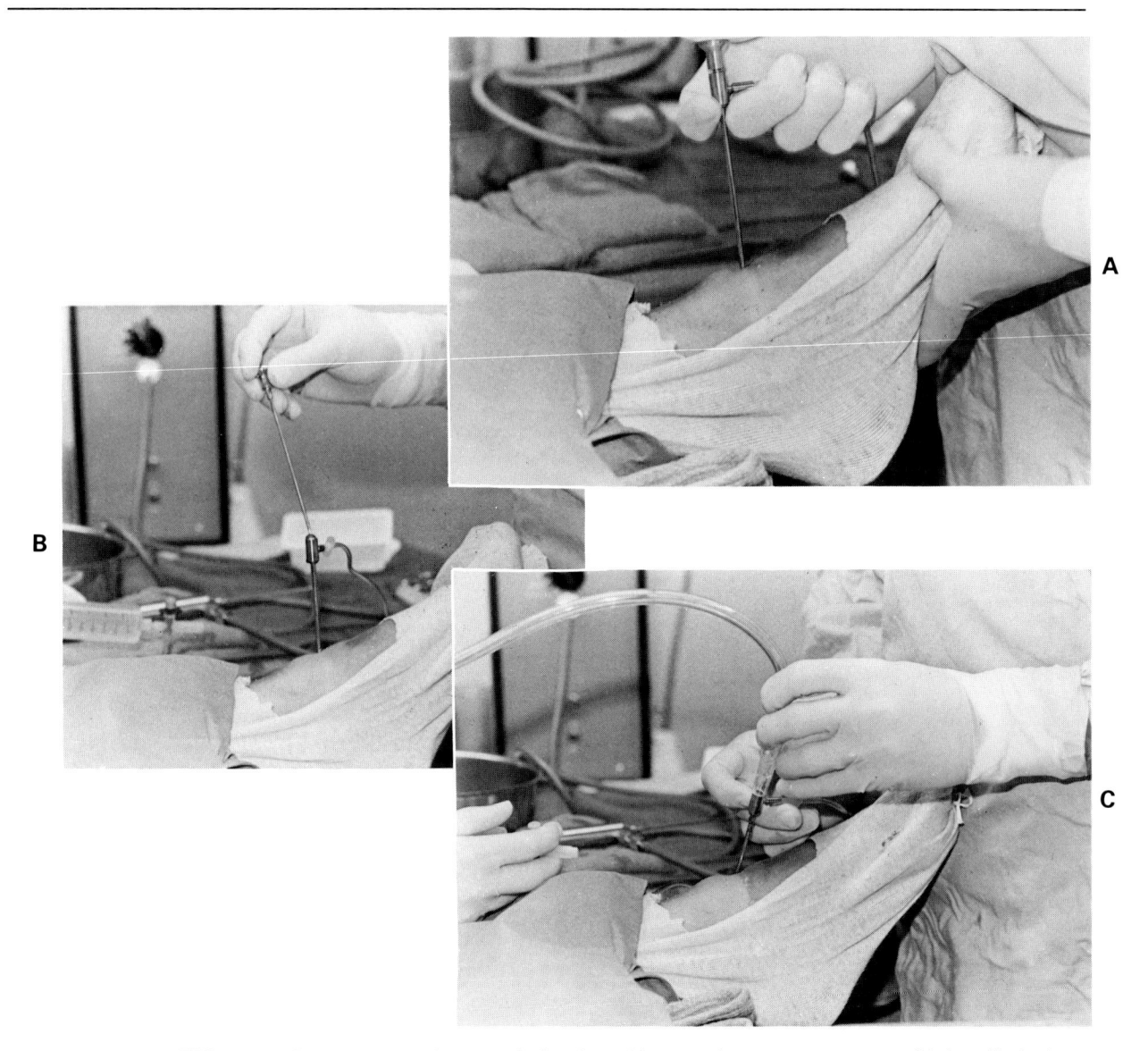

Diagnostic and surgical arthroscopy: other joints

FIG. 27-3. A, Arthroscopic cannula is placed in anterior compartment of joint. **B,** Arthroscopic cannula is removed. **C,** Joint is vacuumed.

FINDINGS

The space between the talus and the tibia is easily identified (Fig. 27-4). These bones should be identified first. Then the surgeon can visualize across the entire talus by manipulation of eversion and inversion, flexion, extension, distension, and distraction. Inspection is then made from the medial facet of the medial malleolus (Fig. 27-5). Then the lateral malleolus and the articulating talar surface are visualized (Fig. 27-6). It should be noted that it is common to find some villi of synovium around both malleolar areas as well as a fat pad (Fig. 27-7).

Ankle joint

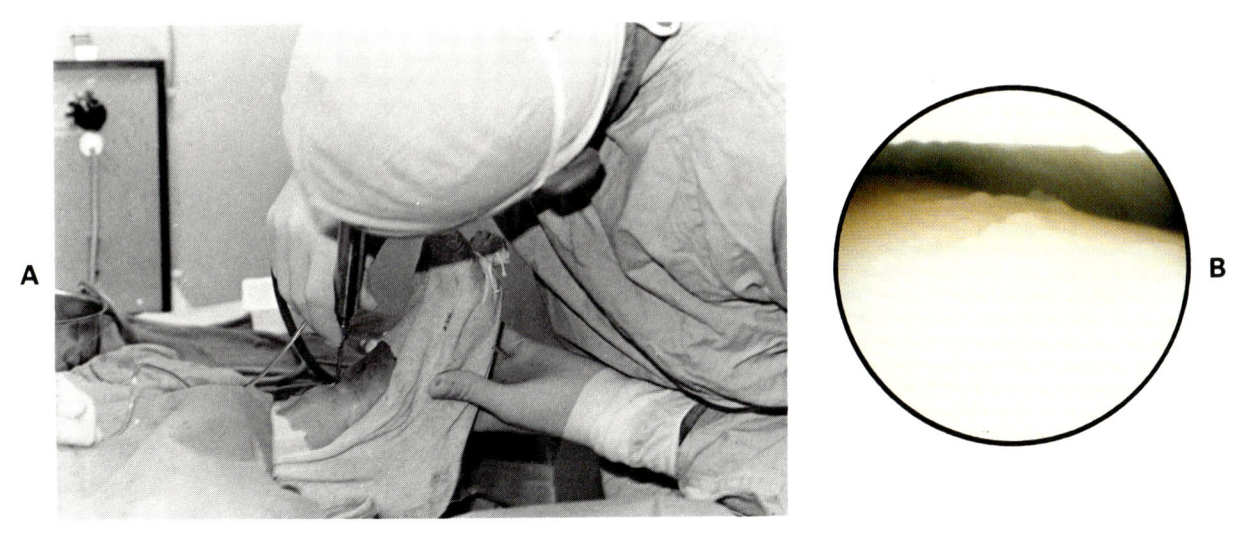

FIG. 27-4. A, Arthroscopic inspection of tibial talar joint. **B,** Arthroscopic view of tibial talar joint with distraction.

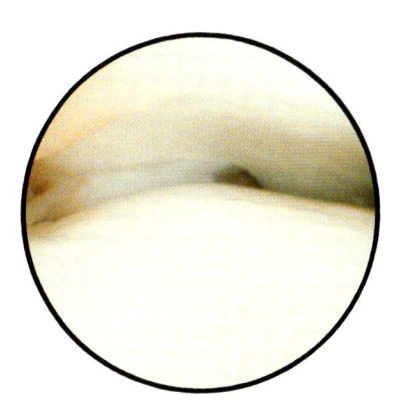

FIG. 27-5. Arthroscopic view of talus and medial malleolus joint. Taken with rod-lens arthroscope.

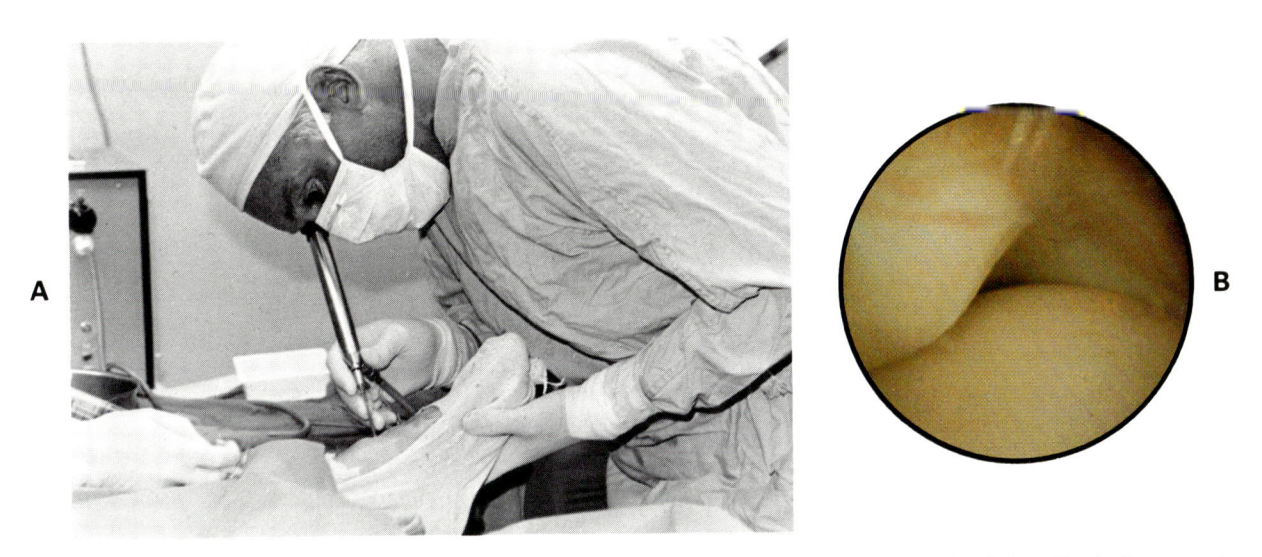

FIG. 27-6. A, Arthroscope moved to lateral portion of tibial talar joint. **B,** Arthroscopic view of talus above and below and fibula in back.

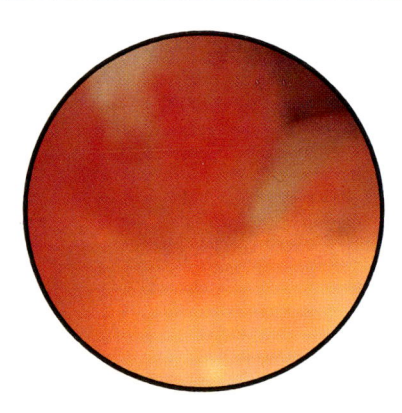

Diagnostic and surgical arthroscopy: other joints

FIG. 27-7. Synovitis is frequently seen in old, previously injured ankle joints.

Osteochondritis dissecans

This lesion is common in the ankle joint. It usually is lateral and occasionally can be medial. Identification is made by x-ray examination (Fig. 27-8). Whether the fragment is intact is best determined by arthroscopic inspection. If the lesion is small and separate, it can be removed arthroscopically. Repeat inspection of the healing at the base of articular defects can be monitored by arthroscopic inspection. Pinning or drilling fragments that are not loosened has not been performed.

Loose bodies

Loose bodies that were not seen on x-ray examination have been visualized inside the joint and have been removed transcutaneously.

Degenerative arthritis

Degenerative changes are not uncommon following fracture and open reduction. A patient may have continued symptoms and discomfort in the joint, and this may be determined by arthroscopic evaluation. Also, removal of loose bodies percutaneously or by vacuuming is possible.

There may also be a perfectly smooth joint surface as well as ankle stiffness following fractures. The lack of motion or pain can be due to intra-articular fibrosis and scar. Fibrous bands have been determined to be pathologic under local anesthesia. Sectioning has relieved symptoms and restored range of motion.

Rheumatoid arthritis

A rheumatoid arthritic patient can profit by inspection or even diagnostic biopsy. I have not performed synovectomy as yet.

Fibrosis and fibrous adhesions

It is very common, even following a simple ankle fracture, to see intra-articular fibrous bands in the area of the medial or lateral malleolus (Fig. 27-9). This can result in discomfort or even ankylosis. These can be incised or resected transcutaneously, yielding a rather dramatic relief.

Ankle joint

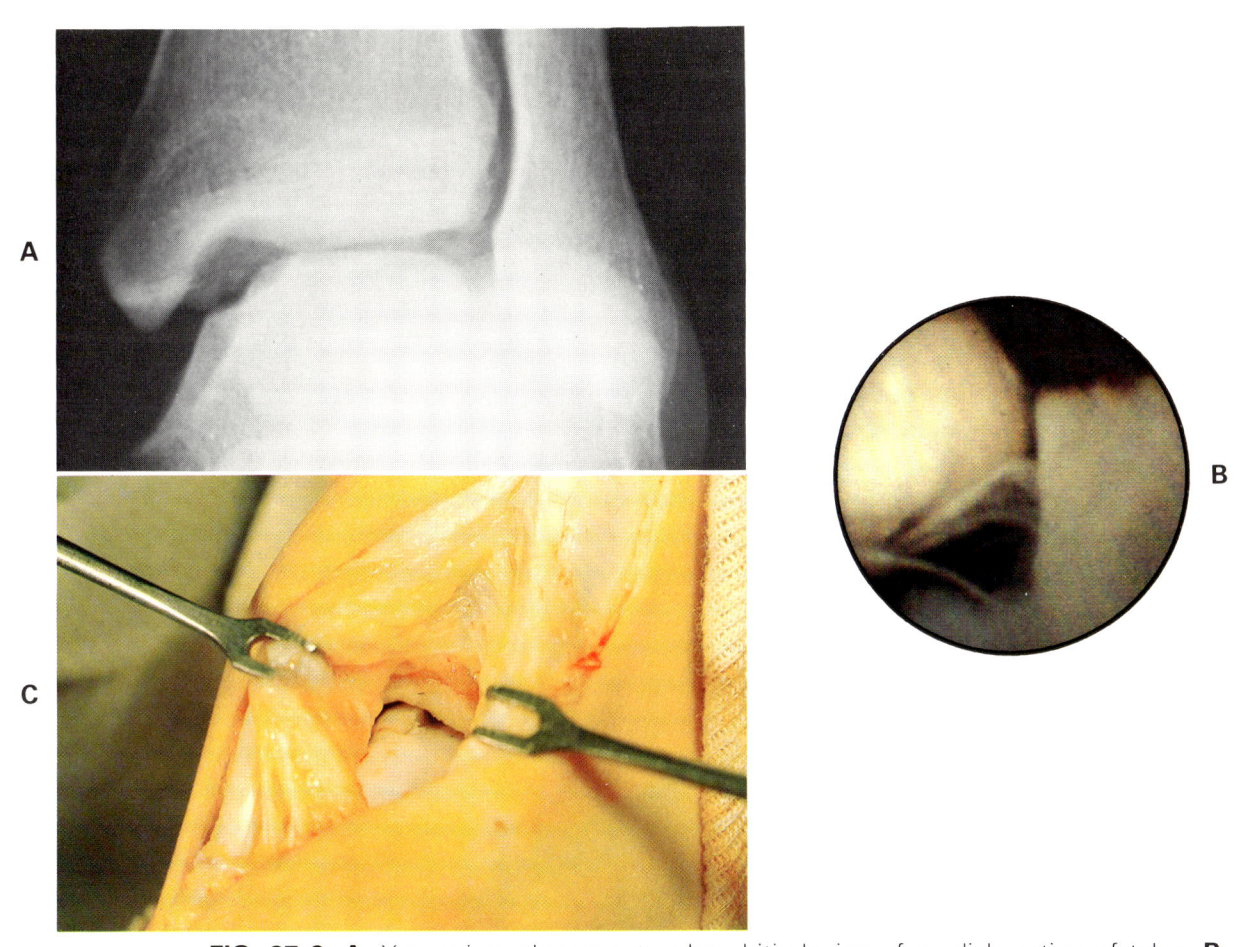

FIG. 27-8. A, X-ray view shows osteochondritic lesion of medial portion of talus. **B,** Arthroscopic view shows separated fragment. **C,** Removal of osteochondritic portion. This can be done by transcutaneous method.

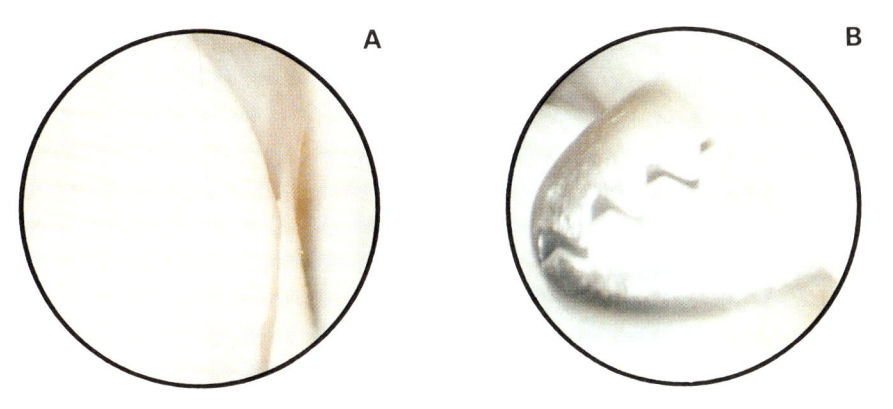

FIG. 27-9. Fibrous bands.

A Arthroscopic view of talus at left and fibula with fibrous bands at right.
B Forceps removal of fibrous bands catching over talus.

Diagnostic and surgical arthroscopy: other joints

Subluxation

Some of the referred diagnostic problems have been in patients who have had subluxation of the talus in the ankle mortise due to a ligamentous injury. This, of course, can be determined by stress x-ray examination and/or perhaps an arthrogram on the peroneal tendon sheath. It is easily determined dynamically and correlates well with the patient's symptoms without as great a stress having to be applied at the time of arthroscopy. Also, any other potential intra-articular loose pieces can be observed.

Degenerative change

It is difficult to determine whether juxta-articular osteophyte formation is intra-articular. An arthroscopic evaluation will help the surgeon decide and also indicate whether there is adjacent synovitis as well as the site of the patient's problems. This would best be determined under local anesthesia; then a subsequent resection can be done. The postoperative treatment includes placement of a sterile dressing; ambulation is indicated; and there is virtually no morbidity from the multiple puncture wounds.

OPERATIVE ARTHROSCOPY

The patient is draped and positioned as for general arthroscopy. The viewing is best from a direct central location. An inflow cannula is inserted from an anteromedial aspect. The cannula should be at least 2.7 mm in its inside diameter. The Intra-articular Shaver can be brought in from a lateral aspect (Fig. 27-10). The location of instrumentation is first determined by palpation and then insertion of the needle and then followed with the Intra-articular Little Shaver. The technique has had considerable benefit in cases of degenerative arthritis with fibrous scars and/or subsequent synovitis in the anterior chamber adjacent to osteophytes. It has been possible to resect the osteophytes as well as fibrous bands by transarthroscopic surgical methods. Also, I have resected osteochondritic lesions and curetted their bases. I have not had any experience with drilling or reattaching osteochondritic lesions to date. Intra-articular chondroplastic shaving has not produced encouraging results.

Ankle joint

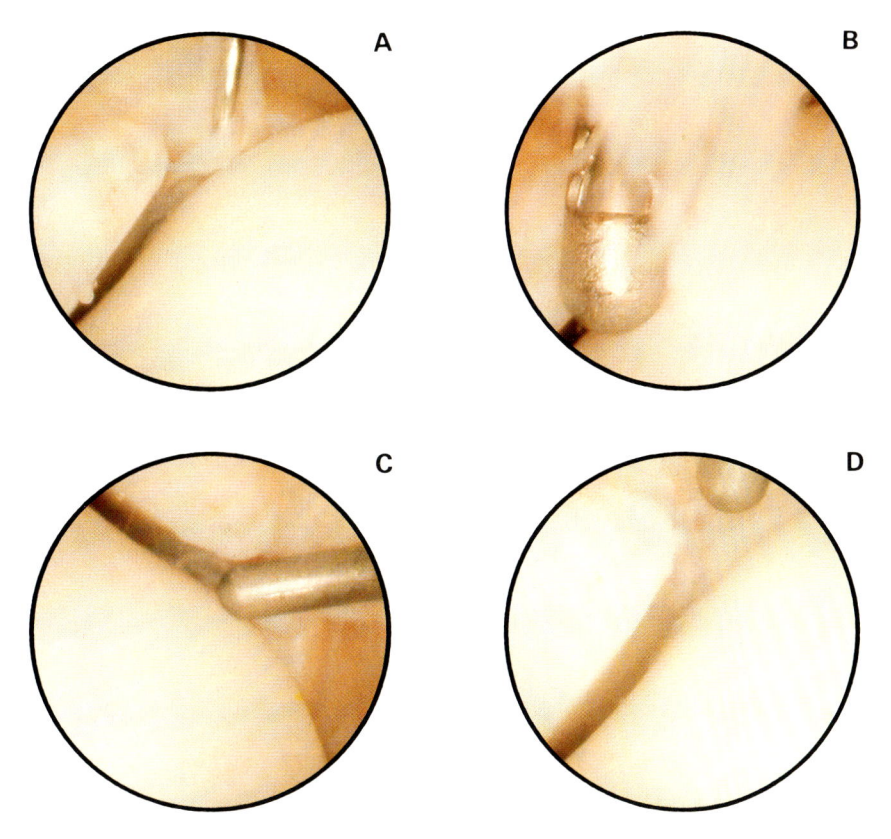

FIG. 27-10

A Arthroscopic view of talus with synovial pileup in lateral sulcus.
B Little Shaver in ankle joint resecting area of synovitis.
C Near completion of arthroscopic resection of area affected by synovitis in lateral compartment of ankle joint.
D Final area of synovium is removed.

APPENDIX

ARTHROSCOPIC INSTRUMENTS AND EQUIPMENT

ARTHROSCOPIC SURGERY

Light source:	Dyonics Model 500
Light cable:	Dyonics 5 mm
Arthroscope:	Storz 4.0 mm, 30°
	Storz 4.0 mm, 70°
	Dyonics Needlescope 1.7 mm
Articulated viewing device:	Storz 5-linked
	Storz 3-linked
Leg holder:	Surgical Assistant, Instrument Makar, Inc.
Television:	Cruse Communications Co.
	Hitachi Camera Model 9017 or GP5
	Sony Recorder
	Sony Trinitron Monitor
Draping:	Johnson & Johnson Surgicos barrier drapes
	Paper shoes (Converters)
	Plastic apron (Converters)
Motor instrumentation:	Dyonics Intra-articular Shaver System
	Cannula system
	Shaver drain case
	Cutter
	Trimmer
	Drill chuck
	Whisker
	Burr
	Synovectomy set
	Battery power source and foot pedal
	Flexible stylette
Hand instruments:	IM probes, Instrument Makar, Inc.
	Oretorp probes (DePuy)
	IM blades, Instrument Makar, Inc., Nos. 711, 747, 761, 764, and 767
	Beaver blades (disposable) Nos. 64 and 67
	Bard-Parker blades Nos. 11 and 15

Appendix

Forceps:	Dyonics Jaws
	Dyonics Jaws Jr.
	Biposy
	Schlessinger (George Tieman)
	Straight and angled
	DePuy basket, 5 mm
	DePuy basket, 3 mm
Scissors:	Eder 3 mm
	Straight Mayo
Spinal needle:	3½ inches, No. 18
Curette:	Zimmer No. 000
Golden Retriever:	Instrument Makar, Inc.

ARTHROSCOPY

Johnson & Johnson hip barrier pack No. 1291
Cloth draw sheet (1)
Mayo cover (1)
Converters apron No. 3175
Green towels (2 packages)
Straight Mayo scissors
Light handle (sterile)
Prep tray
Cysto Y-tubing, Travenol Co., Deerfield, Ill.
3000-ml saline bags, Travenol Co., Deerfield, Ill.
Beaver No. 11 blade
Bard-Parker No. 15 blade for removal of loose bodies
5 & 1 connector
4-inch web
Pyrex suction bottle (5-gallon capacity Kimax Nos. B7601-5 and B7600-5, American Hospital Supply Corp., 1430 Waukegan Rd., McGaw Park, Ill. 60085)
Disposable specimen bag No. GL-8050, V. Mueller Co., 6600 W. Touhy Ave., Chicago, Ill. 60648
Cysto pan
Gomco rubber stopper for bottle
Cidex

LOOSE BODY SET

Adson forceps
Needle holder
Suture scissors
U.S. Army retractors (2)
Senn retractors (2)
2-0 and 3-0 Dexon suture

Index

A

Achilles tendon, monitoring tension in, in diagnostic arthroscopy of knee, 37, 38, 65
Alkaptonuria, arthroscopic diagnosis of, 209, *211*
Anesthesia
  for arthroscopy
    of ankle, 412
    of elbow, 390, *391*
    of finger joint, 404
    of hip, 405
    of shoulder, 376
    of temporomandibular joint, 373
    of wrist, 400
  for diagnostic arthroscopy of knee, 61-68
    choice of, 75-76
    complications of, 67-68
    general, 67
    local, 6-8, 61-67; *see also* Diagnostic arthroscopy of knee with local anesthetic
      patient instructions for, 63-65
      patient monitoring for, 65
      patient selection for, 65
      technique for, 62-63
Ankle
  arthroscopic diagnosis and surgery of, 412-419
  degenerative arthritis of, arthroscopic diagnosis and management of, 416
  fibrous adhesions in, arthroscopic management of, 416, *417*
  loose bodies in, arthroscopic detection of, 416
  osteochondritis dissecans of, arthroscopic evaluation and management of, 416, *417*
  rheumatoid arthritis of, arthroscopic diagnosis of, 416
  subluxation of, arthroscopic evaluation and management of, 418
Ankylosis of knee
  arthroscopic evaluation of, 195
  arthroscopic surgery for, 357-358
Anterior chambers of knee, arthroscopic surgery on, positions for, 271
Anterolateral compartment of knee
  arthroscopic evaluation of, 48, 118-119
    multiple puncture technique for, 119
    normal arthroscopic appearance of, *116*
Anteromedial approach to diagnostic arthroscopy of knee, 43-46
Anteromedial compartment of knee, arthroscopic evaluation of, 49-50, 122-123
  multiple puncture technique for, 123
Arthritis
  degenerative; *see* Degenerative arthritis

Page numbers in *italics* indicate illustrations.

Arthritis—cont'd
  gouty, acute, of knee, arthroscopic diagnosis of, 206-207
  psoriatic, of knee, arthroscopic diagnosis of, 209
  rheumatoid; *see* Rheumatoid arthritis
Arthrography versus arthroscopy for knee evaluation, 72
Arthroscope(s)
  coherent bundle system, 16
  for diagnostic arthroscopy of hip joint, 206
  entry of, for diagnostic arthroscopy of knee, 29-30, *31*
  graded refractory index system, 16
  light guides for, 17-20
  light sources for, 17
  manipulation of, in diagnostic arthroscopy of knee, 33
  operating, 235
  pistoning of, in diagnostic arthroscopy of knee, 35
  placement of
    for comprehensive arthroscopic surgical technique, 272-274
    for diagnostic arthroscopy of knee, 28
  redirection of, for diagnostic arthroscopy of knee, 31
  replacement of, for diagnostic arthroscopy of knee, 28-29
  rod-lens system, 14, *15*
  rotation of, in diagnostic arthroscopy of knee, 35-36
  selection of, 13
  self-focusing, development of, 4-5
  sterilization and disinfection of, 22-24
  for surgery of knee, 221-222
  sweeping with, in diagnostic arthroscopy of knee, 36-37
  thin-lens system, 14
  types of, 14-16
Arthroscopic surgery
  of ankle, 412-419
  of elbow, 396-399
  of finger, 404
  of hip, 405-411
  instruments and equipment for, 421-422
  of knee
    articulated viewing device in, *220*, 222
    chondral, 338-350
    comprehensive technique for, 263-284
      for patella and patellofemoral shaving, 283-284
      patient positioning and preparation in, 264-269
      placement of arthroscope in, 272-274
      placement of inflow cannula in, 269-271
      positions for, 271-272
      preoperative arthroscopic diagnostic examination for, 275-278
      probing in, 278-279
      puncture sites for instruments in, 279-283
    draping for, 227
    expectations for, 244
    extrasynovial, 352-359
    Golden Retriever for, 239

423

Index

Arthroscopic surgery—cont'd
  of knee—cont'd
    hand cutting instruments for, 233-235
    hand tools for, 227-233
    instrumentation for, 215-239; *see also* Instrumentation for arthroscopic surgery of knee
    Intra-articular Shaver System for, 235-239
    joint irrigation for, 243
    learning, 241-242
    meniscal, 285-315; *see also* Meniscectomy, arthroscopic
    operating arthroscopes for, 235
    patellar, 317-337; *see also* Patella, arthroscopic surgery on
    patient selection and preparation for, 244-246
    principles of, 241-284
    saline flow devices for, 225-227, 243
    Surgical Assistant for, 223-225
    synovial, 360-370
    team approach to, 248
    technical concepts in, 246-248
    techniques for, 246
    television in, 222
    triangulation in, 242-243
  of shoulder, 385-389
  of temporomandibular joint, 373-375
  of wrist, 400-403
Arthroscopic synovectomy for pigmented villonodular synovitis, 204
Arthroscopy
  diagnostic; *see* Diagnostic arthroscopy
  instruments and equipment for, 422
  of joints other than knee, 74
  surgical, of knee, 213-370; *see also* Arthroscopic surgery of knee
Arthrotomy
  quadriceps exercises following, complications of, 168-169
  synovitis following, arthroscopy for, 168
Articular cartilage
  of knee
    damage to, postoperative arthroscopic evaluation of, 185
    degenerative changes in, *180-181*, 182
    disease of, arthroscopic diagnosis of, 180-185
    healing of, arthroscopic evaluation of, 154-156
    loose fragments of
      arthroscopic detection of, 182, *183*
      arthroscopic removal of, 340-343
      in patellar dislocation, 173, *174*
    meniscus in service of, 145
    normal arthroscopic appearance of, 113
  of wrist, fracture of, arthroscopic diagnosis of, 403
Articular disease, arthroscopic evaluation of, 147
Articular surfaces of knee, defects of
  arthroscopic diagnosis of, 184, 338-339
  arthroscopic surgery for, 339-340
Articulated viewing device for arthroscopic surgery of knee, *220*, 222
Assistants, responsibilities of
  in comprehensive arthroscopic surgical technique, 269
  in diagnostic arthroscopy of knee, 40-41
Autoclaving for arthroscope, 22-23

B

Baker cysts, arthroscopic diagnosis of, 194
Basket forceps for arthroscopic surgery of knee, 233, *234*
Beaulieu cameras for movie documentation of diagnostic arthroscopy of knee, 106, 108
Beaver knife blades
  for arthroscopic meniscectomy, 291
  for arthroscopic surgery of knee, 228, *229*
Biceps tendon
  arthroscopic inspection of, *378*, *379*
  ruptured, arthroscopic diagnosis of, 383
Biopsy forceps, small, 22
Bupivacaine for lateral release technique, *258*, 261

C

Cables, light, for arthroscopes, 17-20
Camera
  for documentation of arthroscopic surgery of knee, 223
  for photographic documentation of diagnostic arthroscopy of knee, 102-104
Cannula(s)
  for diagnostic arthroscopy of knee, 20
  inflow, for comprehensive arthroscopic surgical technique, placement of, 269-271
  for vacuuming of joint, 34-35
Capsular tissue of knee, fibrosis of, arthroscopic diagnosis of, 148-149
Cartilage, articular; *see* Articular cartilage
Chart for documentation of diagnostic arthroscopy of knee, 99, *100*
Chondral conditions, arthroscopic surgery for, 338-350
  indications for, 338-340
Chondromalacia of patella
  arthroscopic diagnosis of, 71, 171-173
    experience with, 89
  arthroscopic intra-articular shaving for, 320-325
Chondronecrosis
  of hip, arthroscopic diagnosis and management of, *408*, 409
  of knee, arthroscopic surgery for, 348
Cidex for disinfection of arthroscope, 23, 41
Cinephotography for documentation of diagnostic arthroscopy of knee, 10, 106, *107*
Clark attachment for comprehensive arthroscopic surgical technique, *264*, 265
Cleansing of joint for diagnostic arthroscopy of knee, 33-35
Condylar disease
  arthroscopic diagnosis of, 145-147, 180-185
    experience with, 79, 83-84, 86
  arthroscopic surgery for, 347-348
  postoperative arthroscopic evaluation of, 185
  preoperative arthroscopic evaluation of, 184-185
Contrast staining for diagnostic arthroscopy of knee, 35
Cruciate ligament
  anterior
    injury of, seen in posterolateral compartment, *127*
    normal arthroscopic appearance of, 114, *115*
    torn
      acute, arthroscopic surgery for, 352-355
      arthroscopic diagnosis of, 79-80, 84-85, 89, 90-91, 148, 186-190
      seen in intercondylar notch, *121*
  posterior
    normal arthroscopic appearance of, *114*, 115

Index

Cruciate ligament—cont'd
  posterior—cont'd
    torn, arthroscopic diagnosis of, 148, 192, *193*
    torn, in knee instability, 193-194
Curettes for arthroscopic surgery of knee, 232, 233
Cysts
  Baker, arthroscopic diagnosis of, 194
  juxta-articular ganglion, arthroscopic diagnosis of, 194-195
  meniscal
    arthroscopic diagnosis of, 194
    arthroscopic resection of, 357

D

Dandy probe for arthroscopic surgery of knee, 227-228
Degenerative arthritis
  of ankle, arthroscopic diagnosis and management of, 416
  of elbow, arthroscopic diagnosis and management of, 394, *395*
  of hip, arthroscopic diagnosis of, 408, 409
  of knee
    accompanying anterior cruciate ligament tear, 188, 190
    arthroscopic diagnosis of, 203, *204*
      experience with, 90
    arthroscopic evaluation of, 182
    with compartmental loss and deformity, arthroscopic surgery for, 349
    in knee instability, 193-194
    after medial meniscectomy, arthroscopic diagnosis of, experience with, 89
    severe, all-compartment shave for, 349-350
    synovitis with, management of, 369
  of shoulder, arthroscopic diagnosis of, 383
Diagnostic arthroscopy
  of ankle, 412-419
  of elbow, 390-395
  equipment distribution for, *39*
  of finger, 404
  of hip, 405-411
  of joints other than knee, 74
  of knee
    anatomy in, 113-141
      normal, 113-117
    anesthesia for, 61-68; *see also* Anesthesia for diagnostic arthroscopy of knee
    anterolateral compartment in, 48, 118-119
    anteromedial approach to, 43-46
    anteromedial compartment in, 49-50, 122-123
    versus arthrography, 72
    cannulas for, 20
    cleansing of joint for, 33-35
    in clinical practice, 69-96
    clinical value of, 8, 95
    compartments in, 43-58, 117-127; *see also* specific compartment, e.g., Anterolateral compartment of knee
    complications of, 58, 60
    contrast staining in, 35
    development of, 3-11
    for differential diagnosis of knee disorder, 71-72
    distension in, 27-28
    documentation of, 9-10, 97-112; *see also* Documentation of diagnostic arthroscopy of knee
    effect of
      on patient management, 70-71
      on surgical design, 72-73

Diagnostic arthroscopy—cont'd
  of knee—cont'd
    enhancement of clinical skills by, 70
    entry of arthroscope in, 29-31
    experience with, review of, 75-92
      analysis of, 76-77
      choice of anesthetic in, 75-76
      classification of patients in, 76
      in Series I, 77-84
      in Series II, 81-85
      in Series III, 86-87
      in Series IV, 87-92
    follow-up for, 58, *59*
    forceps for, 21-22
    free hand activity in, 37-38
    hand control in, 31-32
    history of, 3-4
    instrumentation for; *see* Instrumentation for diagnostic arthroscopy of knee
    intercondylar notch in, 48-49, 120-121, 136-137; *see also* Intercondylar notch of knee
    lateral compartment in, 138-139
    learning, 95-96
    light for, 26-27
    light guides for, 17-20
    light sources for, 17
    with local anesthetic, 6-8
      clinical judgment in, 66-67
      physician-patient relationship in, 66
      tourniquet in, 66
      value of, 66
    manipulation of scope in, 33
    medial compartment in, 132-133
    for meniscal diseases, 158-169
    modified Gillquist approach to, 58, 128-141; *see also* Gillquist technique for diagnostic arthroscopy of knee, modified
    palpation in, 32
    patella in, 46-47
    for patellar diseases, 170-179
    pathologic findings in, 142-156
    in patient management routine, 92-95
    pistoning in, 35
    placement of arthroscope in, 28
    posterolateral compartment in, 53-55, 126-127, 140-141; *see also* Posterolateral compartment of knee
    posterolateral puncture routine for, 8-9
    posteromedial compartment in, 50-53, 124-125, 134-135; *see also* Posteromedial compartment of knee
    posteromedial puncture routine for, 8
    for postoperative evaluations, 168-169
    preoperative, for comprehensive arthroscopic surgical technique, 275-278
    probing in, 32
    procedure for, *41-42*, 43
    redirection of arthroscope in, 31
    rehabilitation and, 73-74
    replacement of arthroscope in, 28-29
    research using, 74-75
    rotation of scope in, 35-36
    scanning horizon in, 35, *36*
    scope sweeping in, 36-37
    suprapatellar approach to, 56-57
    suprapatellar pouch in, 46-47, 130-131

425

Index

Diagnostic arthroscopy—cont'd
  of knee—cont'd
    suprapatellar puncture routine for, 9
    team approach to, 38-43
    technical concepts in, 26-38
    techniques for, 25-60
      development of, 6-9
    transpatellar tendon approach to, 57-58
    vacuuming of joint for, 33-35
  of shoulder, 376-385
  of temporomandibular joint, 373-375
  of wrist, 400-403
Dialdehyde solution, activated, for disinfection of arthroscope, 23, 41
Dictated narrative for documentation of diagnostic arthroscopy of knee, 97-99
Disinfection of arthroscopic equipment, 22-24
Dislocation
  of patella
    arthroscopic chondroplasty for, 336-337
    arthroscopic diagnosis of, 173-174
      experience with, 89-90
    congenital, recurrent, lateral release for, 334
    patellar shave in, 331
    seen in anterolateral compartment, *119*
  of shoulder, arthroscopic diagnosis of, *379*, *380*, 382
Distension of joint for diagnostic arthroscopy of knee, 27-28
Documentation of diagnostic arthroscopy of knee, 97-112
  chart in, 99, *100*
  dictated narrative in, 97-99
  movie photography in, 106-108
  still photography in, 99-106
  television in, 108-112
Draping
  for arthroscopic surgery of knee, 227
  for arthroscopy of shoulder, 376, *377*
  for comprehensive arthroscopic surgical technique, *266*, 267
Drilling
  for articular defects, 339-340
  of osteochondritic defects, 343-346
Dyonics Model 500 light source for arthroscopes, 17
Dyonics rod-lens system, endoscopic photography with, *104*, 105

E

Ektachrome ASA-64 film for photographic documentation of diagnostic arthroscopy of knee, 104-105
Ektachrome ASA-160 film for photographic documentation of diagnostic arthroscopy of knee, 105
Ektachrome ASA-400 film for photographic documentation of diagnostic arthroscopy of knee, 105
Elbow
  anatomy of, normal arthroscopic views of, *393*, *394*
  arthroscopic diagnosis and surgery of, 390-399
  degenerative arthritis of, arthroscopic diagnosis and management of, *394*, *395*
  fracture of, arthroscopic assessment of, 394-395
  loose bodies in, arthroscopic removal of, *396*, *397*
  rheumatoid arthritis of, arthroscopic diagnosis and management of, 394
  tennis, arthroscopic evaluation and management of, 394
Ethylene oxide gas for sterilization of arthroscope, 22-23

Exercises, quadriceps, following arthrotomy, complications of, 168-169
Extrasynovial lesions
  arthroscopic diagnosis of, 186-195
    experience with, 79-81, 84-85, 86-87, 90-91
  arthroscopic surgery for, 352-359
  preoperative arthroscopic evaluations of, 195
Extremity, control of, for patellar shaving, 251-255

F

Femoral condyle, defects on, arthroscopic surgery for, 347
Fibrosis
  in ankle, arthroscopic management of, 416, *417*
  capsular, in knee joint, arthroscopic diagnosis of, 148-149
Film for photographic documentation of diagnostic arthroscopy of knee, 104-106
Finger joints, arthroscopic diagnosis and surgery of, 404
Flap tear of meniscus, 293, *294*
Forceps
  basket, for arthroscopic surgery of knee, 233, *234*
  for diagnostic arthroscopy of knee, 21-22
  guillotine, for arthroscopic surgery of knee, *234*, 235
Fracture
  of articular cartilage of wrist, arthroscopic diagnosis of, 403
  of elbow, arthroscopic assessment of, 394-395
  intra-articular, arthroscopic evaluation of, 180, 182
  of patella
    acute, arthroscopic evaluation of, 175-176
    old, arthroscopic evaluation of, 176

G

Gillquist technique for diagnostic arthroscopy of knee, 57-58
  modified, 58, 128-141
    for intercondylar notch, 136-137
    for lateral compartment, 138-139
    for medial compartment, 132-133
    for posterolateral compartment, 140-141
    for posteromedial compartment, 134-135
    for suprapatellar pouch, 130-131
Glenohumeral ligament, arthroscopic inspection of, 380, *381*
Golden Retriever for arthroscopic surgery of knee, 239
Gout of knee
  arthroscopic diagnosis of, 206-207
  synovitis in, arthroscopic irrigation for, 366
Graspers for arthroscopic surgery of knee, 231, *232*
Guillotine forceps for arthroscopic surgery of knee, *234*, 235

H

Halo light for arthroscopes, *18*, 19
Hands, control of, in diagnostic arthroscopy of knee, 31-32
Harpoon, miniature, for arthroscopic surgery of knee, 231
Hauser reconstruction of knee, postoperative arthroscopic evaluation of, 177, *178*
Hemangioma of knee, arthroscopic diagnosis of, 208
Hemarthrosis, diagnostic arthroscopy and, 70-71, 195
Hematoma complicating lateral release, 335
Hemorrhage
  in anterior cruciate ligament injury, 188
  synovial, arthroscopic diagnosis of, 209, *210*
Hill-Sach lesion of head of humerus in dislocated shoulder, *379*, 380

Index

Hip
    arthroscopic diagnosis and surgery of, 405-411
    aseptic necrosis of, arthroscopic diagnosis of, 411
    degenerative arthritis of, arthroscopic diagnosis of, 408, 409
    reconstructive surgery on, arthroscopic evaluation for, 410, 411
    trauma to, arthroscopic diagnosis of, 409

I

IM knife blades
    for arthroscopic meniscectomy, 291
    for arthroscopic surgery of knee, 229, 230, 231
Infection(s)
    of prosthetic knee, exacerbation of, complicating diagnostic arthroscopy of knee, 58, 60
    synovial
        arthroscopic diagnosis of, 212
        arthroscopic management of, 370
Instrumentation
    for arthroscopic surgery of knee
        positioning of, 223
        powered
            development of, 215-221
            history of, 215-217
        visual, 221-223
    for diagnostic arthroscopy of knee, 13-24; see also Arthroscope(s)
    care of, between patients, 41
    development of, 4-6
    new developments in, 10
    sterilization and disinfection of, 22-24
Intercondylar notch of knee
    arthroscopic evaluation of, 48-49
        before comprehensive arthroscopic surgical technique, 275
        modified Gillquist technique for, 136-137
        multiple puncture technique for, 120-121
    arthroscopic surgery on, position for, 271
    normal arthroscopic appearance of, 114
Intra-articular Shaver System
    for anterior cruciate ligament tear, 352-353, 354
    for arthroscopic meniscectomy, 289-292
    for arthroscopic surgery of knee, 235-239
        development of, 217-221
        saline flow devices for, 243
    for chondromalacia patellae, 320-334
    for chondronecrosis, 348
    for loose body removal, 342
    for synovial adhesions, 365
    for synovial plica resection, 363, 364
Intra-articular shaving of patella, 248, 249-258, 320-334; see also Shaving, patellar
Isometric quadriceps exercises following arthrotomy, 168-169

J

Jaws forceps, 21
Jaws Jr. forceps, 21, 22
Joint(s)
    ankle, arthroscopic diagnosis and surgery of, 412-419; see also Ankle
    elbow, arthroscopic diagnosis and surgery of, 390-399; see also Elbow

Joint(s)—cont'd
    finger, arthroscopic diagnosis and surgery of, 404
    hip, arthroscopic diagnosis and surgery of, 405-411; see also Hip
    knee; see Knee
    patellofemoral, degenerative changes in
        arthroscopic chondroplasty for, 336-337
        intra-articular shaving for, 333
    shoulder, arthroscopic diagnosis and surgery of, 376-389; see also Shoulder
    temporomandibular, arthroscopic diagnosis and surgery of, 373-375
    wrist, arthroscopic diagnosis and surgery of, 400-403
Juxta-articular ganglion cysts, arthroscopic diagnosis of, 194-195
Juxta-articular loose body, arthroscopic removal of, 358-359
Juxta-articular osteophyte formation in ankle, arthroscopic evaluation of, 418
Juxtachondral synovitis, arthroscopic resection for, 369

K

Knee
    ankylosis of
        arthroscopic evaluation of, 195
        arthroscopic surgery for, 357-358
    arthrography of, versus arthroscopy, 72
    arthroscopic compartments of, 43-58
    arthroscopic surgery of, 213-370; see also Arthroscopic surgery of knee
    articular surface of, defects of, arthroscopic diagnosis of, 184
    cleansing of, for diagnostic arthroscopy, 33-35
    contusion of, arthroscopic examination of, 177
    degenerative arthritis of; see Degenerative arthritis of knee
    diagnostic arthroscopy of, 1-212; see also Diagnostic arthroscopy of knee
    extra ossicles of, arthroscopic resection of, 358-359
    gout of
        arthroscopic diagnosis of, 206-207
        synovitis in, arthroscopic irrigation for, 366
    hemangioma of, arthroscopic diagnosis of, 208
    instability of, chronic
        arthroscopic evaluation of, 192-194, 355-356
        arthroscopic surgery for, 355-357
    prosthetic, infection of, exacerbation of, complicating diagnostic arthroscopy of knee, 58, 60
    pseudogout of, arthroscopic diagnosis of, 207
    replacement of, total, arthroscopic evaluation of candidate for, 184-185
    vacuuming of, for diagnostic arthroscopy, 33-35
Knives
    for arthroscopic meniscectomy, 291
    for arthroscopic surgery of knee, 228-231

L

Labrum, anterior, avulsed and displaced, arthroscopic resection for, 384
Lateral compartment of knee
    arthroscopic evaluation of
        before comprehensive arthroscopic surgical technique, 276
        modified Gillquist technique for, 138-139
        puncture sites for surgical instrumentation in, 282, 283

Index

Lateral release
  indication for, 334
  technique for, 258-263
Lateral synovial plica, arthroscopic evaluation of, 362
Lidocaine
  for diagnostic arthroscopy of knee, 62; *see also* Anesthesia
    for diagnostic arthroscopy of knee, local
  for lateral release technique, 261
Ligament(s)
  anterior cruciate
    injury of, seen in posterolateral compartment, 127
    normal arthroscopic appearance of, *114*, 115
    torn
      acute, arthroscopic surgery for, 352-355
      arthroscopic diagnosis of, 79-80, 84-85, 89, 90-91, 148, 186-190
      seen in intercondylar notch, *121*
  cruciate, torn, in knee instability, 193-194
  glenohumeral, arthroscopic inspection of, 380, *381*
  posterior cruciate
    normal arthroscopic appearance of, *114*, 115
    torn, arthroscopic diagnosis of, 148, 192, *193*
  tibial collateral
    normal arthroscopic appearance of, *114*, 115
    torn, arthroscopic diagnosis of, 148, 190-192
      experience with, 80, 84
Light for diagnostic arthroscopy of knee, 26-27
Light guides for arthroscopes, 17-20
Light sources for arthroscopes, 17
Light wand for arthroscopes, 19, *20*

M

Marcaine for lateral release technique, *258*, 261
Medial compartment of knee
  arthroscopic evaluation of
    before comprehensive arthroscopic surgical technique, 275
    modified Gillquist technique for, 132-133
  arthroscopic surgery on, positions for, 271
  normal arthroscopic appearance of, *114*
  puncture sites for surgical instrumentation in, 279-283
Medial shelf (plica)
  arthroscopic evaluation of, 198, *200*, 201
  arthroscopic resection of, *361*, 362-363
Medic III television system for documentation of diagnostic arthroscopy of knee, 110-111
Meniscal cysts, arthroscopic diagnosis of, 194
Meniscectomy
  amount of material removed by, 285-286
  arthroscopic, 285-315
    case reports on, 312-315
    complications of, 311
    postoperative management of, *310*, 311
    surgical principles of, 288-293
  arthroscopic evaluation of need for, 194
  incisions for, 285
  indications and contraindications for, 145, 158, 161
  at level of vascularity, 165-166
  open, diagnostic arthroscopy after, 73-74
  partial, disadvantages of, 287
  selective, 288
  subtotal, ideal, 287-288
Meniscoid lesion of wrist, arthroscopic diagnosis of, *402*, 403
Meniscoresis for peripheral detachment of meniscus, 162

Meniscus(i)
  arthroscopic surgery on, 285-315; *see also* Meniscectomy, arthroscopic
  bucket-handle tear of, arthroscopic diagnosis of, 167
  cysts of
    arthroscopic diagnosis of, 194
    arthroscopic resection of, 357
  degenerative changes in, 161
    arthroscopic appearance of, 142-143, *144*, 145
    normal, 115
  discoid, 164
  disease of, arthroscopic diagnosis of, 158-169
  disorders, of, arthroscopic diagnosis of, experience with, 77-78, 81-83, 86, 88
  healing of, arthroscopic evaluation of, 151, *152-153*
  hypermobile, arthroscopic diagnosis of, 71-72, 168
  injury of, without tear, 143, 145
  lateral, tears of, 302
    accompanying anterior cruciate ligament tear, 189-190
    arthroscopic diagnosis of, experience with, 77, 82, 88, 89
    bucket-handle, arthroscopic meniscectomy for, 309
    complex, arthroscopic meniscectomy for, 308
      case report on, 312-313
    degenerative flaps, arthroscopic meniscectomy for, 306
    discoid meniscal, arthroscopic meniscectomy for, 304
    incomplete posterior horn, arthroscopic meniscectomy for, 305
    posterior horn, from periphery, arthroscopic meniscectomy for, 307
    transverse, arthroscopic meniscectomy for, 303
  medial
    posterior horn tear of, seen in posteromedial compartment, 125
    tears of
      accompanying anterior cruciate ligament tear, 189
      arthroscopic diagnosis of, experience with, 77, 82, 88
      bucket-handle, arthroscopic meniscectomy for, 314-315
      complex, arthroscopic meniscectomy for, 300
      flap, arthroscopic meniscectomy for, 298
      parrot-beak, arthroscopic meniscectomy for, 295
      peripheral, arthroscopic meniscectomy for, 299
      transverse, arthroscopic meniscectomy for, 296
      vertical, arthroscopic meniscectomy for, 297
  normal, 158
    arthroscopic appearance of, 113, 115, *116*
  pathologic arthroscopic findings of, 142-145
  peripheral detachment of, 162, *163*
  posterior, retained, 165-166
    arthroscopic diagnosis of, experience with, 77-78, 82-83, 85
    seen in posteromedial compartment, 125
  posterior medial horns of, abnormal, in knee instability, 193-194
  posterolateral, torn, seen in posterolateral compartment, 127
  posteromedial horn tear of, seen in posteromedial compartment, 125
  rounded inner border of, in torn meniscus, 159, *160*
  in service of articular cartilage, 145
  tears of
    accompanying anterior cruciate ligament tears, 188, 189-190

Index

Meniscus(i)—cont'd
  tears of—cont'd
    arthroscopic diagnosis of, 71
    bucket-handle, 294
    circumstantial signs of, 159, *160*
    complex, 294
    flap, 293, *294*
    horizontal, 293, *294*
    parrot-beak, 293, *294*
    peripheral, 294
    repeat arthroscopy for diagnosis of, 143, 161
    seen in posterolateral compartment, *127*
    transverse, 293, *294*
    types of, 293-309
    vertical, 293-294
Methylene blue dye
  for diagnostic arthroscopy of knee, 35
  for evaluation of osteochondritis dissecans, *183*, 184
Movie photography for documentation of diagnostic arthroscopy of knee, 106-108

N

Narrative, dictated, for documentation of diagnostic arthroscopy of knee, 97-99
Needle for arthroscopic surgery of knee, 227
Needlescope
  for arthroscopy of ankle, 412
  development of, 5-6
  Model III, endoscopic photography with *104*, 105
  1.7-mm diameter, advantages of, 13
  2.2-mm diameter, for arthroscopy of hip joint, 406
  for visualization of posterolateral loose bodies, 343
Nurse, circulating, responsibilities of
  in diagnostic arthroscopy of knee, 40
  in patellar shaving, 250

O

Ochronosis in alkaptonuria, 209, *211*
Olecranon fossa, arthroscopic inspection of, 390, *392*, 393
Olympus OM-2, 35-mm, for photographic documentation of diagnostic arthroscopy of knee, 102, *103*, 104
Olympus Pen F, 35-mm, for photographic documentation of diagnostic arthroscopy of knee, 102
Oretorp basket forceps for arthroscopic surgery of knee, 233, *234*
Oretorp probe for arthroscopic surgery of knee, 227-228, 270
Oretorp retractable blade system for arthroscopic surgery of knee, 228, 229
Osgood-Schlatter disease
  arthroscopic evaluation of, 195
  arthroscopic surgery for, 358-359
Osteochondral defects, arthroscopic diagnosis of, 184
Osteochondritis dissecans
  of ankle, arthroscopic evaluation and management of, 416, *417*
  of elbow, arthroscopic evaluation and management of, 395
  of hip, arthroscopic diagnosis of, 409
  of knee
    arthroscopic evaluation of, 147, 175, *183*, 184
      experience with, 79
    arthroscopic surgery for, 343-346
    natural history of, arthroscopic research on, 74

Osteochondromatosis
  arthroscopic diagnosis of, 206
    experience with, 85
  arthroscopic surgery for, 369
Osteophytes
  arthroscopic surgery for, 359
  juxta-articular, formation of, in ankle, arthroscopic evaluation of, 418
Osteotomy, tibial
  arthroscopic evaluation of, 184
  high, for chondronecrosis, 348

P

Palpation in diagnostic arthroscopy of knee, 32
Panner disease, arthroscopic evaluation and management of, 395
Parrot-beak tear of meniscus, 293, *294*
Patella
  arthroscopic evaluation of, 46-47
  arthroscopic surgery on
    intra-articular shaving as, 320-334; *see also* Shaving, patellar
    lateral release as, 334-337
    standard procedures for, 317, *318-319*
  bipartite, arthroscopic diagnosis of, 179
    experience with, 83
  chondromalacia of, 71, 171-172; *see also* Chondromalacia of patella
  diseases of, arthroscopic diagnosis of, 170-179
  dislocation of; *see* Dislocation of patella
  disorders of, arthroscopic diagnosis of, experience with, 78-79, 83, 86, 89-90
  fracture of
    acute, arthroscopic evaluation of, 175-176
    old, arthroscopic evaluation of, 176
  normal arthroscopic appearance of, 113, *114*
  osteochondritis dissecans of; *see* Osteochondritis dissecans of knee
  prosthesis for, metallic, postoperative arthroscopic evaluation of, 177
  ruptured tendons of, arthroscopic evaluation of, 176
  shaving of, basic setup for, *248*, 249-258; *see also* Shaving, patellar
  subluxation of; *see* Subluxation of patella
Patella baja, postoperative arthroscopic evaluation of, 177, *179*
Patellectomy
  postoperative arthroscopic evaluation of, *178*, 179
  subtotal, postoperative arthroscopic evaluation of, 177
Patellofemoral joint, degenerative changes in
  arthroscopic chondroplasty for, 336-337
  intra-articular shaving for, 333
Patient(s)
  classification of, in review of diagnostic arthroscopy experience, 76
  management of, diagnostic arthroscopy in, 92-95
  positioning of, for comprehensive arthroscopic surgical technique, 264-269
  preparation of
    for arthroscopic surgery of knee, 244-246
    for comprehensive arthroscopic surgical technique, 264-269
  selection of, for arthroscopic surgery of knee, 244-246

429

Index

Pedunculated nodular synovitis, arthroscopic diagnosis of, 212
Peripatellar synovitis
  arthroscopic diagnosis of, 179
  arthroscopic resection for, 369
Photography for documentation of diagnostic arthroscopy of knee
  movie, 106-108
  slide, 9, 99-106
  still, 99-106
Physician-patient relationship in diagnostic arthroscopy of knee under local anesthesia, 66
Pigmented villonodular synovitis
  arthroscopic diagnosis of, 204, 205
  arthroscopic surgery for, 365, 366, 368
Pin for fixation of osteochondritic defects, 344-346
Pistoning of scope in diagnostic arthroscopy of knee, 35
Plica
  lateral, arthroscopic evaluation of, 362
  medial
    arthroscopic evaluation of, 198, 200, 201
    arthroscopic resection of, *361*, 362-363
  suprapatellar
    arthroscopic evaluation of, 198, 201
    arthroscopic resection of, 362
  synovial, 198-201
    arthroscopic surgery for, 360-365
Popliteus tendon
  avulsion of, arthroscopic diagnosis of, 192
  normal arthroscopic appearance of, 115, *116*
Posterolateral compartment of knee
  arthroscopic evaluation of, 53-55
    before comprehensive arthroscopic surgical technique, 276, 277, 278
    modified Gillquist technique for, 140-141
    multiple puncture technique for, 126-127
    normal arthroscopic appearance of, *116*
    puncture sites for surgical instrumentation in, 284
Posterolateral puncture routine for diagnostic arthroscopy of knee, 8-9
Posteromedial approach to comprehensive arthroscopic surgical technique, 284
Posteromedial compartment of knee
  arthroscopic evaluation of, 50-53
    before comprehensive arthroscopic surgical technique, 277, 278
    modified Gillquist technique for, 134-135
    multiple puncture technique for, 124-125
    normal arthroscopic appearance of, *114*
Posteromedial puncture routine for diagnostic arthroscopy of knee, 8
Probe for arthroscopic surgery of knee, 227-228
Probing
  in comprehensive arthroscopic surgical technique, 278-279
  in diagnostic arthroscopy of knee, 32
Prosthesis
  knee, infection of, exacerbation of, complicating diagnostic arthroscopy of knee, 58, 60
  patellar, metallic, postoperative arthroscopic evaluation of, 177
Pseudogout of knee
  arthroscopic diagnosis of, 207
  synovitis in, arthroscopic irrigation for, 366

Psoriatic arthritis of knee, arthroscopic diagnosis of, 209

Q

Quadriceps exercises following arthrotomy, complications of, 168-169
Quadriceps tendon, ruptured, arthroscopic evaluation of, 176

R

Rehabilitation of knee, diagnostic arthroscopy enhancing, 73-74
Reiter syndrome, arthroscopic diagnosis of, 208
Research using diagnostic arthroscopy of knee, 74-75
Rheumatoid arthritis
  of ankle, arthroscopic diagnosis of, 416
  of elbow, arthroscopic diagnosis and management of, 394
  of knee
    arthroscopic diagnosis of, 201-203
    with synovitis, arthroscopic synovectomy for, 366
  of shoulder with synovitis, arthroscopic assessment and management of, 384-385
Rotator cuff injuries in shoulder, arthroscopic diagnosis of, 380, 382

S

Saline
  for distension of joint for diagnostic arthroscopy of knee, 27-28
  inflow of
    for arthroscopic surgery
      of knee, 225, *226*, 243
      of shoulder, 385, *386*
    cannula placement for, for comprehensive arthroscopic surgical technique, 269-271
  outflow of
    for arthroscopic surgery of knee, 225-227, 243
    system for, in patellar shaving operation, 255-258
Saphenous vein, damage to, complicating diagnostic arthroscopy of knee, 58
Schlessinger Grasper for arthroscopic surgery of knee, 231
Scissors for arthroscopic surgery of knee, 233, 235
Shaving
  all-compartment
    for chronic instability of knee, 357
    indications for, 349-350
  intra-articular, 320-334; *see also* Shaving, patellar
  patellar
    arthroscopic, 184, 320-334
      adequacy of resection in, 329-333
      anesthesia for, 324
      complications of, 325
      in patellofemoral degeneration, 333
      postoperative management of, 333-334
      results of, 326-329
    assistants in, 250-251
    basic setup for, 248, 249-258
    circulating nurse in, 250
    comprehensive arthroscopic surgical technique for, 283-284
    control of extremity for, 251-255
    patient positioning and preparation for, 249
    postoperative instructions for, 257
  patellofemoral, comprehensive arthroscopic surgical technique for, 283-284

Index

Shoulder
  arthroscopic diagnosis and surgery of, 376-389
  degenerative arthritis of, arthroscopic diagnosis of, 383
  dislocation of, arthroscopic diagnosis of, *379*, 380, 382
  frozen, arthroscopic examination and management of, 384
  loose bodies in, arthroscopic diagnosis of, 383
  rheumatoid arthritis of, with synovitis, arthroscopic assessment and management of, 384-385
  rotator cuff injuries in, arthroscopic diagnosis of, 380, 382
  subluxation of, arthroscopic diagnosis of, 382
Slide photography for documentation of diagnostic arthroscopy of knee, 9
Staining, contrast, for diagnostic arthroscopy of knee, 35
Sterilization of arthroscopic equipment, 22-24
Storz flash generator, endoscopic photography with, *104*, 105-106
Storz-Hopkins rod-lens system, endoscopic photography with, *104*, 105-106
Storz scope for arthroscopy of hip joint, 206
Storz xenon arc illuminator for arthroscopes, 17
Subluxation
  of ankle, arthroscopic evaluation and management of, 418
  of patella
    arthroscopic diagnosis of, 175
      experience with, 89-90
      chondromalacia of patella in, 330
      lateral release for, 334-335
  of shoulder, arthroscopic diagnosis of, 382
Suctioning for loose body removal, 340, 342
Suprapatellar approach to diagnostic arthroscopy of knee, 56-57
Suprapatellar plica
  arthroscopic evaluation of, 198, 201
  arthroscopic resection of, 362
Suprapatellar pouch
  arthroscopic evaluation of, 46-47
    before comprehensive arthroscopic surgical technique, 275, *276*
    modified Gillquist technique for, 130-131
  arthroscopic surgery on, positions for, 271
  normal arthroscopic appearance of, *114*
Suprapatellar puncture routine for diagnostic arthroscopy of knee, 9
Surgical Assistant
  for arthroscopic surgery of knee, 223-225
    development of, 219, 220
  for comprehensive arthroscopic surgical technique, 264-267
Sylvania 300/16 light bulb as illumination source for arthroscope, 17
Synovectomy, arthroscopic
  indications for, 366
  for pigmented villonodular synovitis, 204
  technique of, 366-368
Synovitis
  of ankle, arthroscopic diagnosis of, 414, *416*
  of hip, arthroscopic diagnosis of, 409
  of knee
    degenerative, arthroscopic diagnosis of, 182
    with degenerative arthritis, management of, 369
    following arthrotomy, arthroscopy for, 168
    juxtachondral, arthroscopic resection for, 369
    localized, arthroscopic surgery for, 365-366
    nodular, pedunculated, arthroscopic diagnosis of, 212

Synovitis—cont'd
  of knee—cont'd
    peripatellar
      arthroscopic diagnosis of, 179
      arthroscopic resection for, 369
    pigmented villonodular
      arthroscopic diagnosis of, 204, *205*
      arthroscopic surgery for, 365, *366*, 368
    rheumatoid, arthroscopic treatment of, 366
  of shoulder with rheumatoid arthritis, arthroscopic assessment and management of, 384-385
  of wrist, arthroscopic diagnosis and management of, 403
Synovium
  of elbow, normal, 393
  of knee
    adhesions of, arthroscopic section of, 365
    diseases of
      arthroscopic diagnosis of, 81, 85, 87, 91, *150*, 151, 197-212
      arthroscopic research on, 74-75
      arthroscopic surgery for, 360-370
      postoperative arthroscopic evaluation of, 212
    folds in, 198-201
      arthroscopic surgery for, 360-365
    foreign bodies in
      arthroscopic diagnosis of, 212
      arthroscopic resection of, 370
    hemorrhagic, arthroscopic diagnosis of, 209, *210*
    infections of
      arthroscopic diagnosis of, 212
      arthroscopic management of, 370
    normal arthroscopic appearance of, *114*, 115, *116*
    pileup of, at synovial-meniscal junction in torn meniscus, 159, *160*
    plica of, 198-201
  of shoulder, reflection of, arthroscopic evaluation of, 380, *381*

T

Team approach
  to arthroscopic surgery of knee, 248
  to diagnostic arthroscopy of knee, 38-43
Television
  in arthroscopic surgery, 222
  for documentation of diagnostic arthroscopy of knee, 10, 108-110
Temporomandibular joint, arthroscopic diagnosis and surgery of, 373-375
Tendon(s)
  Achilles, monitoring tension in, in diagnostic arthroscopy of knee, 37, *38*, 65
  biceps
    arthroscopic inspection of, *378*, 379
    ruptured, arthroscopic diagnosis of, 383
  patellar, ruptured, arthroscopic evaluation of, 176
  popliteus
    avulsion of, arthroscopic diagnosis of, 192
    normal arthroscopic appearance of, 115, *116*
  quadriceps, ruptured, arthroscopic evaluation of, 176
Tennis elbow, arthroscopic evaluation and management of, 394
Tibial collateral ligament
  normal arthroscopic appearance of, *114*, 115
  torn, arthroscopic diagnosis of, 148, 190-192

Index

Tibial collateral ligament—cont'd
  torn, arthroscopic diagnosis of—cont'd
    experience with, 80, 84
Tibial osteotomy
  evaluation of, arthroscopy in, 184
  high, for chondronecrosis, 348
Tourniquet in diagnostic arthroscopy of knee under local anesthesia, 66
Transpatellar tendon approach to diagnostic arthroscopy of knee, 57-58
Triangulation in arthroscopic surgery of knee, 242-243

V

Vacuuming of joint
  for diagnostic arthroscopy of knee, 33-35

Vacuuming of joint—cont'd
  for loose body removal, 340, 342
Vein, saphenous, damage to, complicating diagnostic arthroscopy of knee, 58
Videotape for documentation of diagnostic arthroscopy of knee, 108-112
Villonodular synovitis, pigmented
  arthroscopic diagnosis of, 204, 205
  arthroscopic surgery for, 365, 366, 368

W

Wrist, arthroscopic diagnosis and surgery of, 400-403